D0085182

ENCYCLOPEDIA OF CHILDBEARING

CRITICAL PERSPECTIVES

Edited by Barbara Katz Rothman

Managing Editor, Donna Lee King

ORYX PRESS
1993

WITHDRAWN
LIBRARY
College of St. Scholastica
Duluth, Minnesota 55811

The rare Arabian Oryx is believed to have inspired the myth of the unicorn. This desert antelope became virtually extinct in the early 1960s. At that time several groups of international conservationists arranged to have 9 animals sent to the Phoenix Zoo to be the nucleus of a captive breeding herd. Today the Oryx population is nearly 800 and over 400 have been returned to reserves in the Middle East.

Copyright © 1993 by The Oryx Press
4041 North Central at Indian School Road
Phoenix, Arizona 85012-3397

Published simultaneously in Canada

All rights reserved
No part of this publication may be reproduced or transmitted in any form or by any means, electronic or mechanical, including photocopying, recording, or by any information storage and retrieval system, without permission in writing from The Oryx Press.

Printed and Bound in the United States of America

♾ The paper used in this publication meets the minimum requirements of American National Standard for Information Science—Permanence of Paper for Printed Library Materials, ANSI Z39.48, 1984

Library of Congress Cataloging-in-Publication Data

Encyclopedia of Childbearing : critical perspectives / edited by
Barbara Katz Rothman.
p. cm.
Includes bibliographical references and index.
ISBN 0-89774-648-1
1. Pregnancy—Encyclopedias. 2. Childbirth—Encyclopedias.
3. Human reproduction—Social aspects—Encyclopedias. I. Rothman, Barbara Katz, II. Title: Encyclopedia of childbearing.
RG525.E52 1992
618.2′ 003—dc20 92-14975
CIP

I take great pleasure in dedicating this volume to my mother, Marcia Katz Berken, who taught me to "look it up," and to the editors of the 1959 *World Book Encyclopedia.*

Contents

Preface

The field of birth studies is at an interesting point in its development: One is tempted to describe it as in its "infancy." While midwifery has an ancient and honorable history, and obstetrics a fully developed body of professional literature, the interest of academic scholars in childbirth is comparatively recent. Much of the work has grown since the 1970s and the current wave of the feminist movement and the development of feminist studies in related fields and disciplines.

This encyclopedia gathers together key people in this field, those whose work has created, shaped, and furthered the study of childbearing. There are, represented in this volume, people from the following fields and more: anthropology; art history; childbirth education; chiropracty; counseling, including abortion, adoption, contraception, genetic and lactation counseling; demography; ethics; history; law; literature; medicine; midwifery; musicology; nursing; philosophy; physical therapy; political science; psychology; social work; sociology; theology; and women's studies.

This list shows not only the enormous diversity of this encyclopedia, but something else as well, something I have grown increasingly impressed by and even fond of as the work progressed: the power of the alphabet as an organizing tool. In the alphabetical list, musicology falls between midwifery and nursing—think of it! Ethics comes between demography and history; history between ethics and the law.

The leveling and integrating effect of the alphabet delights me over and over: in the list of contributors, the list of entries, and the list of organizations and resources. The most astonishing things come together, the most wondrous, intriguing, absurd, and challenging connections made.

And *that* is the power, as well as the weakness, of an encyclopedia, any encyclopedia. Everything and anything can become an entry. Where every other piece of intellectual work I have ever done involved pulling together, weaving and integrating diverse ideas and concepts into a coherent whole, editing this encyclopedia has meant facing a whole—the field of childbearing studies—and breaking it down into 250 or so separate entries and alphabetizing them.

And yet—the process has been a continuous movement back and forth between the integrative and the compartmentalizing, putting it together and pulling it back apart again. While the articles can and do stand alone, they are also each part of a larger context. To see if a subfield was complete, or at least coherent, I would have to reach in and pull out all of the related articles and read them together, as if they were a chapter. But then, with whatever missing pieces assigned and redundancies edited out, the articles would be scattered back into their places in the alphabet. This process was repeated, over and over again, as the encyclopedia grew more complex and more complete.

Of course, it never does get completed: I urge you never to edit an encyclopedia if you have no tolerance for the unfinished. There are my oversights; there are the articles eternally promised and never delivered; there are all kinds of missing pieces. I continue to come across a new book, a reference, a newspaper article, even a song, and think: That ought to be an encyclopedia entry. But my focus cannot be on what is not here—other than for the purpose of starting a file for a next edition. While much may be missing, nothing is extra. Each piece makes its contribution; each is part of the growing whole.

The job of an editor of an encyclopedia goes beyond deciding which articles belong and attempting to get them written. Decisions also have to be made about entry length: The pages allotted to a book are finite, and longer articles must mean fewer articles. I think it is fair to say that there is not a single author here who did not feel constrained by the word limitations I had to impose: Most of these articles are, in fact, the subject of many book-length treatments in themselves. Do not make the mistake of thinking that the length of an article reflects its "importance." I thought all of these articles were important or I would not have included them. Some articles are very short just because it is possible to keep them short: for example, the various positions of the fetus can described in relatively few words, as can the practice of daily fetal movement counting. Both of these articles (under 500 words each, thanks to the skill of their authors) are about literally life and death issues. Some articles are kept short because they cover material that has already been extensively researched, allowing the entries to serve as both a brief summary and a guide to further research: The article on family-centered maternity care typifies this approach. Some articles are longer because the ideas are inherently difficult to express succinctly. Some of the more theoretical articles, such as the one on feminist ethics of abortion, or the one on Chodorow's theory of the reproduction of mothering, or the one on the anthropology of ritual in birth, exemplify this. These articles are not only relatively long, but also make for rather dense reading. They are "packed" into their space.

In a few cases, an article is given somewhat more space because it is unique to this encyclopedia: Such is the case with the articles on maternity clothing and childbirth in science fiction. These articles, and especially this last, along with all of the other articles on childbearing in the arts and in literature, add to the larger theme that infuses this encyclopedia: Pregnancy, childbirth, and motherhood are social constructions, and the practices, imagery, and technology a culture develops, or even in the case of science fiction, imagines developing, grow out of this cultural grounding.

Nowhere is this point made more clearly, nor the problems of selectivity more obviously highlighted, than in the choice of societies to include—and to exclude—for cross-cultural comparison. There is no inherently good reason for leaving out any particular country: There is also no possible way to include them all. The simplest criterion is to ensure geographical diversity, and that was done. But more profoundly, these countries were chosen for what the North American reader could learn from them. Each presents implicit or explicit contrast with American practices, systems, values, or beliefs. The article on Sweden, for example, one of the longer pieces in this volume, shows what it is like to give birth in a country that offers social support for women, children, and families. Others—Mexico and Uganda especially—show what birth is like with far fewer economic resources. Some—notably Israel and Japan—show birth in as highly a technological mode as the United States, yet with different social supports; while the article on the Netherlands presents a very different model, one of success with a modern home birth system. So in this grouping of articles as in the encyclopedia as a whole, while much could be added, nothing is extra. Each inclusion makes its contribution to the whole.

The parts of an encyclopedia, the articles or pieces, are often called "entries," and that is the best word of all. Because that is precisely what they are; each piece is an entry into the whole. Looking up one topic frequently pulls the reader on to another, either directly, with the editor's "see also" references, indirectly, through the power of the alphabet to call the preceding and following articles to attention, or even more indirectly as a word or a picture catches the eye on the way to the topic one seeks. Look up one thing, be drawn to another—and find yourself thinking about the whole from which they are drawn.

Some of the work of making these connections is done for you, in the "Guide to Related Topics." When an entry is related to others, the reader will find not only referrals to other specific entries, but also a referral to the appropriate Guide. Different editors might well have put these Guides together differently: Probably the most interesting work in preparing this encyclopedia was having long and thoughtful discussions with Donna King about how to construct these guides. What does, after all, constitute a pregnancy complication? Which technologies of procreation are "new?" Which issues are "psychological?" These are not simple administrative or clerical decisions, but represent a world view: a social, political, and ethical framework that shapes this encyclopedia.

An encyclopedia of childbearing should answer the question: What is childbearing? The diversity of the encyclopedia is the answer to that question. Childbearing is, as you will see in this volume, the having and not having of children—see entries on contraception, abortion, and infertility as well as pregnancy and labor. It is an event in the lives of families—see entries on fathers and on siblings at birth, on matrescence and patrescence. It is an event in the lives and bodies of women, ever grounded in our bellies and our experiences. Childbearing is a political, a legal, a religious, a cultural event—all that and more.

Use each entry as an entry. But use the encyclopedia itself as an entry. The "Resources" section that concludes each entry contains references and suggestions for further reading. A guide to organizations and resources can be found in the appendix.

I learned from this project—and I also had enormous fun with it. I hope it brings you, too, both the learning and the fun.

✻ BARBARA KATZ ROTHMAN

Acknowledgments

It is hard to imagine what this project would have been like without the assistance, insights, and support of its managing editor, Donna King. I wish to express my deep appreciation to her and to the Professional Staff Congress, City University of New York Research Award, which enabled her participation. Clerical help was provided by Segundo Pantojera, for which I thank the City University of New York Department of Sociology, and by Leah Colb Rothman and Daniel Colb Rothman. Not too much interference was provided by Alexander Bowden and Victoria Colb Rothman, thanks in no small part to the work of Alan Bowden, Daniel Colb Rothman, Mary White, and Herschel Rothman, for which Donna King and I express our continuing gratitude.

Contributor Profiles

Richard Alford is associate professor and department chair of Sociology at East Central University, Ada, Oklahoma. He is author of *Naming and Identity: A Cross-Cultural Study of Personal Naming Practices* (HRAF Press, 1988).

Max Allen is author of *The Birth Symbol in Traditional Women's Art from Eurasia and the Western Pacific* (The Museum for Textiles, 1981).

Julia Allison is a lecturer at the University of Nottingham, where she is preparing a Ph.D. thesis on the life and work of district nurses in Nottingham, England. She worked as a district midwife in Nottingham until 1986.

Howard Altstein is professor and dean, University of Maryland, School of Social Work, Baltimore. He is coauthor, with Rita James Simon, of five books on transracial and intercountry adoption, most recently *Intercountry Adoption: A Multinational Perspective* (Praeger Publishing, 1991).

Rima D. Apple is a member of the Women's Studies Program at the University of Wisconsin at Madison. She is author of *Mothers and Medicine: A Social History of Infant Feeding, 1890-1950* (University of Wisconsin Press, 1987) and editor of *Women, Health and Medicine in America: A Historical Handbook* (Garland, 1990; forthcoming in paperback from Rutgers University Press).

Rita Arditti is an editor of *Issues in Reproductive and Genetic Engineering: Journal of International Feminist Analysis*. She is coeditor of *Test Tube Women: What Future for Motherhood* (Pandora Press, 1984 and 1989) and *Science and Liberation* (South End Press, 1980). She is a faculty member in the graduate program of the Union Institute, Cincinnati, Ohio.

Janet Isaacs Ashford is a writer, illustrator, and graphic designer in Solana Beach, California. She is author of *Mothers and Midwives: A History of Traditional Childbirth* and other slide series, available from Childbirth Resources (see organizations listings), and is editor of *The Whole Birth Catalog* (1983).

Hani K. Atrash is an obstetrician/gynecologist, medical epidemiologist, and chief of the Pregnancy and Infant Health Branch of the Division of Reproductive Health, Center for Chronic Disease Prevention and Health Promotion, Centers for Disease Control, Atlanta, Georgia. His research interests include pregnancy-related morbidity and mortality and the black/white gap in infant mortality.

Kathleen G. Auerbach is a medical sociologist, researcher, writer, and board-certified lactation consultant. She operates Lectures Unlimited, a company providing presentations to professional and lay groups on breastfeeding and lactation, childbearing, and family issues. She is editor-in-chief of the *Journal of Human Lactation*.

Rahima Baldwin is a midwife and childbirth educator. She is author of *Special Delivery* (Celestial Arts, 1979; revised 1986) and *You Are Your Child's First Teacher* (Celestial Arts, 1989). She is founder of Informed Homebirth/Informed Birth and Parenting, and codirector of the Garden of Life Birth Center in Dearborn, Michigan.

Elizabeth Balkite is a member of the National Society of Human Genetics and is nationally certified as a genetic counselor by the American Board of Medical Genetics. She is in private practice in Stamford, Connecticut, and serves as consultant to the graduate program in human genetics at Sarah Lawrence College.

Diane Barnes is a registered nurse and midwife. She operates a freestanding birthing center in Missouri and has counseled families coping with central closure disorders. She is president of the Midwives Alliance of North America.

Sandra Barnhill is an attorney and executive director of Aid to Imprisoned Mothers, Inc., in Atlanta, Georgia.

Ellen Becker works as a freelance writer and editor in Santa Fe, New Mexico.

Terry Beresford is a free-lance consultant in family planning. She is cofounder and former president of the National Abortion Federation and was the 1989 recipient of the Christopher Tietze Humanitarian Award for her contributions to women's health and reproductive rights.

Vangie Bergum is associate professor, Faculty of Nursing, and associate faculty, Division of Biomedical Ethics and Humanities, Faculty of Medicine, University of Alberta, Canada. She is author of *Woman to Mother: A Transformation* (Bergen & Garvey Publishers, 1989) and coeditor, with Jane Ross, of *Through the Looking Glass: Children and Health Promotion* (Canadian Public Health Association, 1990).

Joan E. Bertin is a lawyer with the Women's Rights Project of the American Civil Liberties Union. She is on the editorial board of *Women and Health*, and served on the advisory panel for the Congressional Office of Technology Assessment report *Reproductive Health Hazards in the Workplace*.

Dawn Beveridge worked as an intern at the Women's Self Help Center and at Advocate Services for Abused Women, both in St. Louis, Missouri, while pursuing her law degree from Washington University in St. Louis.

Robin J.R. Blatt is author of *Prenatal Tests: What They Are, Their Benefits and Risks, and How to Decide to Have Them or Not* (Vintage Books, 1988). She is the education coordinator for the Massachusetts Genetics Program, Massachusetts Department of Public Health, and is founder and coeditor of *The Genetic Resource*, a publication developed to update medical professionals and consumers on developments in human genetics.

Renate Blumenfeld-Kosinski is associate professor of French at Columbia University. She is author of *Not of Woman Born: Representations of Caesarean Birth in Medieval and Renaissance Culture* (Cornell University Press, 1990) and *The Writings of Margaret of Oingt, Medieval Prioress and Mystic* (Focus Press, 1990).

Janet Carlisle Bogdan is a faculty member of the Department of Sociology, Le Moyne College, Syracuse, New York.

Heather D. Boonstra served as an intern for the National Women's Health Network. Currently she is working as an admissions counselor for the University of Oregon, where she advises students and coordinates publications.

Datha Clapper Brack served on the National Women's Health Network from 1979-87, chairing the Network Committee on Infant Feeding and representing the Network on the International Nestle Boycott Committee. She writes on women's health issues for *New Directions for Women*.

Thomas Burgess studies anthropology at the Graduate School of the City University of New York. He has spent several years on Lakota Indian reservations as a liaison with Women of All Red Nations. WARN successfully organized opposition to forced sterilization, uranium mining, and toxic wastes.

Cathryn L. Caldwell is an obstetric nurse at the Baptist Medical Center—Montclair in Birmingham, Alabama, where she is also active in the childbirth movement.

Muktai Jain Campion is a writer and documentary filmmaker with a special interest in parenting issues. She is author of *The Baby Challenge: A Handbook on Pregnancy for Women with a Physical Disability* (Routledge, 1990). Forthcoming books include *Who Is Fit to Be a Parent?* (Routledge, 1992) and *The Good Parent Guide*. She is active in improving support and access to information and services for pregnant women with disabilities in Great Britain.

Allison Carter is an instructor of sociology at Glassboro State College, Glassboro, New Jersey. She is writing her dissertation on "Realism in Feminist Social Theory" for York University, Toronto.

Mary Beth Caschetta is an editor of AIDS medical information, a free-lance writer, and a student of feminist theory.

Carol J. Castellano is a prematurity prevention activist and a founding member of SCAMP, a parents' support and information group. She is also a member of the National Federation of the Blind, Parents of Blind Children Division, and vice-chair of the Consumer Advisory Board of the New Jersey Commission for the Blind and Visually Impaired.

Rebecca Chalker is editor of *A New View of a Woman's Body* (Simon & Schuster, 1981) and *How to Stay Out of the Gynecologist's Office* (Peace Press, 1981). She is author of *The Complete Cervical Cap Guide* (Harper & Row, 1987) and coauthor of *Overcoming Bladder Disorders* (HarperCollins, 1990).

David B. Chamberlain is a psychologist in practice in San Diego. He is vice president of the Pre and Perinatal Psychology Association of North America (PPPANA). He is author of over a dozen scholarly articles on birth memory reliability and the capabilites of fetuses and newborns. He is author of *Babies Remember Birth* (Ballantine Books, 1990).

R. Alta Charo is assistant professor of law and medical ethics at the University of Wisconsin Schools of Law and Medicine. She was an American Association for the Advancement of Science Diplomacy Fellow at the U.S. Agency for International Development, and a legal analyst at the Office of Technology Assessment, U.S. Congress. Her work on bioethics and law has been widely published in legal and scholarly journals.

Phyllis Chesler is the author of six books: *Women and Madness; Women, Money and Power; About Men; With Child: A Diary of Motherhood; Mothers on Trial: The Battle for Children and Custody*, and, most recently, *Sacred Bond: The Legacy of Baby M.* Many of her books have been translated into several foreign languages. She is a founder of the Association for Women in Psychology, a member of the American Psychology Association's task force on custody, and professor of psychology and women's studies at the College of Staten Island, City University of New York.

Nancy J. Chodorow is professor of sociology at the University of California, Berkeley. She is author of *The Reproduction of Mothering: Psychoanalysis and the Sociology of Gender* (University of California Press, 1978) and *Feminism and Psychoanalytic Theory* (University of California Press, 1989). She has a psychoanalytic clinical practice in Berkeley.

Nancy Wainer Cohen is coauthor of *Silent Knife: Cesarean Prevention and Vaginal Birth After Cesarean* (Bergin & Garvey, 1983) and author of *Open Season: A Survival Guide for Natural Childbirth and VBAC in the 90's* (Greenwood Publishing Group, 1991). She is cofounder of C/Sec Inc. and a member of the education committee of the National Cesarean Prevention Movement.

Karen Cosner is a staff nurse-midwife in a full-scope nurse-midwifery practice in Ocala, Florida.

Ruth Schwartz Cowan is professor of history, State University of New York at Stony Brook. She is author of *More Work for Mother: The Ironies of Household Technology from the Open Hearth to the Microwave* (Basic Books, 1983).

Aileen Crow is a therapist and bodyworker in private practice in New York City.

Diane D'Alessandro is a registered nurse currently enrolled in the Ph.D. program in sociology at the Graduate School and University Center of the City University of New York.

Elizabeth Davis is author of *Heart and Hands: A Midwife's Guide to Pregnancy and Birth* (Celestial Arts, 1987), *Energetic Pregnancy* (Celestial Arts, 1988), and *Women's Intuition* (Celestial Arts, 1990). She has been a regional representative to the Midwives Alliance of North America and was instrumental in developing the certification process for the California Association of Midwives.

Robbie Davis-Floyd is a cultural anthropologist specializing in the anthropology of reproduction, gender studies, and symbolic and cognitive anthropology. She has published and lectured widely on the subject of ritual and technology in childbirth, and currently teaches at the University of Texas at Austin. She is author of *Birth as an American Rite of Passage* (University of California Press, 1992) and *American Rites of Passage* (Waveland Press, 1992).

Jeanne F. DeJoseph is assistant professor and codirector of the Nurse-Midwifery Program at the University of California, San Francisco.

Pat de la Fuente is cochair of the New Jersey affiliate of the National Women's Health Network and a member of the American Medical Writers' Association. She is a free-lance writer and editor, specializing in women's health.

Diane E. Depken is a member of the faculty at Buffalo State College, New York. She recently completed a doctoral dissertation in which she designed and implemented a program of exercise and stress reduction for pregnant urban adolescents.

Tamie L. Dixon is a chiropractor in private practice in Palm Bay, Florida.

Mary Donahue is a doctoral student in art history at the Graduate School and University Center of the City University of New York.

Paula Dressel is assistant professor of sociology, Georgia State University, Atlanta.

Andrea Boroff Eagan is a health writer whose work includes *The Newborn Mother* (Holt) and *Why Am I so Miserable If These Are the Best Years of My Life?* (Avon).

Pamela S. Eakins is an affiliated scholar at the Institute for Research on Women and Gender, Stanford University, Stanford, California, where she directs the Birth Research Project. She is editor of *The American Way of Birth* (Temple University Press, 1986) and has written numerous articles on childbirth.

Murray W. Enkin is professor emeritus, Departments of Obstetrics and Gynecology, and Clinical Epidemiology and Biostatistics, McMaster University, Ontario, Canada. Among his many scholarly publications is coeditorship, with Keirse and Chalmers, of *A Guide to Effective Care in Pregnancy and Childbirth* (Oxford University Press, 1989).

Jacqueline Fawcett is professor, School of Nursing, University of Pennsylvania. She is the author of several scholarly books on theory and research in nursing.

Barbara Feldman is director of the Fertility Awareness Center in New York City. She conducts workshops on natural birth control, offers private sessions on achieving pregnancy naturally, and provides pre- and post-abortion counseling. She also writes the column "Reproductive Health Line" in *To Your Health* magazine.

Judy Lobo Ferry holds a bachelors of science degree in nursing, and is currently a childbirth educator in Louisville, Kentucky. She is president of the Kentucky Alliance for the Advancement of Midwifery and mother of four—including one set of twins.

Thais R. Forbes is a medical anthropologist and childbirth educator. She teaches classes in home safety and pediatric CPR for parents and day care providers in Hillsborough County, Florida.

Judi Lowenburg Forman is a certified childbirth educator and past president of the Childbirth Education Association of Metropolitan New York.

Karen Joy Fowler is a science fiction writer who has written for numerous magazine publications as well as a collection of short stories entitled *Artificial Things* (Bantam, 1986). She is the 1987 winner of the John W. Campbell Award for best new writer in science fiction, and is author of a novel, *Sarah Canary* (Henry Holt, 1991).

Margery B. Franklin is a developmental psychologist on the faculty of Sarah Lawrence College in New York. She is coeditor of *Developmental Processes* (International Universities Press, 1978), *Symbolic Functioning in Childhood* (Erlbaum, 1979), and *Child Language* (Oxford University Press, 1988). She is currently working on a study of artistic development.

Anne Frye is a practicing midwife and author of *Understanding Lab Work in the Childbearing Year* (Labrys Press, 1990).

Ina May Gaskin is a practicing midwife and founder of The Farm Midwifery Center in Summertown, Tennessee. She is author of *Spiritual Midwifery* (Book Publishing Company, 1975) and editor-publisher of *The Birth Gazette*.

Alice Gilgoff is a labor and delivery staff nurse, certified childbirth educator, La Leche League leader, and president of Mother Nurture, Inc., a postpartum home-care service. She is author of *Home Birth* (Coward, McCann and Geoghegan, 1978) and *Home Birth: An Invitation and a Guide* (Bergin & Garvey, 1989).

Linda Gordon is professor of sociology, University of Wisconsin, Madison. She is author of many scholarly publications on women's history, and her most recent book is the revised edition of her classic *Woman's Body, Woman's Right: Birth Control in America* (Penguin, 1990).

Nicole J. Grant is a member of the sociology faculty at Ball State University in Muncie, Indiana. She is author of *The Selling of Contraception: The Dalkon Shield Case, Sexuality and Women's Autonomy* (Ohio State University Press, 1992).

Karen Greene is a licensed clinical psychologist in private practice in New York City. She specializes in the treatment of postpartum disorders and distress related to stillbirth, miscarriage, and abortion.

Arthur L. Greil is professor of sociology and associate dean of the College of Liberal Arts and Sciences at Alfred University, Alfred, New York. He is author of *Not Yet Pregnant: Infertile Couples in Contemporary America* (Rutgers University Press, 1991). His work on infertility has been widely published in academic journals.

Jeanne Harley Guillemin is professor of sociology at Boston College. Her many scholarly publications include coauthorship, with Lynda Lytle Holmstrom, of *Mixed Blessings: Intensive Care for Newborns* (Oxford, 1986).

Doris B. Haire is director of the American Foundation for Maternal & Child Health in New York City, and chair of the Committee on Maternal Child Health, National Women's Health Network. Her many publications include the pamphlet, "The Cultural Warping of Childbirth."

Gail Hanssen is a doctoral student at the Heller School for Advanced Studies in Social Welfare at Brandeis University in Waltham, Massachusetts. She was a founding member and an officer of the Board of Concerned United Birth Parents.

Harriette Hartigan has been photographing childbirth since 1975. She is a midwife, writer, and teacher who leads seminars and workshops on women, birth, and photography. She is the president of Artemis, a company that produces art and educational materials about the childbirth experience, including *The Birth Disc*, an interactive laser disc of 10,000 of Hartigan's photographs.

Cynthia Lee Henthorn is a doctoral student in art history at the City University of New York. Her interests include the impact of colonialism on the female body, as well as the social history of commercial art and popular culture.

Helen Bequaert Holmes is a geneticist who works on feminist technology assessment and ethical analysis of reproductive medicine. She is editor of *Birth Control and Controlling Birth: Women-Centered Perspectives* (Humana Press, 1981), author of *The Custom-Made Child? Women-Centered Perspectives* (Humana Press, 1981) and *Feminist Medical Ethics* (Indiana University Press, 1992), and consultant to the 1988 Office of Technology Assessment report on "Risks of Infertility Diagnosis and Treatment."

Linda Janet Holmes is founder and executive director of the Traditional Midwives Center International. She has conducted extensive interviews with indigenous black midwives in Alabama, and is currently a doctoral student in Public Health and Anthropology at Columbia University.

Lynda Lytle Holmstrom is professor of sociology at Boston College. Her many scholarly publications include coauthorship, with Jeanne Harley Guillemin, of *Mixed Blessings: Intensive Care for Newborns* (Oxford, 1986).

Elizabeth Hormann has been involved in breastfeeding education since 1967. She serves as area professional liaison for the English Speaking La Leche League in Germany and leads both English and German La Leche League groups. She is a lactation consultant, training health care providers through the Breastfeeding Promotion Project (Arbeitsgruppe Babynahrung, e.V./Aachen) funded by the European Economic Community, and in Africa through the International Babyfood Action Network. She is author of *After the Adoption* (Revell, 1987).

Ruth Hubbard is professor emerita of biology, Harvard University. Her many published works include *The Politics of Women's Biology* (Rutgers University Press, 1990).

Sherry Hurwitz is a graduate student in the Department of Anthropology at Michigan State University. She is pursuing training in nutrition and agricultural practices and policies, with an emphasis on gender issues.

Paula Hyde is a shoe designer and vice-president of research and development at a prominent children's shoe company.

Sherokee Ilse is cofounder of The Pregnancy and Infant Loss Center in Wayzata, Minnesota, a nonprofit organization. She is author of *Empty Arms: Coping with Miscarriage, Stillbirth and Infant Death* (Wintergreen Press, 1990).

Sandra Jamrog is a certified childbirth educator and registered movement therapist. She is founder and past president of the Childbirth Education Association of Metropolitan New York, and is a practitioner and teacher of Body-Mind Centering. She is in private practice in New York City.

Carole Joffe is professor of sociology, University of California, Davis. She is author of *The Regulation of Sexuality: Experiences of Family Planning Workers* (Temple University Press, 1986).

Joy Johnson is codirector of Centering Corporation, a nonprofit organization specializing in publishing supportive literature for bereaved families.

Diana Jones is a graduate student in sociology at Emory University in Atlanta, Georgia. Her interests include the political economy of the world system, women in development, and delinquency research.

Joy M. Jones is a registered nurse, a childbirth educator, and a doula/labor assistant. She is director of Perinatal Support Services in Evanston, Illinois, and has authored brochures and magazine articles on pregnancy health issues.

Donna Jordan is a graduate student in anthropology at the Graduate School and University Center of the City University of New York.

Robbie Pfeufer Kahn is assistant professor of sociology at the University of Vermont. She is author of *The Language of Birth: Female Generativity in Western Tradition* (University of Illinois Press, forthcoming).

Jeffrey P. Katz is a social worker and director of the Ocean State Adoption Resource Exchange in Providence, Rhode Island.

Karen E. Katz is a certified nurse midwife currently on the faculty at the University of Medicine and Dentistry of New Jersey, School of Health-Related Professions in Newark. She is also a clinician in a full scope nurse-midwifery practice.

Linda G. Katz is a graduate of the New England School of Law, where she wrote a *New England Law Review* article on wrongful birth and wrongful life cases. She has practiced as a government lawyer in the Boston area since 1978.

Robert T. Keegan is a psychologist on the faculty of Pace University in New York. He is coeditor of the Special Issue of the *Journal of the History of the Behavioral Sciences* on Charles Darwin and the human sciences.

Amy King is a semi-retired childbirth educator who works in a large bookstore in Portland, Oregon.

Donna Lee King teaches sociology and psychology at Orange County Community College in Middletown, New York. She is a doctoral candidate in sociology at the Graduate School and University Center of the City University of New York, where she is writing her dissertation on children and the environmental crisis. She is managing editor of *The Encyclopedia of Childbearing: Critical Perspectives* (Oryx Press, 1992).

Sheila Kitzinger is a social anthropologist and member of the advisory board of England's National Childbirth Trust. Her many books include *Your Baby, Your Way; Birth at Home; The Complete Book of Pregnancy and Childbirth; Women's Experience of Sex;* and *Women as Mothers.*

Allen G. Kleiman is doing research and graduate work at the Graduate School and University Center of the City University of New York on the impact of advanced technology on sensory impaired persons.

Aliza Kolker is associate professor of sociology at George Mason University in Fairfax, Virginia, and author of numerous articles on the psycho-social implications of prenatal diagnosis.

Susan Kolod is assistant clinical professor, Derner Institute of Advanced Psychological Studies, Adelphi University, Adelphi, New York. She is a certified sign language interpreter and a clinical psychologist in private practice in Brooklyn, New York.

Lisa M. Koonin is a family nurse practitioner and epidemiologist and chief, surveillance unit, Statistics and Computer Resources Branch of the Division of Reproductive Health, Centers for Chronic Disease Prevention and Health Promotion, Centers for Disease Control, Atlanta, Georgia. Her research interests include reproductive health issues such as pregnancy-associated mortality, particularly the black/white gap in maternal mortality.

Sharon Krummel is author of "Refugee Women and the Experience of Cultural Uprooting" (World Council of Churches, 1988).

Rosalind Ekman Ladd is professor of philosophy, Wheaton College, Norton, Massachusetts, and lecturer in pediatrics, Brown University Program in Medicine. She is coauthor, with E.N. Forman, of *Ethical Dilemmas in Pediatrics: A Case Study Approach* (Springer-Verlag, 1991).

Barbara Ursenbach Lamb is a certified childbirth educator in private practice in West Cape May, New Jersey.

Judith N. Lasker is professor of sociology at Lehigh University in Bethlehem, Pennsylvania. She is coauthor, with Susan Borg, of *When Pregnancy Fails: Coping with Miscarriage, Stillbirth and Infant Death* (Beacon, 1981) and *In Search of Parenthood: Coping with Infertility and High Tech Conception* (Beacon, 1987).

Sharon Lebell is author of *Naming Ourselves, Naming Our Children: Resolving the Last Name Dilemma* (Crossing Press, 1988).

Marie Leduc is coordinator, Family-Child Program, Department of Community Health, The Montreal General Hospital, Montreal, Canada.

Susan Goodrich Lehmann is a Ph.D. candidate in sociology at Harvard University, where she is writing a dissertation on the causes and state responses to Russian low fertility.

Betty Wolder Levin is a medical anthropologist, and assistant professor in the Department of Health and Nutrition Sciences, Brooklyn College of the City University of New York. Her main areas of interest are maternal and child health and bioethics. She has been studying decision-making in neonatal intensive care units since 1977 and is currently doing research on ethical issues in pediatric AIDS.

Caroline T. Lewis is a statistician at the National Center for Health Statistics, Hyattsville, Maryland. She is author of, among other scholarly works, *Prenatal Care in the United States, 1980-1988* (National Center for Health Statistics, forthcoming).

Adrienne B. Lieberman is author of *Easing Labor Pain* (Doubleday, 1987).

Joan Liebmann-Smith is a sociologist and medical writer. Her publications include *In Pursuit of Pregnancy* (Newmarket, 1987).

Juliette Liesenfeld was born and raised in West Germany, and now resides in the United States. She has a master's degree in liberal studies with a specialization in translation. Her English-to-German translations include *The Tentative Pregnancy* by Barbara Katz Rothman and *Prenatal Diagnosis* by Robin Blatt.

Hanny Lightfoot-Klein is author of *Prisoners of Ritual: An Odyssey into Female Genital Circumcision in Africa* (Haworth Press, 1989) and *A Woman's Odyssey into Africa, Tracks Across a Life* (Haworth Press, 1991). Her work on female genital circumcision has been widely published in scholarly journals.

Petra Liljestrand was born and raised in Sweden, and is currently a research fellow at the Alcohol Research Group, Berkeley, California. She is author of *Rhetoric and Reason: Donor Insemination Politics in Sweden* (unpublished doctoral dissertation, 1990) and "Children Without Fathers: Handling the Anonymous Donor Question," *Out/Look*, Fall 1988.

Priscilla Rachun Linn is a social anthropologist specializing in material culture. She has planned, researched, and curated several exhibitions for the Smithsonian Institution, including "Generations," a show about birth and the first year of life.

Abby Lippman is associate professor, epidemiology department, and research associate, Department of Humanities and Social Studies in Medicine, at McGill University, Montreal, Canada.

Martha Livingston is a social psychologist, certified childbirth educator, and long-time health activist. She is on the faculty of Community Health, Biological Sciences, State University of New York at Old Westbury.

Meria Loeks (formerly Long) is the editor of the birth, midwifery, and breastfeeding departments of *Mothering* magazine. She is a licensed midwife and joint author of *Midwifery and the Law* (Mothering, 1991).

Ehrick Long is a doctoral student in musicology at The Graduate School and University Center of the City University of New York, where he is writing his dissertation on popular music.

Judith Lorber is professor of sociology and women's studies at the Graduate School and University Center, and at Brooklyn College, the City University of New York. Her many scholarly publications include *Women Physicians: Careers, Status and Power* (Tavistock, 1984). She is founding editor of *Gender & Society*.

Ruth Watson Lubic is general director of the Maternity Center Association in New York City. Her many honors include being named National Nurse of the Year (1985) by the March of Dimes Birth Defects Foundation, and Maternal and Child Health Nurse of the Year (1985).

Dana Luciano works as a family planning counselor. She has been involved in women's health activism and abortion clinic defense for several years. She currently works with Women's Health Action and Mobilization (WHAM!), a New York City-based direct action women's health advocacy organization.

Cassie Luhrs is a certified childbirth educator in South Carolina. She is cofounder of B.A.B.I.E.S. (Birth and Babies Information, Education, Support), a local support group for expecting and new parents.

Marian MacDorman, Ph.D., is a demographer/statistician in the Mortality Statistics Branch, Division of Vital Statistics, National Center for Health Statistics, Hyattsville, Maryland. Her research interests include fetal and perinatal mortality and trends in infant mortality by cause of death.

Margaret E. Malnory is a perinatal clinical nurse specialist at Sinai Samaritan Medical Center in Milwaukee, Wisconsin.

Jutta Mason is a La Leche League leader in Toronto, Canada, where she is a veteran activist in the Canadian midwifery and childbirth movement.

Patricia Maybruck is a psychologist in private practice in San Francisco and St. Helena, California. She is author of *Pregnancy and Dreams* (Tarcher, 1989) and *Romantic Dreams* (Pocket Books, 1991).

Peggy McGarrahan is a doctoral candidate in anthropology at the Graduate School and University Center of the City University of New York. She is completing research on the care of HIV patients in New York City.

Susan McKay is professor of nursing at the University of Wyoming in Laramie. Her publications include *The Assertive Approach to Childbirth* (International Childbirth Education Association, 1986).

Joan McTigue is a woman's health care practitioner in Gainesville, Florida. She is a physician's assistant in obstetrics and gynecology, a licensed midwife, and a registered nurse.

Ann V. Millard is associate professor of anthropology at Michigan State University. She has published articles on breastfeeding and weaning, pediatric advice, and women and international development.

Mary Ann Miller is a member of the faculty in the Department of Advanced Nursing Science at the University of Delaware. She is author of "Psychosocial Factors Related to Cigarette Smoking during Pregnancy," (unpublished doctoral dissertation, Temple University, 1990).

Marilyn Fayre Milos is a registered nurse, founder and executive director of the National Organization of Circumcision Information Resource Center in California, and coordinator of the International Symposia on Circumcision. She is the recipient of the California Nurses' Association's Maureen Ricke Award.

Joya Misra is a doctoral student at Emory University in Atlanta, Georgia. She is presently working on a project linking Catholic political and economic institutions to the processes of unionization.

Eileen Geil Moran is a sociologist at The Center for Labor and Society at Queens College of the City University of New York, and former director of Women's Survival Space, the first shelter for battered women and their children in Brooklyn, New York.

Carolyn Morell is a graduate student at Eugene Lang College of The New School for Social Research in New York City.

Janice M. Morse is on the faculty of nursing at the Pennsylvania State University, University Park, Pennsylvania. She has many scholarly publications in the area of breastfeeding.

Marian J. Morton is professor of history at John Carroll University in Cleveland, Ohio. Her publications include *New World, New Roles: A Documentary History of Women in Pre-Industrial America* (Greenwood Press, 1986), coedited with Sylvia Frey.

Richard Moskowitz has practiced family medicine since 1967 and specializes in classical homeopathy. His principal articles include "Homeopathic Reasoning" (1980), "The Case against Immunizations" (1983), and "Some Thoughts on the Malpractice Crisis" (1988).

Margaret Muwonge was born and raised in Uganda, the daughter of a prominent midwife. She currently resides in the Washington, DC area.

Patricia Mynaugh is assistant professor of nursing, College of Nursing, Villanova University, Villanova, Pennsylvania.

Carol Wright Napier is a recent graduate of the Washington University School of Law and the George Warren Brown School of Social Work. Her article "Civil Incest Suits: Getting beyond the Statute of Limitations" was recently published in the *Washington University Law Quarterly.*

Elizabeth Noble is an obstetric physical therapist and childbirth educator. She is the founder of the obstetrics and gynecology section of the American Physical Therapy Association, and is director of the Maternal and Child Health Center in Cambridge, Massachusetts. Her publications include *Childbirth with Insight* (Houghton Mifflin, 1980), *Having Your Baby by Donor Insemination* (Houghton Mifflin, 1987), *Essential Exercises for the Childbearing Year* (3rd edition, Houghton Mifflin, 1988), and *Having Twins* (2nd edition, Houghton Mifflin, 1991).

Margaret Nofziger is author of *Signs of Fertility: The Personal Science of Natural Birth Control* (MND Publishing, 1988).

Judy Norsigian is a coauthor of *Our Bodies, Ourselves* and *The New Our Bodies Ourselves.* She is codirector of the Boston Women's Health Book Collective and has served on the Board of the National Women's Health Network.

Michel Odent developed the maternity unit in Pithiviers, France, which became a focal point for new consciousness about birth. He has created the Primal Health Research Center in London, England. His publications include *Entering the World: The Demedicalization of Childbirth* (New American Library, 1984), *Birth Reborn* (Pantheon, 1984), *Water and Sexuality* (Penguin, 1990), and *The Ecology of Birth and Breastfeeding* (Bergin Garvey, 1992).

Gabrielle Palmer is a member of the Baby Milk Action Coalition, and the International Baby Food Action Network. She is author of *The Politics of Breastfeeding* (Pandora Press, 1988).

Ann Pappert is a journalist specializing in health issues. She is the first recipient of the Atkinson Fellowship in Public Policy, and is writing a book on in vitro fertilization.

Alison Parra is a midwife in private practice in Mexico. She is author of a column on alternative medicine for the newsletter *Informed Homebirth,* and is a regional representative to the Midwives Alliance of North America.

Kathryn A. Patterson is a nurse-midwife and assistant professor at the University of Hawaii School of Nursing. Her scholarly works include "The Social Construction of the Pregnancy Experience by Black Women at Risk for Preterm Birth" (unpublished doctoral dissertation, Ann Arbor, Michigan, University Microfilms International, 1990).

Paulina G. Perez is a perinatal registered nurse, a certified childbirth educator, and a monitrice in private practice in Katy, Texas. She is author of *Special Women: The Role of the Professional Labor Assistant* (Pennypress, 1990).

Rosalind Pollack Petchesky is professor of political science and women's studies at Hunter College of the City University of New York. She is author of *Abortion and Woman's Choice* (Northeastern University Press, 1990).

Gayle Peterson is a psychotherapist specializing in perinatal psychology and family development. Her publications include *Birthing Normally* (Shadow and Light Publications, 1984) and *An Easier Childbirth: A Mother's Workbook during Pregnancy and Delivery* (Tarcher, 1991).

Kate Prager is a demographer/statistician in the Mortality Statistics Branch, Division of Vital Statistics, National Center for Health Statistics, Hyattsville, Maryland. She is project director of the NCHS project to develop a national linked birth and infant death data set. Her research interests include infant and maternal mortality.

Margaret R. Primeau is the perinatal clinical nurse specialist for the Medical Center of Central Massachusetts in Worcester, Massachusetts. She is president-elect of the Massachusetts Perinatal Association, a member of the Nursing Association of the American College of Obstetrics and Gynecology, and a member of the Consumer Education Committee—NAACOG.

Deborah Raines is a doctoral student in nursing administration and information systems at Virginia Commonwealth University, Richmond. She has worked as a perinatal clinical nurse specialist and held positions as clinician, educator, and manager in a variety of acute care, outpatient, and academic settings.

Dana Raphael is director of the Human Lactation Center in Westport, Connecticut. Her publications include *Only Mothers Know: Patterns of Infant Feeding in a Hungry World* (Greenwood Press, 1984) and *The Tender Gift: Breastfeeding* (Schocken Books, 1976).

Shana Reed is a certified nurse midwife who practices in a hospital-based service providing prenatal, intrapartal, and postpartal care to indigent women and their families in Reading, Pennsylvania.

Katherine Reese is a fellow of the American College of Obstetricians and Gynecologists, working at the Yale University Health Services. She is a clinical instructor in obstetrics and gynecology at Yale Medical School and Yale-New Haven Hospital.

Margaret Regan is a graduate student in sociology at the Graduate School and University Center of the City University of New York.

Shulamit Reinharz is professor of sociology and director of women's studies at Brandeis University in Waltham, Massachusetts.

Pat Richter is prevention coordinator at Prevention Resources, a grant project funded by the New York State Developmental Disabilities Planning Council and New Horizons for the Retarded, Inc., in Millbrook, New York.

Kathy Rosenberg is a nurse-midwife in clinical practice at the Health Science Center of the State University of New York at Brooklyn.

Barbara Katz Rothman is professor of sociology, Baruch College and the Graduate School and University Center, City University of New York. Her publications include *In Labor: Women and Power in the Birthplace* (Norton, 1982 and 1991), *The Tentative Pregnancy: Women's Experience with Amniocentesis and Prenatal Diagnosis* (Norton, 1993), and *Recreating Motherhood: Ideology and Technology in a Patriarchal Society* (Norton, 1989), which received the 1991 Jessie Bernard Award of the American Sociological Association.

Joan Rothschild is professor of political science, University of Lowell, Lowell, Massachusetts. Her publications include *Machina Ex Dea: Feminist Perspectives on Technology* (Pergamon Press, 1983), *Teaching Technology from a Feminist Perspective* (Pergamon, 1988), and *Engineering Birth* (Indiana University Press, forthcoming).

Ruth Rubinstein is associate professor of sociology at the Fashion Institute of Technology in New York.

Sara Ruddick teaches philosophy and women's studies at Eugene Lang College, New School for Social Research in New York City. She is coeditor of two anthologies: *Working It Out* (Pantheon, 1977) and *Between Women* (Beacon Press, 1984). She is author of *Maternal Thinking: Toward a Politics of Peace* (Beacon Press, 1989).

Sheryl Burt Ruzek is associate professor of health education at Temple University, Philadelphia, Pennsylvania. She is a member of the National Women's Health Network, the Maternity Care

Coalition of Philadelphia, and the Food and Drug Administration Obstetrics and Gynecology Devices Panel. She has edited the *Health, Society and Policy Series*, with Irving Kenneth Zola, for Temple University Press since 1984. Her books include *The Women's Health Movement, Feminist Alternatives to Medical Control* (Praeger, 1978).

Carol Sakala is codirector of the Women's Institute for Childbearing Policy, a public interest group promoting transformation of maternity care arrangements. She is a Pew Health Policy Fellow at Boston University, where she is completing a doctorate in health policy.

Deirdre Colby Sato is a recent graduate of the master's program in higher education administration at New York University, and is active in the DES movement.

Diana Scully is associate professor of sociology and coordinator of women's studies at Virginia Commonwealth University. Her publications include *Men Who Control Women's Health: The Miseducation of Obstetrician-Gynecologists* (Houghton Mifflin, 1980) and *Understanding Sexual Violence: A Study of Convicted Rapists* (HarperCollins Academic, 1990).

Brenda Seals is assistant professor of sociology, Tulane University, New Orleans, Louisiana, and author of many articles on reproductive issues.

Barbara Seaman is cofounder of the National Womens Health Network and author of *The Doctors' Case against the Pill* (1969); *Free and Female* (1972); *Women and the Crisis in Sex Hormones* (1977); and *Lovely Me: The Life of Jacqueline Susann* (1987).

Althea Seaver is a midwife and nutritionist in private practice in Eugene, Oregon. She writes a nutrition column for *Midwifery Today*.

Nancy C. Sharts-Engel served on the Maternal-Infant Nursing Faculty at St. Luke's College of Nursing, Tokyo. She is associate professor in the College of Nursing at Villanova University, Villanova, Pennsylvania.

Beth Shearer is a founder and director of C/Sec Inc., Cesarean/Support Education and Concern, in Framingham, Massachusetts.

Pamela Shrock is director of psychosomatic obstetrics and gynecology at Winthrop University Hospital, Mineola, New York. She is a psychotherapist and sex therapist in private practice.

Wendy Simonds is assistant professor of sociology at Emory University in Atlanta, Georgia. Her publications include coauthorship, with Barbara Katz Rothman, of *Centuries of Solace: A Comparative Analysis of Maternal Consolation Literature* (Temple University Press, 1992) and *Women and Self Help Culture: Reading Between the Lines* (Rutgers University Press, 1992).

Sharleen H. Simpson is a nurse/anthropologist specializing in maternal/child and women's health. Currently she is assistant professor at the University of Florida College of Nursing, and an affiliate faculty member in Latin American Studies.

Mary Ann M. Smith is a certified nurse midwife practicing at The Birth Center of Gainesville, Florida, where she does birth center and home births.

Ann Snitow, writer and feminist activist since 1970, teaches literature and women's studies at Eugene Lang College of The New School for Social Research in New York City. She coedited *Powers of Desire: The Politics of Sexuality*, and is currently publishing parts of her work in progress, *A Gender Diary*, which includes a chapter on feminism and motherhood.

Jill Stanzler-Katz is a social worker and therapist in private practice in the Boston area.

Carolyn Steiger is a midwife in private practice in Oregon. She has served on several state task forces related to maternal-infant health and is author of *Becoming a Midwife* (Hoogan House, 1987).

B. Collene Stout is a social worker, childbirth educator, and psychotherapist specializing in family life issues who practices in New Jersey.

Frederic Suffet is a researcher with the Center for Comprehensive Health Practice in New York City, whose programs include the Pregnant Addicts and Addicted Mothers programs. He is also a member of the faculty of the Department of Psychiatry and Behavioral Science of New York Medical College.

Deborah Sullivan is professor of sociology at Arizona State University and coauthor, with Rose Weitz, of *Labor Pains: Modern Midwives and Home Birth* (Yale University Press, 1988).

Meredith Dingman Sutton holds a master's degree in art history from Hunter College, The City University of New York. She works at the Archer M. Huntington Art Gallery, University of Texas at Austin.

Marlene Sweeney is a childbirth educator advocate, a La Leche League leader, and managing editor of *New Beginnings*, the La Leche League's breastfeeding journal.

Jane C. Szczepaniak is a childbirth educator in private practice in Maryland. She is author of "So You Have Just Had a Cesarean" and "So You're Thinking about VBAC" (International Childbirth Education Association pamphlets).

Selma Taffel is a health statistician at the National Center for Health Statistics, Hyattsville, Maryland. She has many scholarly publications in the area of health-related aspects of natality data. She is the 1983 recipient of the National Center for Health Statistics Director's Award for statistical reporting, and the 1990 recipient of the Elijah White Memorial Award for major contributions to the field of public health statistics.

Tine Thevenin is author of *The Family Bed: An Age-Old Concept in Childrearing* (originally published in 1976; re-issued in 1987 by Avery).

Wenda R. Trevathan is associate professor of anthropology at New Mexico State University. She has received midwifery training, and is the recipient of the 1990 Margaret Mead Award of the American Anthropology Association and the Society for Applied Anthropology. Her publications include *Human Birth: An Evolutionary Perspective* (Aldine de Gruyter, 1987).

Julia Ann Upton is associate professor of theology at St. John's University in New York. She is author of *A Church for the Next Generation: Sacraments in Transition* (Liturgical Press, 1990) and *Journey into Mystery* (Paulist Press, 1986).

Joanna Varadi is a certified nurse-midwife in practice in Gainesville, Florida. Her work has emphasized re-empowering women in childbirth and their daily lives.

Stephanie J. Ventura is a statistician/demographer at the National Center for Health Statistics, Hyattsville, Maryland, researching birth statistics from vital registration data. Her many publications include *Advance Report of Final Natality Statistics; Trends and Variations in First Births to Older Women, 1970-86;* and several analytic reports on births of Hispanic parentage.

Sandra Waldman is a senior associate and deputy in the office of communications of the Population Council, and manager of public information. Prior to joining the Council, she worked for the Associated Press and CBS News and was a principal in her own public relations firm.

Barbara G. Walker is the author of many books, including *The Woman's Encyclopedia of Myths and Secrets* (Harper and Row,

1983), *The Crone* (Harper and Row, 1987), *The Skeptical Feminist* (Harper and Row, 1987), *The I Ching of the Goddess* (Harper and Row, 1986), and *Women's Rituals* (Harper and Row, 1990). She is also the designer of *The Barbara Walker Tarot Deck* (U.S. Games Systems, 1986).

Doris B. Wallace is a developmental psychologist and family therapist working in New York City. She is coeditor of *Creative People at Work* (Oxford University Press, 1989) and is working on a book about siblings and creativity.

Edward Wallerstein is author of *Circumcision: An American Health Fallacy* (Springer Publishing Company, 1980), a recipient of the American Medical Writers' Award in 1981.

Alison Ward is an adoption reform advocate and former vice-president and director of Concerned United Birth Parents (CUB).

Alan J. Weisbard is associate professor of law and of medical ethics at the University of Wisconsin Schools of Law and Medicine in Madison. He has served as executive director of the New Jersey Bioethics Commission and as assistant director for legal studies with the President's Commission on Ethics in Medicine and Research. He is a fellow and former adjunct associate of the Hastings Center for Biomedical Ethics, Hastings on Hudson, New York.

Rose Weitz is professor of sociology at Arizona State University. She is author of *Life with AIDS* (Rutgers University Press, 1991) and coauthor, with Deborah Sullivan, of *Labor Pains: Modern Midwives and Home Birth* (Yale University Press, 1988).

Dorothy C. Wertz is senior scientist at the Eunice Kennedy Shriver Center for Mental Retardation, and research professor at Boston University School of Public Health. She is author of *Ethics and Human Genetics: A Cross-Cultural Perspective* (Springer-Verlag, 1989), and coauthor, with Richard W. Wertz, of *Lying-in: A History of Childbirth in America* (expanded edition, Yale University Press, 1989).

Helen Wessel is founder and president of Apple Tree Family Ministries, Artesia, California. She is a former president of the International Childbirth Education Association and is an honorary life member. She is author of *Natural Childbirth of the Christian Family* (ATFM, 1991), *Under the Apple Tree, Marrying, Birthing, Parenting* (ATFM, 1992), and coeditor, with Harlan Ellis, M.D., of *Childbirth Without Fear* (HarperCollins, 1984).

Caroline Whitbeck is senior lecturer in mechanical engineering and senior research scholar at the Center for Technology, Policy, and Industrial Development in Cambridge, Massachusetts. She was elected fellow of the American Association for the Advancement of Science (AAAS) for her work in engineering ethics and serves on the AAAS Committee on Scientific Freedom and Responsibility. She is completing a book on ethics in science and engineering, titled *Ethics in the Works* (forthcoming).

Linda M. Whiteford is associate professor of anthropology at the University of South Florida. Along with Marilyn Poland, she edited *New Approaches to Human Reproduction: Social and Ethical Dimensions* (Westview Press, 1989), and is currently working on a book with Lois Gonzalez on the social construction of infertility, to be called *Infertility: The Hidden Burden* (Westview Press, 1992).

Ahuva Windsor was born and raised in Israel, where she worked for several years in research, planning, and evaluation of health care facilities and services in the public and private sectors, as well as with grassroots organizations aimed at improving the state of women's health in Israel. She lives in London, England.

Margarete Yard is a doctoral student in sociology at The Graduate School and University Center of the City University of New York. She is a registered nurse with extensive background in medical administration policy and program development, specializing in substance abuse, physician and allied health practices, and quality assurance and cost containment.

Diony Young is editor of *Birth: Issues in Perinatal Care and Education*. She serves on the New York State Department of Health Prenatal/Perinatal Advisory Council and Consumer Health Information Council, was a member of the National Institutes of Health Expert Panel on the Content of Prenatal Care, and is a consultant for the International Childbirth Education Association. Her publications include *Changing Childbirth: Family Birth in the Hospital* (Childbirth Graphics Limited, 1982).

Laura Zeidenstein is a nurse-midwife in clinical practice at University Hospital, Health Science Center, Brooklyn, New York.

Meg Zweiback is a pediatric nurse practitioner and an assistant clinical professor of nursing at the University of California, San Francisco. She specializes in behavioral pediatrics and has a private practice consulting with families and schools. She is a contributing editor to *Parents Press*, and author of *Keys to Preparing and Caring for Your Second Child* (Barron's Educational Series, 1991) and *Keys to Parenting Your One-Year-Old* (Barron's Educational Series, 1992).

Alphabetical List of Articles

Guide to Related Topics

Abortion

Abortion: Feminist Ethical Analyses
Abortion, Politics of
Abortion Counseling
Abortion Rights Groups
Menstrual Extraction
Problem Pregnancy Counseling
Roe v. Wade
RU486
Selective Abortion
Webster v. Reproductive Health Services

Adoption

Adoption, Closed
Adoption, Intercountry
Adoption, Open
Adoption, Special Needs Children
Adoption, Transracial
Birthmothers
Lactation, Induced
Maternity Homes
Problem Pregnancy Counseling

Baby Care

Apgar
Baby Diaries: The History of Child Development
Baptism, Infant
Circumcision, Male
Circumcision Surgery
Colic
Comfort Objects
Diapers: Environmental Concerns
Eye Prophylaxis
The Family Bed
Genital Mutilation, Female
Infant Carriers
Infant Feeding and Care: Nineteenth and Twentieth Centuries, United States
Infant Movement
Jaundice, Newborn
Leboyer Method
Lullabies and Cradle Songs
Naming Practices: Given Names
Naming Practices: Surnames
Newborn Intelligence
Newborn Pain
Newborn Senses
Pediatrics, History of
Rooming-In
Shoes for Babies
Spock, Dr. Benjamin
Swaddling
Toys for Babies
Vaccinations

Caregivers and Practitioners

Chiropractic Care
Doula
Evolution of Human Birth
Labor Assistants
Labor Partners
Midwife Licensing
Midwife-Attended Births
Midwifery: Overview
Midwifery and the Law
Midwives, Southern Black
Nurse-Midwifery: History in the United States
Obstetrics, History of
Pediatrics, History of
Social Science Research on American Childbirth Practices
Witch Midwives

Childbirth Practices and Locations

Birth Centers
Bradley Method: Husband-Coached Childbirth
Breath Control in Labor
Cesarean Birth: Indications and Consequences
Cesarean Birth: Social and Political Aspects
Cesarean Birth: Trends in the United States
Childbirth Practices in American History
Electronic Fetal Monitoring
Epidural Anesthesia
Episiotomy
External Cephalic Version
Family-Centered Maternity Care
Home Birth
Hospital Birth: An Anthropological Analysis of Ritual and Practice
Hypnosis for Childbirth
Labor: Overview
Leboyer Method
Obstetric Drugs: Their Effects on Mother and Infant
Pain Relief in Labor: Non-Drug Methods
Posture for Labor and Birth
Psychoprophylactic Method (Lamaze)
Read Method: Natural Childbirth
Siblings at Birth
Social Science Research on American Childbirth Practices
Twilight Sleep
Underwater Birth

Contraception

The Cervical Cap
Condoms
Contraception: Defining Terms
Depo-Provera
The Diaphragm
IUD: Intrauterine Device
Natural Family Planning
Norplant
The Pill
RU486
Sanger, Margaret

Cross-Cultural Perspectives

Germany
Hispanics: United States
Israel
Japan
Mexico
Midwives, Southern Black
The Netherlands
Soviet Union, Former
Sweden
Uganda

Infant Feeding

Breastfeeding: Historical Aspects
Breastfeeding: Physiological and Cultural Aspects
Breastfeeding beyond Infancy
Breastfeeding Patterns
Doula
Formula Marketing
Infant Feeding and Care: Nineteenth and Twentieth Centuries, United States
Lactation, Induced
Nipples, Artificial
Nipples, Human
Relactation
Weaning

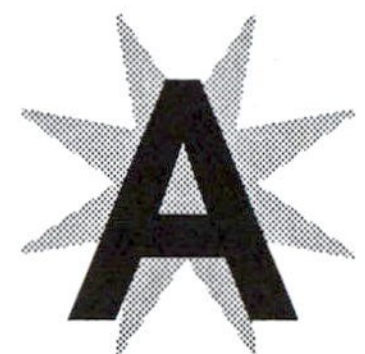

ABORTION: FEMINIST ETHICAL ANALYSES

In deriving grounds for ethical decision making, feminists locate themselves along different points of a continuum between two poles variously labeled self-determination and nurturance, particularity and solidarity, or interest and beneficence. These poles correspond to the tension at the psychic level between individuation and identity and at the social level between the claims its members have on the community and their obligations to serve communal needs. The two poles necessarily remain in a dialectical relation, that is, neither is dispensable. This means, first, that individuals' moral decisions have to be made from the standpoint of their own particular embodiment—who they are in the material situation (including their bodies but also their social conditions) in which they find themselves.

To assert the legitimacy of an ethic of the body—by definition "interested" and "particular"—has special historical significance for feminists. From the early 19th century, "moral woman" has been confined to the ethics of nurturance. Associating her with bodily self-determination represents a dialectically determined stance of resistance.

At the same time, whether out of their socialization or their inventiveness, women have persistently reclaimed the ethic of nurturance and solidarity and tried to turn it to useful purposes. From Victorian feminists and moral reformers to 20th-century peace activists to the abortion patients interviewed by Carol Gilligan (1982), women have understood their goals in terms less of self-liberation than of concern with, and responsibility to, others.

Feminist moral thinking seeks a complex position with regard to abortion decisions. While the standpoint of embodiment represents a radical position from which to make an ethical decision, women's practice, if not feminist theory, belies the very possibility of a totally isolated decision about a pregnancy; women's bodies exist in social contexts, and their decisions almost always reflect their relations with significant others. Neither the decision to get an abortion nor the decision to bear a child is inherently moral or immoral; it all depends on the circumstances and the reasons involved. Of course, this argument rests on the assumption that fetuses are not persons.

The Fetus Is Not a Person. In a framework of biological determinism, antiabortionists attempt to prove "fetal personhood" in terms of biochemistry and genetics, thereby reducing humanity to chemical bits. The notion of personhood, a metaphysical, moral idea, is transmogrified into a crude expression of the fetus as "baby," along with a Calvinist doctrine of predestination ("the individual is whoever he [*sic*] is supposed to become from the moment of impregnation") inserted into the randomness of human fertilization and genetic pairing.

The most striking fallacy in the genetic arguments of antiabortionists is their leap from the *fact* of genetic individuality—a characteristic not only of humans but of all living things—to the *value* of human personhood. This is a problem, in part, of confusing the self, the person, with her or his genetic basis, ignoring the enormously complex interaction between genes, environment, and development that ultimately determines who or what an actual person becomes. To say that who a person is is codified from the moment of conception is to deny most people's common-sense assumptions about who they are and their selfhood and its roots in conscious experience. It also confuses genetic *potentiality* with *actual* human personality and character, which are highly influenced by culture.

Thus, the broader problem with the idea that the fetus is a "person" from conception has to do with the concept of personhood, or even humanity, for it either rests on a theological premise—"ensoulment"—or it reduces to a crude, mechanistic biologism. In legal and moral terms, this means that the concept of "person" (moral) is totally collapsed into the concept of "human life" (biological, genetic).

The beginning of human life is not the issue, for it can be argued that fetuses, even if they are "human life," are still not human persons. That the fetus is human and may even have a "right to life" does not prove that abortion is "morally (im)permissible," because being "human in the genetic sense" is distinct from being "human in the moral sense"—that is, from being a person. The fetus is not a human person in this latter sense; therefore, whatever rights it may have "could not possibly outweigh the right of a woman to obtain an abortion, since the rights of actual persons invariably outweigh those of any potential person whenever the two conflict" (Warren, 1979, p. 48). To deny that the fetus is a "full human person" does not necessarily mean denying that the fetus, as a *potentially* human and presently sentient being, is morally deserving of consideration, or even that it can make moral or emotional claims on those in charge of its care—mainly pregnant women. The problem is that whatever those claims may be, they frequently come into conflict with the rights and needs of women and others with whom they are connected who *are* (in the opinion of feminists and humanists) full human persons. But the "right-to-life" position either denies such conflict or dissolves the abortion issue into a definition of "motherhood" that makes the fetus's life determinant of the woman's.

The Ethic of Woman's Embodiment. How individual women ought to think about an abortion or childbearing decision, the kinds of values or concerns they ought to bring to bear, is so enmeshed in their particular situation that to attempt ethical prescriptions seems presumptuous, if not pointless. Even if our moral stance as feminist is weighted toward the pole of nurturance—"responsibility to others"—we still have to ask, "Which others?" Who is our community and how do we best determine its needs?

An ethic of embodiment requires and permits the grounding of a decision about abortion or childbirth in the actual conditions of a woman's life, conditions not usually freely chosen but imposed instead by society. The absence of social supports, income, skills, prenatal care, all affect powerfully a woman's decision making regarding childbearing or the termination of pregnancy. Any woman seeking (in a particular time, in a particular country) to make a moral decision about abortion must take these realities into account. Doing so, she is not merely engaging in some kind of utilitarian cost-benefit analysis but is making her decision squarely within the constraints that will determine its consequences for herself and others—the essence of moral praxis.

The absence of social and material support does not, on the other hand, give the pregnant woman a moral duty to have an abortion. Instead it presents her with a kind of negative social contract—without these supports, the society has no basis whatever for telling her she has a moral duty to bear a child. The woman who believes the fetus is not a person can *choose* to either have an abortion or renounce her other life projects in favor of its life, as a kind of gift, however burdensome. But no one can compel her to do so, and a woman needs to consider very carefully that her body and life course have moral value and deserve her respect, as well as others'. Even in the (unlikely) event of radical social changes in which priority is given to the needs of *all* children and the people who nurture them, a situation demanding compulsory motherhood could still never be morally justified.

From the standpoint of embodiment, particular circumstances of many sorts may motivate an abortion decision and have moral weight. In a conservative political and cultural climate, every abortion on some level represents a woman's assertion of her moral right to be sexual. A complicated question arises within this framework of embodiment: Is there ever a situation where abortion may be unethical, or at least morally ambiguous, from the standpoint of a woman's particularity, her self and its morally legitimate needs?

Situations exist where a woman has to weigh material circumstances—lack of money or a job, lack of a loving partner, lack of social services to accommodate physical disability (her own or her fetus's)—against a strong desire to have a child. In this dilemma she may experience a deep sense of injustice that indeed reflects something morally and socially askew in the world. But the wrong here is not in her decision but in the circumstances that prompt it; society, not the woman, is to blame.

The more difficult case is the woman who decides to abort a fetus on the basis of its sex or possible impairment. But the reasons why such cases may be ambiguous—and why the woman ought to or does weigh her decision more carefully—do not have to do with the moral status of the fetus. Rather, they have to do with the reinforcement her decision gives to cultural stereotypes that emphasize gender division, devalue daughters, or stigmatize disability. Despite this dilemma, compelling circumstances in the particular case, along with the society's failure to support disabled children or to abolish gender inequality, may justify an abortion.

On the other hand, the prevalent moral discourse about abortion seldom recognizes that a decision to go through with a pregnancy may be just as "selfishly" motivated as a decision to abort. Here, too, the legitimacy of self-determination as a moral ground for the decision will depend on the particular circumstances. A poor woman who decides to have another baby despite her oppressed social conditions may be claiming one small space where she has some control and the possibility of pleasure.

There are cases, however, where the morality of a decision to bear a child may be problematic. Why one wants this child, what one intends to do with it, and how one plans to care for it are legitimate questions (although this is not to suggest that their resolution should be made through state or legislative intervention). Is bearing a child in order to keep a man, to prove one's adulthood, or to have a live doll to love necessarily a nurturant act, or a moral one?

The Ethic of Nurturance. While a woman's own situation remains a legitimate and compelling vantage point from which to make a decision about pregnancy, the fact is that she rarely makes such a decision in a vacuum. Because she is a social being, and one who has been socialized to think relationally, the pull of others' needs, interests, and desires will permeate her thinking about what is "best." In this process, the ethic of nurturance, or beneficence, will make its claims, and in ways that feminists must respect.

An ethic of nurturance stipulates that the provision of one's body—whether in maternity, sex, or national defense—is always a *gift*, never a *duty*. A gift, by definition, cannot be coerced; it must be voluntary. The woman herself, out of her own feelings of love and fidelity, must determine the uses she will make of her body and the communities or loved ones it will serve. Any other determination, whether by national leaders, priests, rabbis, ayatollahs, or husbands, is servitude.

The gift relation, the relation of love and caring, may also be the basis of an abortion decision. When a black woman under slavery or a political prisoner in a fascist jail aborts her fetus, she is giving the gift of death to a potential child whose life, if it survived, would be a living death. This relation might also apply to cases where a fetus is diagnosed as having Tay-Sachs disease or a condition that causes similar terrible pain and early death. To relieve from gratuitous suffering is to act from an ethic of nurturance. These decisions are never entirely altruistic, for no gift is ever completely free of self-interest. The purpose of a gift is to articulate the relation between the self and another, not to obliterate the self.

An abortion may also be motivated by concern not only, or primarily, for the fetus but for others to whom one is responsible. Many abortions reflect moral decisions by women not to risk the well-being of existing children, or of other persons to whom they owe care, for the sake of a child not born. From the standpoint of nurturance, these women too act out of solidarity.

Ultimately, certain life-and-death decisions must be entrusted to the people whose bodies and/or caretaking activities are most intimately involved. The further such decisions are separated from personal relations, the more remote and irrelevant they become from either the ethics of embodiment or the ethics of nurturance, and the less they deserve women's trust.

✱ ROSALIND POLLACK PETCHESKY, Ph.D.

See also: Abortion, Politics of; Problem Pregnancy Counseling; The Reproduction of Mothering; Selective Abortion

See **Guide to Related Topics:** Abortion

Resources

Gilligan, Carol. (1982). *In a Different Voice.* Cambridge, MA: Harvard University Press.

Murray, Thomas. (1986) "The Ownership and Disposal of Body Parts." Unpublished talk, The Hastings Center, Hastings On Hudson, NY, June 13.

———. (1986, Jan-Feb). "Who Owns the Body? On the Ethics of Using Human Tissue for Commercial Purposes." vol. 8 *IRB*.

Petchesky, Rosalind Pollack. (1980). "Reproductive Freedom: Beyond A Woman's Right to Choose". In C.R. Simpson & E.S. Person (Eds.) *Women, Sex and Sexuality.* Chicago: University of Chicago Press, pp. 92-116.

———. (1986, Jul) "A Framework for Choice." *Christianity and Crisis 14*: 247-50.

———. (1990). *Abortion and Woman's Choice.* Boston: Northeastern University Press.

Warren, Mary Anne. (1979). "On the Moral and Legal Status of Abortion." In Richard A. Wasserstrom (Ed.) *Today's Moral Problems.* New York: MacMillan, pp. 35-50

ABORTION, POLITICS OF

Social attitudes about abortion as a political or legislative issue have varied considerably over time and from place to place along with changing ideas about the appropriateness of government or church intervention, fertility rates and the popularity of eugenic ideologies, medical authority, women, fetuses, and motherhood. Whether legal or not, abortion has always been a method women have used to stop pregnancy; today, over half of the abortions performed in the world are illegal, and it has been estimated that 84,000 women die each year as a result of illegal abortions.

In the United States, it was not until the mid-1800s that laws restricting abortion were first enacted, as physicians sought to amplify their control over pregnancy. Doctors' decisions about whether or not abortions are deemed appropriate or necessary have remained central to the formulation and enforcement of laws restricting abortion. Even now, pollsters ask people whether or not they believe a woman *and her doctor* should have the right to decide about abortion.

In the political battle that has raged in this country since *Roe v. Wade* made abortion a right-to-privacy issue in 1973, organizations opposing abortion have been dominated by Catholics and fundamentalist Christians (who have labeled themselves "pro-life"), while organizations supporting access to abortion (that label themselves "pro-choice") have grown as part of mainstream feminism. Feminist support for abortion has shifted from a call to de-legislate abortion and repeal abortion laws (before *Roe v. Wade*) to an insistence on maintaining legal access to abortion. In the 1992 Supreme Court decision on the Pennsylvania case, the court upheld the states' ability to restrict access to abortion, including provisions for parental notification, and waiting periods, but not husband notification.

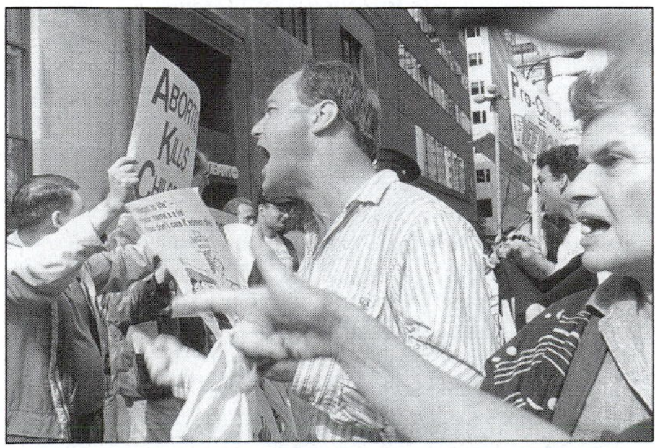

The National Right to Life Committee's "Chain of Life" is confronted by 6,000 pro-choice demonstrators, New York City, September 29, 1991. © Meryl Levin/Impact Visuals.

The language being used to evaluate abortion shows that the debate involves competing moral frameworks: those opposed to abortion focus on the fetus as innocent life that must be protected from misguided women, while those who support access to abortion focus on women's rights to control procreation (since it takes place within—or as a part of—their bodies). Ironically, both groups' ideological stances stem from their notions of what womanhood should be and what mothering should mean.

General support for the continued availability of abortion has hovered at around 70 percent during the past 15 years. But when abortion is diced up into various "what if?" hypothetical scenarios, this majority commitment begins to fall apart. People are most likely to see abortion as appropriate when a woman's life is endangered by pregnancy; when her pregnancy results from rape or incest; and when the fetus is "defective." Support for legal abortion wanes (ranges from less than half to one-quarter of those polled) if a woman "cannot afford any more children"; if she "does not want to marry the man"; and if the "pregnancy would interfere with [her] work or education." So, while support for legal abortion remains consistent over time in many circumstances, support for women's decision making does not. People's willingness to conceive of abortion as the result of women's irresponsibility or cavalier attitude toward pregnancy indicates that the rhetoric of anti-abortion activists has been successful.

Support for abortion is correlated with education (the more schooling, the more likely a person is to support legal abortion); with political orientation (people who define themselves as "liberals" and "moderates" are more likely to support legal abortion than "conservatives"); with knowing someone—or being someone—who has had an abortion; with age (younger people are more likely to support abortion); and with marital status (unmarried people are more likely to support abortion). One of the biggest predictors of opposition to abortion is religiosity; people to whom religion is very important are much more likely to oppose abortion than those to whom religion is not so important.

The actions of anti-abortion protesters, which grew more violent during the 1980s, and included bombing clinics and forcibly blocking women from entering clinics, has focused media attention on abortion over the past decade. The avowed pro-life stances of Ronald Reagan and George

Bush have had—and will no doubt continue to have—far-reaching effects on how people think about abortion, and indeed, upon whether or not abortion remains legal in this country.

Access to abortion in the United States has diminished in recent years, with broad cuts in Medicaid funding, but the number of abortions performed has remained relatively stable since 1980 (approximately 1.6 million annually). The vast majority (more than 98 percent) of abortions are performed in metropolitan areas. The number of hospitals providing abortions declined by 13 percent between 1985 and 1988, while clinics offering abortion services increased by only four percent during this time. Most abortions now take place in clinics, a radical change since 1973, when the majority of abortions were performed in hospitals. It becomes increasingly difficult for abortion-providing facilities to find doctors who will perform abortions. Certainly within the medical profession, abortion has retained its status as "dirty work."

The Supreme Court, in its *Webster* decision of 1989, allowed states to enact legislative restrictions on abortion, despite a wave of public protest. Access to abortion has already been diminished by the implementation of parental notification restrictions in several states. Those involved in the fight to keep abortion legal point to bills already introduced or expected to be introduced that would limit the availability of abortion to women whose lives are endangered by their pregnancies, who have been the victims of rape or incest, or whose fetuses are "deformed/handicapped"; reformulate clinic licensing (to make providing abortion much more difficult or impossible); institute "viability tests" on fetuses aborted during the second trimester; impose spousal consent regulations; and stipulate wait periods (between the pregnancy test and the abortion). The Supreme Court's 1991 decision to uphold Title 10, which denies clinics federal money if their staffs discuss abortion with clients, will certainly hamper women's access to abortion.

In the 1992 Supreme Court decision on the Pennsylvania case, the court upheld the states' ability to restrict access to abortion, including provisions for parental notification and waiting periods, but not husband notification.

Interviews conducted with people who work to provide abortion show that they are frightened about the future. They think that the right to an abortion is slowly being chipped away. Abortion advocates and workers do express hope that, should abortion become criminalized, a "better underground" would develop because abortion has been legal since 1973 and so many people now have knowledge of the relatively simple technique (dilation and evacuation) used to perform first trimester abortions, as well as of menstrual extraction. Even so, they say, access to abortion has increasingly become a class-based privilege with Medicaid cuts, and this situation would worsen if abortion were prohibited by law.

✷ WENDY SIMONDS, Ph.D.

See also: Abortion Rights Groups; Roe v. Wade; Webster v. Reproductive Health Services

See **Guide to Related Topics:** Abortion

Resources

Callahan, Sidney & Callahan, Daniel. (Eds.) (1984). *Abortion: Understanding Differences.* New York: Plenum Press.

Ginsburg, Faye. (1989). *Contested Lives: The Abortion Debate in an American Community.* Berkeley, CA: University of California Press.

Luker, Kristin. (1984). *Abortion and the Politics of Motherhood.* Berkeley, CA: University of California Press.

Messer, Ellen & May, Kathryn E. (1988). *Back Rooms: Voices from the Illegal Abortion Era.* New York: St. Martin's Press.

Rothman, Barbara Katz. (1989). *Recreating Motherhood: Ideology and Technology in a Patriarchal Society.* New York: W.W. Norton.

Simonds, Wendy. "Is Progress a Thing of the Past?: Abortion Workers on the Politics of Abortion." Work in progress.

Singer, Gail. (Author and Director). (1985). "Abortion: Stories from North and South" (film).

Note: The author thanks the Alan Guttmacher Institute, the National Abortion Federation, and Planned Parenthood for providing information about survey data and the incidence and availability of abortions.

ABORTION COUNSELING

In 1971, when the District of Columbia legalized abortion, the first outpatient clinic, Preterm Center for Reproductive Health, developed a model for preabortion counseling and counselor-assisted procedures. When the Supreme Court's *Roe v. Wade* decision made abortion legal everywhere in the U.S., outpatient abortion clinics commonly used the Preterm model for counseling. The model provided for one-to-one counseling with a trained lay counselor, who also accompanied the woman through the surgical procedure to provide support and assistance in pain management. Today, after nearly two decades of legal, safe abortion, most clinics provide education for their clients in a group setting and only offer individual counseling when requested or when clinic staff identify a problem; procedure room support may be provided by a counselor, a specially trained aide, or a nurse. It is desirable for a pregnant woman and her partner or other involved family member to make decisions jointly when possible. The counselor can assist them in examining their feelings and resolving conflict. If resolution is impossible within the time constraints posed by the pregnancy, it is the woman who ultimately makes the decision on whether or not to abort the pregnancy.

The goals of preabortion counseling are (1) to ensure that the woman has considered her alternatives and has made an uncoerced choice for abortion; (2) to secure informed consent by explaining the procedure and its risks and complications to the clients; (3) to assess the suitability of an outpatient procedure for the client, and, when appropriate, to refer her for an inpatient procedure; (4) to assist the woman in reviewing her decision, her feelings, and her ability to handle mixed emotions engendered by the pregnancy, her circumstances, and the choice of abortion; (5) to prepare the woman for the procedure by reducing her anxiety and providing her with relaxation and pain management techniques; and (6) to discuss with the woman her contraceptive history and assist her in making an appropriate contraceptive choice to use after her abortion.

In meeting these goals, the counselor acts as a surrogate for the operating physician, enabling more extensive education and counseling about abortion, contraception, and fertility management to be offered by clinics as part of routine service and without additional charge. Counselors are usually lay personnel, given training in short-term counseling skills, abortion and contraceptive technology, and related subjects by their own clinics or through the National Abortion Federation, a professional association for abortion providers.

While many woman are well able to make a decision about their unplanned or unwanted pregnancies and to handle the abortion procedure adequately without a counseling intervention, the widespread use of woman-to-woman counseling has meant that nearly all women experience their abortions as nontraumatic, many citing it as an important learning and growth experience as well. For some women, the choice of abortion constitutes their first entry into the health care system, and the counselor is also able to make referrals for other kinds of preventive care and medical services.

Repeated attempts by abortion providers to offer postabortion counseling or support groups has shown that few women who had preabortion counseling feel the need for additional counseling afterward, although some women will seek help elsewhere for other sexual, health, or relationship problems for which the abortion was not a remedy.

✱ TERRY BERESFORD

See also: Problem Pregnancy Counseling

See **Guide to Related Topics:** Abortion

Resources

Baker, Anne. (1985). *The Complete Book of Problem Pregnancy Counseling*. Granite City, IL: The Hope Clinic for Women.

Benderly, Beryl Lieff. (1984). *Thinking about Abortion*. Garden City, NY: The Dial Press.

Beresford, Terry. (1979). "Abortion Counseling." In Gerald I. Zatuchni, John J. Sciarra, & J. Joseph Speidel, (Eds.) *Pregnancy Termination*. New York: Harper and Row.

———. (1988). *Short Term Relationship Counseling: A Self-Instructional Manual for Family Planning Clinics*. Baltimore: Planned Parenthood of Maryland.

Hern, Warren. (1990). *Abortion Practice*. Philadelphia: J.B. Lippincott.

Saltzman, Lori et.al. (1988). *Pregnancy Counseling*. San Francisco: Planned Parenthood of San Francisco/Alameda.

ABORTION RIGHTS GROUPS

Abortion rights groups have long been active in the United States at both the national and local levels. Before the *Roe v. Wade* decision, which decriminalized abortion in 1973, a number of groups worked to make abortion legal: physicians, clergy, public health workers, and, most significantly, thousands of "average" women who mobilized on behalf of abortion rights. After legalization in 1973, the abortion rights movement went into somewhat of a quiescent phase, but with changes in the composition of the Supreme Court as a result of the Reagan and Bush administrations, the movement has recently been able to galvanize the formerly complacent, and draw in many new supporters. This has been especially true since the summer of 1989, when the Supreme Court handed down its *Webster* decision, which permitted states to significantly restrict the delivery of abortion services, and again in the summer of 1992 when the ruling in the Pennsylvania case extended the restrictions.

Nationally, the most important abortion rights groups are the National Abortion Rights Action League (NARAL) and Planned Parenthood Federation of America. Unlike NARAL, the latter is not a single-issue organization (the major activity of Planned Parenthood clinics nationwide is the delivery of contraceptive services and education), but the past president of Planned Parenthood, Faye Wattleton, has emerged as a leading spokesperson for the pro-choice movement, and the organization has devoted much effort to mobilizing public opinion in favor of protecting abortion rights. The National Organization of Women (NOW) has also played a highly visible role at the national level in the defense of reproductive freedom, e.g., organizing demonstrations in Washington and other cities and raising funds for litigation against anti-abortion groups that participate in clinic blockades. Some other important national abortion rights groups are religiously based, such as Catholics for a Free Choice, and the Religious Coalition for Abortion Rights, as well as many pro-choice caucuses that exist within various Protestant and Jewish organizations. The National Abortion Federation is an organization of abortion providers who offer information and services to its members (mostly physicians in private practice and staffs of abortion clinics) but also have a hotline service for the public with abortion information and referrals in particular communities.

The most important group that works on the legal aspects of abortion is the Reproductive Freedom Project of the American Civil Liberties Union. Lawyers associated with this project have argued the key abortion cases before the Supreme Court as well as before lower courts and have played a leadership role in legal battles to defend abortion facilities against attacks by anti-abortion groups.

The Alan Guttmacher Institute, a research organization, is an excellent source of information on various social and medical aspects of abortion. In particular, the AGI has been at the forefront of groups in the U.S. that have tried to bring to public attention the suppression of RU486 ("the abortion pill" which also has other medical uses) by anti-abortion groups. The National Women's Health Network and the Center for Population Options also offer useful information on various facets of abortion.

Abortion rights activity at the local level occurs in a number of ways. Perhaps the most important of such activities recently have been various forms of support offered to abortion facilities under siege by militant anti-abortion activists. Sometimes organized by local NOW chapters, pro-choice supporters will form escort services for patients of abortion clinics who must face a gauntlet of anti-abortionists in order to enter the clinic. In other cases, abortion rights supporters will organize mass demonstrations at the site of a clinic in order to physically prohibit a "blockade" by anti-abortionists.

Additionally, abortion rights activists in a number of communities have organized funds that either subsidize free abortions or offer no-interest loans to poor women who cannot afford the cost of an abortion. Another focus of local pro-choice activism, particularly since *Webster* has been to work on the electoral campaigns of pro-choice candidates for city, regional, and state office—especially when such pro-choice candidates are running against an opponent who is identified as strongly anti-abortion. The impact of the pro-choice movement as a voting bloc was particularly evident in the fall 1989 elections (the first elections after the *Webster* decision) when abortion rights proponents were widely credited as being decisive elements in the gubernatorial races in New Jersey and Virginia.

Useful sources on abortion rights activity before *Roe* are Lader (1966, 1973), Mohr (1978), Luker (1984), Smith-Rosenberg (1985), National Women's Health Network (1989), and Petchesky (1990). On present-day activism, see Luker (1984) and Petchesky (1990). An especially useful discussion of the complex relationship between abortion rights and other reproductive issues can be found in Freid (1990). Joffe (1986) discusses the relationship between "front line" workers in abortion clinics and the larger movement for abortion rights. A very moving discussion of abortion ferment within the contemporary Catholic Church can be found in Ferraro and Hussey (1990), an account by two nuns of their struggle with the Vatican hierarchy because of the signing of an open letter that claimed a diversity of viewpoints on the abortion issue within the Church.

✱ CAROLE JOFFE, Ph.D.

See also: Abortion, Politics of; Anti-Abortion Movement; Roe v. Wade; Webster v. Reproductive Health Services

See **Guide to Related Topics:** Abortion

Resources

Ferraro, Barbara & Hussey, Patricia, with O'Reilly, Jane. (1990). *No Turning Back: Two Nuns' Battle with the Vatican over Women's Right to Choose.* New York: Poseidon Press.

Freid, Marlene G. (Ed.) (1990). *From Abortion to Reproductive Freedom: Transforming a Movement.* Boston: South End Press.

Joffe, Carole. (1986). *The Regulation of Sexuality: Experiences of Family Planning Workers.* Philadelphia: Temple University Press.

Lader, Lawrence. (1966). *Abortion.* Boston: Beacon Press.

———. (1973). *Abortion II: Making the Revolution.* Boston: Beacon Press.

Luker, Kristin. (1984). *Abortion and the Politics of Motherhood.* Berkeley, CA: University of California Press.

Mohr, James. (1978). *Abortion in America: The Origins and Evolution of National Policy, 1800-1900.* New York: Oxford University Press.

National Women's Health Network. (1989). *Abortion Then and Now: Creative Responses to Restricted Access.*

Washington, DC: National Women's Health Network.

Petchesky, Rosalind Pollack. (1990). *Abortion and Woman's Choice: The State, Sexuality and Reproductive Freedom.* Boston: Northeastern University Press.

Smith-Rosenberg, Carroll. (1985). "The Abortion Movement and the AMA, 1850-1880." In C. Smith-Rosenberg (Ed.) *Disorderly Conduct: Visions of Gender on Victorian America.* New York: Alfred A. Knopf, pp. 217-44.

ADOPTION, CLOSED

Closed adoption, or traditional adoption, is a system of adoption that specifies that parents placing a child for adoption and parents adopting the child remain anonymous to one another. Typically, the birth and adoptive parents are told very little about one another and have no personal contact. During the adoption process, the adoption agency or agent acts as an intermediary for the transmission of any necessary information (such as medical histories) and seeks to assure each party confidentiality and protection from one another. In closed adoption, birth parents are typically denied any information about the child after he or she is surrendered and are not expected to play any continuing role in the child's life. Adoptive parents are often unable to obtain any further information on the birth family, including updated medical information, once the adoption is finalized. The adopted child (even as an adult) is denied access to detailed or identifying information about his or her birth family.

Closed adoption procedures developed in an era when there was a very great stigma attached to the infertility of adoptors, to the fertility of women outside of marriage, and to the so-called illegitimacy of the individual born "out of wedlock." The secrecy of the closed adoption was intended to protect all parties.

The current thrust in social science research and in social work practice has been to support greater openness in communication in all areas of family life, including adoption. Specifically in the area of adoption, research, along with anecdotal reports and the growing social movements of both adult adoptees and of birthmothers, has begun to reveal the consequences of closed adoption for all involved. Identity conflicts; genealogical bewilderment; insecurity; a sense of rootlessness; an exaggerated need to be obedient and to please; a sense of isolation; a lack of self-confidence and self-esteem; heightened vulnerability to loss, abandonment, or rejection; increased "acting out" behavior during adolescence (particularly sexual and running away behaviors); and a general overrepresentation in the psychiatric population are problems found among some adoptees by a number of researchers (Paton, 1954; Kirk, 1964; Kittson, 1968; Triseliotis, 1970; Fisher, 1974; Lawrence, 1976; Baran, Pannor, and Sorosky, 1976, 1978; and Lifton, 1984).

Research addressing the long-term consequences for birth parents, both birthmothers and biological fathers, of losing a child to (closed) adoption have been outlined by researchers such as Baran, Pannor, and Sorosky (1976, 1978), Burnell and Norfleet (1979), Lifton (1979), Silverman (1981), Rynearson (1982), Deykin, Campbell, and Patti (1984), and Deykin and Ryan (1988). The research indicates that such loss can affect future fertility, subsequent parenting, and heterosexual relationships, and can result in prolonged mourning, pain and loss, continued caring for the lost child, depression, and restitution fantasies. Researchers have found that birth parents raising later children are sometimes overprotective, worry compulsively over children's health, have difficulty in accepting the growing independence of their children, and experience heightened valuation of and involvement in their children's lives (Rynearson, 1982; Deykin, Campbell, and Patti, 1984). Closed adoption can color marital interactions between a birth parent and spouse by accentuating issues of allegiance, commitment, and jealousy of prior relationships (Deykin, Campbell, and Patti, 1984). Birth parent couples who subsequently marry are particularly vulnerable to issues of blame, guilt, and the ever-present, unresolved loss (Silverman, 1981). In addition, many birth parents report that their sense of identity is put in question by closed adoption, as their parental status is unclear (Hanssen, forthcoming). Compounding the ongoing pain experienced by birth parents as a result of never knowing the fate or well-being of the surrendered child is a sense of helplessness stemming from being denied any legitimate means to alleviate their concerns. Once the surrender is taken, the birth parents have no legal right to any further information about the child.

Research indicates that infertile couples who adopt children through closed adoption may suffer a host of emotional and psychological consequences affecting identity and relationships to children. Baran, Pannor, and Sorosky (1978), Simons (1982), and Mazor and Simons (1984) reviewed a total of 19 other studies that addressed the emotional and psychological consequences of infertility. Issues of concern included guilt and ambivalence toward adopted children, failure to develop a sense of (or security in) parental identity, anxiety, guilt, overprotectiveness toward children, overindulgence toward children, overreaction toward children's aggressive or sexual feelings, unrealistic and rigid expectations of the children's development, and problems with children's independence.

Adoptive parents who are sensitive to the enormity of the loss birth parents suffer may feel guilt for their reciprocal gain. On the other hand, in spite of their willingness to adopt, ambivalence toward the child as it grows up may be experienced by adoptive parents who hold negative images of birth parents, particularly birthmothers, as immoral women, prostitutes, drug users, or child abusers. Because they do not know the birth parents ar "real people," fantasies are free to develop. Adoptive parents may fear that the adopted child will follow in the birth parent's (imagined) footsteps and grow up to be a "bad seed"; fears that the adopted child will become sexually promiscuous may lead the adoptive parents to overreact to the child's developing sexuality (Baran, Pannor, and Sorosky, 1978).

Closed adoption prohibits adoptive parents from being the primary source of information for their children about their birth and background. Since closed adoption most often does not allow them access to the information their children may want or need, including medical family histories, adoptive parents are not fully enabled as parents.

Because many adoptees and birth parents are not content to live under the constraints of the closed adoption system, they sometimes search for and meet one another. Closed adoption makes any attempts at reconciliation difficult, emotionally draining, and potentially disappointing. A great deal of psychological adjustment and accommodation are required, as years of fantasy, fear, and worry are replaced by reality.

In light of the greater social acceptability of both infertility and of childbirth outside of marriage, the need for protection against stigma has lessened. And in light of the growing research on the consequences of secrets in families in general, and the consequences of closed adoption policies in particular, even the most traditional adoption agencies have begun moving towards some increase in openness. Many now permit a single meeting, without the exchange of last names, between birth mothers and potential adoptors. Many agree to forward photographs of the child to the birthmother: in some agencies this is done only for the first months after placement, and in some for as long as the adoptive parents wish. Some agencies now agree to maintain files on the birth family, and forward the information to the adoptee, on request, at adulthood. And a growing number of agencies are willing to continue to act as intermediary in the rare event of emergency medical situations requiring the exchange of information. Finally, some agencies promote the sharing of identifying information and the development of an ongoing personal relationship between birth and adoptive families.

This is a period of rapid change in adoption procedures, and the fully "closed" adoption, with its complete anonymity and secrecy, may soon be a thing of the past. ✱ GAIL HANSSEN, M.A.

See also: Adoption, Open; Birthmothers

See **Guide to Related Topics:** Adoption

Resources

Baran, Annette, Pannor, Reuben & Sorosky, Arthur. (1978). *The Adoption Triangle.* New York: Anchor/Doubleday.

Baran, Annette, Sorosky, Arthur & Pannor, Reuben. (1976, Mar). "Open Adoption." *Social Work XXI.*

Burnell, G. & Norfleet, N. (1979). "Women Who Place Their Infants for Adoption: A Pilot Study." *Patient Counsel and Health Education 1*: 169-72.

Deykin, E., Campbell, L., & Patti, P. (1984, May). "The Post Adoption Experience of Surrendering Parents." *American Journal of Orthopsychiatry 54* (2).

Deykin, E. & Ryan, J. (1988, May). "The Post Adoption Experience of Surrendering Fathers." *American Journal of Orthopsychiatry 58* (2).

Fisher, Florence. (1974). *The Search for Anna Fisher.* Greenwich, CT: Fawcett Publications.

Hanssen, Gail. (forthcoming). *Participation of Adoptive Parents in Open vs. Closed Adoption.* Dissertation in progress. Waltham, MA: The Heller School, Brandeis University.

Kirk, H. David. (1964). *Shared Fate.* New York: Abington Press.

Kittson, Ruthena Hill. (1968). *Orphan Voyage.* Cedaredge, CO: Country Press.

Lawrence Margaret. (1976). "Inside, Looking Out of Adoption." Paper presented at the annual meeting of the American Psychological Association, Washington, DC.

Lifton, J.J. (1979). *Lost & Found.* New York: Dial Press.

Mazor, Miriam & Simons, Harriet. (Eds.) (1984). *Infertility: Medical, Emotional and Social Considerations.* New York: Human Services Press.

Paton, Jean. (1954). *The Adopted Break Silence.* Cedaredge, CO: Orphan Voyage.

Rynearson, Edward K. (1982). "Relinquishment and Its Maternal Complications: A Preliminary Study." *American Journal of Psychiatry 139*: 338-40.

Silverman, Phyllis. (1981). *Helping Women Cope with Grief.* Beverly Hills, CA: Sage Publications.

Simons, Harriet. (1982). "Infertility as an Emerging Social Concern." Unpublished manuscript. Waltham, MA: The Heller School, Brandeis University.

Triseliotis, Paul. (1970). *In Search of One's Origins.* Toronto, Ontario: Routledge, Kegan Paul.

ADOPTION, INTERCOUNTRY

Since the end of World War II, hundreds of thousands of families in the West, particularly in the United States, have adopted non-native-born children. In the United States alone, the decade ending 1987 saw 77,908 foreign-born children adopted. In a single year, 1987, 10,097 non-native-born children were adopted in the United States (*Statistical Yearbook*, 1987). This unique type of child placement is known as intercountry adoption (ICA) and is being defined as a "target of opportunity" by the approximately two million Americans who want to adopt.

On the surface, one would imagine that ICA shares certain similar dynamics to transracial adoption. The latter is a distinctly North American phenomenon whereby whites adopt native-born African-American and Native-American children. It was and continues to be a highly controversial type of adoption. (See "Adoption, Transracial.")

The fact is that in any society foreign-born adoptees differ in fundamental ways from native-born adoptees, no matter what the latter's racial group. Whereas native-born adoptees, even if racially different from the majority, share an overall common cultural heritage, foreign-born children, and especially those coming from Third World countries, have no historic connection to the country into which they have been brought. The large majority share neither the traditions, values, religion, nor language of their adopted country. What most foreign-born adoptees share with their transracially adopted counterparts is a minority status based on race.

Agency-sponsored ICA first began at the end of World War II when European and, to a somewhat lesser extent, Asian orphans (particularly from Germany, Greece, and Japan) were adopted by American families. This turned out to be the first and shortest "era" of ICA, lasting only about five years (1948-53). It comprised the neediest children who were orphaned, primarily as a result of World War II and the Greek civil war, which began in 1946.

The second phase of ICA and the one which now appears to be slowly waning began in the early 1950s, again as a Western response to children left parentless by an international conflict. This time, however, the conflict took place on the Asian continent. It was the Korean War and the children at issue were Korean. The adoption of these children by Westerners presaged an era in child placement that differed from the traditional practice of placing children with racially similar adoptive parents. For the first time in history, relatively large numbers of Western (American) couples were adopting children racially and culturally different from themselves.

Between 1953 and 1962, approximately 15,000 foreign-born children were adopted by American citizens (Weil, 1984). The following 11 years, 1965-76, saw an additional 37,469 foreign-born children adopted, of which about 65 percent were Asian, the largest group of which was from the Republic of Korea (ROK). During this period, of the West European children adopted by Americans, some 60 percent were born in West Germany or Italy (Weil, 1984, p. 282). It is interesting to note that, while Western Europe as a whole adopts many non-European-born children, West Germany continued to send orphans abroad for adoption purposes until as recently as 1981. From 1976-81, 304 West German-born children were adopted by Americans. One explanation is that many of these children were racially mixed, the products of African-American U.S. servicemen stationed in Germany, and would have a difficult time being fully accepted into mainstream German society.

From the 1950s until the early 1970s, ROK was the main provider of healthy infants to the West. For some 30 years it allowed almost unrestricted adoption by foreigners of its orphaned and abandoned children. Although no exact figures exist, it is estimated that during the 30-year period between the early 1950s and 1980s, in excess of 100,000 Korean children were adopted by Western families (Maass, 1988).

For a number of reasons, including the ending of the war in Vietnam, an overall improvement in the economies of Asian countries, and the development of domestic child welfare programs that encouraged domestic adoptions, the 1970s saw changes in the pattern of ICA from Asia. Important too in reducing the numbers of Korean children adopted by Westerners was 1980 ROK legislation liberalizing the availability of abortion services in ROK.

While Asia remained a prime source of adoptees for Western couples, the relationship between the sending and receiving countries, particularly from the Asian perspective, was never a totally comfortable one. Asia's reliability as a permanent source of children was therefore questionable, and for good reason (Melone, 1976). As a result of the events in ROK, Western interest was directed closer to the borders of the United States, toward Latin America, where civil wars and economic conditions similar to those in Asia were present.

By 1987, Latin America accounted for 23 percent of all children entering the United States for purposes of adoption. This figure represents an increase of 15 percent over 1973.

Adoption figures continue to indicate America's interest in this type of transfer. The decade 1977-87 saw an additional 77,908 foreign-born children adopted. In only a three-year span, 1984-87, 37,655 foreign-born children entered this country for adoption purposes, 60 percent from ROK (U.S. Bureau of the Census, 1990). In 1987 alone, 10,097 foreign-born children were adopted in the U.S., a figure that is almost twice as high as the number in 1975. It is worth noting that while ICA involves thousands of children, when considered along with national adoption figures, these numbers are still comparatively small. For example, it is estimated that until recently there were approximately 150,000 adoptions per year in the United States. However, that number is falling. Some attribute this reduction to abortion rates (Cole, 1988; McGrory, 1990; Henshaw et al., 1987). Others argue that a combination of factors appears to be operating, namely infertility rates, greater use of contraception, and lifestyle changes sanctioning unwed parenthood (Cole, 1987).

There is, however, another side to the ICA coin, the side representing the positions of countries allowing their children to be adopted in the West. From the 1960s, Third World countries have had a surplus population of healthy infants. Removing these surplus infants to be adopted was seen as an easy solution to the problem of childlessness in Western societies. What could be more humane, most Westerners reasoned, than to remove seemingly unwanted, even discarded children from what looked to be lives of misery and poverty to an environment in which material comfort and social opportunity abounded? All would benefit. The childless couple's desire for a child would be fulfilled, and the adopted children would be given unprecedented opportunities.

What the West for the most part viewed as charitable, humane, even noble behavior, developing countries have come to define as "imperialistic," self-serving, and a return to a form of colonialism in which whites exploit and steal their natural resources (Miller, 1971). In the 1970s, 1980s, and 1990s their children were the natural resource that was being exploited and of which they were being cheated.

Whether ICA has thus far been successful, in terms of these children's adjustments to their adopted families and society, has only recently begun to receive scientific scrutiny. Several studies concerned with policy issues were conducted in the 1970s and to a lesser extent in the 1980s (Joe, 1978). The range of focus in the medical literature went from the fact that intercountry adoptees could suffer from such simple maladies as sleeping problems to the possibility that these children might be carriers of infectious diseases such as hepatitis B and tuberculosis. In some instances, particularly if it were known that a child was born to an HIV-positive mother or had a history of hemophilia, it was recommended that the child be screened for AIDS, especially if he or she was born in Brazil, Venezuela, Haiti, or Honduras (Jenista and Chapman, 1987).

Until very recently, when empirical pieces did appear they were usually relatively limited examinations, restricted in scope and size to (very) small numbers, and in most instances using case study designs. In 1991 Altstein and Simon published the first comprehensive study of ICA that described the experiences of 80 families and 96 children (Altstein and Simon, 1991). Their findings strongly suggest that children who are adopted as infants make positive adjustments to their new environments. Parents are eager to have them, and the children perceive themselves as fully integrated family members. Most parents make strong efforts to maintain multiethnic environments in their homes.

✱ HOWARD ALTSTEIN, Ph.D.

See also: Adoption, Special Needs Children; Adoption, Transracial

See **Guide to Related Topics:** Adoption

Resources

Altstein, Howard & Simon, Rita J. (1991). *Intercountry Adoption: A Multinational Perspective.* New York: Praeger Publishing.

Cole, Diane. (1987, Aug 9). "Cost of Entering the Baby Chase." *New York Times Business Section, 9.*

———. (1988, Apr 28). "The Cost of Entering the Baby Chase." *New York Times. C8.*

Henshaw, Samuel K., Forrest, Jacqueline Darroch, & Van Vort, Jennifer. (1987, Mar/Apr). "Abortion Services in the United States, 1984 and 1985." *Family Planning Perspectives 19*: 63-70.

Jenista, Jerri Ann & Chapman, Daniel. (1987, Mar). "Medical Problems of Foreign Born Children." *American Journal of Diseases of Children 141:* 298-302.

Joe, Barbara. (1978, Mar). "In Defense of Intercountry Adoption." *Social Service Review 52*: 1-20.

Maass, Peter. (1988, Dec 12). "Orphans: Korea's Disquieting Problem." *Washington Post, 1.*

McGrory, Mary. (1990, Apr 22). "The Adoption Option." *Washington Post B1.*

Melone, Thomas. (1976, Jun). "Adoption and Crisis in the Third World: Thoughts on the Future." *International Child Welfare Review 29*: 20-28.

Miller, Helene. (1971, Summer). "Korea's International Children." *Lutheran Social Welfare*: 12-23.

Statistical Yearbook. (1987). Washington, DC: Government Printing Office, Immigration and Naturalization Service, Statistical Analysis Branch.

U.S. Bureau of the Census. *Statistical Abstract of the United States*. (1990). Washington, DC: U.S. Government Printing Office.

Weil, Richard H. (1984, Feb). "International Adoptions: The Quiet Migration." *International Migration Review XVIII*: 276-93.

ADOPTION, OPEN

Adoption is one way in which children born as a result of untimely pregnancies are given the families and homes they need. Historically, society seemed to view adoption as the process by which "unwanted" children were placed with deserving, infertile, middle-class couples, solving two painful problems in one efficient transaction. The pain felt by birth parents who were cut off from any knowledge or contact with their child was believed justifiable: the prevailing view was that the parents were only reaping the consequences of their behavior. Every procedure in an adoption was justified by the phrase "best interests of the child."

Since the late 1960s, debate in the adoption world has centered on the subject of open records: whether adoptees and birth parents have the right to find one another. The "search" or "adoption reform" movement explores both the relationships between adoptee and their birth families and the relationship between birth and adoptive families. It questions the need for confidentiality that has been the cornerstone of U.S. adoptions for the previous three generations and proposes a more open system, sensitive to the needs of all members of the adoption triangle.

Traditional Adoption. Traditional, or confidential, adoption has worked reasonably well for many families, but the system is far from perfect. It has three major shortcomings: (1) its commitment to secrecy; (2) the handling of vital information; and (3) the insistence on retaining complete control over the adoption experience.

Originally, adoption records in the U.S. were open. They were closed in the early part of this century to protect adoptees, birth parents, and adoptive parents from the stigmas of illegitimacy, out-of-wedlock pregnancy, and infertility. The need for such secrecy no longer exists in most cases since society has become increasingly accepting of these conditions. Secrecy begets an atmosphere in which fear may thrive and presumes that birth and adoptive parents are natural adversaries who must be protected from one another.

Another flaw in the closed adoption system is the manner in which it gathers and transmits information. It has tended to underestimate the importance of information, both social and medical, and has not been diligent in collecting and updating these vital data. Information about genetic diseases and conditions that later develop in either adoptees or birth parents is not exchanged. Since the traditional form considers it important that birth and adoptive families be kept separate, there is no opportunity for communication and little chance for an ongoing exchange of information.

Open Adoption. In 1976 the concept of open adoption was formally proposed by West Coast researchers Baran, Pannor, and Sorosky. By 1980 several agencies and lawyers had changed their approach from confidential to open adoption. "Open" means many different things; there are degrees of openness and a wide spectrum of differences. All proponents of open adoption, however, agree that there is little advantage in severing all ties between birth and adoptive families, and they assume they are inextricably connected emotionally, medically, and psychologically. Open adoption ranges from "semi-open" or "identified" (similar to traditional adoption, in which there is some exchange of information and minimal contact at the time of placement but little ongoing contact) to "cooperative adoption," where there is co-parenting, similar to the agreement between divorced parents with joint custody.

Open adoption can enable birthmothers, and those fathers who are involved in the decision making, to resolve guilt and grief, since they know the child is safe and that the adoptive parents are loving. It can allow adoptive parents to replace fantasies about their children's background with accurate information, and to deal more honestly with themselves and their children about the adoption. The adoptees can come to terms with their identity by knowing their biological roots and the reasons they were placed for adoption.

Research on parents involved in open adoption shows that they share these characteristics: They tend to see the world in positive terms; genuinely like other people and are able to identify with them; are open-minded; are self-confident and willing to take risks; accept the fact that adoption is different from having children born to them and are enthusiastic about the child's prior heritage; and do not see children as possessions.

Children placed through open adoption have come to understand what it means to have two families. There has been concern that adoptees with two families will have confusion of parental authority and that the child will experience competition for his or her love. This is not what happens: The families share a common vision—the love and welfare of their children, and this is usually enough to protect the child from such conflict.

Enough adoptees have suffered from confusion about their identities through confidential adoption that a phenomenon of "geneological bewilderment" has been identified. Adoptees face unusual challenges in development which are often misdiagnosed as problems. Open adoption is seen by its supporters as a way to benefit all parties, especially the child whose best interests must be served.

Openness Is No Panacea. Where advocates for open adoption see value, proponents of traditional adoption see risk. For birthmothers, the message is that it is possible to place a baby without needing to entirely separate from it; the risk to adoptive parents is that they may feel threatened by the relationship with the birthmother. For some adoptees, contact with the birthmother can be stressful and disappointing. For birth parents, open adoption is a complex and sometimes deceptive choice, leading to relationships for which there is insufficient social precedent. Without legal support, open adoption is an unenforceable agreement, made and kept at the whim of the adoptive parents. Proponents of open adoption protest the manner in which some lawyers and other intermediaries use open adoption as a marketing tool, luring birthmothers with promises of openness they cannot guarantee. These entrepreneurs are motivated by profit and basically unregulated.

Conclusion. For all of its optimism, open adoption is based on the premise that any adoption is second best—that ideally all children should be with their families of birth. When that is not possible, life with adoptive parents should not cut a child off from his or her biological roots and history. While all adoption may entail fear and the inevitable sense of loss, increased openness can be helpful in resolving these feelings positively.

✱ ALISON WARD

See also: Adoption, Closed; Birthmothers

See **Guide to Related Topics:** Adoption

Resources

Arms, Suzanne. (1983). *To Love and Let Go.* New York: Knopf.

Campbell, Lee H. (1978). *Understanding the Birthparent.* Milford, MA: Concerned United Birthparents.

Dusky, Lorraine. (1979). *Birthmark.* New York: Evans & Company.

Gritter, James L. (1989). *Adoption without Fear.* San Antonio, TX: Corona Publishing Company.

Krementz, Jill. (1982). *How It Feels to Be Adopted.* New York: Knopf.

Lifton, Betty Jean. (1988). *Lost and Found.* New York: Harper & Row.

Rillera, Mary Jo & Kaplan, Sharon. (1984). *Cooperative Adoption.* Westminster, CA: Triadoption Publications.

Sorosky, Arthur D., Baran, Annette, & Pannor, Reuben. (1979). *The Adoption Triangle.* Garden City, NY: Doubleday Anchor Books.

ADOPTION, SPECIAL NEEDS CHILDREN

In the context of adoption, a child with special needs is generally defined as having one or more of the following characteristics:

- being between 6 and 16 years of age;
- having physical, intellectual, or emotional disabilities;
- needing to be placed with one or more biological siblings into an adoptive home;
- being a member of a racial or ethnic minority.

As a practical matter, "special needs" can be considered synonymous with "hard-to-place." According to the National Committee for Adoption, there were 13,568 adoptions of children with special needs in the United States in 1986 (National Committee for Adoption, 1989, p. 63). As with all areas of adoption, within the category of special needs, there is a bias toward younger, healthier, and lighter-skinned children. Of special needs children waiting to be adopted in 1985, only 30 percent were under the age of 6; however 48 percent of children adopted that year were under the age of 6 (National Committee for Adoption, 1989, p. 63). In the same year, 38 percent of waiting children were black; however only 25 percent of children adopted were black (National Committee for Adoption, 1989, p. 191).

There are no national data collection systems for adoption: there are therefore no national data available on special needs children awaiting adoption (Toshio Tatara, American Public Welfare Association, January 1992). What is known is that white children under the age of six are rarely available for placement with any state agencies.

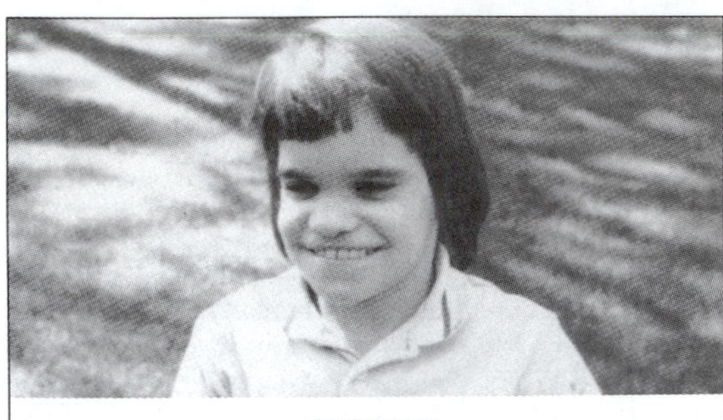

ROBIN

Robin, 10 years old, has been waiting for a very long time for a family of her own. She is a courageous child who has been able to overcome tremendous setbacks. She has surprised many of the adults who know her by the significant gains she has been able to make.

Robin is a child challenged by multiple handicaps. She has a seizure disorder which is controlled by medication. Robin was shunted at birth to manage her hydrocephaly. She also has spastic quadraplegia. These conditions have contributed to Robin's significant developmental delays.

Robin attends a specialized school for 240 days per year where she receives personal attention and educational programming, including speech, physical and occupational therapy. She lives in an excellent foster home. Because of the coordinated efforts between school and home, Robin is progressing well. She is able to walk independently with the assistance of a walker. She has also learned to speak several words, although she expresses her needs best by using sign language. It is possible to learn enough sign to communicate with Robin in a matter of days.

Robin has been in state care since birth. Prior to entering her first foster home, she spent two years in a pediatric nursing home.

Robin is an affectionate child who is expected to do well in an adoptive home. All families willing to provide the care and nurturing Robin needs will be considered.

Ocean State Adoption Resource Exchange   September, 1990   (RI)   page 362

A page from the photo listing manual of available children. Robin has been in the book each year of her life. Photo courtesy of Ocean State Adoption Resource Exchange.

Special needs children, with or without physical disabilities, are generally older and/or nonwhite.

Common disabilities among children with special needs include attention deficit disorder, learning disabilities, and emotional problems. These are by definition disabilities of older children, and are frequently related to the neglect or abuse which brought them into the adoption system.

Children in need of adoptive homes have generally gone through a legal process that has resulted in a termination of parental rights. Although termination of parental rights is sometimes voluntary, in most instances it involves a long legal struggle resulting in involuntary termination. This process typically includes an initial report of child abuse or neglect, removal of the child from parental care into state custody, implementation of a reunification plan, and, failing a satisfactory reunification, the permanent termination of parental rights. In 85 percent of cases, parents of children in substitute care eventually have their parental rights maintained (National Committee for Adoption, 1989, p. 187).

While the legal issues of custody are being resolved, approximately 69 percent of children in substitute care are in foster homes. Most of the remainder are in group homes or other child care facilities (National Committee for Adoption, 1989, p. 187). Because the legal process for terminating parental rights is lengthy, it is not uncommon for foster parents to adopt their foster children. In 1985, 39 percent of all adoptions of children with special needs involved adoption by unrelated foster parents (National Committee for Adoption, 1989, p. 190). The primary benefit of foster care adoption is the continuity of caretakers for the child. Negative aspects include the perpetuation of temporary decisions, i.e., continued separation of siblings into different foster homes.

Beginning in 1958, a national network of adoption exchanges was developed for the purpose of recruiting adoptive families. Typical recruitment activities include profiling waiting children on local television and in newspapers, publication and distribution of "photolisting" books, and use of a national computer network to search for "matches." ✱ JEFFREY P. KATZ, M.S.W.

See also: Adoption, Intercountry; Adoption, Transracial

See **Guide to Related Topics:** Adoption

Resources

Jewett, Claudia L. (1978). *Adopting the Older Child.* Boston: The Harvard Common Press.

National Committee for Adoption. (1989). *1989 Adoption Factbook: United States Data, Issues, Regulations and Resources.*

ADOPTION, TRANSRACIAL

Whether the inception of adoption is credited to the Romans or the Egyptians, it began as the transfer of poor children to rich families. In the overwhelming majority of cases this ancient social class exchange (rich families/poor children) still characterizes adoption as we know it. With transracial adoption (TRA), that transfer takes on the added dimension of race. The link now is between poor black children and wealthier white families. In America today, this is not a gentle mix.

Holding class issues aside for the moment, why should this type of arrangement be an anathema to so many? The U.S. has long been a multiracial society. Centuries before the birth of our republic, racial mixing occurred and, with societal approval and encouragement, continues up until today. Yet when it comes to sanctioning TRAs, there is often strong opposition, even in the face of data that indicate TRAs can be and are often successful. Even some respected social investigators do not consider TRA as an option for parentless minority children and see the modern day equivalent to orphanages as the only alternative to foster care or reunion with ill-prepared birth families (Ladner, 1989).

Since at best, conventional (i.e., in-racial) adoption is a highly complex arrangement of genetic, environmental, emotional, and psychological factors, TRA would seem all the more so. Much therefore should be known about the lasting consequences (positive and negative) this type of placement may have on the adoptees and their families.

Few if any responsible organizations or individuals blindly support TRA as a placement of first choice. Were there sufficient black families for all black children, Latino families for Latino children, Asian families for Asian children, etc., there would be no need for TRA. Adoptive agencies and experts support increased efforts to locate minority families, and especially black families, for minority children legally available for adoption. "Traditional" agency policies and practices, often based on by-gone white middle-class assumptions, need to be altered to meet current realities of non-white communities, thereby increasing the likelihood that larger numbers of potential minority adopters will be located ("Adoption Agency Rules Called Unfair to Blacks," 1987).

Most if not all who see TRA as a viable arrangement see it only when a child's options are less permanent types of placements such as foster care or group homes. In fact arguments are rarely, if ever, heard in favor of TRA that do not define it as "second best" to permanent in-racial placement and do not also include strong support for community agencies to vigorously recruit minority adoptive parents.

By the beginning of the 1990s it is quite clear that major child welfare and adoption organizations remain strongly committed to the idea of recruiting minority adoptive parents for minority children. These agencies would no longer advocate TRA if there were sufficient racially similar parents to accommodate waiting non-white children.

The position of the National Association of Black Social Workers (NABSW) on TRA in 1991 remains consistent with its original repudiation of it in 1972. At that time the NABSW stated:

> Black children should be placed only with Black families whether in foster care or adoption. Black children belong physically, psychologically and culturally in Black families in order that they receive the total sense of themselves and develop a sound projection of their future....Black children in White homes are cut off from the healthy development of themselves as Black people. (1972).

In some cases, organizations doggedly cling to the questionable policy that race should be *the* primary determinant of a child's placement even if the child has already been placed with and integrated successfully into a family of another race. In such successful placements, support for the concept of in-racial placement as the only adoption option would seem to work to the detriment of the child's best interests.

Over the decades social scientists and those interested in child welfare have been examining the effects of cross-race adoption not only upon the adoptees themselves but on their adoptive parents and adopted/birth siblings as well (Grow and Shapiro, 1974; Feigelman and Silverman, 1983; McRoy and Zurcher, 1983). The work of Simon and Altstein represents the best available longitudinal data to date on this type of adoption. Their findings indicate quite positive results. Evidence supports the position that this type of placement "works" many more times than it does not. It works in the sense that all involved appear to be satisfied and happy. The adoptees themselves are well integrated into their respective worlds (social, familial, educational, etc). They do well in school, have established meaningful peer relationships, feel closer to their families, and are optimistic about their futures. They do not seem racially confused or angry about why they were adopted by families of another color. The families too appear satisfied and express very few regrets about their decision to adopt a child of a different race. Certainly, there are problems, a few of which are serious. But the overwhelming evidence seems to support this type of placement (Simon and Altstein, 1977, 1981, 1987).

The fact that transracial placements are as stable as other more traditional adoptive arrangements was reinforced by data presented at a North American Council on Adoptable Children (NACAC) meeting on adoption disruption held in 1988. There it was reported that the rate of adoption disruption (adopted children removed from their homes) averages about 15 percent. Of particular note here is the recognition that TRAs have no greater rate of disruption than in-racial placements. In fact several other factors that define a special needs placement also, by and large, have no effect on the disruption rate. For example, disruptions did not appear to be influenced by the adoptees' race, gender, or the fact that they were placed as a sibling group. When examining adoptive parent characteristics neither their religion, race, marital status, length of time married, educational achievement, or income seemed predictive of adoption disruption (FACE Facts, 1989).

Thus, the research on transracial adoption continues to demonstrate that it can be a viable, successful option for both adoptees and adoptive parents. Transracial adoptees do not seem to be losing their racial identities, they do not appear to be racially unaware of who they are, nor do they display negative or conflicted racial attitudes about themselves. In fact, it appears that transracially placed children and their families are doing as well as their counterparts have done in the past, living quite normal and satisfying lives.

✱ HOWARD ALTSTEIN, Ph.D.

See also: Adoption, Intercountry; Adoption, Special Needs Children

See **Guide to Related Topics:** Adoption

Resources

"Adoption Agency Rules Called Unfair to Blacks." (1987, Feb 2). *New York Times, C11.*

FACE Facts. (1989, Jan/Feb): 35.

Feigelman, William & Silverman, Arnold. (1983). *Chosen Children: New Patterns of Adoptive Relationships.* New York: Praeger Publishing.

Grow, J. Lucille & Shapiro, Deborah. (1974). *Black Children-White Parents: A Study of Transracial Adoption.* New York: Child Welfare League of America.

Ladner, Joyce. (1989, Oct 29). "Bring Back the Orphanages." *Washington Post.*

McRoy, Ruth & Zurcher, Louis. (1983). *Transracial and Inracial Adoptees.* Springfield, IL: Charles C. Thomas.

National Association of Black Social Workers. (1972, Apr). Position Paper.

Simon, Rita J. & Altstein, Howard. (1977). *Transracial Adoption.* New York: John Wiley and Sons.

———. (1981). *Transracial Adoption: A Follow-up.* Lexington, MA: Lexington Books.

———. (1987). *Transracial Adoptees and Their Families: A Study of Identity and Commitment.* New York: Praeger Publishing.

A.F.P. *See instead* MATERNAL SERUM ALPHA-FETOPROTEIN SCREENING

AMNIOCENTESIS, HISTORY OF

Amniocentesis has had a complex and rather ironic history. The technique has six component parts (ultrasound examination; amniotic tap; biochemical assay of amniotic fluid; culturing of fetal cells; karyotyping and chromosomal analysis of fetal cells; and abortion), and each of these has evolved on a somewhat different path.

Although it is very startling to the patient, the amniotic tap—removal of amniotic fluid—is the simplest part of the procedure—and the one with the longest history. Since at least the 1930s it has been standard practice for physicians to remove some of the excess fluid of hydroamniotic patients (women who produce vastly too much amniotic fluid) by inserting a hollow needle through the abdominal wall and into the uterine cavity. Done late in pregnancy the procedure was regarded as reasonably safe, both for the mother and the fetus.

In the early 1950s, D.C.A. Bevis began a series of clinical studies in which he attempted to assess the degree of incompatibility between Rh-negative mothers and their Rh-positive fetuses by examining the concentration of certain blood pigments in amniotic fluid during the last trimester of pregnancy. Bevis's technique, which required amniotic taps of afflicted mothers, turned out to be very useful; in 1963, A.W. Liley demonstrated that intrauterine blood transfusions could save the lives of fetuses when the severity of Rh disease was estimated by Bevis's technique. Thus, sometime in the middle years of the 1960s, amniotic tapping became a routine aspect of clinical training and clinical practice in obstetrics.

In 1949, a Canadian physician, M.L. Barr, discovered that the cells of female and male mammals could be distinguished from each other by the presence or absence, not of sex chromosomes (which, in those years, were very difficult to see under the microscope), but of a very small dark spot near the nuclear membrane, which has since been named after him: the Barr body. Females have it and males don't; as long as a technician has a fairly large sample of cells under a microscope, the Barr body is reasonably easy to see, and a fairly accurate guess can be made about the sex of the organism that produced the cells.

In those years (the 1950s) there was a very small group of medical specialists who were very interested in making accurate guesses about the sex of fetuses: medical geneticists. Patients from families in which there was a hereditary disease might be sent to a medical geneticist for a consultation. The medical geneticist had no diagnostic technique to offer except the construction and analysis of an often faulty family medical history. In most cases the diagnosis was little more than a probability statement: "The chances are 50-50 that your child will be afflicted," or "The chances are very slim that your partner will carry the same recessive gene that you do." Not surprisingly, both patients and specialists found this a tragically frustrating enterprise.

One of the few hereditary diseases that was reasonably well understood in those days was hemophilia, which was known to be sex-linked, carried on the X chromosome. This meant that females were much less likely to be hemophiliacs (since they have two X chromosomes and the hemophilia gene is recessive) than males. Thus—

and this was the crucial point—if a mother had been identified as a carrier of the gene and if the sex of her fetus could be determined *in utero*, then the geneticist could predict, with much greater certainty, whether the child, when born, would be a hemophiliac. Once that prediction was made, if the parents wished it, an abortion could be performed; although such abortions were illegal in some of the United States, they were being performed in others, and in some countries (particularly in Scandinavia) they were legal.

Four different groups of researchers are credited with the discovery, in 1955, that the sex of human fetuses could be predicted through analysis of fetal cells in amniotic fluid, and a short while later a team of physicians in Copenhagen (F. Fuchs and P. Riis) became the first to report that they had performed an abortion in order to prevent the birth of a hemophiliac child.

It can be reasonably assumed (although this is difficult to document) that between the mid-1950s and the late-1960s amniocentesis was only performed in a few medical research centers and only on a very limited number of pregnant women: those who had been referred to specialists because of a familial history of a known sex-linked hereditary disease. Toward the end of the 1960s, this situation began to change, however. In 1966 two different groups of researchers announced that they had succeeded in culturing human fetal cells derived from amniotic fluid. The fact that human fetal cells could be cultured meant that, after a week or two of culturing, a microscopist could see hundreds of cells in active division—chromosomes are only visible when cells are in the process of dividing—and this meant that the number and morphology of the chromosomes could be determined. Medical geneticists already knew that there were certain hereditary conditions that were caused by abnormalities either in the number or in the morphology of chromosomes (one form of Down's syndrome, for example, is called trisomy 21, because there are three, rather than two, copies of the 21st chromosome). Now that it was possible to culture fetal cells, an accurate diagnosis, rather than a statistical probability, could be made for at least a small number of very serious genetic conditions. In 1968 three physicians from Brooklyn, New York (C. Valenti, E.J. Schutta, T. Kehaty), announced that they had performed an abortion that ended a pregnancy in which the fetus had been diagnosed, through amniocentesis and culturing, as having Down's syndrome.

The pressure on physicians to provide amniocentesis services, and on patients to submit to the procedure, increased very rapidly after that. By the early 1970s, many women who became pregnant in their late 30s and in their 40s were being recommended for amniocentesis because the frequency of Down's syndrome births increases as the age of the parents increases. Also in the early 1970s, D.J.H. Brock and his colleagues in Edinburgh, Scotland, discovered that spina bifida and other neural tube defects could be diagnosed prenatally if a sample of amniotic fluid was tested biochemically for the presence of alpha-fetoprotein—an additional reason for offering amniocentesis to a wide population of patients. By the mid-1970s, abortion was legal—and therefore relatively safe—in many countries. In addition, hospitals and clinics had started to acquire ultrasound machines which, when used to provide a visual guide to the person doing the amniotic tap, diminished the risk that either the fetus or the placenta would be touched by the needle. In the mid 1970s, in both Canada and the United States, the results of fairly large-scale clinical trials were announced, and amniocentesis was pronounced safe enough and accurate enough to be used in general clinical practice. Also by the mid-1970s in the United States, several lawsuits had been brought by parents who claimed that their children had been born "wrongfully" since their physicians had not offered them prenatal diagnostic services; several of these suits were successful in court, which meant that increasingly large numbers of American physicians began encouraging their patients to have amniocentesis in order to avoid malpractice claims.

Over the ensuing two decades, the use of amniocentesis has expanded. Some groups of feminists object to prenatal diagnosis on the grounds that it can be used to discriminate against female fetuses, that it is potentially eugenic, and that it discriminates against the disabled. All activists opposed to legalized abortion also object to amniocentesis on the grounds that it increases the reasons why women request abortions. These objections have not carried very much weight either with the vast majority of physicians in the developed countries or with the vast majority of patients. In many countries with socialized medical services, patient demand for amniocentesis exceeds the supply of laboratory time and facilities. As the result of new techniques of chromosomal analysis, the list of diagnosable conditions increases with every passing year. Since 1980, new diagnostic techniques have been developed: Fetoscopy, for example, can permit a physician to draw a blood sample directly from a fetus; chorionic villus sampling can allow genetic diagnosis to be done much earlier in a pregnancy; maternal blood can be tested for alpha-fetoprotein. At this time, however, none of these procedures is as safe and as accurate and as wide-ranging as amniocentesis, and so it is likely to be the diagnostic procedure most likely to be offered to pregnant women for the foreseeable future. ✱ RUTH SCHWARTZ COWAN, Ph.D.

See also: Childkeeping and Childbearing; Chorionic Villus Sampling; Eugenics; Genetic Counseling; Imaging Techniques; Maternal Serum Alpha-Fetoprotein Screening; Prenatal Diagnosis: Overview; Selective Abortion; Wrongful Birth and Wrongful Life

See **Guide to Related Topics:** New Procreative Technologies; Prenatal Diagnosis and Screening

Resources

Brock, D.J.H. (1982). *Early Diagnosis of Fetal Defects.* Edinburgh: Churchill Livingston.

Powledge, T.M. & Fletcher, J. (1979). "Guidelines for the Ethical, Social and Legal Issues in Prenatal Diagnosis: A Report from the Genetics Research Group of the Hastings Center, Institute of Society, Ethics and the Life Sciences." *New England Journal of Medicine, 300:* 168-72.

Rothman, Barbara Katz. (1986). *The Tentative Pregnancy: Prenatal Diagnosis and the Future of Motherhood.* New York: Viking Press.

Sandler, Merton. (1981). *Amniotic Fluid and Its Clinical Significance.* New York: Wiley.

Valenti, Carlo, Schutta, Edward J., & Kehaty, Tehila. (1968, Jul). "Prenatal Diagnosis of Down's Syndrome." *Lancet 27:* 220.

ANTI-ABORTION MOVEMENT

The first national anti-abortion movement in the United States was led in the mid-19th century by the same two groups—medical professionals and feminists—that one century later spearheaded the wave of pro-choice activism that crested with *Roe v. Wade*, the 1973 U.S. Supreme Court decision that guaranteed women the right to end an unwanted pregnancy.

At the beginning of the 19th century, no U.S. state considered abortion a crime if performed before quickening, or the point at which fetal movements can be felt. Nineteenth-century doctors initiated a crusade against abortion in an attempt to establish a "professional morality" that would distinguish them from the midwives and apothecaries who made up much of the burgeoning U.S. abortion industry at the time. In campaigning against abortion, doctors succeeded not only in distinguishing themselves morally as champions of the fetus, but also in securing a monopoly on abortion procedures: Doctors were granted control over the few abortions permitted by the restrictive legislation their crusade put in place (Mohr, 1978).

The doctors obtained little support for their campaign from organized religion; nineteenth-century church leaders, unlike many of their twentieth-century counterparts, were unwilling to take part in public debate about the regulation of abortion. Nineteenth-century feminists, however, did join doctors in condemning abortion. These women considered abortion a crime against womanhood and a perversion of "natural" femininity, which was essentially chaste, pure, and devoted to maternity. They feared that the ready availability of abortion and contraception would diminish women's authority within the family and would encourage male promiscuity.

Modern-day anti-abortion activists worked to strengthen anti-abortion laws in the years prior to the Roe ruling. Trained lobbyists visited state legislators to try to dissuade them from sponsoring or supporting legislation that would overturn the strict prohibitions on abortion that states put in place during the nineteenth century. The movement's use of fetal imagery—alternating between placid representations of fetuses *in utero* and bloody images said to be the result of abortions—also arose during this period. These pictures were intended to establish the existence of the fetus as a separate entity, which, the anti-abortionists argued, must obviously be endowed with the same rights as the woman who carried and sustained it. Early practitioners of this method included Father Paul Marx, who traveled with a fetus preserved in a jar, and Dr. Jack Willke and his wife, Barbara, authors of *Handbook on Abortion*. These and other campaigners attempted to reverse the rise of the pro-choice movement in the U.S.

In the wake of *Roe*, anti-abortion fervor initially directed itself at the most visible signs of abortions' legality—the facilities where abortions were performed, the medical professionals who provided them, and the women who had them. Picketers marched outside clinics, greeting women having abortions with cries of "Murderer!" and "Please don't kill your baby!" Behind the scenes, well-organized anti-abortion lobbyists dedicated themselves to chipping away at abortion rights by targeting vulnerable areas such as public funding for abortions, parental consent for minors, and late abortions. By attempting to surround the procedure with hostility and shame and maintaining a constant assault on its legal status, the movement endeavored to prevent women from growing accustomed to the right to abortion.

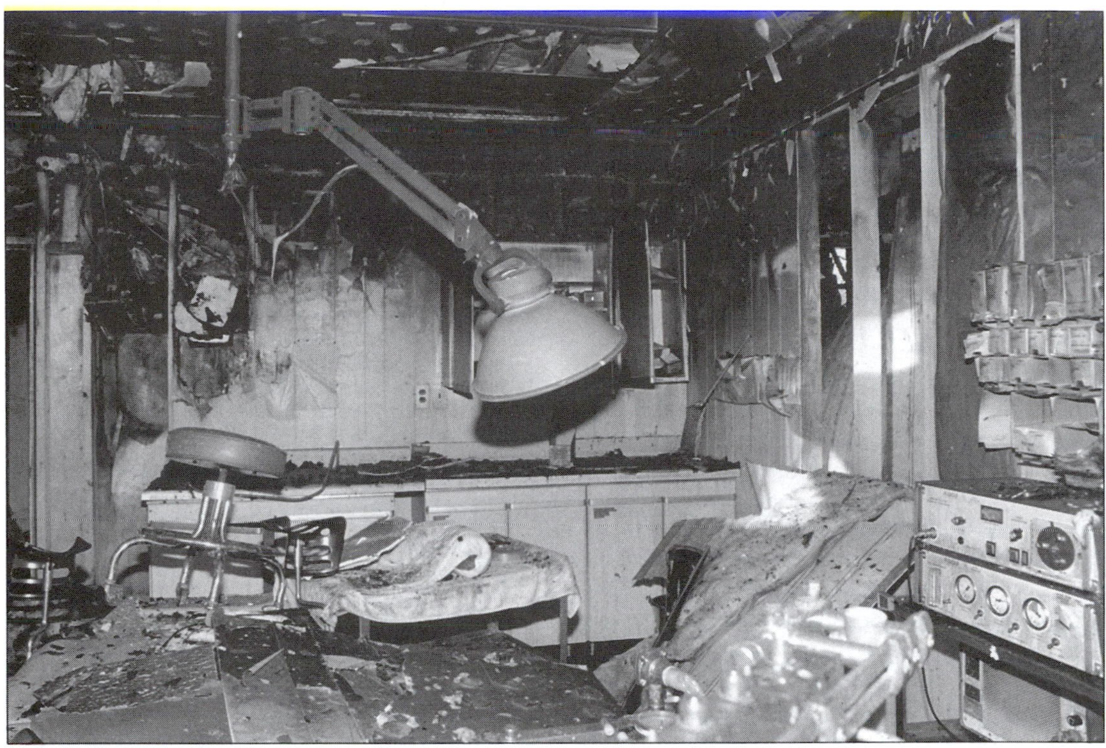

Abortion clinic in Woodbridge, New Jersey, burned down by arson, Monday, May 22, 1991. © Meryl Levin/Impact Visuals.

As the 1970s gave way to the conservatism and neo-traditionalism of the 1980s, the anti-abortion movement flourished and became more aggressive. Anti-abortion literature, such as Joseph Scheidler's *Closed: Ninety-Nine Ways to Stop Abortion*, recommended such tactics as picketing the private residences of doctors who performed abortions and harassing women leaving clinics after terminations. Activists set up "counseling" services, which attempted to represent themselves as clinics, advertising pregnancy tests or help with problem pregnancies; women who used these agencies found themselves aggressively "counseled" or shown a slide show about the horrors of abortion while waiting for the results of their pregnancy test.

Violence against abortion providers also increased sharply in the 1980s. Vandalism and bombings of clinics and in a few cases, assault or kidnapping of clinic staff, became the newest tactics used by those opposed to legal abortion. The founding of "Operation Rescue" in 1986 by Randall Terry, a former used-car salesman turned evangelical preacher, brought the use of civil disobedience to the movement. Terry's organization mobilized hundreds of anti-abortion protesters to barricade the doors of abortion facilities, blocking access with their bodies until they were cleared away and arrested by police. While the tactics of the radical wing of the anti-abortion movement were often deplored by such moderates as the National Right to Life Committee, their activism effected a renewed surge of anti-abortion campaigning, and brought substantial media attention.

The movement also began to expand on what was perhaps its most effective tactic, the use of fetal imagery in the elaboration of the ideology of fetal personhood. Fetal imagery has become such a cornerstone of the anti-abortion movement that a 1990 Volvo commercial featuring a sonogram image of a fetus was criticized by abortion opponents for "commercializing the unborn." Anti-abortion picketers carry posters of both fetuses and babies in an attempt to elide the difference between the two. The visual rhetoric of the fetus-as-person was taken to a new level by the 1985 video *The Silent Scream*. Produced by the National Right to Life Committee and hosted by Dr. Bernard Nathanson, a former board member of the National Abortion Rights Action League turned anti-abortion supporter, the half-hour video purported to represent "the point of view of the fetus" by showing a sonogram image of a 12-week fetus supposedly struggling and screaming during an abortion. Fetal imaging bolstered anti-abortionists' attempts to depict theirs as a new civil rights movement, for in separating the fetus from pregnancy, they were then able to present it as an autonomous individual deserving of legal protection. However, images of women, especially pregnant women, rarely appear in anti-abortion materials; such images would counter the efforts of the movement to shift the terms of the debate away from women's rights and onto the question of the fetus' alleged humanity.

The anti-abortion movement's successes have been due in large part to its diversity of tactics; its strategies have ranged from simple prayer vigils and memorial masses for the "unborn" to such traditionally leftist tactics as civil disobedience, tax resistance, and boycotts of corporations that support pro-choice organizations such as Planned Parenthood. Its efforts have been aided by generous funding from churches, corporations, and individuals sympathetic to its ideology. Most important, the anti-abortion movement has been relentless in its assault on public opinion. While many pro-choice activists moved on to other issues after *Roe v. Wade*, assuming that the right to abortion was now secure, the "right-to-lifers" endeavored to keep the U.S. population from growing accustomed to, and comfortable with, that right.

Less than two decades after *Roe v. Wade*, the anti-abortion movement has succeeded in changing the political context in which abortion takes place. In a move now supported by the 1992 Supreme Court decision in the Pennsylvania case, many states have enacted laws limiting abortion rights, requiring parental consent for minors, imposing strict regulations on second-trimester terminations, or even banning most abortions altogether. Federal funding for abortions was cut off in 1976, with most states following suit soon thereafter. With the Supreme Court having begun to restrict *Roe*, and a committed, well-organized, generously funded anti-abortion lobby, the continued legality of abortion itself is in doubt.

* DANA LUCIANO

See also: Abortion, Politics of
See **Guide to Related Topics:** Abortion

Resources

Critical Perspectives

Condit, Celeste Michelle. (1990). *Decoding Abortion Rhetoric: Communicating Social Change.* Urbana, IL: University of Illinois Press.

Conover, Pamela Johnston & Gray, Virginia. (1983). *Feminism and the New Right: Conflict Over the American Family.* New York: Praeger.

Dubinsky, Karen. (1985). *Lament for a 'Patriarchy Lost'? Anti-feminism, Anti-abortion and R.E.A.L. Women in Canada.* Ottawa: Canadian Research Institute for the Advancement of Women.

Ginsburg, Faye. (1989). *Contested Lives: The Abortion Debate in an American Community.* Berkeley, CA: University of California Press.

Luker, Kristin. (1984). *Abortion and the Politics of Motherhood.* Berkeley, CA: University of California Press.

Merton, Andrew. (1981). *Enemies of Choice: The Right-to-Life Movement and Its Threat to Abortion.* Boston: Beacon Press.

Mohr, James C. (1978). *Abortions in America: The Origins and Evolution of National Policy 1800-1900.* New York: Oxford University Press.

Petchetsky, Rosalind Pollack. (1990). *Abortion and Woman's Choice: The State, Sexuality and Women's Freedom.* Boston: Northeastern University Press.

———. (1987). "Foetal Images: The Power of Visual Rhetoric in the Politics of Reproduction." In Michelle Stanworth (Ed.) *Reproductive Technology: Gender, Motherhood and Medicine.* Minneapolis, MN: University of Minnesota Press. pp. 57-80.

Anti-Abortion Literature

Horan, Dennis J. (Ed.). (1987). *Abortion and the Constitution: Reversing* Roe v. Wade *Through the Courts.* Washington, DC: Georgetown University Press.

The Human Life Review: Journal of the Human Life Foundation. (1975-). New York.

Nathanson, Bernard N. (1979). *Aborting America.* Garden City, NY: Doubleday.

———. (1983). *The Abortion Papers: Inside the Abortion Mentality.* New York: Frederick Fell Publishers.

Scheidler, Joseph M. (1985). *Closed: Ninety-Nine Ways to Stop Abortion.* Westchester, IL: Crossway Books.

Sisterlife Journal: Newsletter of Feminists for Life. (1974-). Columbus, OH.

Storer, Horatio. (1866). *Why Not? A Book For Every Woman.* Boston: Lee and Shephard.

Reagan, Ronald. (1984). *Abortion and the Conscience of the Nation.* Nashville, TN: Thomas Nelson Press.

Willke, Jack & Willke, Barbara. (1985). *Handbook on Abortion.* Cincinnati, OH: Hayes Publishing Co.

APGAR

The Apgar test is a scoring system that is applied to newborns, one minute after delivery and again at five minutes, to assess the condition of the baby immediately following birth. It evaluates the baby from 0 to 2 in five areas. (See Table 1 below.) The 5 numbers are summed for the Apgar score.

The physical signs evaluated are listed on the table in order of importance. Heart rate is of most importance and is checked by the birth attendant by using a stethoscope on the newborn's chest or observing the pulsation of the umbilical cord. Respiratory effort evaluates how well the baby is breathing on his or her own. Good muscle tone is noted by observing if the newborn keeps his or her arms and legs well flexed and resists efforts to extend them. Reflex irritability measures a baby's response to poking and prodding. Color is evalu-

Table 1. Apgar Scoring System

SIGN	SCORE		
	0	1	2
Heart rate	absent	slow (less than 100)	over 100
Respiratory effort	absent	slow, irregular	good lusty cry
Muscle tone	limp	some flexing of arms and legs	active motion
Reflex irritability*	absent	frown, grimace	grimace, sneezing, crying, coughing
Color	blue pale	body pink, extremities blue	entirely pink

*Response to flick of finger against foot or catheter inserted into nostril.

ated by the length of time it takes before the baby's entire body is pink.

An Apgar score of 7 to 10 indicates a baby who requires no treatment. A score of 4 to 6 may indicate a need for resuscitation. A score of 0 to 3 is an indication of an infant who needs immediate assistance. This evaluation is not meant to act as a predictor of the child's health but merely to provide an indication of how the baby is doing at the moment.

This scoring system was developed by Virginia Apgar in 1953 while she was a professor of anesthesiology at Columbia-Presbyterian Medical Center. Dr. Apgar went on to earn a master's degree in public health from Johns Hopkins University and become the director of the medical program on birth defects for The National Foundation-March of Dimes. She received numerous awards for her contributions as a physician, teacher, and humanitarian before her death on August 7, 1974, at the age of 65.

✱ MARLENE SWEENEY, C.C.E.

See **Guide to Related Topics:** Baby Care

Resources

Apgar, Virginia & Beck, Joan. (1972). *Is My Baby All Right?* New York: Trident Press, p. 9.

Ashford, Janet Isaacs. (1983). *The Whole Birth Catalog.* New York: Crossing Press, p. 167.

Wilson, Christine Coleman & Hovey, Wendy Roe. (1980). *Cesarean Childbirth.* New York: Dolphin Books, p. 107.

ART AND BIRTH METAPHORS: NATURE-CULTURE DICHOTOMIES

Within Western culture, the female body has been used as a visual metaphor or emblem of nature. The womb, the pregnant belly, the lactating breasts, and the ability to give birth have been equated with the life-giving processes of nature. In addition, the enigmatic and unpredictable wilderness of nature has been associated with the woman's sexuality, which, due to its internal location, has been perceived as a mysterious "dark continent." The male, on the other hand, has been associated with reason, civilization, and progress. These cultural manifestations emphasize the intellect, rather than the body. According to this perception, the man is aligned with intellectual, active, and aggressive processes of culture, while the woman represents those passive, physical ones of nature.

Of course, both women and men are neither entirely "Nature" nor "Culture." But, because the human procreative function is specific to the female body, this aspect aligns the woman closer to nature and appears to free her male counterpart from the responsibilities and activities that are the consequence of this function, allowing him to focus more on the activities of culture. Since his creativity is pursued externally and "artificially," the male becomes associated with the products of technology and civilization (Ortner, 1974).

Based on this assumption, western civilizations are built by subduing nature. In this respect, culture attempts to harness nature, and this sets the two in opposition to each other; one dominates while the other submits. Thus, the nature/culture dichotomy results from the associations of men and women with their basic, yet stereotypical, social and biological functions and these two poles of masculinity and femininity have been used within the Western world as metaphors to represent the essence of "Nature" and "Culture."

Although the association between woman's reproductive cycle and nature has existed for hundreds, if not thousands of years, within the Judeo-Christian tradition the association of the female with nature and the male with culture finds its origins in this tradition's creation myth. In Genesis, man is given control over all the earth and its animal population. Such responsibilities award him the right to name all that is under his supervision. Man possesses language and power, which have been divinely sanctioned by the deity in whose image man was made. From this act, culture is born and, along with it, the justification for man's domination over nature. Later in the story, woman is created from man to assuage his loneliness, and he names her as he did the rest of the animals under his domain. In this respect, woman, like the rest of nature, becomes the possession of man. The Western world's hierarchy of man over woman and nature was sanctioned and perpetuated by a belief in the Genesis myth, which, ultimately, justified the growth of culture at the expense of nature (MacCormack and Stathern, 1980).

Western culture eventually pursued this "divinely" sanctioned destiny in its colonization of "New," or non-Western, worlds. The indigenous peoples and natural resources of the "New" lands were appropriated and used for the sake of commercial profits and Western progress. In order to reap the benefits of these untapped "riches," imperialists rationalized that they, as more superior in their civilized state, possessed the responsibility to control the people and the resources of the "New" lands.

Because these lands were perceived as wild, untamed, and bountiful, they were regarded in feminine terms. These vanquished lands not only shared with women the state of subordination to the powers of Western male culture, but they also had in common fertility and nurturance—the ability to sustain and bring forth life. The metaphors of "Mother" and "Virgin" were used to describe and identify these "New" lands. As Mother, the land provided a womb to generate a new culture and breasts to feed it (Kolodny, 1975). As Virgin, the land was an unpenetrated and succulent paradise. Taken by force, the land, like the woman, was raped and overpowered by Western culture.

In art (as well as literature) the allegory of nature, as it is personified in the female body, has been used to metaphorically represent the lands of the non-Western world. For example, in a 1589 print by Jan van der Straet (Ioannes Strandanus), entitled *Discovery of America: Vespucci Landing in America*, Western culture is personified by the clothed, standing male, while the colonized, "New" land, in this case America, is represented by the nude female, reclining on the hammock. Her hand reaches toward him like a nurturing mother, while her legs spread for entry. He holds the symbols of Western reason and progress; his retinue of ships behind him represent the advanced and superior technology of this civilization. To the right of the female is the technology of her culture—a spear—and behind her are the

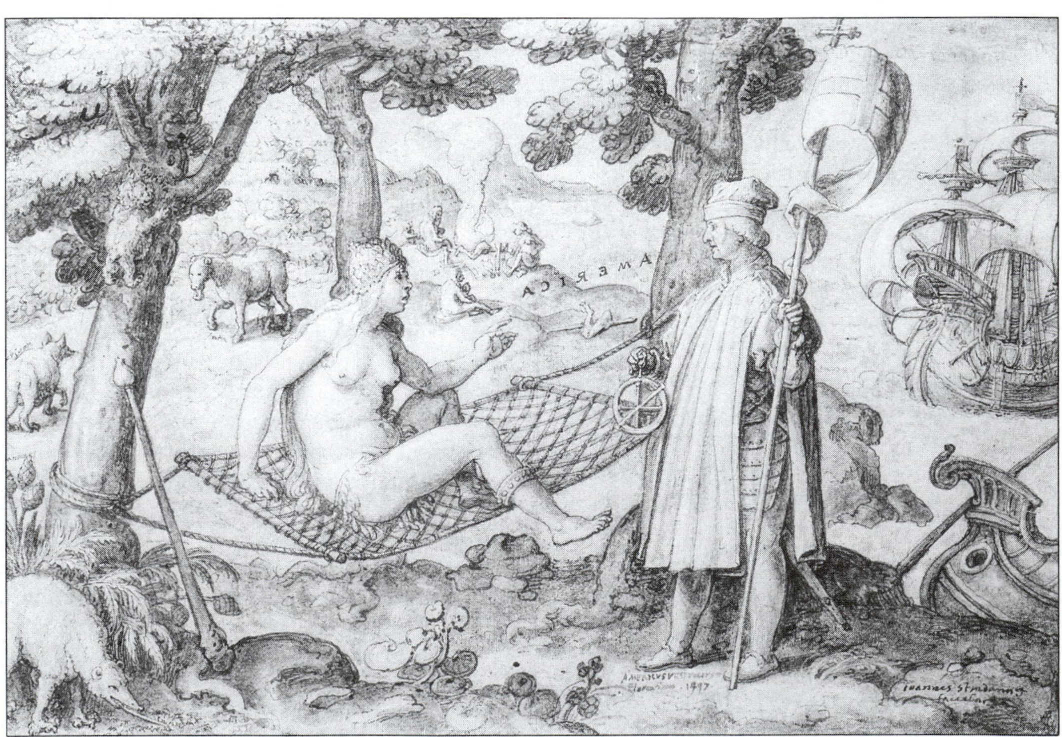

Discovery of America: Vespucci Landing in America by Ioannes Strandanus (1523-1605). [Pen and brown ink, heightened with white. H.: 7½; W.: 10⅝ inches (19 x 26.9 cm). The Metropolitan Museum of Art, New York, gift of the estate of James Hazen Hyde, 1958.] All rights reserved, The Metropolitan Museum of Art.

bounties of paradise as well as the mysteries of the untamed wilderness.

This metaphor also appears in Jean-Baptiste Carpeaux's 1872 bronze monument "Les Quatre Parties du Monde Soutenant la Sphére" [The four parts of the world supporting the globe] (Paris, Jardins du Luxembourg, Fontaine de l'Observatoire). Here, four female nudes support a sphere—symbol of the world—upon their shoulders. These female figures (an African, Asian, European, and Native American woman) not only personify the four continents, but they also represent colonized lands subject to the French Empire (Honour, 1989).

The history behind such metaphors indicates that the woman was put in a subordinate position to man on the basis of her body's ability to give birth. Accordingly, her body was perceived as an extension of the fertility and nurturance associated with nature. These metaphors express an attitude that positions "Culture" (male) over "Nature" (female), consequently revealing why "New" lands, because of their affinity with the female body, were perceived as both an untamed, virgin paradise and a fertile, nurturing motherland. As a result, the "New" lands were exploited and dominated by the civilizations of Western culture, suffering a similar fate as the female body and nature as a whole.

✱ CYNTHIA LEE HENTHORN

See also: The Birth Symbol; Creation Stories in Western Culture; Goddess Imagery

See **Guide to Related Topics:** Literature and the Arts

Resources

Honour, Hugh. (1975). *The European Vision of America.* Cleveland: Cleveland Museum of Art.

———. (1975). *The New Golden Land: European Images of America from the Discoveries to the Present Time.* New York: Random House.

———. (1989). *Image of the Black in Western Art.* Cambridge, MA: Harvard University Press.

Kolodny, Annette. (1975). *The Lay of the Land: Metaphor as Experience and History in American Life and Letters.* Chapel Hill, NC: University of North Carolina Press.

MacCormack, Carol P. & Stathern, Marilyn. (Eds.). (1980). *Nature, Culture and Gender.* Cambridge, MA: Cambridge University Press.

Mies, Maria, Benholdt-Thomsen, Veronika, & von Werlhof, Claudia. (1988). *Women: The Last Colony.* London and Atlantic Highlands, NJ: Zed Books Ltd.

Ortner, Sherry B. (1974). "Is Female to Male as Nature Is to Culture?" In Michelle Zimbalist Rosaldo & Louis Lamphere (Eds.) *Woman Culture and Society.* Stanford, CA: Stanford University Press.

ARTIFICIAL INSEMINATION. *See instead* DONOR INSEMINATION

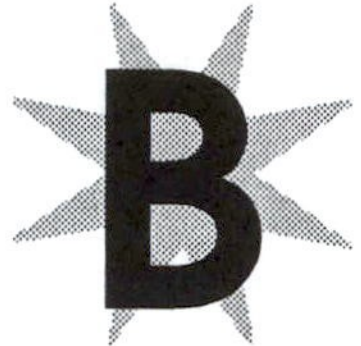

BABY DIARIES: THE HISTORY OF CHILD DEVELOPMENT

Baby diaries—the recorded observations of the behavior of babies—have been kept for centuries (Franklin, Wallace, and Keegan, in progress). Often, such diaries were kept by men and women with professional interests—educators, philosophers, psychologists, evolutionists, and others. They reveal changing ideas about infancy and childhood, child care, education, and development. Diarists had different goals: to know what behaviors and capacities were present at birth; to discern patterns of development; and to assess the influence of child-rearing practices.

The Early Diarists. The first diaries to focus exclusively on infant development appeared in Germany in the late eighteenth century. The diary kept by the philosopher Dietrich Tiedemann (1787) of his son's first three years became the model for a century. Tiedemann's observations touched on his son's social behavior, emotional expression, and early language.

Other diarists of this period were interested in educational reform, seen as developing abilities present at birth. Lacking reliable information about these abilities, the study of babies was important. Dillenius (1789), a teacher, observed his daughter from birth to 12 months. He identified several instincts present at birth or soon after—the instinct for survival, curiosity, and so on. Von Winterfeld (1789, 1790, 1791) was interested in child rearing. Following Rousseau's advice, he kept his daughter unswaddled in an unheated room and bathed her in cold water from birth. Both men discuss their babies' brushes with illness and death, and their medical treatment. Indeed, these were central issues since close to half of all children did not survive to age eight.

Diaries were also published to encourage mothers to develop their young children's characters. The diary of Mrs. Willard (1835), an English infant school teacher, is one such document. John Abbott (1833), in the United States, used mothers' diaries to explore the best methods, including harsh punishment, to control the young child's temper, ensure obedience, and encourage proper moral development.

Darwin and His Contemporaries. Just as Tiedemann's diary served as a model, so did Darwin's. The impetus for Darwin to publish came from an article by the French intellectual Hyppolyte Taine (1877).

Taine's account of his daughter's language development during her first 18 months of life included comparisons of her achievements with those of animals and "primitive" humans. Taine supported the view of the evolution of language in humans proposed by Darwin in *Descent of Man*. The article led Darwin to review and write a summary of a diary of the development of his first child, kept 37 years earlier (Darwin, 1877).

Darwin's observations of his son's first two years of development included motor, sensory, emotional, moral, and intellectual functioning. This brief, influential publication was a clear demonstration of how careful observation of an individual child could yield substantive developmental information.

Over the next four years, the journal *Mind* published three additional articles relying on diary records of infant development (Pollack, 1878; Sully, 1880; Champneys, 1881). In France, Perez's (1878) *The First Three Years of Childhood* appeared; in Germany, Preyer (1882) published *The Mind of the Child*. In both works, diary records of their sons' first three years provided the material for discussion of child development. Preyer also set forth requirements for systematic scientific observation. These works were highly influential in Europe and the U.S. and gave further impetus to the diary method in the emerging scientific study of the child.

Developmental Psychology Takes Shape. In 1881, Emily Talbot (1882) of the American Social Science Association issued a call to parents to record observations of their young children and thereby contribute to the scientific understanding of early development. Talbot's program coincided with the beginnings of the child study movement, initiated by educated women convinced that new scientific findings would provide a basis for optimal child rearing. This movement, based on a view of the child as requiring thoughtful nurturance rather than harsh discipline, was supported by John Dewey and G. Stanley Hall. James Sully supported a similar movement in Britain.

More than 30 diary accounts of infancy and early childhood were published between 1890 and 1915. Many explicitly followed those requirements spelled out earlier by Preyer. For the founders of developmental psychology in the U.S. and Britain—G. Stanley Hall, James Mark Baldwin, and James Sully—systematic diary records provided essential data. Baldwin (1894) and Sully (1896/1977) observed their own children, as Wilhelm Stern (1914/1924) did some years later. Among the most widely cited studies of this period is Milicent Shinn's (1893-1899/1966; 1907/1966), which focused on the development of her niece's sensory capacities. Kathleen Carter Moore (1896) traced her daughter's early intellectual growth and language in addition to her sensory and motor development. Louise E. Hogan (1898/1975), a teacher and follower of Pestalozzi and Froebel, provided a chronological account of her child's first communications, exploratory activity, drawing, and imaginative play.

The Modern Era. The 1920s were marked by a growing divergence of U.S. and European approaches to theory and research in developmental psychology. As child psychology became established in the U.S., observation of children moved out of the privacy of the home into the school and laboratory.

Nevertheless Fenton (1925) published a diary record of her son's first two years. Referring to Preyer, Shinn, Moore, and other predecessors, Fenton's book is a well-informed account of the child's sensory development, motor coordination, and play. This book, which includes guidelines for observation, was intended to provide mothers with "a more understanding appreciation of the nature and needs of babyhood," but was also seen as an appropriate text for students of child psychology and education. It may be the last baby diary in English directed to these two audiences.

Among the most prominent developmental theorists of the twentieth century, Heinz Werner in Germany and Jean Piaget in Switzerland drew extensively on diary records to create their theories of child development.

The diary has continued to be used to gather observations on language development. As a method for studying other aspects of development, the baby diary has virtually disappeared. Its critical historical role is only now being recognized.

✱ DORIS B. WALLACE, Ph.D., MARGERY B. FRANKLIN, Ph.D., and ROBERT T. KEEGAN, Ph.D.

See also: Pediatrics, History of

See **Guide to Related Topics:** Baby Care

Resources

Abbott, John S.C. (1833). *The Mother at Home.* New York: Crocker and Brewster.

Baldwin, James M. (1894). *Mental Development in the Child and the Race.* New York: Macmillan.

Champneys, F.H. (1881). "Notes on an Infant." *Mind* 6: 104-07.

Darwin, Charles R. (1877). "A Biographical Sketch of an Infant." *Mind,* 2: 285-94.

Dillenius, Friedrich W.J. (1789). "Fragmente eines Tagebuchs über die Entwickelung der körperlichen und geistigen Fähigkeiten und Anlagen eines Kindes." *Braunschweigisches Journal philosophischen, philologischen und padagogischen Inhalts* 3: 320-42.

Fenton, J.C. (1925). *A Practical Psychology of Babyhood.* New York: Houghton Mifflin.

Franklin, Margery B., Wallace, Doris B., & Keegan, Robert T. (In progress). *The Developing Mind: 200 Years of Baby Diaries.* New York: Oxford University Press.

Hogan, Louise E. (1975). *A Study of a Child.* New York: Arno Press (Classics in Child Development). Original work published in 1898.

Moore, Kathleen C. (1896). "The Mental Development of a Child." *Psychological Review* (3), Monograph Supplement.

Perez, N. (1878). La Psychologie de l'Enfant: Les Trois Premières Années. Paris: Alcan. See also F. Louis Soldan (Trans). (1890). *Record of an Infant Life.* Syracuse, NY: C.W. Bardeen.

Pollack, F. (1878). "An Infant's Progress in Language." *Mind,* 3: 392-401.

Preyer, Wilhelm. (1882). *Die Seele des Kindes.* Leipzig: Grieben. See also H.W. Brown (Trans). (1890). *The Mind of a Child, Parts 1 and 2.* New York: Appleton.

Shinn, Milicent, W. (1966). *Notes on the Development of a Child, I.* University of California Studies, Vol. I. New York: Johnson Reprint Corporation. Original work published in 1893-99.

———. (1966). *Notes on the Development of a Child, II.* University of California Studies, Vol. IV. New York:

Johnson Reprint Corporation. Original work published in 1907.

Stern, Wilhelm. (1924). *Psychology of Early Childhood, Supplemented by Extracts from the Unpublished Diaries of Clara Stern*. A. Barwell (Trans). New York: Holt. Original work published in 1914.

Sully, James. (1880). "Mental Development in Children." *Mind 5*: 385-86.

———. (1977). "Studies of Childhood." In D.N. Robinson (Ed.) *Significant Contributions to the History of Psychology, 1750-1920*. New York: University Publications of America. Original work published in 1896.

Taine, Hyppolyte A. (1877). "Taine on the Acquisition of Language in Children." *Mind 2*: 252-59.

Talbot, Emily (Ed.) (1882). "Papers on Infant Development." *Journal of Social Science 15*: 1-52.

Tiedemann, Dietrich. (1787). "Boebachtungen über die Entwicklung der Seelenfahigkeiten bei Kindern." *Hessische Beitrage zur Gelehrsamkeit und Kunst 2*: 313-15 and *3*: 486-88. See also Murchison, Carl & Langer, Suzanne (Trans). (1927). "Tiedemann's Observations on the Development of the Mental Faculties of Children." *The Pedagogical Seminary 34* (1): 205-30.

von Winterfeld, M.A. (1789). "Tagebuch eines Vaters über sein neugeborenes Kind." *Braunschweigisches Journal 5*: 404-41.

———. (1790). "Beantwortung einiger Einwürfe des Herausgeber des Tagebuchs eines Vaters im Auguststücke von dem Verfasser dieses Tagebuchs." *Braunschweigishes Journal 7*: 311-32.

———. (1791). "Fortsetzung des Tagebuchs eines Vaters." *Braunschweigishes Journal 12*: 476-84.

Willard, Mrs. (1835). *"Appendix" to Progressive Education, Commencing with the Infant by Mme. Necker de Saussure*. Boston: William D. Ticknor.

BABY DOE

On April 9, 1982, an infant who became known as "Baby Doe" was born in Bloomington, Indiana. He had Down's syndrome and intestinal defects. Treatment could be expected to correct the intestinal defects, but nothing could prevent the developmental delays associated with Down's syndrome. After considering the advice of their obstetrician, who presented the option of withholding treatment and allowing the baby to die, and the advice of their pediatrician, who recommended surgery, Baby Doe's parents decided against an operation. Without surgery, he could not eat or drink; he received no nutrition or fluids. He was sedated and moved to a private room. Many nurses and physicians were disturbed by the decision. The hospital petitioned the courts for permission to treat. The Indiana courts upheld the parents' right to refuse surgery. Six days after his birth, while efforts were being made to bring the case to the U.S. Supreme Court, Baby Doe died. The media attention that followed this case and subsequent attempts by the federal government to regulate the treatment of newborns led to the emergence of "Baby Doe decisions" as a public issue.

Baby Doe decisions are choices about care for infants who are both likely to die without life-sustaining treatment and likely to have disabilities if they survive. Such choices have always been faced by families and birth attendants concerned with the care of catastrophically ill newborns. For example, the ancient Greek physician Soranus, in his text *Gynecology*, described how a midwife might recognize an infant "not worth rearing." Traditionally, treatment choices were seen as private dilemmas, to be faced by a baby's family and caretakers. However, technological, political, and social developments of the 20th century set the stage for a wider societal controversy.

At one time, there was little treatment available to sustain the lives of infants born critically ill. However, since World War II, there have been rapid technological developments in treatment for babies born prematurely or with other congenital impairments. In addition, economic and organizational developments, such as health insurance and the regionalization of medical care, led to the establishment of neonatal intensive care units (NICUs) by the 1960s. These specialized units delivered state-of-the-art care to critically ill newborns.

For most infants, neonatal intensive care was clearly beneficial. However, some clinicians felt that their technological interventions did more harm than good for some infants. By the late 1960s and early 1970s, articles advocating decisions to withhold treatment when an infant would have a poor quality of life began to appear in the clinical literature. At the same time, as the field of bioethics developed, philosophers, lawyers, and others often focused on questions of care for newborns as they discussed such issues as care of the dying and protection of vulnerable patients. Bioethicists debated "Which babies should be treated?" and "Who should decide?" Also, at the time, political and ideological battles raged on issues of relevance to Baby Doe decisions, such as the appropriate use of technology; the separation of church and state; the rights of people with disabilities; the rights of professionals, parents, and children; and the appropriate role of the state versus federal governments.

Previously, there were no specific laws pertaining to treatment of newborns. Generally, child abuse and neglect statutes were used when efforts were made to override parental decisions. Court decisions appeared inconsistent; sometimes parents' positions were supported, other times they were overruled. All were handled on an individual basis. However, some members of the Right-to-Life movement came to see such decisions as part of a wider attack on the "sanctity of life." They believed that government involvement was needed. In response to pressure from this organized lobby following the case of Baby Doe, President Reagan issued a directive, based on a disability rights law, stating that the "discriminatory failure to feed and care for handicapped infants . . . is prohibited by Federal Law."

At first the regulation received little notice. However, in 1983, perhaps in an effort to maintain the support of the New Right, Reagan publicly announced plans to enforce the directives. Hospitals would be required to hang signs with the law in prominent places, a "Baby Doe Hotline" was to be established, and squads of federal investigators would be sent to investigate claims of discriminatory denials of treatment. This catapulted the issue into the national spotlight.

The "Baby Doe Directives" were applauded, not only by "Right to Life" advocates, but also by liberal members of civil rights and disability rights groups, who felt that the directives provided needed protection for infants with disabilities. Other civil rights groups, women's health groups, and organizations of health care professions opposed the regulations, seeing them as an infringement on the privacy of the physician/patient relationship, on the rights of parents, and on the right of patients or their proxy decision makers to refuse treatment. Some parents and physicians felt compelled to provide treatments that they did not believe were in the infants' best interests. The regulations were successfully challenged in court; revised regulations were issued.

Later, in 1983, a girl who was known as Baby Jane Doe was born in New York. She had spina bifida, a defect that causes paralysis and is often associated with developmental delays. Her parents refused neurosurgery. Right-to-Life activists tried unsuccessfully to have the state courts order treatment. In pursuing the case, they also tried to use the revised federal directives. A lower court decision to invalidate these directives was upheld by the U.S. Supreme Court in 1986. The Court noted that treatment decisions have traditionally been the province of parents and physicians, or in exceptional cases, child welfare authorities; there was no specific ruling on the appropriateness of withholding treatment in this case (*Bowen v. the United Hospital Association et al.*, 1986).

While the directives were under review in the courts, compromise legislation was passed by Congress. Amendments to child abuse laws stated that treatment could only be withheld if an infant was irreversibly comatose, if treatment would be futile in terms of survival, or if treatment would be "virtually futile" and the treatment itself would be inhumane. The amendments also encouraged the establishment of hospital-based committees to review cases in which life-sustaining treatments are withheld (U.S. Congress, 1984). Advocates who supported government intervention believed the act would prevent the withholding of treatments from infants with disabilities; those who opposed the directives thought the amendments would allow the withholding of intrusive treatments from hopelessly ill newborns.

For now the political controversy surrounding Baby Doe decisions has subsided, but the issue has not been resolved definitively. Many people do not agree with the requirements under the law. For example, some people reviewing the case of an infant with severe heart defects whose only chance for survival would entail a number of complex surgeries or a heart transplant would believe that treatment would be required while others would think the treatments would be virtually futile and inhumane. Different opinions also exist concerning the benefits of aggressive treatment for very small premature infants, infants with HIV, and some infants requiring intensive care who would be expected to have a very poor quality of life. During the next few years, it is likely that parents, health professionals, and activists with varied political interests will again be embroiled in political debates over Baby Doe decisions. ✱ BETTY WOLDER LEVIN, Ph.D.

See also: Decision Making: Newborn Care; Ethics Committees

See **Guide to Related Topics:** Legal Issues; Special Needs Infants

Resources

Anspach, Renee R. (Forthcoming). *Life and Death Decisions in Neonatal Intensive Care: A Study in the Sociology of Knowledge*. Berkeley, CA: University of California Press.

Asch, Adrienne & Rothman, Barbara Katz. (1986). "The Question of Baby Doe." *Health/PAC Bulletin 16* (6): 5-13.

Bowen v. American Hospital Association et al. (1986). Supreme Court of the United States. No. 84-1529. Argued Jan 15, 1986. Decided June 9, 1986.

Caplan, Art et al. (1987). "Imperiled Newborns." *The Hastings Center Report 17* (6): 5-32.

Fox, Daniel M. (Ed.) (1986). "Special Section on the Treatment of Handicapped Newborns." *Journal of Health Politics, Policy and Law 11* (2): 195-304.

Guillemin, Jeanne & Holmstrom, Lynda Lytle. (1986). *Mixed Blessings: Intensive Care for Newborns*. New York: Oxford University Press.

Lantos, John. (1987). "Baby Doe Five Years Later." *New England Journal of Medicine 317* (7): 444-47.

Levin, Betty Wolder. (1988). "The Cultural Context of Decision Making of Catastrophically Ill Newborns: The Case of Baby Jane Doe." In Karen Michaelson (Ed.) *Childbirth in America: Anthropological Perspectives.* South Hadley, MA: Bergin and Garvey, pp.178-93.
Lyon, Jeff. (1985). *Playing God in the Nursery.* New York: W.W. Norton and Company.
Moss, Kathryn. (1987). "The 'Baby Doe' Legislation: Its Rise and Fall." *Policy Studies Journal 15* (4): 627-51.
U.S. Congress. (1984). Child Abuse Amendments of 1984. Public law 98-457.
Weir, Robert. (1984). *Selective Nontreatment of Handicapped Newborns.* New York: Oxford University Press.

BABY FOOD. *See instead* WEANING FOOD

BAPTISM, INFANT

Birth, a most sacred event to the religions of the world, is celebrated with rites and festivities, some of which appear to be inconsistent in many religions. Although mothers of newborn children are regarded as participating in the sacred event by having brought forth a new being into the world, among the Israelites and Zoroastrians they themselves are seen as ritually unclean, probably a result of the presence of blood at birth, the loss of which would symbolize the loss of some of the life-sustaining force. Among the Kikuyu of eastern Africa, mother and child symbolically die and rise again during and after a ceremony of seclusion, after which a feast is held in which a goat is sacrificed and prayers are said. The whole community joins in the celebration to rejoice that the new child has become part of the family of humankind.

Modern Christian baptism is deeply rooted in the religious traditions of the Roman Catholic, Orthodox, and Reformed churches. In the Orthodox church, Christian initiation for children is generally completed in a single ceremony, while the other Christian churches tend to separate the initiation rites over the course of childhood. The ceremonies of the initiation rites include tracing the sign of the cross on the forehead of the child; giving a Christian name; saying prayers of exorcism; immersing the infant in or infusing the infant with water; anointing with perfumed oil (chrism); laying on of hands; and sharing the sacred meal.

For induction into Christianity, initiation is not regarded as a "birthright" but is predicated on the presence of faith. Since infants, for obvious reasons, cannot make a personal profession of faith, the Christian church's understanding of faith includes the "incipient" faith of the child; the matured faith of the parent(s); and the corporate faith of the particular Christian community. Should one dimension of faith be lacking, the presence of the other two is generally considered sufficient for proceeding with initiation.

Infant baptism places heavy educative and formative obligations on both the family and the faith community, as expressed by the Faith and Order Commission of the World Council of Churches. Nevertheless, infant baptism is often little more than a social convention or a ritual adhered to because it is presumed to have quasi-magical powers. Some people believe that once baptized, infants will sleep through the night. Others maintain theological misconceptions such as the belief, that without baptism, a child who should die would be doomed to limbo or suffer some pain of spiritual loss.

For most Christian faiths, baptism serves as a ritual means of incorporating the infant into a theocentric community and acts to help counter the effects of "original sin" in his or her own life.

✱ JULIA ANN UPTON, R.S.M.

See **Guide to Related Topics:** Baby Care

Resources

Aland, K. (1963). *Did the Early Church Baptize Infants?* G.R. Beasley-Murray (trans). Philadelphia: Westminster Press.
Barth, K. (1948). *The Teaching of the Church Regarding Baptism.* E. Payne (trans). London: SCM Press.
Covino, P. (1982). "The Postconciliar Infant Baptism Debate in the American Catholic Church." *Worship 56*: 240-60.
Jeremias, J. (1962). *Infant Baptism in the First Four Centuries.* David Cairns (trans). Philadelphia: Westminster Press.
———. (1963). *Origins of Infant Baptism.* Dorothese M. Barton (trans). Volume 1: Studies in Historical Theology. London: SCM Press.
Jewett, P.K. (1978). *Infant Baptism and the Covenant of Grace.* Grand Rapids, MI: Eerdmans.
Kavanagh, A. (1978). *The Shape of Baptism: The Rite of Christian Initiation.* New York: Pueblo.
Murphy Center. (Ed.) (1976). *Made not Born.* Notre Dame, IN: University of Notre Dame Press.
Philibert, P. (1989, Mar). "Children's Ritual Enculturation: What, How and Why?" *Catechumenate 11*: 27-44.
Riley, H. (1974). *Christian Initiation: A Comparative Study of the Interpretation of the Baptismal Liturgy.* Washington, DC: Catholic University of America Press.
Yarnold, E. (1971). *The Awe-Inspiring Rites of Initiation.* Slough, MN: St. Paul Publications.

BIBLICAL AND TALMUDIC IMAGES OF CHILDBIRTH

The concept of pain in childbirth, the so-called curse of Eve, cannot be traced to Scripture in the original languages, or to early Judaism. Genesis 3:16 is used as proof that pain is inevitable, ordained by the Creator as a punishment for Eve's sin. The word translated as "sorrow" or "pain" is the Hebrew word *etzev*. However *etzev* is *also* used for Adam in the following verse, Genesis 3:17, a fact most translators have overlooked! The Hebrew Bible with English translation reads as follows: "Unto the woman he said, I will greatly multiply thy *sorrow* (*etzev*) and thy pregnancy: in *pain* (*etzev*) thou shall bear children....And unto Adam he said,...cursed is the ground for thy sake; in *toil* (*etzev*) shalt thou eat of it all the days of thy life" (*Hebrew Bible*, 1965).

When the *same* Hebrew word is translated as "pain" for the woman and "toil" for the man, it is clear that the translator's cultural beliefs have biased his judgment as a scholar of the text. The best description of giving birth is toil, or labor. When Eve's first child Cain was born there is no mention of pain or any kind of difficulty in the birth, but only the joyful statement, "I have obtained a man [from] the Eternal" (Genesis 4:1). In the Talmud, Eve's "curse" is divided into 10 parts, embracing the whole of a woman's life. Adam's "curse" is paired with Eve's, and divided into 10 parts also.

Even a casual reading of Scripture reveals expressions of joy, not pain, from mothers at the births. Sarah named Isaac "laughter" (Genesis 21:6). Leah expressed praise at the birth of each of her six sons, naming the fourth one Judah, "praise," saying at the birth of the fifth, "God has rewarded me," and at the birth of the sixth, "God has presented me with a precious gift" (Genesis 29:31-35, 30:17-21).

When Rachel's first son was born, she exclaimed happily, "Lord give me another son!" (Genesis 30:24) But when she gave birth to her younger son, Benjamin, the word used to describe her labor is the Hebrew word *qashah*, "hard, difficult, fierce." It is used only this once in the entire Bible to describe a birth. Benjamin's birth appears from the text to have been an abnormal one, with the baby presenting in a complicated breech or transverse position. The midwife succeeded in getting the child delivered, but Rachel died (Genesis 35:16-18).

In Exodus, the Pharaoh complains that the midwives are not killing the baby boys of the Israelites as he had commanded. The midwives explain that the Hebrew women gave birth so quickly that the babies were born before they could get there. Their statement was unchallenged, as it was credible.

Only one other death at childbirth is mentioned in the Bible. Eli's daughter-in-law was near the due date of her *second* child. When she heard the news that her father-in-law had died, her husband killed in battle, and the ark of God stolen by the Philistines, the shock sent her into labor. The women around tried to comfort her showing her the baby as she lay dying. "But she answered not, neither did she regard it. And she named the child Ichabod, saying, 'The glory is departed from Israel, for the ark of God is taken!'" (1 Samuel 4:19-22)

There are two Hebrew words used that relate to birth: *chul* and *yalad*. *Yalad* is used to refer to a father begetting as well as a mother giving birth. But when it refers to the mother, the translations often read "pangs," "travail," or "anguish" rather than simply "to give birth." *Chul* is sometimes used of God "*shaping* (*chul*)" the unborn child in the womb, or of "making the hinds to *calve* (*chul*)" or as "*making* (*chul*) a man," or as "*forming* (*chul*) the earth." But when used in relation to a woman giving birth, the translators' bias and misconceptions are evident in words like "anguish" or "pangs" (Wessel, 1983).

Scripture teaches that having children is a blessing, a sign of God's favor (Psalms 127:3). One of the stated results of disobedience to God's laws is the inability to have children: "Give them, O Lord, what wilt thou give? Give them a miscarrying womb and dry breasts...for all their wickedness" (Hosea 9:4). None of the prophets used the word *etzev* in regard to childbirth. They used words to describe labor such as *yapeach*, (Jeremiah 4:31) which means gasping, or "to breathe oneself out." Another word is *tsarah*, (2 Kings 6:1) commonly translated as distress or anguish when used to describe labor, but which conveys the idea of constriction, or narrowness (Isaiah 28:20). And surely, the child being born is in a "narrow" place. The prophets also mention sighing, groaning, fatigue, constriction, and fear. They are not describing any particular birth. Some of these are normal adjuncts of labor and do not mean the woman is in pain.

The Greek translation of the Hebrew Bible made by 70 scholars nearly 300 years before Christ uses the Greek word *lupe* to translate the Hebrew word *etzev* in Genesis 3:16. The word *lupe* refers only to an emotion. Three Greek words are used to translate *chul* and *yalad*. These words are *gennao*, *tikto*, and *odino*. *Gennao* means to have a child and is used of either parent. *Tikto* simply means "to give birth." *Odino* means to labor in birth. These same three simple words are found in the Greek New Testament. But again, translators have too often imposed on them the false assumption of pain or anguish in birth, even though the Bible describes the bearing of children as one of the most rewarding and joyous experiences of a woman's life. ✱ HELEN WESSEL

See also: Baptism, Infant

See **Guide to Related Topics:** Literature and the Arts

Resources

Hebrew Bible. (1965). Tel Aviv: Sinai Publishing.
Wessel, Helen. (1983). *Natural Childbirth and the Christian Family, 4th edition.* New York: Harper & Row.

BILIRUBIN. *See instead* JAUNDICE, NEWBORN

BIRTH CENTERS

Birth centers, also known as freestanding birth centers, FSBCs, and childbearing centers, have been defined as "nonhospital facilities organized to provide family-centered maternity care for women judged to be at low risk of obstetrical complications" (Rooks et al., 1989). The first birth centers in the United States served isolated rural areas. In the mid-1970s, however, birth centers began to proliferate in cities. According to the National Association of Childbearing Centers, at least 240 were operating by 1987. These centers, diverse in size, style, structure, and service area, were established as for-profit or non-profit medical centers or office practices by certified nurse-midwives, physicians, investors, and interested laypersons. The goal was to provide more supportive, less technologically oriented maternity care (Eakins and Richwald, 1986).

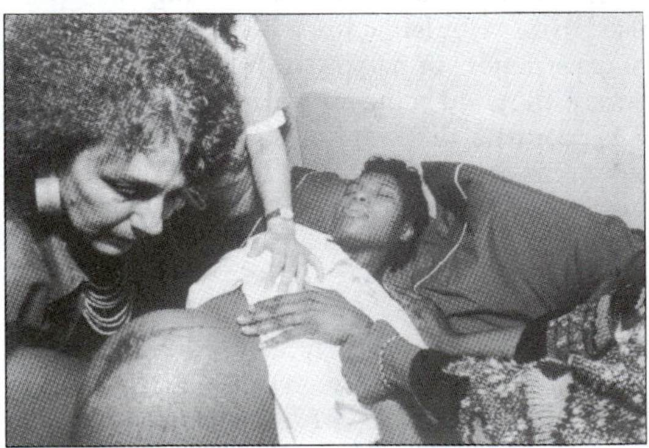

Birth at a birth center. Photo courtesy of Zakiyyah S. Madyun.

Birth centers spearheading the out-of-hospital birth movement differed philosophically from hospitals. First, unlike hospitals, birth centers stressed minimal technical intervention, believing such intervention was unnecessary for women classified as low-risk. Birth center personnel frequently believed that technological birth was physiologically and psychologically damaging to women and their babies. At a time when deliveries by cesarean section had skyrocketed to nearly 30 percent nationwide, birth centers endorsed one-on-one care, claiming that providing gentle guidance, understanding, and protection for pregnant women would reduce the need for cesarean section. According to several medical studies, the overall cesarean rate among birth center users has ranged from 2 to 6.6 percent (Eakins, 1989a; Rooks et al., 1989).

Second, birth centers supported family participation. The Maternity Center Association, a birth center in New York City, stressed sibling involvement. It was felt that childbirth, constituting a major rite of passage in family life, was an arena that could strengthen family ties, and this, in an era when the American divorce rate was higher than it had ever been.

Third, birth centers raised issues with regard to women's rights. The Birth Place of Menlo Park, California, actively supported "a woman's *right* to design and control her own birth experience." These centers catered to women's desires, claiming that the nature of the birth experience had a critical impact on a birthing mother's subsequent psychological health. Birth centers billed themselves as safer and more humane than hospitals.

Birth centers greatly affected the nation's philosophy of maternity care. Since they were capable of having an enormous economic effect as well, whether or not they were "medically safe" became the major political focal point. In 1979, the American Public Health Association concluded that "births to healthy mothers can occur safely outside the setting of an acute care hospital" and adopted guidelines for freestanding birth center licensure and regulation (American Public Health Association, 1983). Conversely, a joint publication by the American Academy of Pediatrics and the American College of Obstetricians and Gynecologists stated, "Until scientific studies are available to evaluate safety and outcome in freestanding centers, the use of such centers cannot be encouraged" (American Academy of Pediatrics and

American College of Obstetricians and Gynecologists, 1983).

In December 1989, two major scientific studies were released, one in the *New England Journal of Medicine*, the other in *The Journal of Reproductive Medicine*. The first, carried out by the National Association of Childbearing Centers in conjunction with Columbia University's School of Public Health, examined 11,814 deliveries at 84 birth centers cross-nationally (Rooks et al., 1989). The second, funded by the California Department of Health and Human Services and executed by the University of California, Los Angeles School of Public Health in association with Stanford University, examined 3,445 consecutive births at 25 birth centers in California (Eakins, 1989b). Both studies concluded that low-risk women delivering at freestanding birth centers were no more likely to have poor birth outcomes than were low-risk women delivering in hospitals. Birth center patients were less likely than hospital patients of comparable risk to deliver by cesarean section. Both studies stated that freestanding birth centers were associated with low neonatal mortality and no maternal mortality. In short, birth centers, with their alternative philosophy, appeared to offer care comparable to hospitals.

As of 1985, 20 states had devised requirements for licensure of nonhospital-based birth centers. These included Arizona, Colorado, Florida, Georgia, Hawaii, Kansas, Kentucky, Maryland, Massachusetts, Mississippi, Nevada, New Mexico, Oregon, Pennsylvania, Rhode Island, Utah, Vermont, Washington, West Virginia, and Wyoming (National Association of Childbearing Centers, 1984-85). Other states were working to adopt requirements.

By 1990, nearly all major health insurance companies covered birth center delivery. Not only were birth centers viewed as safe and philosophically attractive, they could deliver care at about two-thirds the cost of hospitals for similar services. The lower cost of birth centers was attributed to (a) lower overhead due to type of facility used; (b) the absence of certain costly medical equipment; (c) the types of practitioners employed—nurse-midwives as opposed to obstetrician-gynecologists; and (d) increased levels of overall efficiency (*Cooperative Birth Center Network News*, 1983; Ermann and Gabel, 1985; Eakins, 1989a).

It is believed that the philosophy and style of practice in birth centers enhances psychological and emotional satisfaction for women and their families while providing a medically safe environment for childbirth. It has been surmised that increased satisfaction is the reason for the exceeding low rate of malpractice lawsuits against freestanding birth centers as compared to hospitals (Shearer and Eakins, 1988). In the 1990s, some hospitals, observing the success of the birth center model, began to incorporate birth center philosophies and methods. Experimental "freestanding birth centers," owned and operated by hospitals, have been built on or near hospital grounds. One of the first to open its doors was established by Washington Hospital of Fremont, California, in 1988. These hospital-based centers, while providing easy access to high-risk medical teams and equipment, emphasize catered birthing with the least possible amount of technical intervention. While they currently serve only those women classified as low-risk, with such systems in place, by the year 2000, hospitals may be able to provide a safe and satisfying birth center-like experience for all women, including those with high-risk obstetric profiles.

✱ PAMELA S. EAKINS, Ph.D.

See also: Nurse-Midwifery: History in the United States

See **Guide to Related Topics:** Childbirth Practices and Locations

Resources

American Academy of Pediatrics and American College of Obstetricians and Gynecologists. (1983). *Guidelines for Perinatal Care*. Evanston, IL.

American Public Health Association. (1983, Mar). "Guidelines for Licensing and Regulating Birth Centers." *American Journal of Public Health 73*: 331-34.

Cooperative Birth Center Network News. 1983:1. Perkiomenville, Pennsylvania.

Eakins, Pamela S. (1988, Mar). "Freestanding Birth Centers: Prospects and Problems." *Birth 15*:(1):25-30.

———. (1989a, Sept). "Obstetric Outcomes at the Birth Place in Menlo Park: The First Seven Years." *Birth 16*:(3):123-29.

———. (1989b, Dec). "Freestanding Birth Centers in California: Program and Medical Outcome." *The Journal of Reproductive Medicine 34*:(12): 960-70.

Eakins, Pamela S. & Richwald, Gary A. (1986). *Freestanding Birth Centers in California: Structure, Cost, Medical Outcome and Issues*. Berkeley, CA: California Department of Health and Human Services.

Ermann, D. & Gabel, J. (1985). "The Changing Face of American Health Care: Multihospital Systems, Emergency Centers, and Surgery Centers. *Medical Care 23*: 401-20.

National Association of Childbearing Centers News. (Winter 1984-85). pp. 2, 3 & 4.

Rooks, Judith P. et al. (1989, Dec). "Outcomes of Care in Birth Centers." *New England Journal of Medicine 321*: 1801-11.

Shearer, Madeleine H. & Eakins, Pamela S. (1988, Mar). "Commentary and Response: The Malpractice Insurance Crisis and Freestanding Birth Centers." *Birth 15*:(1): 30-32.

BIRTH CERTIFICATES

Most governments collect and publish vital statistics based on legal registration of births, marriages, and deaths. While this is done primarily for administrative purposes, "bills of mortality" have been used since the 18th century to study medical causes of death (Barron and Thomson, 1983). The World Health Organization has provided standard forms of birth and death certification as well as international classifications of diseases, injuries, and causes of death (World Health Organization, 1975).

Because of a concern with infant mortality rates, many states are now including data related to pregnancy outcome on the birth certificate. This information may include the month when prenatal care began, the number of visits made, tobacco and alcohol use, the weight gained during pregnancy, maternal medical history, complications of pregnancy, obstetric procedures used, and condition of the baby. Social and demographic data such as marital status, educational level, and race/ethnicity are also usually included.

To maintain confidentiality, the top part of the certificate contains information of public record, e.g., names of the mother and father, addresses, and date and place of birth. The bottom portion contains the information related to pregnancy outcome, which is available for medical and health use only to persons engaged in health research who have special permission. (See Figure 1.)

In recent years, with the advent of computers that are able to process large amounts of data, many researchers have begun to use the information from birth certificates to look at such problems as the changes in birth weight over time, across generations, and among different ethnic groups (Kessel et al, 1984; Klebanoff et al., 1984; Shiono et al., 1986). Some of these studies have suggested that a woman's birth weight, and her subsequent growth and development, may influence the outcome of her pregnancy when she becomes an adult (Hackman et al., 1983). Other studies have shown a relationship between birth weight, infant mortality, and childhood morbidity (McCormick, 1985).

A recent study used birth certificate data to compare the adequacy of prenatal care in two Florida counties (Carson and Simpson, 1990). The two counties were similar in terms of socioeconomic status and rate of low birth-weight babies, but one had a much higher neonatal mortality rate. In the state of Florida birth certificate data includes the number of prenatal visits as well as the month of pregnancy when prenatal care began. This study used an instrument developed by the Institute of Medicine called the Maternal Health Care Index (Kessner, 1973), which classifies prenatal care as adequate, inadequate, or intermediate based on the month when care began and the number of visits. Early initiation of care and more visits mean adequate care while late registration and few visits mean inadequate care.

Birth certificate information, which had been put on computer tapes, was available through the University of Florida library, an official repository for vital statistics data for the state of Florida. This information was recorded, using only identification numbers to ensure confidentiality. Analysis determined that although the two rural counties appeared similar in socioeconomic status and racial composition, women in the county with the high neonatal mortality rate were more often black, unmarried, and less educated. They also started prenatal care later in pregnancy, received fewer prenatal visits, and delivered lower birthweight infants than women in the other county.

Such a study illustrates the accessibility and usefulness of birth certificate data. Its analysis makes it possible to suggest some possible reasons for the high neonatal mortality rates, as well as strategies for improving prenatal care. Thus, this information has many useful applications beyond verification of place and time of birth.

✱ SHARLEEN H. SIMPSON, A.R.N.P., Ph.D.

See **Guide to Related Topics:** Legal Issues

Resources

Barron, S.L. & Thomson, A.M. (1983). "Epidemiology of Pregnancy." In S.L. Barron & A.M. Thomson (Eds.) *Obstetrical Epidemiology*. New York: Academic Press, 1-24.

Carson, Elizabeth C. & Simpson, Sharleen H. (1990). "Prenatal Care and Neonatal Mortality Rates in Two Florida Counties." *Florida Journal of Public Health* 2 (3): 33-37.

Hackman, E. et al. (1983). "Maternal Birth Weight and Subsequent Pregnancy Outcome." *JAMA 250* (15): 2016-19.

Kessel, Samuel S. et al. (1984). "The Changing Pattern of Low Birth Weight in the United States, 1970 to 1980." *JAMA 252* (15): 1978-82.

Kessner, D. (1973). "Infant Death: An Analysis by Maternal Risk Factor and Health Care." In *Contrasts in Health Status*. Volume I, pp. 6-143. Institute of Medicine, Washington, DC: National Academy of Sciences Press.

Klebanoff, Mark A. et al. (1984). "Low Birth Weight across Generations." *JAMA 252* (17): 2423-27.

McCormick, Marie C. (1985). "The Contribution of Low Birth Weight to Infant Mortality and Childhood Morbidity." *The New England Journal of Medicine 312* (2): 82-90.

Figure 1. State of Florida Birth Certificate Form

State of Florida, Department of Health and Rehabilitative Services, Vital Statistics.

TYPE OR PRINT IN BLACK INK

CERTIFICATE OF LIVE BIRTH
FLORIDA 109—

LOCAL FILE NO.

BABY# ____________

MOM# ____________

CHILD

1. CHILD'S NAME *(First, Middle, Last)*
2. DATE OF BIRTH *(Month, Day, Year)*
3. TIME OF BIRTH M
4. SEX
5. CITY, TOWN OR LOCATION OF BIRTH
6. COUNTY OF BIRTH
7. PLACE OF BIRTH: ☐ HOSPITAL ☐ FREESTANDING BIRTHING CENTER ☐ CLINIC/DOCTOR'S OFFICE ☐ RESIDENCE ☐ OTHER
8. FACILITY NAME *(If not institution, give street and number)*
9. INSIDE CITY LIMITS? *(Yes or No)*

CERTIFIER

10. I CERTIFY THAT THIS CHILD WAS BORN ALIVE AT THE PLACE AND TIME AND ON THE DATE STATED.
SIGNATURE: ▶
11. DATE SIGNED *(Month, Day, Year)*
12. CERTIFIER'S NAME AND TITLE *(Type/Print)*
NAME ____________
☐ M.D. ☐ D.O. ☐ HOSPITAL ADMIN. ☐ C.N.M. ☐ OTHER MIDWIFE
☐ OTHER *(Specify)*

ATTENDANT

13. ATTENDANT'S NAME AND TITLE *(If other than certifier) (Type/Print)*
Name ____________
☐ M.D. ☐ D.O. ☐ C.N.M. ☐ OTHER MIDWIFE ☐ OTHER
☐ Specify if other:
14. ATTENDANT'S MAILING ADDRESS *(Street and Number or Rural Route Number, City or Town, State, Zip Code)*

CENSUS TRACT

15. REGISTRAR'S SIGNATURE ▶
16. DATE REGISTERED BY REGISTRAR *(Month, Day, Year)*

MOTHER

17a. MOTHER'S NAME *(First, Middle, Last)*
17b. MAIDEN SURNAME
18. DATE OF BIRTH *(Month, Day, Year)*
19. BIRTHPLACE *(State or Foreign Country)*
20a. RESIDENCE — STATE
20b. COUNTY

STATE FILE NO. FOR DEATH UNDER 6 YEARS OF AGE

20c. CITY, TOWN, OR LOCATION
20d. STREET AND NUMBER
20e. APT. NO.
20f. INSIDE CITY LIMITS? *(Yes or No)*
20g. MOTHER'S MAILING ADDRESS *(If same as residence, enter Zip Code only)*

FATHER

21. FATHER'S NAME *(First, Middle, Last)*
22. DATE OF BIRTH *(Month, Day, Year)*
23. BIRTHPLACE *(State or Foreign Country)*

SIGN:

24. PARENT(S) REQUEST THAT A SOCIAL SECURITY NUMBER BE ISSUED FOR THIS CHILD ☐ YES ☐ NO
25. PARENT(S) AUTHORIZE RELEASE OF CHILD'S SOCIAL SECURITY NUMBER TO THE OFFICE OF VITAL STATISTICS ☐ YES ☐ NO

INFORMANT

26a. I CERTIFY THAT THE PERSONAL INFORMATION PROVIDED ON THIS CERTIFICATE IS CORRECT TO THE BEST OF MY KNOWLEDGE.
SIGNATURE OF PARENT: ▶

SOCIAL SECURITY NUMBER
26b. MOTHER
26c. FATHER

INFORMATION FOR MEDICAL AND HEALTH USE ONLY

	OF HISPANIC OR HAITIAN ORIGIN? *(Specify No or Yes IF YES, SPECIFY HAITIAN, CUBAN, MEXICAN, PUERTO RICAN, ETC.)*	RACE — AMERICAN INDIAN, BLACK, WHITE, ETC. *(Specify below)*	EDUCATION *(Specify only highest grade completed)* ELEMENTARY/SECONDARY (0 - 12)	COLLEGE (1 - 4 or 5 +)
MOTHER	27a. ☐ NO ☐ YES *(Specify)*	28a.	29a.	
FATHER	27b. ☐ NO ☐ YES *(Specify)*	28b.	29b.	

PREGNANCY HISTORY *(Complete each section)*

31. IS MOTHER MARRIED? ☐ YES ☐ NO
32. DATE LAST NORMAL MENSES BEGAN *(Month, Day, Year)*

PARITY: ____________

LIVE BIRTHS *(Do not include this child)*

30a. NOW LIVING — Number ___ ☐ None
30b. NOW DEAD — Number ___ ☐ None

OTHER TERMINATIONS *(Spontaneous and induced at any time after conception)*

30d. Number ____________ ☐ None

33. MONTH OF PREGNANCY PRENATAL CARE BEGAN — First, Second, Third, etc. *(Specify) (If none, so state)*
34. PRENATAL VISITS — Total Number *(If none, so state)*
35. BIRTH WEIGHT *(Specify unit)*
36. CLINICAL ESTIMATE OF GESTATION *(Weeks)*
37a. PLURALITY — Single, Twin, Triplet, etc. *(Specify)*
37b. IF NOT SINGLE BIRTH — Born First, Second, Third, Etc. *(Specify)*

PHONE: ____________

30c. DATE OF LAST LIVE BIRTH *(Month, Year)*
30e. DATE OF LAST OTHER TERMINATION *(Month, Year)*

OTHER HISTORY FACTORS FOR THIS PREGNANCY *(Complete all items)*

38a. TOBACCO USE DURING PREGNANCY Yes ☐ No ☐ Average number of cigarettes per day ____
38b. ALCOHOL USE DURING PREGNANCY Yes ☐ No ☐ Average number of drinks per week ____
38c. WEIGHT GAINED DURING PREGNANCY ____ lbs.

APGAR SCORE
39a. 1 MINUTE
39b. 5 MINUTES

MEDICAL AND HEALTH INFORMATION

40. MEDICAL HISTORY FACTORS FOR THIS PREGNANCY *(Check all that apply)*

01 ☐ Anemia (Hct. <30/Hgb. <10)
02 ☐ Cardiac disease
03 ☐ Acute or chronic lung disease
04 ☐ Diabetes
05 ☐ Genital herpes
06 ☐ Hydramnios/Oligohydramnios
07 ☐ Hemoglobinopathy
08 ☐ Hypertension, chronic
09 ☐ Hypertension, pregnancy-associated
10 ☐ Eclampsia
11 ☐ Incompetent cervix
12 ☐ Previous infant 4000 + grams
13 ☐ Previous preterm or small-for-gestational-age infant
14 ☐ Renal disease
15 ☐ Rh sensitization
16 ☐ Uterine bleeding
00 ☐ None
17 ☐ Other - Specify ____________

41. COMPLICATIONS OF LABOR AND/OR DELIVERY *(Check all that apply)*

01 ☐ Febrile (>100°F. or 38°C.)
02 ☐ Meconium, moderate/heavy
03 ☐ Premature rupture of membrane (> 12 hours)
04 ☐ Abruptio placenta
05 ☐ Placenta previa
06 ☐ Other excessive bleeding
07 ☐ Seizures during labor
08 ☐ Precipitous labor (<3 hours)
09 ☐ Prolonged labor (>20 hours)
10 ☐ Dysfunctional labor
11 ☐ Breech/Malpresentation
12 ☐ Cephalopelvic disproportion
13 ☐ Cord prolapse
14 ☐ Anesthetic complications
15 ☐ Fetal distress
00 ☐ None
16 ☐ Other - Specify ____________

42. METHOD OF DELIVERY *(Check all that apply)*

01 ☐ Vaginal
02 ☐ Vaginal birth after previous C-Section
03 ☐ Primary C-Section
04 ☐ Repeat C-Section
05 ☐ Forceps
06 ☐ Vacuum

43. OBSTETRIC PROCEDURES *(Check all that apply)*

01 ☐ Amniocentesis
02 ☐ Electronic fetal monitoring
03 ☐ Induction of labor
04 ☐ Stimulation of labor
05 ☐ Tocolysis
06 ☐ Ultrasound
00 ☐ None
07 ☐ Other - Specify ____________

44. ABNORMAL CONDITIONS OF THE NEWBORN *(Check all that apply)*

01 ☐ Anemia (Hct. <39/Hgb. <13)
02 ☐ Birth injury
03 ☐ Fetal alcohol syndrome
04 ☐ Hyaline membrane disease/RDS
05 ☐ Meconium aspiration syndrome
06 ☐ Assisted ventilation <30 min.
07 ☐ Assisted ventilation ≥ 30 min.
08 ☐ Seizures
00 ☐ None
09 ☐ Other - Specify ____________

45. CONGENITAL ANOMALIES OF CHILD *(Check all that apply)*

01 ☐ Anencephalus
02 ☐ Spina bifida/Meningocele
03 ☐ Hydrocephalus
04 ☐ Microcephalus
05 ☐ Other central nervous system anomalies
06 ☐ Heart malformations
07 ☐ Other circulatory/respiratory anomalies
08 ☐ Rectal atresia/stenosis
09 ☐ Tracheo-esophageal fistula/esophageal atresia
10 ☐ Omphalocele/Gastroschisis
11 ☐ Other gastrointestinal anomalies
12 ☐ Malformed genitalia
13 ☐ Renal agenesis
14 ☐ Other urogenital anomalies
15 ☐ Cleft lip/palate
16 ☐ Polydactyly/Syndactyly/Adactyly
17 ☐ Club foot
18 ☐ Diaphragmatic hernia
19 ☐ Other musculoskeletal/integumental anomalies
20 ☐ Down's Syndrome
21 ☐ Other chromosomal anomalies
00 ☐ None
22 ☐ Other - *Specify* ____________

HRS Form 511
Jan 89 (obsoletes previous editions)

Shiono, Patricia H. et al. (1986). "Birth Weight among Women of Different Ethnic Groups." *JAMA 255* (1): 48-52.

World Health Organization. (1975). *International Classification of Diseases.* 9th revision. Geneva: World Health Organization.

BIRTH CONTROL. *See instead* CONTRACEPTION: DEFINING TERMS

THE BIRTH PROJECT

The Birth Project, organized by American artist-writer Judy Chicago, is a multimedia needlework portrayal of the experience of childbirth. Chicago was inspired by the knowledge and techniques learned during the production of her monumental triangle-shaped tribute to famous women in history, "The Dinner Party." Funding for the project came from a grant from the California Arts Council, as well as through donations and gifts from friends and supporters of the project.

The Birth Project Collection is owned by Through the Flower, a nonprofit corporation, which had a small paid staff to administer the project during the five years (1980-85) it took to complete it. The early plan of the project was to include over 150 pieces; however, many were never completed. Today Through the Flower is totally committed to and responsible for the 80 works that were produced. Continued care and protective maintenance have been ensured to allow for the continuation of this traveling exhibit with its wide and varied distribution of stunning art works and historical documentation.

As a series of individual works intended to symbolize and represent the designs of Chicago, The Birth Project was created by many highly skilled needlework volunteers, each devoting hundreds of hours to producing the faultlessly majestic works that make up this textile art collection. Projects were designed using the traditional forms of needlework updated and expanded to fit each individual scene. Crafters worked in crochet, knit, quilting, embroidery, filet crochet, needlepoint, lace with smocking and/or weaving, and other techniques. Throughout history women have worked with the arts, in medieval workshops, all-female Renaissance guilds, and 19th-century quilting bees. The Birth Project has used this historical link with the past to bring out and celebrate the most central and uniting aspect of women's lives—birth.

Frequently graphic, the images of childbirth, with all the blood and soul-wrenching pain, are not easily accepted by a society used to seeing only images of sweetly dressed infants and modestly covered maternal figures. It is the process of giving birth that the artist values and celebrates with stark, powerful portraits of mother with child first together, their separation, and then mother with her child.

Among the works is "Birth Trinity," which took two years to produce and portrays a mother giving birth, with the child leaving the womb with support from the father or midwife. The quilted and embroidered piece "The Crowning," completed by Gwen Glesmann, offers a beautiful image of the beginning moments of pushing the baby forth.

Another theme of the project presents the clothes that women have worn during different times and stages of pregnancy and at the time of birth. Women's bodies until recently (and still in some cultures) were carefully hidden when swollen by pregnancy, camouflaged with corsets or loose clothing, depending upon family class. Considerable research went into uncovering information concerning wearing apparel for the mother-to-be, since history gives it little mention. One design that blends quilting and humor with other media shows society's influence on the clothes and behavior of women, sometimes shaming them for their bodies, which were viewed as too "gross" for public viewing.

The Birth Project intention is to suggest to men and women the need to celebrate life-giving, so they will begin to honor the process of pregnancy and birth. ✱ MARGARET REGAN, M.S.

See also: The Birth Symbol

See **Guide to Related Topics:** Literature and the Arts

Resources

Chicago, Judy. (1985). *The Birth Project.* Garden City, NY: Doubleday.

THE BIRTH SYMBOL

The birth symbol is an ancient textile pattern, still used across Europe and Asia, throughout Indonesia, and in the Phillipines. It originally represented The Great Goddess. The pattern, in its simplest form, consists of a diamond with pairs of lines projecting like arms and legs from its top and bottom vertices. Often the diamond, representing the female torso, encloses a cross-shaped figure; sometimes additional pairs of curved or hooked lines project from the edges or side vertices of the diamond, elaborating the pattern.

The earliest religious practices involved the veneration of the female principle; in the beginning, God was a woman. Traditionally, the art of women—almost universally rendered in textiles—has been concerned with the preservation and communication of spiritual and cultural values. Eccentric, individualistic expression has taken second place in traditional societies to conservative representation, to giving physical form to shared ideas of continuity, nurturance, and regeneration. Art history has ignored the special aesthetic productions of women, labeling them "crafts." Similarly, psychoanalytic studies of art have missed women's work almost entirely. Phallic symbolism has been widely analyzed, but women's conceptions of the reproductive force have remained mostly invisible to scholars. In spite of the fact that the birth symbol is still the most frequently occurring iconic motif in Eurasia and Indonesia, it was not systematically described before 1981 (Allen, 1981).

The geographical spread of the symbol follows the track of known migrations and cultural diffusions. The 8000-year-old Anatolian town of Catal Huyuk yields evidence of the birth symbol. Its very early west-to-east spread, from areas north and west of the Danube eastward to Southeast Asia, was followed more than 2,000 years ago by diffusion throughout Southeast Asia and Indonesia. At about this same time, the birth symbol also appears on Jomon ceramics in Japan.

The birth symbol was and is widely distributed, but this distribution is neither random nor unbounded. Arguments that ancient geometric patterns were initially nonrepresentational and technically determined can be shown not to apply to the birth symbol. The pattern appears only where it might be expected to be from historically documented cultural movements (for example, it does not appear in Chinese or African or Indian textiles); and it is found rendered in at least 17 structurally distinct techniques. As a rule, its iconography is encoded in predictable ways; yet in its easternmost incarnation, in the Phillipines, no attempt whatsoever is made to disguise its meaning: mother with child. The birth symbol is graphically too complicated to be adventitious and too old to be nonrepresentational. What it represents is humanity's earliest conception of the cosmos as the Mother of Us All.

It is difficult *not* to notice the birth symbol in weaving and embroidery because it is central to the design vocabularies of so many textile traditions. So the oriental rug literature often refers to

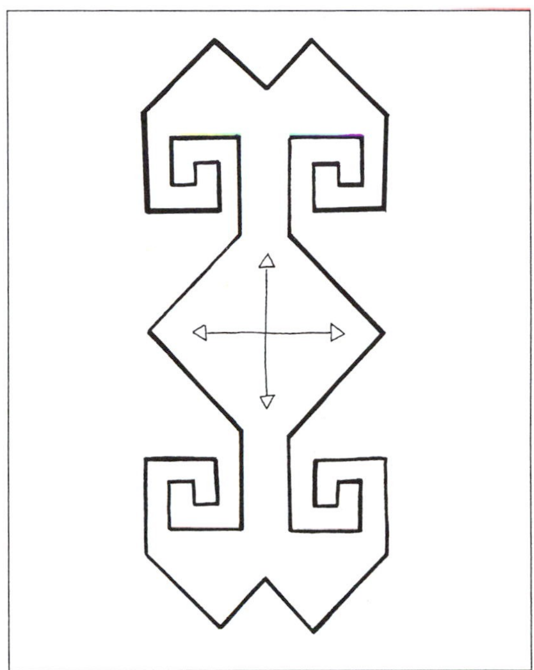

Birth Symbol. Illustration courtesy of Linda G. Katz.

it in various ways, and weavers today in Indonesia, for example, realize it is an important motif and have many names for it. But because the motif has been in use for more than 400 generations, it does not look exactly alike every time it appears. The problem is to find the basic configuration and fundamental significance behind all of this variety.

Over its immensely long history, the birth symbol has accumulated a variety of names; it has been disguised and dressed up; it has encountered a myriad of foreign traditions and been accommodated to them; it has at different times and in different places moved from abstract to realistic to nonrepresentational—looking sometimes like a crab and sometimes like a flower; it has been passed from the hands of grandmothers to granddaughters since the time of the invention of agriculture and at least a third of the way around the world. At its center lies a diamond, a rhomb, according to the Cirlot the universally recognized symbol of female sexuality. ✱ MAX ALLEN

See also: Art and Birth Metaphors: Nature-Culture Dichotomies; The Birth Project; Goddess Imagery

See **Guide to Related Topics:** Literature and the Arts

Resources

Allen, Max. (1981) *The Birth Symbol in Traditional Women's Art from Eurasia and the Western Pacific*. Toronto: The Museum for Textiles.

BIRTHMOTHERS

Women who conceive and give birth to one or more children and subsequently surrender them for adoption placement are birthmothers. Sometimes referred to by the less preferred terms "biological," "natural," or "real" mothers, birthmothers may seek adoption placement for their children voluntarily or may acquire their birthmother status by court order terminating parental rights as a result of a finding of chronic abuse or neglect. Birthmothers may be of any age, race, or socioeconomic status, and may be married or single. However, since (voluntary) adoption is largely a white, middle-class phenomenon, very poor, very wealthy, and minority birthmothers are less prevalent. This is due to: (1) greater familiarity with alternative means of support among the poor; (2) greater access to abortion historically available to the more affluent; and (3) the common practice within the black culture of "shared parenting," or informal, family "adoption." Use of the term "birthmother" is unrelated to the circumstances of impregnation. Thus, women presently referred to as "surrogate mothers," who conceive and bear a child and surrender the child for adoption by the child's (biological) father and his wife (or by others) according to a prearranged plan are birthmothers as well.

The term does not apply to noncustodial mothers, i.e., mothers who retain their parental rights while children reside with their father or other substitute parents. Neither does the term apply to mothers who give birth to and raise their children. It is surrender that confers birthparent status.

Because accurate figures regarding the number of adoptions completed nationwide have not been maintained, it is difficult to speak with precision about the number of birthmothers in the United States. However, it is estimated that there are approximately eight million birthmothers in this country—approximately two percent of the total population.

Although it is sometimes assumed that birthmothers place their children for adoption out of a lack of caring, and then forget about them, neither is generally the case. Birthmothers usually place their children for adoption because their personal circumstances (age, earning power, support systems) will not allow them to meet a standard of parenting they feel is acceptable for their children. Research and anecdotal reports (Baran, Pannor, and Sorosky, 1978; Burnell and Norfleet, 1979; Deykin, Campbell, and Patti, 1984; Silverman, 1981) have indicated that many (if not most) birthmothers suffer negative consequences from the adoption loss, including prolonged mourning for the lost child and negative effects on self-esteem, future relationships with men, and parenting of later children. For some birthmothers, these consequences are lifelong.

Historically, birthmothers placed their children for adoption and then became "strangers" to them. They were allowed no role in the child's life, and often kept the pregnancy, birth, and adoption a secret from everyone. They almost never learned anything of the fate of the surrendered child.

Over the last 15 years, however, it has become fairly common for birthparents or adult adoptees, with the assistance of mutual-help groups, to seek out their counterparts in adoption. If an ongoing relationship develops after reunion, the birthmother commonly plays a role similar to an aunt or close family friend, while the relationship between adoptee and adoptive parents continues as usual. Of course, individual cases may vary, depending on the needs and wants of the people involved.

In recent years, alternative forms of adoption have developed, most notably fully open adoption, wherein birth and adoptive parents are known to one another prior to the child's placement and maintain an ongoing relationship during the child's early years. In this type of adoption, the birthmother's role, similar to a close family friend or an aunt, begins immediately at placement, rather than after years of separation followed by reunion. The child knows the birthmother as his or her birthmother and his or her adoptive parents as "Mom" and "Dad."

Although biological fathers (unless married to the birthmother) were not allowed to take part in adoption planning or accorded any legal rights toward their children until recent years (following *Stanley v. Illinois*), every adopted child certainly has a biological father. Because some women choose not to tell the father of the child of their pregnancy, some men are unaware of their status. Others, however, have come forward in recent years to speak about consequences similar to those experienced by birthmothers (Deykin, Patti, and Ryan, 1988). ✱ GAIL HANSSEN, M.A.

See also: Adoption, Closed; Adoption, Open; Maternity Homes; Problem Pregnancy Counseling

See **Guide to Related Topics:** Adoption

Resources

Baran, Annette, Pannor, Reuben, & Sorosky, Arthur. (1978). *The Adoption Triangle*. New York: Doubleday.

Burnell, G. & Norfleet, M. (1979). "Women Who Place Their Infants for Adoption: A Pilot Study." *Patient Counsel and Health Education* 1: 169-72.

Campbell, Lee (Ed.). (1977). *Understanding the Birthparent*. Milford, MA: Concerned United Birthparents, Inc.

Deykin, Eva, Campbell, Lee, & Patti, Patricia. (1984, Apr). "The Post Adoption Experience of Surrendering Parents." *American Journal of Orthopsychiatry: 54* (2): 271-80.

Deykin, Eva, Patti, Patricia, & Ryan, Jon. (1988, Apr). "Fathers of Adopted Children: A Study of the Impact of Child Surrender on Birthfathers." *American Journal of Orthopsychiatry: 58* (2): 240-48.

Dusky, Lorraine. (1979). *Birthmark*. New York: M. Evans & Company.

Musser, Sandra Kay. (1979). *I Would Have Searched Forever*. Bala Cynwyd, PA: Jan Enterprises.

Rynearson, Edward K. (1982). "Relinquishment and Its Maternal Complications: A Preliminary Study." *American Journal of Psychiatry: 139*: 338-40.

Silverman, Phyllis. (1981). *Helping Women Cope with Grief*. Beverly Hills, CA: Sage Publications.

Stanley v. Illinois, 405 U.S. 645 (1972).

BODYWORK

Moving or having a person move in a particular manner can help that person learn how to move more comfortably, efficiently, consciously, healthfully, and/or prevent injury. Bodywork, movement therapy, sensory motor education, somatic movement education, and therapy are terms for the various approaches to educating the body. Practitioners use touch, imagery, movement, and technical information. Specific touch techniques can help a person establish a new sensory engram, that is, a new way of sensing, feeling, moving, and behaving. Heightened body awareness and control may be enhanced by understanding physical functioning in emotionally laden images and/or accurate technical information. Movement is both an expression of the inner person and an important input of sensory information into that person. A change in movement can reflect a change in the inner person and a change in movement can in fact change the sensory environment in that inner person.

Bodywork, during pregnancy and postpartum, can be used: (1) to help women become more aware of and more comfortable with the profound physical and emotional changes that occur and (2) to alleviate the discomforts of pregnancy and postpartum that are related to movement patterning, stress, habit, belief system, and inaccurate physical information, e.g., muscle ache or muscle spasm in the upper or lower back, coccyx, shoulders, and calf may be exacerbated by postural and weight changes and may be aided by specific touch/movement work and stress reduction. Brachial plexus and carpal tunnel syndrome, particularly postpartum, may be due to habitual faulty movement patterns associated with the stress of picking up and carrying the baby (as well as edema) and may be alleviated by changing those movement patterns. There is tremendous shifting of the organs during pregnancy and a relaxation of the supporting ligaments. Postpartum, there are bodywork techniques that can aid in rebalancing those organs. Pelvic floor dysfunction is another area that is often amenable to bodywork techniques.

Bodyworkers/movement therapists are generally trained and certified by a particular school. One organization, the International Movement Therapy Association, registers several schools. Certification requirements vary. One excellent, very specific technique requires a minimum of 100 hours of classroom training, 50 hours of hands-on clinical training, and practical and written evaluations. Another organization encompassing a very broad approach requires a minimum of 700 hours of classroom work over four semesters, plus written case studies; a final project; additional college or graduate-level courses in anatomy, physiology, and kinesiology; and 500 hours of personal practices, including counseling; movement; bodywork; music, voice, or art; nutrition; and mind/spiritual practices for their minimum certification of practitioner. To prevent teacher stasis requires the fulfillment of many additional requirements. ✱ SANDRA JAMROG, C.C.E., R.M.T.

See also: Chiropractic Care; Common Complaints of Pregnancy; Exercise Physiology in Pregnancy; Pelvic Muscles

See **Guide to Related Topics:** Pregnancy, Physical Aspects

Resources

Bartenieff, Irmgard & Lewis, Doris. (1980). *Body Movement: Coping with the Environment*. New York: Gordon and Breach.

Bertherat, Therese & Bernstein, Carol. (1989). *The Body Has Its Reasons*. Rochester, VT: Healing Arts Press.

Cohen, Bonnie Bainbridge. (1987). "The Action in Perceiving." *Contact Quarterly 12* (3): 22-24.

———. (1989). "The Alphabet of Movement, Part 1." *Contact Quarterly 14* (2): 23-38.

———. (1989). "The Alphabet of Movement, Part 2." *Contact Quarterly 14* (3): 23-38.

Ed Feitis, Rosemary. (1978). *Ida Rolf Talks about Rolfing and Physical Reality*. New York: The Rolf Institute.

Feldenkrais, M. (1972). *Awareness through Movement*. New York: Harper & Row.

Haberly, Helen J. (1990). *Reiki Hawayo Takata's Story*. Salem, OR: Blue Mountain Publications.

Iyengar, B.K.S. (1987). *Light on Yoga*. New York: Schocken.

Iyengar, Getta S. (1983). *Yoga: A Gem for Women*. New Delhi: Allied Publishers, Put.

Jones, Frank Pierce. (1978). *Body Awareness in Action: A Study of the Alexander Technique*. New York: Schocken Books.

Menta, S., Menta, M., & Menta, S. (1990). *Yoga: The Iyengar Way*. New York: Alfred Knopf.

Montague, Ashley. (1971). *Touching*. New York: Harper & Row.

Norman, Laura. (1988). *Feet First: A Guide to Foot Reflexology*. New York: Simon & Schuster.

Ohasi, Wataru & Hoover, Mary. (1983). *Natural Childbirth the Eastern Way: A Healthy Pregnancy and Delivery through Shiatsu*. New York: Ballantine Books.

———. (1985). *Touch for Love: Shiatsu for Your Baby*. New York: Ballantine Books.

Rubenfeld, Ilana. (1991). "Ushering in a Century of Integration." *Somatics* 7 (1): 59-63.

Saltonstall, Ellen. (1988). *Kinetic Awareness: Discovering Your Bodymind*. New York: Kinetic Awareness Center.

Sweigard, L. (1974). *Human Movement Potential*. New York: Harper & Row.

Todd, M.E. (1968). *The Thinking Body*. New York: Dance Horizons.

BONDING

In the mid 1970s, in a series of highly influential journal articles and then in a book called *Maternal-Infant Bonding*, Marshall Klaus and John Kennell, two Cleveland pediatricians, asserted that there is a specific and very short period just after birth when mothers "attach" to their infants. They argued that separating mothers from their babies after delivery interferes with the mother's ability to love her infant, with possibly dire long-term consequences, such as the mother's failure to care properly for her baby and the baby's failure to thrive. While no sensible person any longer believes that there is any excuse for trundling a newborn off to the nursery "for observation" moments after it is born, Klaus and Kennell's theory of bonding has had some dire consequences of its own: The study on which they based their conclusions was seriously flawed. Controls were not properly selected and no account was taken of the effects of class, culture, family structure, or poverty on the behavior of the mothers. Nonetheless, the study's conclusions were widely disseminated, offering as they did a simple answer to a number of social problems. Today, in delivery rooms across the country, women are scored on such factors as whether they gaze at their baby or touch it or make the proper sounds when the baby is first handed to them, on the delivery table, within a minute or so of birth.

This research on bonding fed the persistent myth that mothers fall in love with their babies in the moment when the baby is first placed in their arms. So widespread is the myth, in fact, that many mothers claim that this is exactly what happened to them. But when interviewing women very soon after delivery, before the birth has been romanticized or distorted by selective amnesia, many mothers report that they were really only mildly curious about the baby, and that once they had ascertained that the infant was healthy, they were happy to have him or her looked after, for a while, by someone else.

Why don't most mothers love their babies at first sight? And why do they say that they do? What is the reason for the lack of overwhelming interest in the baby? And why is there such distortion in mothers' reporting of their first response?

Heavy, tired, waiting, and tired of waiting, a woman at the end of her pregnancy is absorbed in herself; whatever claims there may be on her attention, there is a part of her that remains focused on herself and the expected baby. She indulges her nesting instinct as well as she can, e.g., by scrubbing all the floors, painting the baby's room, readying the clothes, and practicing special breathing for labor. The woman about to deliver will also speculate obsessively about the impending event of childbirth. There is little that can shake a woman at this stage from her preoccupation, and the number of things that can distract her dwindles as the days pass. She did not arrive at this state of self-absorption all at once; nor will she emerge from it all at once. The state persists, and even intensifies, during labor and delivery and does not end with the birth of the baby.

In the early stages of labor, a woman is usually quite capable of carrying on a conversation, doing household chores, or reading between contractions. As labor accelerates, her focus narrows. She will not notice noises from the street outside. In the late stages, she will be largely unaware of events in the same room. Birth attendants often find it necessary to shout their instructions to the laboring woman, just to get through to her.

In the last few minutes of labor, unless someone does interfere, a woman's energy and attention become centered deeply on her body and the powerful events taking place within it. Even when a mirror is available so that the woman can watch the birth, a surprising number keep their eyes shut, unwilling to break that intense internal focus. In the very last moment, the self-absorption, the concentration is total.

Often overwhelming the woman, too, at this moment, is the fear of death. Just as the self-absorption of the last stage of delivery is an extension of the growing self-involvement of late pregnancy, the terror that seizes many women during delivery seems to be the culmination of the massive anxiety of late pregnancy. T. Berry Brazelton has reported that interviews with a group of pregnant women "uncovered anxiety which often seemed to be of pathological proportions." He believes these feelings are normal and "become a force for reorganization, for readjustment to her important new role." The themes of death and birth are closely linked in psychology and myth, and it may be that the only possible metaphor for the loss of so large a part of oneself as the baby is death.

A woman's sense of physical self is likewise diminished during labor as she sheds any identity save that of laboring woman. Many women have commented, often with surprise, on their lack of physical modesty during childbirth. It is as if, in the late stages of labor, the centering of attention on the inside of the body is so complete that the outside of the body ceases to matter. Disheveled hair, streaming sweat, water, blood, excreta are of no consequence whatever. Concern for appearance, so much a part of the psyche of most women, does not reappear for some time—hours or even days. The woman's personal boundary has collapsed inward to the womb and reextends itself only gradually. One minute after the baby's birth, or two, or five, the woman's self is not yet large enough to encompass the child. She remains within herself and the infant seems alien.

The act of giving birth, mysterious and most private, is kept so by the woman's capacity for shutting out everything but the essence of the process. The need to be undisturbed (though not alone) may explain at least in part the rage and sense of violation that so many women express concerning standard hospital practices. The lights, the noise, the restraints, the orders, the examinations, the air of crisis that exists in even the most routine of hospital births are brutal intrusion on a woman's need to enwomb herself.

The myth of the maternal instinct implies that a woman will be overcome by feelings of love when she holds her infant in her arms for the first time, but real life belies the myth. Love at first sight, whether for a handsome stranger or a newborn baby, is rare indeed. Many women, recognizing that they are being observed for a "proper" reaction when the baby is first placed in their arms, will make a valiant attempt to smile and look interested. What they are really feeling, however, may be quite different. "I was so busy worrying about whether I was still alive that it was hard to get interested in this kid," confided one mother shortly after the deliver of a much-wanted first child, "except that the kid was alive, too."

✱ ANDREA BOROFF EAGAN

See also: Fathers at Birth; Labor: Overview; Matrescence and Patrescence; Motherhood as Transformation

***See* Guide to Related Topics:** Pregnancy, Psychological Aspects

Resources

Eagan, Andrea Boroff. (1976). *Why Am I So Miserable, If These Are the Best Years of My Life?* New York: Avon.

———. (1985). *Newborn Mother*. New York: Holt.

Klaus, Marshall et al. (1972). "Maternal Attachment: Importance of the First Postpartum Days." *New England Journal of Medicine 286*: 460-63.

Klaus, Marshall & Kennell, John. *Maternal-Infant Bonding*. (1976). St. Louis: C.V. Mosby Co.

BRADLEY METHOD: HUSBAND-COACHED CHILDBIRTH

Dr. Robert A. Bradley (1917-), an American obstetrician and an early and enthusiastic supporter of Grantly Dick-Read's method of natural childbirth, attributes that support to his wife's influence; just as he was finishing his obstetrical training, "and knew just about everything" (Bradley, 1965, p. 9), she was reading Read (1944). Bradley started to use Read's natural childbirth techniques in 1947 and evolved a popular new form of childbirth preparation, called "husband-coached childbirth," from it. When he started practicing natural childbirth, fathers were not included in the process, but an experience in the delivery room in which a new mother reached up and joyfully kissed Bradley jolted him into realizing that the father really should have been there to receive the kiss. Bradley then made the father's support such a key aspect of his method that his book (Bradley, 1965; 3rd ed., 1981) is addressed to fathers, not to mothers.

The strength and popularity of the Bradley Method lie in Bradley's staunch vision of birth as a natural physiological event, albeit one often conducted in a hospital. Using other mammals' birthing as a model, Bradley finds their need for darkness, solitude, quiet, physical comfort, relaxation, controlled breathing, closed eyes, and the appearance of sleep similar to the needs of human mothers. In placing the husband in the role of comforter and supporter, Bradley exhorts him to be a real man and get the woman out of the fix in the same way he got her into it—by touching her lovingly and whispering sweet nothings in her ear. "Play the lover role," he says, "during the glorious climax to your act of love—the birth of your baby" (1965, p. 43). Bradley is no feminist, and is clearly of the opinion that men's and women's roles in life are very different, as illustrated by this piece of advice to new fathers (Bradley, 1965, p. 148):

> Males are good labor coaches but make frustrated, pitiful housewives. You may be entertaining martyr-like thoughts of doing the housework yourself. Don't. Go back to your employment as a breadwinner and let a female take over.

The flip side of this attitude, however, is unmixed, unmitigated awe at the female's power to do naturally what she was put on earth to do—bear children—and humility in the face of this power.

Enthusiastic supporters Marjie and Jay Hathaway, after using the method successfully during the birth of their fourth child, founded the American Academy of Husband-Coached Childbirth (P.O. Box 5224, Sherman Oaks, California 91413) in 1970 to train childbirth educators in the method. Consistent with their view of birth, Bradley instructors are, for the most part, mothers and other health care consumers. Arms (1975, pp. 185-86) believes that the success of the Bradley method lies in the fact that, with the husband running interference with hospital personnel and providing the kind of support necessary to keep the woman calm, she can achieve something like natural childbirth in a U.S. hospital setting. Many Bradley instructors, however, encourage expectant couples to seek birthing environments more hospitable to the Bradley natural childbirth principles. ✱ MARTHA LIVINGSTON, Ph.D.

See also: Labor: Overview; Read Method: Natural Childbirth

See **Guide to Related Topics:** Childbirth Practices and Locations

Resources

Arms, S. (1975). *Immaculate Deception: A New Look at Women and Childbirth.* New York: Bantam Books.

Bradley, R.A. (1965). *Husband-Coached Childbirth.* 1st ed. New York: Harper & Row.

———. (1981). *Husband-Coached Childbirth,* 3rd ed. New York: Harper & Row.

Hathaway, M. et al. (1989). *The Bradley Method Student Workbook.* Sherman Oaks, CA: American Academy of Husband-Coached Childbirth.

McCutcheon-Rosegg, S. & Rosegg, P. (1984). *Natural Childbirth the Bradley Way.* New York: E.P. Dutton.

Read, G.D. (1944). *Childbirth without Fear.* New York and London: Harper and Brothers.

BRAXTON HICKS CONTRACTIONS

The intermittent uterine contractions that regularly occur throughout pregnancy, from the very early stages on through the last trimester, are known as Braxton Hicks contractions. It is now understood that the uterus, as a muscular organ, is in a continuous state of contractive motion throughout the childbearing years—whether or not the woman is pregnant. The phenomenon during pregnancy of alternately contracting and relaxing uterine activity was first described by John Braxton Hicks, a 19th-century English gynecologist, and is now known by his name.

In the first trimester of pregnancy, beginning in the earliest weeks, the uterus contracts in a sporadic, nonrhythmic manner. Although these early contractions are painless and generally go unnoticed, they may be palpable when enhanced by massage. By the second trimester, Braxton Hicks contractions are often detectable by bimanual examination in which the uterus is palpated externally with one hand while the cervix is felt internally with the other. At this point in the pregnancy, the contractions may also become perceptible to the pregnant woman who has previously given birth, as she may be more sensitive to the uterine activity occurring and as the contractions of the enlarging uterus become stronger.

The Braxton Hicks contractions of the third trimester will generally increase in both frequency and intensity; what was previously felt as a rhythmic tightening may, in the last few weeks of pregnancy, be considered more painful or irritating. The recurring episodes of contractions as term nears are possibly quite regular and intense, and are frequently (and understandably) confused with the beginning of labor. While the term "false labor" is commonly used in reference to the periods of Braxton Hicks contractions, a more positive and accurate characterization might be "practice" contractions.

Although the theories on what purpose Braxton Hicks contractions serve in pregnancy are quite numerous and varied, all share a positive and beneficial view. The belief that continuous contractions contribute to the preparation of the uterus for both pregnancy and birth is the basis for most theories. It is quite reasonable to accept that, through regularly contracting and relaxing, the muscles of the uterus are gradually allowed to enlarge and therefore accommodate the growing fetus (Reeder, Mastroianni, and Martin, 1983). Braxton Hicks contractions may also be responsible for increasing the uterine segment and facilitating blood flow to the placental site, as well as developing the lower uterine segment (Myles, 1975). It is commonly held that frequent episodes of Braxton Hicks contractions in the last few weeks of pregnancy serve to prepare or "ripen" the cervix, thus beginning the softening and dilation process; the contractions preparatory to labor are therefore considered normal and beneficial (Kitzinger, 1977). The intermittent squeezing and releasing of the uterus positively affects the baby within, as the lungs are stimulated and prepared for dilation and breathing (Bradley, 1981). That "false labor" or "practice" contractions are often viewed as mere annoyances is quite contrary to the actual role that the contractions play in preparation for birth. Their presence throughout pregnancy and as the birth nears serves to heighten awareness of the dynamic and productive energy of the uterus. ✷ BARBARA URSENBACH LAMB, C.C.E.

***See* Guide to Related Topics:** Pregnancy, Physical Aspects

Resources

Bradley, Robert A. (1981). *Husband-Coached Childbirth.* New York: Harper & Row.

Kitzinger, Sheila. (1977). *Education and Counseling for Childbirth.* New York: Schocken Books.

———. (1984). *The Experience of Childbirth.* New York: Penguin Books.

Myles, Margaret F. (1975). *Textbook for Midwives, 8th edition.* New York: Churchill Livingstone.

Pritchard, Jack A. & MacDonald, Paul C. (1980). *Williams Obstetrics, 16th edition.* New York: Appleton-Century-Crofts.

Reeder, Sharon J., Mastroianni, Luigi, & Martin, Leonide L. (1983). *Maternity Nursing, 15th edition.* Philadelphia: J.B. Lippincott Co.

Thomas Clayton L. (Ed.) (1977). *Taber's Cyclopedic Medical Dictionary, 13th edition.* Philadelphia: F.A. Davis Co.

BREASTFEEDING: HISTORICAL ASPECTS

While breastfeeding is the rule in preliterate cultures, as societies increase in complexity, alternatives to the milk of the baby's own mother become socially accepted—wet nurses, animal milk, various milk substitutes, and in modern society, commercially prepared formulas and infant foods.

In western society over the past several centuries, infant feeding practices have followed a recognizable pattern. Prior to industrialization most women breastfed their infants, although women in leisured classes generally were expected not to. For these elite women, norms proscribing maternal nursing frequently were very strong. In the southern United States, black women servants nursed the children of privileged whites, and in preindustrial Europe wet nurses, often peasants brought in from the countryside, breastfed babies for the aristocracy. With industrialization, breastfeeding rates fell for whole societies, falling first among the middle classes, then later among the poor. However, in advanced industrial societies, rates currently are rising, with the increase predominantly among educated middle- and upper middle-class women; rates remain low in the lower classes (Auerbach, 1975; Berg, 1977).

These general tendencies are modified by cultural factors such as rural-urban residence, ethnicity, education, and so on. Whether or not women work is not as critical as whether the work separates mother from baby, as western industrial labor policies tend to do. Early in the 20th century, for example, a study by the U.S. Department of Labor Children's Bureau showed that breastfeeding decreased among women factory workers in New England who were expected to return to work soon after a baby was born, but remained high among women who worked long hours doing piecework at home.

A marked decline in breastfeeding began late in the 19th century as urbanization and modernization progressed. The decline accompanied the transformation of childbirth management as birthing moved from home to the hospital, and male physicians displaced female midwives as birth attendants. It also accompanied significant changes in lifestyles, kin support systems, and women's social roles, as the extended family gave way to the nuclear unit.

Typically, the decline in breastfeeding occurred before cities established safe water supplies, public sanitation systems, and efficient transportation and refrigeration. Consequently breastmilk substitutes, insufficient nutritionally for the most part, also were open to contamination and spoilage. Dramatic increases in infant mortality and morbidity invariably accompanied decreases in maternal nursing, stimulating widespread concern. Vigorous public health campaigns were mounted in Europe late in the 19th century and in the U.S. early in the 20th century that blamed bottle feeding for high infant death rates and exhorted women to breastfeed their babies. However as the standard of living rose in the expanding middle classes, improved public hygiene and home refrigeration made bottle feeding safer, and knowledge about formula preparation made it more nutritious; consequently, infant mortality and morbidity rates stabilized despite continued bottle feeding, at least for the middle class (U.S. Department of Labor, 1913-1937). By the 1930s and 1940s in the U.S., many pediatricians were advocating bottle feeding because it allowed the baby's food intake to be "scientifically" managed, and obstetricians discouraged breastfeeding on the grounds that it interfered with their patients' rest. At the same time, a gradually developing baby food industry used modern technology to make bottle feeding more convenient and persuasive marketing techniques to make it more appealing. Bottle feeding became the accepted middle-class norm, a norm eventually adopted by the lower class as well. During this time, breastfeeding rates appeared to have fallen in the U.S. and also to have fallen lower than they did in the rest of the western world. Studies in the late 1950s and early 1960s showed about 20 percent of babies breastfed upon discharge from the hospital; only 10-15 percent of these for two months or more. Negative attitudes about breastfeeding during this period were very strong. Even mentioning it caused more shock and embarrassment than talking about sex, and women who breastfed did so in strict privacy, even in their own homes (Brack, 1979).

However as overall rates were declining during the 1950s, breastfeeding rates among middle-class women began to increase, albeit slowly. (They continued to drop among the poor.) Several factors contributed to this change. One was the Birth Reform Movement, which developed during this same period among middle-class women. Birth reform activists were extremely critical of the medical model for childbirth that involved routinely medicating and anesthetizing women during delivery, then separating them from their babies after birth—practices that interfered with breastfeeding (Haire, 1972). A second factor was the La Leche League, a grassroots association begun late in the 1950s by middle-class breastfeeding women. La Leche has grown into an international organization, quietly successful in its mission to inform, support, and encourage breastfeeding women—a function performed by kin and neighbors in earlier times. But probably more important was the gradual resurgence of feminist consciousness and the development of the Women's Health Movement in the early 1970s; they fostered a climate that encouraged women to know and accept their own bodies and body functions, to share their experiences with other women, to be more knowledgeable about childbirth, and to assert more control over decisions that affected their health and the health of their children.

Ironically, during this same period, public policy has led to poorer perinatal care for women in disadvantaged groups. Today these women are least likely to receive childbirth care that promotes breastfeeding, and few of them have the kind of control over their everyday lives that would allow them to continue nursing their babies easily. Health statistics for their babies are distressingly poor, and worsening. These are the babies who would benefit most from breastfeeding and are least likely today to receive it.

✱ DATHA CLAPPER BRACK, Ph.D.

See also: Formula Marketing; Infant Feeding and Care: Nineteenth and Twentieth Centuries, United States; Pediatrics, History of

See **Guide to Related Topics:** Infant Feeding

Resources

Auerbach, Kathleen G. (1975). "The Ecological, Clinical and Sociological Aspects of Worldwide Lactation Failure." In *Fourth International Congress of Psychosomatic Obstetrics and Gynecology, Tel Aviv, 1974.* Tel Aviv: Karger Basel.

Berg, Alan. (1977, Jan-Feb). "The Crisis in Infant Feeding Practices." *Nutrition Today: 18-23.*

Brack, Datha C. (1979). Why Women Breastfeed: The Influence of Cultural Values and Perinatal Care on Choice of Infant Feeding Methods and Success at Breastfeeding. Ann Arbor, MI: University Microfilms International.

Eiger, Marvin S. & Olds, Sally Wendkos. (1987). The Complete Book of Breastfeeding. New York: Bantam Books.

Haire, Doris. (1972). The Cultural Warping of Childbirth. Milwaukee, WI: The International Childbirth Education Association.

Jelliffe, Derick B. & Jelliffe, E.F. Patrice. (1971). "Overview in Symposium on the Uniqueness of Human Milk." *American Journal of Clinical Nutrition* (24): 1012.

Mead, Margaret & Newton, Niles. (1967). "Cultural Patterning of Perinatal Behavior." In Stephen A. Richardson & Alan F. Guttmacker (Eds.) *Childbearing: Its Social and Psychological Aspects.* Baltimore: Williams and Wilkins, pp. 142-244.

Newton, Michael. (1961). "Human Lactation." In S. Kon & A.T. Cowie (Eds.) *Milk: The Mammary Gland and Its Secretion.* Vol. I. New York: New York Academic Press.

Newton Michael & Newton, Niles. (1972). "Lactation: Its Psychological Components." In John G. Howells (Ed.) *Modern Perspectives in Psycho-Obstetrics.* New York: Brunner/Mazel, pp. 385-410.

Population Reports: Breastfeeding—Aid to Infant Health and Fertility Control. (1975). George Washington University Medical Center, Department of Medical and Public Affairs Series J. No. 4, Washington, DC.

U.S. Department of Labor, Children's Bureau. (1913-1937). Bureau Publications No. 2-9 Report on Save the Baby campaigns; Bureau Publications No. 2-243 Infant Mortality Series. (Washington, DC: Government Printing Office).

BREASTFEEDING: PHYSIOLOGICAL AND CULTURAL ASPECTS

Breastfeeding: A woman giving a baby milk from her breast; nursing a baby; suckling.

In all mammal species including humans, the mother's mammary glands produce milk (lactation) when she gives birth to offspring. Suckling and lactation are normal biological functions, but in humans they may be inhibited or altered by the organization of social life and by cultural expectations for women's behavior.

The Physiology of Lactation. During pregnancy three hormones—estrogen, progesterone, and lactogen—stimulate the proliferation of milk glands and milk ducts in the woman's breasts, preparing them for milk secretion after the baby is born. Estrogen and progesterone are produced mainly by the placenta, and lactogen entirely so. Additionally, the pituitary gland increases production of prolactin, a hormone that signals milk sacs (alveoli) in the mammary glands to produce milk. However, before the baby is born, high levels of estrogen inhibit the action of prolactin.

After the placenta is delivered, estrogen and progesterone levels decline rapidly in the mother's body; prolactin begins to take effect, and lactation begins within 24 to 48 hours. At first the breasts secrete colostrum, a high-protein substance containing antibodies and thymic cells that help immunize the baby against infections. By the fourth or fifth day, the breasts secrete milk (Newton, 1961).

A healthy newborn comes equipped with a strong sucking reflex; when its cheek is brushed by the mother's nipple, the baby will turn its mouth to the nipple, grasp it, and suckle. This activates nerve receptors in the mother's breast, signaling her brain to release the milk-producing prolactin. Milk production is maintained by regular and complete emptying of the breasts; the longer the baby stays at the breast and the stronger its suckling, the more plentiful the milk supply. The supply adjusts to the needs of the baby, increasing as the baby takes more milk (mothers of twins may easily nurse both babies), and diminishing as the older child takes solid food and nurses less at the breast. Although a poorly nourished mother may be able to nurse, milk production will deplete her own body. A nursing woman needs an abundance of nutritious food and fluids.

Oxytocin, another hormone released by the brain in response to breast stimulation, governs the flow of milk from the breast. As the baby begins to nurse, oxytocin reaches the breast within 30 seconds or so, causing myoepithelial cells surrounding the milk alveoli to contract and force milk into ducts and sinuses under the areola (the darker-colored skin area surrounding the nipple). This is the milk ejection, or "let down" reflex, experienced by the mother as a tingling physical sensation in her breast. After the reflex is well established, it may be set off by other stimuli such as the baby's crying, the mother's thinking of her baby, or stimulation during bathing or sexual intercourse (Newton and Newton, 1972).

The benefits of breastfeeding for babies are well documented. Immunological properties in human milk protect infants against infections from staphylococcus, polio virus, Coxsackie B. virus, two types of colon bacilli that can cause fatal infant diarrhea, and pathogenic strains of E. Coli—infections to which infants usually are most susceptible. Breastfed babies have lower rates of respiratory and gastrointestinal infections, and have a natural immunity to almost all common childhood diseases for at least six months. Human milk also contains species-specific nutritional elements, among them proteins and minerals that are uniquely suited to human growth and physical development. Breastfed babies have a lower incidence of neonatal tetany, iron deficiency, celiac syndrome, food allergies, skin disorders, and future tooth decay (Jelliffe and Jelliffe, 1975; *Population Reports*, 1975).

Mothers also benefit from breastfeeding. Oxytocin, which triggers milk ejection, also stimulates the uterus to contract, minimizing the danger of uterine hemorrhage if the baby is put to breast directly after delivery, and, as nursing continues, helping the uterus to expel excess tissue and return to pre-pregnant size. These uterine contractions, commonly called "afterpains," may be surprisingly strong in a woman who has had several deliveries. Many women say that nursing makes them feel particularly close to their babies and that it is a relaxing and calming, even a sensuous, experience (Eiger and Olds, 1987).

Social and Cultural Factors Influencing Breastfeeding. Medical authorities agree that very few women have physical conditions preventing successful lactation. Anthropologists report that lactation failure is virtually unknown in simpler societies unless women are severely undernourished; yet failure to produce milk, or to produce enough of it to nourish a baby, is common in modern societies. There is ample evidence that urban industrial lifestyles, contemporary medical childbirth practices, and cultural definitions of women all influence women's ability to breastfeed (Mead and Newton, 1967).

Nursing a baby involves establishing psychobiological response patterns that are maintained by a woman's desire to nurse; confidence in her body's ability to do so; and a relaxed, intimate relationship with her baby. Her desire to nurse may be thwarted by discouragement from her physician, friends, or family members, or by her own discomfort about her body and the act of nursing. In our society, cultural definitions of women's breasts as sex objects contribute to these negative feelings. A woman's confidence may be undermined by hospital routines and policies that interfere with her first attempts at breastfeeding and by lack of knowledgeable support from hospital personnel. Stress or physical exhaustion disrupts the peaceful emotional state most conducive to milk production and milk ejection. Even successfully nursing mothers "lose" their milk, or give less of it, under adverse circumstances; an inexperienced mother may fail despite a strong desire to succeed (Brack, 1979).

Furthermore, modern life is certainly not arranged with mothers and babies in mind. The breastfeeding relationship flourishes best when the mother has close and continuous contact with her baby and develops an easy rhythm between her body and the baby's needs for food and comfort. But in contemporary society babies are not easily tolerated in public places or in social gatherings, and provision for them in the workplace is rare. Neither clock schedules nor clothing styles are designed to accommodate a nursing baby. Out of necessity, many of today's mothers lead lives that do not mesh with breastfeeding.

✱ DATHA CLAPPER BRACK, Ph.D.

See also: Doula; Infant Feeding and Care: Nineteenth and Twentieth Centuries, United States; Nipples, Human

See **Guide to Related Topics:** Infant Feeding

Resources

Auerbach, Kathleen G. (1975). "The Ecological, Clinical and Sociological Aspects of Worldwide Lactation Failure." In *Fourth International Congress of Psychosomatic Obstetrics and Gynecology, Tel Aviv, 1974.* Tel Aviv: Karger Basel, pp. 415-18.

Berge, Alan. (1977, Jan-Feb). "The Crisis in Infant Feeding Practices." *Nutrition Today*: 18-23.

Brack, Datha C. (1979). *Why Women Breastfeed: The Influence of Cultural Values and Perinatal Care on Choice of Infant Feeding Methods and Success at Breastfeeding.* Ann Arbor, MI: University Microfilms International.

Eiger, Marvin S. & Olds, Sally Wendkos. (1987). *The Complete Book of Breastfeeding.* New York: Bantam Books.

Haire, Doris. (1972). *The Cultural Warping of Childbirth.* Milwaukee, WI: The International Childbirth Education Association.

Jelliffe, Derick B. & Jelliffe, E.F. Patrice. (1975, Aug). "Overview in Symposium on the Uniqueness of Human Milk." *American Journal of Clinical Nutrition* (24): 1012.

Mead, Margaret & Newton, Niles. (1967). "Cultural Patterning of Perinatal Behavior." In Stephen A. Richardson & Alan F. Guttmacker (Eds.) *Childbearing: Its Social and Psychological Aspects.* Baltimore: Williams and Wilkins, pp. 142-244.

Newton, Michael. (1961). "Human Lactation." In S. Kon & A.T. Cowie (Eds.) *Milk: The Mammary Gland and Its Secretion.* Vol. I. New York: New York Academic Press, pp. 281-321.

Newton, Michael & Newton, Niles. (1972). "Lactation: Its Psychological Components." In John G. Howells (Ed.) *Modern Perspectives in Psycho-obstetrics.* New York: Brunner/Mazel, pp. 385-410.

Population Reports: Breastfeeding—Aid to Infant Health and Fertility Control. (1975). George Washington University Medical Center, Department of Medical and Public Affairs Series J. No. 4, Washington, DC.

U.S. Department of Labor, Children's Bureau. (1913-1937). Bureau Publications No. 2-9 Report on Save the Baby campaigns; Bureau Publications No. 2-243 Infant Mortality Series. (Washington, DC: Government Printing Office).

BREASTFEEDING BEYOND INFANCY

Until recently, women in traditional societies nursed long after the birth of a baby, sometimes into the third year of life or longer. For health reasons, extended nursing still is considered preferable to bottle-feeding in the Third World. The World Health Organization recommends nursing for at least the first two years of life. In North America, with the exception of La Leche League International, extended nursing is seldom discussed (Bumgarner, 1982; La Leche League International, 1987).

To North American women, extended nursing may be seen to conflict with joining or rejoining the workforce postpartum, but women all over the world, and throughout history have nursed their young children while doing productive work. Emphasis upon shared parenting encourages minimizing differences between father and mother, for like birth, breastfeeding is something only women can do (Chodorow, 1980). But institutions like medicine and the infant formula market have tried not only to take away a woman's ability to give birth by her own powers (through hospital births) but also take away her ability to feed her child from her own body (through availability of infant formula). The Nestlé formula campaign is such an example (Van Esterik, 1989). Political protests against the Nestlé company have

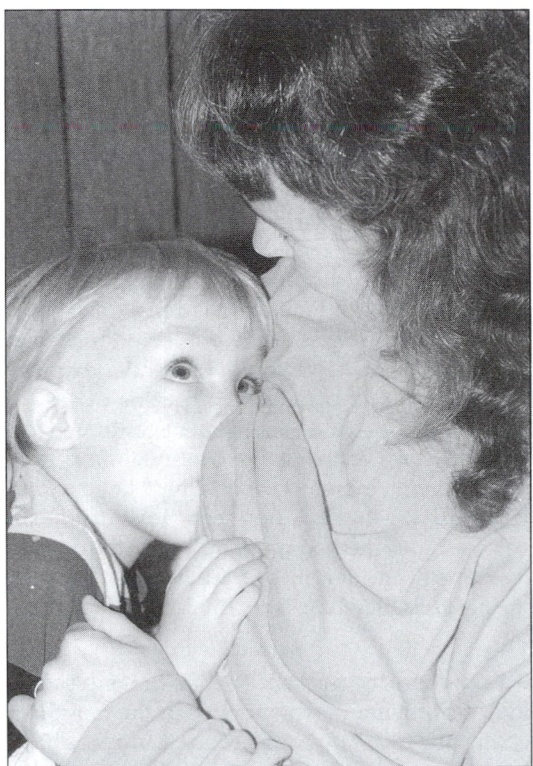

Three-year-old nursing child. Photo courtesy of Jason and Shirley Warren.

taken the form of critiques of capitalism and concern over the health of the babies (admittedly of great importance) rather than emphasis on protecting women's ability to breastfeed in developing countries. Some might even say that women's right to nurse in the North American context is even less considered. [Editor note: See Formula Marketing]

In extended nursing, advantages to the baby include good oral-facial development (the baby uses facial muscles more vigorously than in bottle-feeding); prevention against thumb-sucking, which distorts the dental arch, requiring correctional orthodontia (for those who can afford it); and a nonallergenic source of nutrition. For the mother, extended nursing may protect against breast cancer and provides a limited form of birth control (La Leche League International, 1987).

Extended nursing can make parenthood easier. For example, the "terrible two's" may be an artifact of early weaning; many mothers find the emotional reversals of children during this period much less acute when they continue to be nursed. Nursing comforts the child, and the mother as well. The hormone prolactin, circulating in the mother's body during lactation, has a soothing effect; and the hormone, oxytocin, which "lets down" the milk (the same hormone that triggers orgasm) provides pleasure to the mother during each nursing interlude. Some believe that these relaxing hormones, prolactin and oxytocin, can help mothers ward off "chronic stress" and depression, two hazards of mothering commonplace in North American culture (Newton, 1971).

Extended nursing calls into question ideas taken for granted in child development theory. Some theorists imagine the baby's realization that the mother is not always present to be a sense of separation as severe as the expulsion from Eden. Further, it is believed that a lifelong yearning for the "good mother," who provides sustenance, and resentment of the "bad mother," who withholds the breast, ensues, with unhappy consequences for attitudes toward women in adult years (Durham, 1985). Perhaps it is early weaning, rather than the mother's intermittent absences, that produces separation trauma. With extended nursing, separations always end with a return to the "Eden" of the mother's body. With extended nursing, mother and child can *negotiate* the separation of weaning through language. Perhaps, then, the all-powerful good and bad mother, if such a model exists, would be softened into a person of human proportions, or more human proportions. The mother, too, might feel easier about intermittent separations when nursing restores the connection, and easier about the separation of weaning if it is mediated through language exchange.

Another aspect of child development theory, the "transition object," also may be an artifact of weaning patterns. Children who nurse longer seem less drawn to breast substitutes such as the teddy bear, blanket, or thumb (Winnicott, 1987). Breast substitutes can be viewed as reinforcing the capitalist value of consumerism, as children learn that an object must satisfy desire for the thing itself. With thumb-sucking, youngsters learn that comfort must be found apart from a human connection.

Extended nursing offers a model of human development based upon affiliation rather than separation, grounded in the body. It challenges Western culture's discomfort with the body as well as the idea that maturity equals autonomy and separation (Miller, 1977; Gilligan, 1983). Extended nursing follows the universal species-specific trait youngsters display: a desire for embodied connection (Cook, 1978). From her child's ever widening circle of departure from, but also *return to*, her body, a nursing mother is exposed to a model of human growth that may cause her to rethink central Western values.

Extended nursing could become part of the childbearing continuum even for women who wish to, or must, work. Suggestions for social reforms include granting all females adequate housing and nutrition; working for what could be called "mixed zoning" of public and private spheres where work places accommodate children; organizing family and work life in fresh ways without erasing differences between fathers and mothers; helping women become comfortable using their breasts (associated with sexuality and male approval) for nurturing children; and helping men release control over their wives' bodies.

✱ ROBBIE PFEUFER KAHN, Ph.D.

See also: Weaning

See **Guide to Related Topics:** Infant Feeding

Resources

Bumgarner, Norma Jane. (1982). *Mothering Your Nursing Toddler.* Franklin Park, IL: La Leche League International.

Chodorow, Nancy Julia. (1980). *The Reproduction of Mothering: Psychoanalysis and the Sociology of Gender.* Berkeley, CA: University of California Press.

Cook, Peter S. (1978, Aug 12). "Childrearing, Culture and Mental Health: Exploring an Ethological-Evolutionary Perspective in Child Psychiatry and Preventive Mental Health with Particular Reference to Two Contrasting Approaches to Early Childrearing." *The Medical Journal of Australia.* Special supplement.

Durham, Margery. (1985). "The Mother Tongue: *Christabel* and the Language of Love." In Shirley Nelson Garner, Claire Kahane, & Madelon Sprengnether (Eds.) *The (M)other Tongue: Essays in Feminist Psychoanalytic Interpretation.* Ithaca, NY; London: Cornell University Press.

Gilligan, Carol. (1983). *In a Different Voice: Psychological Theory and Women's Development.* Cambridge, MA: Harvard University Press.

Kahn, Robbie Pfeufer. (1989). "Mother's Milk: The 'Moment of Nurture' Revisited." *Resources for Feminist Research 18* (3): 29-36.

La Leche League International. (1987). *The Womanly Art of Breastfeeding.* 4th revised edition. New York: New American Library.

Miller, Jean Baker. (1977). *Toward a New Psychology of Women* Boston: Beacon Press.

Newton, Niles. (1971). "Psychologic Differences Between Breast and Bottle Feeding." *American Journal of Clinical Nutrition 24*: 993-1004.

Van Esterik, Penny. (1989). *Beyond the Breast-Bottle Controversy.* New Brunswick, NJ: Rutgers University Press.

Winnicott, Donald W. (1987). *The Child, The Family and the Outside World.* Reading, MA: Addison-Wesley.

BREASTFEEDING PATTERNS

Generally, infant feeding is described as one of three broad patterns: total breastfeeding (where the infant is not given supplementary or complementary feedings); mixed feeding (where the infant is given formula and/or solid foods to supplement, complement, or replace breastfeeding); and bottle feeding (when the infant is not breastfed, but is fed formula and other foods from an infant feeding bottle).

The advantages of combining breast and bottle feeding for the mother are obvious. The infant is less dependent on the mother, who may be absent from the infant at least for one feeding per day. The infant may gradually learn to make the transition from the breast to the bottle and/or table foods, which makes weaning a gentle learning experience rather than a difficult time of severance. Further, breastfeeding may be continued for social reasons, enabling the continuation of the mother-infant "nursing relationship" beyond the time that breastmilk is necessary for nutritional reasons. Three methods or patterns of mixed feeding have been identified: partial breastfeeding, flexible breastfeeding, and minimal breastfeeding.

Partial Breastfeeding. Partial breastfeeding involves nursing the infant once in the morning, feeding the infant by bottle or cup during the day, and then nursing the infant as often as he or she wishes during the night. This pattern is continued even when the mother is available to nurse during the day, for example, when a working mother is at home on weekends. During the day, when the mother is not feeding her infant, she does not express her breasts; rather, the breasts "adjust" to the pattern of breastfeeding.

Flexible Breastfeeding. Flexible breastfeeding involves totally breastfeeding the infant for a few days, for example during a weekend, and then reverting to partial breastfeeding during the week when the mother is at work. Mothers who use this pattern of breastfeeding report that their breasts may leak on the first day they return to work each week, but that they quickly adjust to the change; again, the women do not express their breasts.

Minimal Breastfeeding. Minimal breastfeeding follows the practice of nursing once or twice per day, usually in the morning and in the evening, without expressing the breasts during the day. It differs from partial breastfeeding in that the number of times that the infant nurses each day is limited.

Until early in the 1980s, it was believed that unless the mother expressed her breast or nursed at least four times per day, the breasts "dried up" and lactation gradually ceased. Although it is now recognized that lactation is more flexible than previously thought, there are still some questions to be answered about mixed feeding. For example, most mothers appear to start mixed feeding when their infant is at least six weeks old—that is, when lactation is well established. It is not known, for example, if mixed feeding can be started when the infant is a few days old and lactation still continue. For this reason, it is recommended that the mother totally breastfeed the infant, making a gradual transition to mixed feeding one or two weeks before returning to work.

✱ JANICE M. MORSE, R.N., Ph.D.

See also: Breastfeeding: Physiological and Cultural Aspects; Breastfeeding beyond Infancy; Infant Feeding and Care: Nineteenth and Twentieth Centuries, United States; Weaning

See **Guide to Related Topics:** Infant Feeding

Resources

Morse, Janice M., Bottorff, Joan L. & Boman, Jeanette. (1989). "Patterns of Breastfeeding and Work: The Canadian Experience." *Canadian Journal of Public Health 80*: 182-88.

Morse, Janice M. & Harrison, Margaret J. (1988). "Patterns of Mixed Feeding." *Midwifery 4*: 19-23.

Morse, Janice M., Harrison, Margaret J., & Prowse, Margaret. (1986). "Minimal Breastfeeding." *Journal of Obstetrical, Gynecological, and Neonatal Nursing 15* (4): 333-38.

BREATH CONTROL IN LABOR

Techniques of breath control are taught, through childbirth education, for both of the two stages of labor. But in reality, these techniques may be more harmful than helpful to both mother and baby. In the first stage, the complexity and speed of breathing patterns are intentionally increased as contractions become more intense. The term "psychoprophylaxis," popularized by French obstetrician Fernand Lamaze, means "mind-prevention"; various combinations of panting and blowing supposedly limit feeling and awareness during childbirth, and this distracts the birthing woman from pain. However, studies show that adequate exchange of blood gases does not occur in the alveoli of the lungs if there is insufficient air intake to traverse the anatomical dead space. Paced respiration cannot, by definition, be normal breathing. Hyperventilation typically results, along with effort and tension, because an involuntary process is being controlled. Hyperventilation causes an oxygen excess, which is potentially harmful. Respiratory alkalosis results when the CO_2 pressure is less than 20 mmHg, or the pH is more than 7.6. Carbon dioxide is clinically more significant than oxygen, and as it is a waste product, it regulates its own removal through vasodilation. When the blood is saturated with oxygen, the vessels are narrowed, carrying less blood, and less oxygen is released from the hemoglobin. The clinical effects of the diminished blood flow include tingling in the periphery of the body, cloudy vision, diminished awareness, and in extreme cases, muscle spasms in the hands and feet.

The average respiratory rate is 12 to 16 breaths per minute, but artificial breathing patterns in active labor can lead to rates of over 100. Prolonged control of respiration ultimately expends energy, disrupts body rhythms, and diminishes relaxation. In contrast, allowing the breath/energy to flow freely and with spontaneous sound is not only more physiologically beneficial but heightens the mother's experience of labor by integrating (instead of attempting to separate) the functions of her body and mind.

Straining with the breath held during the second stage (the pushing phase) of labor is also commonly taught. This forced effort with a closed glottis is known as the Valsalva maneuver. If prolonged beyond five or six seconds, maternal and fetal physiology become disturbed. A closed pressure system is formed within the body that initially results in elevation of blood pressure, but this falls as venous return to the heart is impeded by high intrathoracic pressure. The subsequent fall in cardiac output affects circulation to the entire body, and significantly, to the placenta. The pelvic floor and the rectus sheath, where the abdominal muscles unite, are both strained. The need for episiotomy is increased as a result of perineal muscle tension. Abnormal electroencephalogram and electrocardiogram changes have been documented. The reduced blood flow to the placenta may result in fetal hypoxia, acidosis, low Apgar scores, and cesarean section.

In contrast, spontaneous pushing efforts last about five seconds and do not begin until the fetal head stimulates the proprioceptors of the pelvic floor. The average of five pushes per contraction, with a normal breath between, maintains normal physiology for mother and child and permits a longer pushing phase should that be necessary.

✱ ELIZABETH NOBLE

See also: Labor: Overview; Pain Relief in Labor: Nondrug Methods

See **Guide to Related Topics:** Childbirth Practices and Locations

Resources

Caldeyro-Barcia, R. (1978). "The Influence of Maternal Position on Labor, and the Influence of Maternal Bearing-down Efforts in the Second Stage of Labor on Fetal Well-being." In P. Simkin & C. Reinke (Eds.)

Kaleidoscope of Childbearing: Preparation, Birth and Nurturing. Seattle, WA: Pennypress, pp. 31-42.
Noble, Elizabeth. (1980). *Childbirth with Insight*. Boston: Houghton Mifflin.
———. (1981, Mar-Apr). "Controversies in Maternal Effort during Labor and Delivery." *Journal of Nurse-Midwifery* 26 (2): 13-22.

BREECH BIRTH. *See instead* FETAL PRESENTATIONS

BREWER PREGNANCY DIET

Introduction. The Brewer diet takes its name from Thomas Brewer, the physician who developed it. This dietary approach reflected the growing concern among many obstetricians, midwives and nutritionists, that the obstetrical approach developed in the 1930s and 1940s, and continued through the 1960s and into the 1970s, of severe weight gain limitation was dangerous for both the mother and the fetus.

The diet evolved through the 1970s, and was primarily geared to the prevention of toxemia, a life-threatening disorder of late pregnancy. The Brewer diet reflects the school of thought that toxemia is primarily a disease of malnutrition. Brewer published his work both for the medical community (1982) and for the general public (with G. Brewer, 1977).

The Brewer Pregnancy Diet consists of 14 food groups from which a mother can choose on a daily or weekly basis. (See Figure 1.) The diet has four basic components: (1) It allows for 2,600 calories to be consumed daily; (2) it allows for 100-120 grams of protein to be consumed; (3) it allows the pregnant woman to salt to taste; and (4) it allows for unrestricted weight gain. Dr. Tom Brewer, an obstetrician, has used the diet to prevent or treat complications of pregnancy such as pre-eclampsia, toxemia, high blood pressure, abruption of the placenta, intrauterine growth retardation, "gestational diabetes," premature labor, anemias, damage of the liver and kidneys, difficult labor, coagulation disorders, and low birth weight (which can cause babies to be hyperactive or infection-prone). According to Brewer, all of these conditions can be caused by food deficiency and low blood volume.

The Importance of Blood Volume. The pregnant body's ability to preserve the pregnancy and nourish the baby depends a great deal on its ability to increase the mother's blood volume. Normally, this blood volume is expected to increase by 50 to 60 percent. To facilitate this blood volume expansion the liver makes albumin, from protein that the mother eats. Albumin has osmotic pressure, which pulls fluid out of the tissues and back into the blood, circulating in the blood vessels. If the mother is trying to restrict her weight gain, much of the protein that she eats will get burned up for calories, and she may have trouble expanding her blood volume adequately. Thus, unrestricted weight gain is seen as a desirable part of this diet.

Salt also has osmotic pressure. While salt restriction may be helpful for pregnant woman who have unhealthy hearts or kidneys, it is *dangerous* in healthy women. The Brewer diet is based on research that shows it is not possible for a healthy pregnant woman to eat too much salt. Her kidneys simply excrete whatever extra salt she eats. It has also been shown that after just two weeks of "salt in moderation," the mother's blood volume can begin to drop (G. Brewer 1988, p. 160).

When the blood volume stops increasing or drops, the same processes begin that occur when the blood volume is dropping due to hemorrhage. The kidneys secrete renin, which causes the blood vessels to constrict. In the absence of hemorrhage, during pregnancy, this blood vessel constriction causes a rise in blood pressure. Attempting to treat this rising blood pressure with salt restriction, weight restriction, or diuretics only causes the blood volume to fall even more, leading to further formation of renin and blood vessels constriction, and a continuing rise in blood pressure.

The kidneys respond to inadequate blood volume by reabsorbing water and salt from the fluid they have filtered out of the blood. This reabsorbed fluid and salt is returned to the circulation. When there isn't enough albumin and salt in the circulation to hold this reabsorbed water, much of it leaks out into the tissues. The kidneys continue reabsorbing water at one end of the process, and water continues leaking out of the capillaries at the other end, causing rapid swelling and rapid weight gain (from water in the tissues), symptoms of pre-eclampsia. If the pregnant woman's nutrition is not improved quickly, or if salt restriction or diuretics (in drugs, herb teas, or homeopathic remedies) are prescribed, her blood volume will continue to drop, and she will develop eclampsia (toxemia). Toxemia can culminate in convulsions, coma, and death. Many sources maintain that there is no known cause of toxemia, and therefore, many practitioners continue to try to treat the symptoms alone, but without success.

Figure 1. The Brewer Diet

The Brewer Diet

You must have, every day, at least:

1. **Milk and milk products**—4 choices
   1 cup milk: whole, skim, 99%, buttermilk
   ½ cup canned evaporated milk: whole or skim
   ⅓ cup powdered milk: whole or skim
   1 cup yogurt
   1 cup sour cream
   ¼ cup cottage cheese: creamed, uncreamed, pot style
   1 large slice cheese (1¼ oz.): cheddar, Swiss, other hard cheese
   1 cup ice milk
   1½ cup soy milk
   1 piece tofu, 3" x 3" x ½" (4 oz.)
2. **Calcium replacements**—as needed (2 per soy exchange from group 1)
   36 almonds
   ⅓ cup bok choy, cooked
   12 Brazil nuts
   1 cup broccoli, cooked
   ⅓ cup collard greens
   ½ cup kale
   2 teaspoons blackstrap molasses
   4 oz. black olives
   1 oz. sardines
3. **Eggs**—2, any style
4. **Meat and meat substitutes**—8 choices
   1 oz. lean beef, lamb, veal, pork, liver, kidney
   1 oz chicken or turkey
   1 oz fish or shellfish
   ¼ cup canned salmon, tuna, mackerel
   3 sardines
   3½ oz. tofu
   ¼ cup peanuts or peanut butter
   ⅛ cup beans + ¼ cup rice or wheat (measured before cooking)—beans: soy beans, peas, black beans, kidney beans, garbanzos; rice: preferably brown; wheat: preferably bulgur
   ⅛ cup brewer's yeast + ¼ cup rice
   ⅛ cup sesame or sunflower seeds + ½ cup rice
   ¼ cup rice + ⅓ cup milk
   ½ oz. cheese + 2 slices whole wheat bread or ⅓ cup (dry) macaroni or noodles or ⅛ cup beans
   ⅛ cup beans + ½ cup cornmeal
   ⅛ cup beans + ⅙ cup seeds (sesame, sunflower)
   ½ large potato + ¼ cup milk or ¼ oz. cheese
   1 oz. cheese: cheddar, Swiss, other hard cheese
   ¼ cup cottage cheese: creamed, uncreamed, pot style
5. **Fresh, dark green vegetables**—2 choices
   1 cup broccoli
   1 cup brussels sprouts
   ⅔ cup spinach
   ⅔ cup greens: collard, turnip, beef, mustard, dandelion, kale
   ½ cup lettuce (preferably romaine)
   ½ cup endive
   ½ cup asparagus
   ½ cup sprouts: bean, alfalfa
6. **Whole grains**—5 choices
   1 waffle or pancake made from whole grain
   1 slice bread: whole wheat, rye, bran, other whole grain
   ½ roll, muffin, or bagel made from whole grain
   1 corn tortilla
   ½ cup oatmeal or Wheatena
   ½ cup brown rice or bulgur wheat
   1 shredded wheat biscuit
   ½ cup bran flakes or granola
   ¼ cup wheat germ
7. **Vitamin C foods**—2 choices
   ½ grapefruit
   ⅔ cup grapefruit juice
   1 orange
   ½ cup orange juice
   1 large tomato
   1 cup tomato juice
   ½ cantaloupe
   1 lemon or lime
   ½ cup papaya
   ½ cup strawberries
   1 large green pepper
   1 large potato, any style
8. **Fats and oils**—3 choices
   1 tablespoon butter or margarine
   1 tablespoon mayonaise
   1 tablespoon vegetable oil
   ¼ avocado
   1 tablespoon peanut butter
9. **Vitamin A foods**—1 choice
   3 apricots
   ½ cantaloupe
   ½ cup carrots (1 large)
   ½ cup pumpkin
   ½ cup winter squash
   1 sweet potato
10. **Liver**—at least once a week
    4 oz. liver: beef, calf, chicken, pork, turkey, liverwurst
11. **Salt and other sodium sources**—unlimited
    table salt, iodized—to taste
    sea salt—to taste
    kelp powder—to taste
    soy sauce—to taste
12. **Water**—unlimited
    Drink to quench thirst, but do not force fluids
    Real juice or milk might make better use of limited stomach space
13. **Snacks and additional menu choices**—unlimited
    More foods from groups 1-11
14. **Optional supplements**—as needed
    Vitamin pills, powders, herbs, yeast, oils, molasses, wheat germ, etc.

Each food you eat may be counted for one group only—e.g., count ¼ cup cottage cheese as 1 milk choice *or* 1 meat and meat substitute choice, not both.

Adapted from *Right from the Start*, by Gail Brewer and Janice Presser Greene, and from *The Brewer Medical Diet for Normal and High-Risk Pregnancy*, by Gail Brewer with Tom Brewer, MD.

Treating Pre-eclampsia. One way to treat pre-eclampsia is to educate the mother about the cause of her illness and put her on the Brewer Diet. Acute cases can be treated with IV albumin and sometimes antibiotics (to lessen the load on the liver by aromatic toxins in the intestines). If there is no doctor available to give IV albumin, the blood pressure may be lowered by including 17

eggs and 2 quarts of milk in the daily diet, for 3 days. This large number of eggs provides the equivalent of the amount of albumin given intravenously.

Weight Gain. The average weight gain on the Brewer Diet is 35-45 pounds. However, if the diet is observed, a weight loss of 5 pounds might be healthy, and a weight gain of 60 pounds (or more, for a multiple pregnancy) could also be healthy. The baby's brain goes through its most rapid rate of growth in the last 2 months of gestation. One problem with limiting a mother to a certain number of pounds is that she will often reach that number before the end of her pregnancy and then feel obligated to starve herself for the rest of the pregnancy.

Some practitioners discourage mothers from using this diet because they believe the weight gain during pregnancy will be difficult to lose after the baby is born. This concern about weight often demonstrates in such practitioners an unfamiliarity with the weight loss usually associated with breastfeeding. They may also be neglecting to apply the "risk vs. benefit" test commonly applied to other therapies, to this nutrition therapy. When this test is applied to the Brewer diet, its advocates conclude that the benefits of avoiding severe complications with the pregnancy, labor, or baby easily outweigh the risk of possibly being slight overweight after the baby's birth.

✱ JOY M. JONES, R.N.

See also: Diabetes: Clinical and Gestational; Premature Birth: Prevention

Resources

Brewer, Gail. (1978). *The Pregnancy after 30 Workbook.* Emmaus, PA: Rodale Press.

———. (1983). *The Brewer Medical Diet for Normal and High Risk Pregnancy.* New York: Simon & Schuster.

———. (1983). *Nine Months, Nine Lessons.* New York: Simon & Schuster.

———. (1988). *The Very Important Pregnancy Program.* Emmaus, PA: Rodale Press.

Brewer, Gail & Brewer, Tom. (1977). *What Every Pregnant Woman Should Know.* New York: Random House.

Brewer, Gail & Greene, Janice Presser. (1981). *Right from the Start.* Emmaus, PA: Rodale Press.

Brewer, Thomas. (1982). *Metabolic Toxemia of Late Pregnancy: A Disease of Malnutrition.* New Canaan, CT: Keats Publishing, Inc., p. 5.

Cronin, Isaac & Brewer, Gail. (1983). *Eating for Two.* New York: Bantam Books.

"Diabetes Mellitus." (1977). In Thorn et al. *Harrison's Principles of Internal Medicine.* 8th edition. New York: McGraw-Hill.

Hodin, Jay & Shanklin, Douglas. (1979). *Maternal Nutrition and Child Health.* Springfield, IL: Charles C. Thomson, Inc.

Jones, Joy. (1990). "The Brewer Pregnancy Diet." Pamphlet. Evanston, IL: Perinatal Support Services.

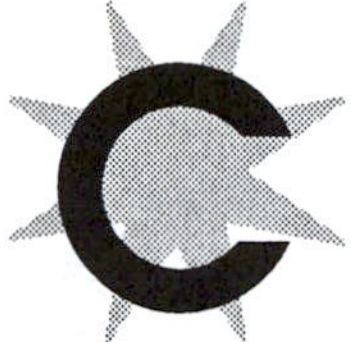

CAUL

The amniotic sac, or bag of waters, is the baglike structure that contains the fetus and the amniotic fluid. The amniotic sac generally ruptures at some point during labor; in some cases, the rupture of the sac (waters breaking) is the first sign that labor has begun. More commonly, the membranes rupture as the labor progresses. In the majority of labors without artificial intervention, the sac ruptures fairly late in the labor. The intact membranes contain the amniotic fluid: the fetus and the cord are consequently cushioned. Electronic fetal monitoring with an "internal" monitor requires the rupture of these membranes, and that is one of the disadvantages of such monitoring. Not only is a pathway to infection opened up, but the cushioning of the waters is no longer available.

When the membranes are not ruptured artificially, they occasionally do not rupture until the time of the birth: the baby is born with the membranes still intact, or with a portion of the membrane still over the baby's face. This portion of the sac, covering the face of the baby, is called the "caul," or the "veil." Being born with a caul, in many cultures throughout the world, is held to have special significance. People born with a caul may be said to have special vision or second sight—the veiling of the physical eye symbolizing the vision of the psychic eye. The Reverend Moses Hastings, an African-American traditional healer in Michigan, cited by Loudell Snow, said: "My mother used to say that I was born with two veils over my face . . . . In other words, they say when you're born with veils over your face you'll be able to discern *spirits*. You'll be able to discern the *inside* of a person."

In addition to this special vision or second sight, the person born with the veil or caul is often credited with special gifts as a healer. Snow says that healers who advertise as spiritual advisors often give having been born with a veil as part of their credentials. ∗ BARBARA KATZ ROTHMAN, Ph.D.

Resources

Dorson, Richard. (1956). *American Negro Folktales*. New York: Fawcett Publications.

Emrich, Duncan. (1972). *Folklore of the American Land*. Boston: Little, Brown.

Forbes, Thomas Rogers. (1966). *The Midwife and the Witch*. New Haven, CT: Yale University Press, pp. 95-97.

Hand, Wayland. (1961). *Popular Beliefs and Superstitions from North Carolina*. (Volume VI of the Frank C. Brown Collection of North Carolina Folklore). Raleigh NC: Duke University Press, pp. 3-68.

Snow, Loudell. (1977). "The Religious Component in Southern Folk Medicine." In Philip Singer (Ed.) *Traditional Healing: New Science or New Colonialism?* Buffalo, NY: Conch Magazine Ltd.

———. Personal Communication, 1991.

CENTRAL CLOSURE DEFECTS

The commonly known central closure defects include spina bifida, meningomyelocele, meningocele, anencephaly, encephalocele, hydrocephalus, cleft lip/cleft palate, and omphalocele. The degree of severity of most of these defects can vary from mild to terminal; most of them can be at least partially repaired surgically. While each of these defects includes an "undesired" opening, they vary in location, severity, ability to be repaired, and potential outcomes.

Neural Tube and Spinal Closure Defects. Spinal closure defects include spina bifida, meningomyelocele, meningocele, hydrocephalus, and encephalocele. Spina bifida is a defect along the spinal column that can vary in degree of severity according to the size and depth. The defect can occur anywhere along the spine and usually results in paralysis of the limbs adjacent to the top of the opening downward. Meningomyelocele is a herniation of the spinal cord and membranes through a midline defect; meningocele is a similar defect but involves only the membranes. Spina bifida occulta is less severe, and is recognized by a tuft of hair or a dimple at the base of the spine. Encephalocele occurs when an opening in the skull allows a portion of the brain to protrude. Hydrocephalus results from an opening within the meninges within the skull, causing a leaking of spinal fluid that causes an enlargement of the skull.

People with open type defects who do not die will be left with long-term disabilities, such as paralysis of the legs, loss of bowel and bladder control, spinal curvatures (scoliosis), hydrocephalus (water on the brain), or mental retardation. The closed defect variations result in death less often, and while there can be impairment in mobility, they render fewer long-term disabilities, and, as a result, individuals with these defects can usually live relatively normal lives.

Anencephaly. Anencephaly is the lack of completion of the skull, and usually includes a lack of full brain development. This condition is incurable and terminal. Many fetuses are terminated following discovery through ultrasound. Babies who are allowed to be born with this condition usually die within hours. No repairs are currently possible. Organ donor programs are considering the ethics of prolonging the life of these babies, in order to use them as donors.

Frontal Closure Defects. Cleft lip/palate and omphalocele are similar and easily repaired. Cleft lip/palate is more familiar to most people because the repair scars can be seen midline on the upper lip of adults who had this birth defect. It occurs when the midline of the upper lip, and sometimes the palate, do not completely form and an open space remains. Omphalocele is an abdominal opening that allows a portion of the intestines to protrude from the abdominal cavity. Both defects can be surgically repaired. The cleft lip/palate repairs are completed by plastic surgeons, who have perfected techniques that make visual identification almost impossible. Ongoing surgery may be required through the growing years to repair the palate, as may orthodontics.

Known and Suspected Causes of Central Closure Defects. Shortly after conception, if the neural tube fails to close properly, or becomes distended and bursts after normal closure, defects can occur. Neural tube defects have more than one cause. The combination of unfavorable genes from both parents could predispose that child to slow neural tube closure. Slow closure, combined with an environmental insult, could result in the manifestation of the defect. Anencephaly and spina bifida combined account for approximately 95 percent of neural tube defects. Causative factors for these defects include: hereditary tendency (whether a family is predisposed to a defect); environmental insults (ranging from pollutants, to poor nutrition—including a diet deficient in ascorbic acid, folate, and zinc, and overheating, such as through hot tubs); medications (prescribed, over-the-counter, or street drugs); and diseases (including Diabetes Mellitus). The frequency of central closure defects is affected by geographical location, race, and ethnic background. The British Isles have the highest overall incidence (4 to 5 per 1,000 births). Other high-frequency areas include Egypt, Pakistan, India, and some Arab countries. In the United States, the frequency is 1 to 2 per 1,000 births, with the highest incidence in the Appalachian region. Countries with the lowest incidence (less than .5 per 1,000 births) include Finland, China, Japan, and Israel. Blacks, Orientals, and Ashkenazi Jews have the lowest occurrence, while the Irish and Sikhs have the highest.

Methods of Detection. Prenatal diagnosis is now possible in some cases. Two tests being used are (1) the alpha-fetoprotein (AFP) test and (2) amniocentesis. Alpha-fetoprotein (AFP) is a maternal blood test taken at 16 to 18 weeks after the last menstrual period. Timing is important, and results are accurate only if the dates are precise. Amniocentesis, which is also done at 16 to 18 weeks, measures the AFP in the amniotic fluid. Approximately 18 percent of these tests have false positive results. Other factors beside inaccurate dates that can affect the results are twin pregnancies, clinical error, and unknown causes. If these tests are positive, then high-resolution ultrasound exam may allow a neural tube defect to be visualized and its severity defined through evaluation.

Possible Prevention Methods. While some factors are unavoidable, nutrition can be improved, drugs and hot tubs can be avoided, and (most often mentioned) multiple vitamins can be taken once a day on a regular basis by all women of childbearing age. Vitamins have been noted in many studies to be the single most important variable in the incidence of central closure defects.

Effects on the Family. Once the possibility of a fetus with a central closure defect arises, the family must make many choices, beginning with the tests available for detection, and then when the outcomes are known, considering an abortion. If the family opts to continue with such a pregnancy, they must prepare to accommodate a special-needs child. The workload increases, financial strains become a reality, and the emotional stress can be overwhelming. There are many support groups available. Overcoming the difficulties can result in making family ties even stronger.

✱ DIANE BARNES, R.N.

See also: Maternal Serum Alpha-Fetoprotein Screening

See **Guide to Related Topics:** Special Needs Infants

Resources

Bobak, Irene M., Jensen, Margaret Duncan, & Zalar, Marianne R. (1989). *Maternity and Gynecologic Care*. St. Louis, MO: C.V. Mosby.

Cohen, Felissa. (1987, Mar/Apr). "Neural Tube Defects." *JOGNN 16*(2): 105-15.

Dickason, Elizabeth J. (1979). *Maternal and Infant Care*. New York: McGraw-Hill.

Erlen, Judith A. & Holzman, Ian R. (1988, Jan/Feb). "Anencephalic Infants: Should They Be Organ Donors?" *Pediatric Nursing 14* (1): 60-64.

Hillard, Paula Adams. (1987, Sept). "Screening for Neural Tube Defects." *Parents 62* (9): 194-96.

Mulinare, Joseph et al. (1988, Dec 2). "Periconceptional Use of Multivitamins and the Occurrence of Neural Tube Defects." *JAMA 260* (21): 3141-45.

THE CERVICAL CAP

Since the beginning of recorded history, medical literature notes a fantastical array of occlusive devices used to keep sperm from entering the cervix: medicated lint tampons, pessaries of every description, sponges, halves of acidic fruit such as lemons or pomegranates, and swatches of waxed fabric or beeswax.

The forefunner of the modern cervical cap, apparently developed by German midwives, was described in a German anatomy text in 1838. Since the 1880s, caps were widely used in Europe, especially in England. Because of Victorian social codes, physicians, instead of women themselves, inserted and removed the caps on a monthly basis. Margaret Sanger was familiar with both the cap and diaphragm and preferred the diaphragm, not because it was superior, but because she saw it as less physician-dependent. Feminists in the U.S. are responsible for rediscovering the cervical cap in the late 1970s, popularizing it, and encouraging the British manufacturer, Lamberts, Ltd., to submit an application to the U.S. Food and Drug Administration (FDA) for approval (Chalker, 1987).

Unlike the diaphragm, which prevents pregnancy by holding spermicide against the cervix, the cervical cap is a true barrier, staying on the cervix by suction and blocking the entry of sperm into the cervical canal. The Prentif cavity rim cervical cap looks like a large rubber thimble, is manufactured by Lamberts, and is the only cap presently available in the United States. Lamberts also makes the bell-shaped Vimule, and the Dumas, which looks like a diaphragm but stays in place by suction. Neither of these caps is approved by the FDA.

Because the cap cannot be felt once it is in place, it can be left on the cervix for an extended period. The FDA recommends keeping the cap on for no more than 48 hours at a time, but since its reintroduction into the U.S., women have left it in place up to seven days with no reported problems. Although some women use the cap without spermicide, it is recommended that a small dollop be placed in the cap dome to serve as a back-up in the unlikely event of a dislodgement. Many cap practitioners have reported a decrease in urinary tract infections after switching to the cervical cap, although no studies have addressed this point definitively.

Because it fits snugly in the back of the vagina, the cap does not interfere with sexual sensation. In addition, the cap can be inserted well before anticipated sexual activity, providing a measure of sexual spontaneity unavailable with any other barrier method. Women in one study reported an increase in both libido and in the frequency of sexual activity (Koch, 1982).

There is a widespread myth that the cervical cap is more difficult to fit than the diaphragm. While it is true that cap fit is more variable than diaphragm fit, it is not inherently difficult. Likewise, insertion and removal are not especially difficult. With patient, supportive instruction, most women can perform these maneuvers in one to three tries.

There are several confounding issues regarding cap fit. The Prentif cap comes in only four sizes, and certain women simply cannot be fit. Factors that may prevent a woman from being fit are a very short, very long, or sharply tapered cervix, or a severely tipped uterus. However, fit is dependent upon other, less objective factors, so it is worthwhile to attempt to fit all women, even if they have a tipped uterus. The percentage of "no fits" varies among practitioners, from 50 to 80 percent. Because of this wide discrepancy in fitting rates, a second opinion on cap fit may be advisable.

The cap has no known health risks. Rather, it has a few annoying problems, including occasional dislodgement, odor inside of the cap, and partner discomfort. None of these problems is serious, and few women stop using the cap because of them.

A study sponsored by the National Institutes of Health found the cap and the diaphragm to be almost equally effective. For women who used their assigned method consistently and correctly for each session of intercourse (except during the menstrual period), there were 6.4 cap failures, or pregnancies, compared to 4.6 for the diaphragm (per hundred women per year). For women who were less consistent in their use, there were 17.4 cap failures and 16.2 diaphragm failures (Bernstein, 1986). The Los Angeles Cervical Cap Study found a 3.8 percent chance of getting pregnant with consistent cap use, and 8.3 percent pregnancy rate for less consistent users (Richwald et al., 1989).

Because of some anomalous data in the NIH study, a controversy arose concerning Pap smear changes in cap users who had had human papilloma virus (venereal warts). Reanalysis of the data revealed serious flaws in both the study's analysis and methodology (Gollub and Sivin, 1990), and at this time, no risk is thought to exist. A custom-fit cap being developed by Dr. James Koch may reach the market by the mid-1990s.

✱ REBECCA CHALKER

See **Guide to Related Topics:** Contraception

Resources

Bernstein, Gerald S. (1986). "Final Report: Use-Effectiveness Study of Cervical Caps. July 1, 1981-Mar. 31, 1986." Contract No. N01-HD—1-2804, Contraceptive Development Branch, Center for Population Research, National Institute of Child Health and Human Development, National Institutes of Health, Bethesda, MD 20892.

Chalker, Rebecca. (1987). *The Complete Cervical Cap Guide.* New York: Harper & Row, pp. 24-27.

Gollub, E.L. & Sivin, I. (1990). "The Prentif Cervical Cap and Pap Smear Results: A Critical Appraisal." *Contraception 40*: 343; "Letters to the Editor" 42 (2): 1990.

Koch, James. (1982). "The Prentif Contraceptive Cervical Cap: Acceptability Aspects and Their Implications for Future Cap Design." *Contraception 25*(2): 165.

Richwald, G.A. et al. (1989). "Effectiveness of the Cavity-Rim Cervical Cap: Results of a Large Clinical Study." *Obstetrics & Gynecology 74*(2): 145.

CESAREAN BIRTH: HISTORY AND LEGEND

Cesarean sections date back to antiquity. A *lex regia* (royal law) proclaimed by a Roman king in 715 B.C. stated that it was unlawful to bury a dead pregnant woman without trying to cut out the child. But ancient medical authorities were silent on the subject of cesarean birth, probably because, for them, procedures performed on dead women did not constitute part of medicine. But Pliny the Elder (A.D. 23-79), the author of the *Natural History*, mentioned cesarean birth in the context of the family name Caesar and thus unwittingly created the mistaken impression that Julius Caesar was born by cesarean section, an idea that was accepted in the Middle Ages and persists to this day. In fact, the term "cesarean section" was coined much later by the French doctor François Rousset

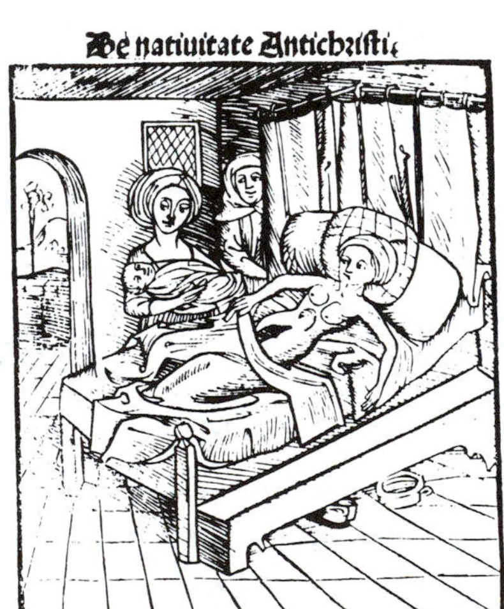

This woodcut from the Pseudo-Methodius's *Revelations* shows the cesarean birth of the Antichrist. Although men already performed cesareans at this time, the sole presence of women here may suggest that they are tied to the Antichrist's evil destiny (Basel, 1498). Stuart Collection, Rare Books and Manuscripts Division, The New York Public Library, Astor, Lenox and Tilden Foundations.

who, at the end of the 16th century, wrote the first treatise about cesareans on living women.

In medieval culture, mentions of cesarean birth first appeared in texts that came out of various Church councils, starting in the late 12th century. These texts insisted on the midwives' duty to try and cut out the fetus and baptize the newborn in case the mother died in childbirth. Regulations like these put an enormous responsibility on the midwives, generally uneducated women who had learned their trade by apprenticeship. Originally, then, it was the midwives who performed cesarean sections: surgical birth, like all other obstetrical procedures, was in the domain of women.

But at the beginning of the 14th century, male surgeons and physicians became interested in cesarean section, and the first medical text discussing cesarean birth appeared at that time. Developments in surgery and the increased use of dissections in medical training paved the way for a consideration of the operation in learned treatises. Bernard of Gordon, a physician from Montpellier in southern France, was the first medical writer to mention cesarean birth. He wrote his *Practica sive lilium medicinae* (The Practice or the "Lily" of Medicine) in 1305. In Book 7, Chapter 15 of this treatise, which named the "humble," that is, novice physicians and surgeons as its target audience, he discusses obstetrics. At the end of the chapter he states that sometimes, even though the mother dies, the fetus may survive, at least for a certain time, through the air that is still in the mother's arteries. In that case, the mother's mouth should be held open and an incision should be made in her abdomen through which the child should be extracted. He also advises that the cervix be held open to ensure the influx of air during the operation. Bernard does not give any clear indication of where the incision is supposed to be located. Medieval medical writers usually relied heavily on ancient authorities and only to a very limited extent on practical observation. But since there is no textual tradition for cesarean birth, one must assume that Bernard received his information from the actual practitioners of the operation, that is, from midwives, although he does not directly address or mention them.

Guy de Chauliac, the great 14th century surgeon and physician, on the other hand, addresses his remarks on cesarean birth directly to midwives. In his *Grande chirurgi* (Great Surgery), written in 1363, he specifies that in case a woman dies during childbirth, one should hold open the mouth and the uterus of the woman and make an incision with a razor along the left side. The child can then be pulled out.

The growing interest in cesarean birth on the part of male physicians marks a step on the way to the medicalization of obstetrics. One important landmark on this way was the moment when, for the first time, a male surgeon, Piero d'Argellata (d. 1423), performed the operation himself. D'Argellata describes in his *Chirurgia* how he himself did a cesarean by using a razor to make an incision along the mother's *linea alba*. From then on surgeons performed the operation with varying success (in most cases, the child died soon after the mother), until in 1581 François Rousset claimed to have witnessed many cesareans with both mother and child surviving. Both his medical expertise and his testimony were doubted by established physicians, such as Ambroise Paré, and finally his treatise was refuted, although the term he invented, "cesarean operation," still endures.

While all the medical writers on cesarean birth were men, in the performance of the operation a distinct changeover from female to male practitioners is visible. Two developments in medievel and Renaissance culture contributed to this restriction in women's medical competency: the professionalization of medicine (women were excluded from the universities and consequently from the practice of medicine) and the witch hunts whose targets were almost exclusively women and frequently midwives (Blumenfeld-Kosinski, 1990, Chapter 3). The textual tradition chronicles the exclusion of women and so does the artistic production of the time. In the images depicting cesarean birth (most of them from the early 13th century manuscripts of the *Faits des Romains* [Deeds of the Romans] showing the birth of Julius Caesar) one can see the change taking place around 1400. Only women perform the operation in the images up to that point; in images created after 1400, only men are shown. The birth scenes, whether portraying women or men performing the operation, are for the most part realistic, showing the mother dead or dying, the practitioner making an incision using the surgical instrument specified in the medical treatises of the time. The medical texts themselves, however, even if they had illustrations, did not depict cesarean births.

In addition to the medical texts there were myths and legends that dealt with heroes born by cesarean. In the Persian tradition it was Rustam, in Greek myth it was Asclepios and Adonis, and in Germanic lore it was Tristan (in the version by Eilhart) who were born this way. One of the most striking images is that of the Antichrist's birth by cesarean in late medieval German woodcuts. This purely pictorial, not textual, tradition, shows dramatically how people in the late Middle Ages thought of cesarean birth as something uncanny and destructive. But there was a compensating, more reassuring tradition as well. In various miracle collections one can read that certain saints and the Virgin performed cesareans in order to save a mother in distress. Cesarean birth could also be an omen of a great destiny or it could pose the ultimate riddle, as in *Macbeth* where McDuff is the one who is "not of woman born."

✱ RENATE BLUMENFELD-KOSINSKI, Ph.D.

See also: Cesarean Birth: Social and Political Aspects

***See* Guide to Related Topics:** Literature and the Arts

Resources

Blumenfeld-Kosinski, Renate. (1990). *Not of Woman Born: Representations of Caesarean Birth in Medieval and Renaissance Culture.* Ithaca, NY: Cornell University Press.

Bullough, Vern. (1966). *The Development of Medicine as a Profession.* New York: Hafner.

Forbes, Thomas. (1966). *The Midwife and the Witch.* New Haven, CT: Yale University Press.

Pundel, J. (1969). *Histoire de l'opération césarienne. Etude historique de la césarienne dans la médecine, l'art et la littérature, les religions et la législation. [History of the Cesarean operation. Historical Study of the Cesarean in medicine, art and literature, religion and the law.]* Brussels, Belgium: Presses Academiques Européennes.

Wyman, A.L. (1984). "The Female Practitioner of Surgery, 1400-1800." *Medical History 28:* 22-41.

Young, John H. (1944). *Caesarean Section: The History and the Development of the Operation from Earliest Times.* London: H.K. Lewis.

CESAREAN BIRTH: INDICATIONS AND CONSEQUENCES

A cesarean section is a birth in which the mother's abdomen and uterus are opened surgically and the baby and placenta removed through the incision. Contrary to popular belief, the operation was not named because Julius Caesar was born this way. At that time surgery was invariably fatal, and Caesar's mother lived many years after his birth. The term may have derived from a Roman law, the *Lex Caesare,* which mandated a cesarean birth if a pregnant woman died, or from the Latin word "cadere," meaning "to cut."

Up until the 20th century, performing a cesarean meant almost certain death for the mother; thus, it was reserved for situations when the mother was dying or dead. Improvements in surgical technique lowered maternal mortality to less than 1 percent by mid-century, allowing obstetricians to resort to the operation in less desperate situations. The cesarean rate increased slowly, from 0.2 percent in 1910 to 4.5 percent in 1968.

Since 1968, however, the cesarean rate in the United States has risen rapidly to its current level of one in four births (24.7 percent in 1988). This dramatic change in obstetrical practice has caused much controversy. Reasons suggested to explain the rising rate include the greater reliance on childbirth technology in general (some technologies, such as electronic fetal monitoring, falsely detect problems with the pregnancy that result in cesareans); a widespread misconception that a cesarean is usually safer for the baby; an increased emphasis on the baby's well-being at the expense of the mother's; fears of malpractice suits; desire for higher reimbursement or time savings by physicians; and women's reluctance to undergo labor.

Although the infant mortality rate has fallen in recent years, there is no evidence that higher cesarean rates have improved outcomes for mothers or babies. Many other factors have contributed to lower infant mortality, particularly the development of neonatal intensive care. The United States was tied for 24th place in the world in infant mortality in 1989; every country with lower infant mortality also has a lower cesarean rate.

Indications for Cesarean. Indications for cesarean section may be divided into three categories.

Definite (must be done to save the mother, baby, or both):

1. Prolapsed cord—when the umbilical cord comes into the vagina ahead of the baby, cutting off the baby's oxygen.
2. Placenta praevia—when the placenta is implanted over the cervix and torn loose as the cervix opens.
3. Placenta abruptio—when the placenta pulls away from the wall of the uterus before the baby is born.
4. Unusual positions of the baby—when the baby's position makes it impossible to come through the pelvis, for example, a transverse (sideways) lie.
5. Severe fetal distress, not responsive to corrective measures—when the baby is not receiving enough oxygen; usually determined by significant changes in the heart rate, or thick meconium (the baby's first bowel movements) in the amniotic fluid.
6. Active herpes—when lesions are present on the mother's genitals; the baby may be infected during a vaginal birth, resulting in death or severe damage.

7. Absolute cephalopelvic disproportion (CPD)—when the mother's pelvis is unusually small or misshapen, or the baby is extremely large.
8. Soft tissue obstruction—when a fibroid tumor or other growth blocks the birth canal.

Relative (needed sometimes but not always):

1. Failure to progress (also called prolonged labor or dystocia)—when the cervix dialates or the baby descends more slowly than usual, usually due to contractions that are too weak or far apart. This may be caused by pain medication, anesthesia, mother's anxiety or depletion of physical resources, or relative CPD (see below). It may also be diagnosed due to impatience, since the guidelines for labor progress represent only an average, not what every woman should do.
2. Relative CPD—when the baby's head is at an unusual angle and/or the mother's pelvis has an unusual shape, slowing labor progress.
3. Breech presentation—when the baby comes buttocks or feet first.
4. Less severe fetal distress—electronic fetal monitoring has increased the use of cesarean for this indication, although many studies have failed to show improved outcomes.
5. Multiple pregnancies.
6. Preterm birth.
7. Maternal illness complicating the pregnancy, such as diabetes or hypertension.

Discredited (no longer considered valid):

1. Previous cesarean delivery—the most common reason for cesarean today; however, the risks of routine repeat cesarean are greater for both mother and baby than the risks of rupture of a cesarean scar.
2. History of herpes without lesions or prodromal symptoms.
3. Suspected large baby, or suspected CPD—there is no safe, accurate way to diagnose CPD without a period of strong, frequent contractions.

Consequences of Cesarean Surgery. Cesarean sections carry all the risks of major abdominal surgery, which are considerably higher than the risks of vaginal birth. The risk of the mother's death, though only about 1/2,500-5,000, is still at least two to four times higher than after vaginal birth. Complications are 5-10 times more common and include infection, excessive blood loss, transfusions, anesthesia complications, blood clots, accidental injury to other organs, abnormal attachment of the placenta in the next pregnancy, and more difficulty conceiving again.

For many women, a surgical delivery has emotional side effects as well, particularly if unexpected. The most important of these is how they felt they were treated during the birth process, a

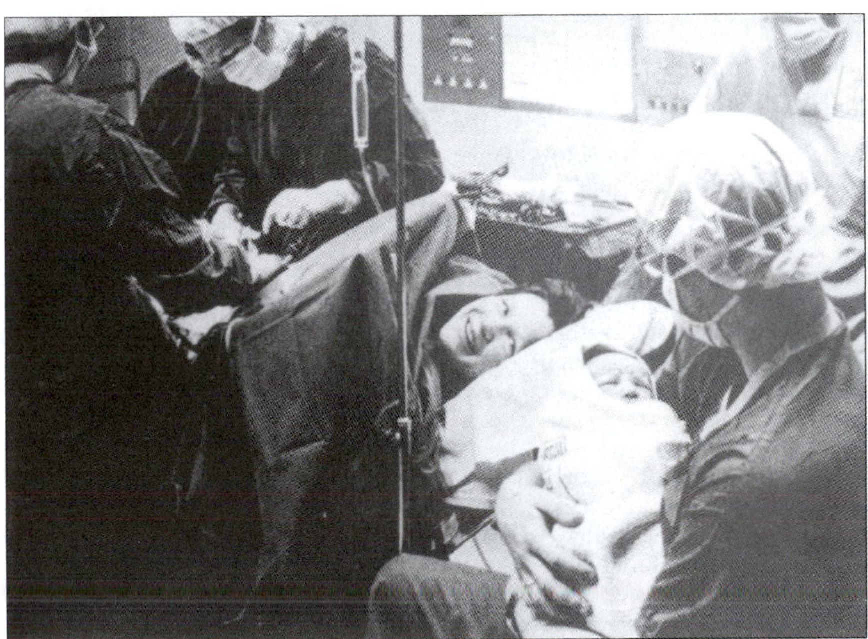

A cesarean birth. Photo courtesy of Kip Kozlowski.

feeling usually quite distinct from feelings about the baby. A surgical delivery inevitably means a longer, more difficult recovery and a longer separation from the newborn, which can undermine a mother's sense of competence in her new role. Many cesarean mothers need to go through a genuine grieving process, even if the baby is healthy.

The most serious risk of cesarean for the baby is respiratory illness if the birth occurs before labor. Even with sophisticated testing, some babies born by scheduled cesarean are accidentally preterm. Labor itself stimulates important changes in the baby's body, such as the absorption of excess fluid from the lungs. The baby may be affected by medications and anesthesia given to the mother, may aspirate fluid and blood, or may be accidentally injured during surgery.

The average total cost of a cesarean birth is about twice that of a vaginal birth in a hospital. The Public Citizen Health Research Group has estimated that over half the cesareans performed in the U.S. are medically unnecessary. In 1987, this resulted in 475,000 unnecessary operations, at an estimated cost of 25-100 maternal deaths; 25,000 serious infections; 1.1 million hospital days; and over $1 billion.

Cesarean Procedures. A cesarean involves all the procedures that accompany any major abdominal surgery, including shaving the abdomen and about an inch of pubic hair, inserting an intravenous (IV) line, and placing a catheter in the bladder. Anesthesia for a cesarean may be regional (spinal or epidural) or general (gas). With regional anesthesia, the mother is numb from approximately her breasts down, but awake. General anesthesia is needed in rare extreme emergencies because it is much faster to administer. However, it carries greater risks for both mother and baby.

The obstetrician will be assisted by a second physician and a nurse, while a second nurse and often a pediatrician are present to attend to the baby. In most U.S. hospitals today, the father or other support person may attend the birth if the parents so wish. He is dressed in surgical scrub gear and usually brought into the operating room after preparations are complete.

The skin incision may be either a midline incision (vertical from the navel to the hairline), or a horizontal "bikini" incision just above the hairline. The latter is more comfortable postoperatively and barely noticeable once the hair grows back. The midline incision is somewhat faster in an extreme emergency. Over 95 percent of uterine incisions are horizontal just above the cervix, called low segment or low cervical incisions. Less common are low verticals (vertical incisions in the lower part of the uterus) or classicals (vertical incisions in the main body of the uterus), used for speed or when more room is needed. Classical incisions present a greater risk of blood loss after the cesarean and of uterine rupture in another pregnancy.

The baby is born within 5-15 minutes. After fluid is suctioned from the air passages, the newborn is usually ready to be wrapped up warmly and brought for the parents to see and hold. Repair of the various layers of muscle tissue takes 30-45 minutes. The mother may feel nausea or pressure when the baby is born and again during the repair, but she should not feel pain. If she is too uncomfortable, medication can be given through the IV as soon as the baby is born. The skin incision is closed with absorbable or removable stitches, or staples. The mother is taken back to a labor room or to a special recovery room until the anesthesia wears off and her vital signs are stable, usually two to four hours. This is the best time to hold or nurse the baby for the first time, before the anesthesia wears off completely.

The usual hospital stay after a cesarean is four to seven days. Almost all women need some postoperative pain relief. Narcotics, first by injection and then by mouth, are most common. Other options include TENS (trans-electrical nerve stimulation) and epidural analgesia, narcotics injected into the lower back. The mother will be helped to her feet within 12-18 hours and encouraged to walk regularly to maintain circulation and stimulate other bodily functions. The digestive tract often slows down or stops after abdominal surgery, resulting in painful intestinal gas. Diet may be limited to liquids at first. Slowly tightening the abdominal muscles during a slow exhale, several times each hour, can help get the intestines moving again. Even after the mother goes home, she will need more rest and help than after a vaginal birth, since she is recovering from both childbirth and major abdominal surgery.

Vaginal Birth after Cesarean (VBAC). For many years, North American physicians followed the adage, "once a cesarean always a cesarean," believing that the risk of rupture of a uterine scar in labor was so great that a woman should have all other children by cesarean. Other countries have never followed such a policy, and many studies have confirmed that vaginal birth after cesarean (VBAC) is safer for both mothers and babies than scheduled repeat cesarean sections. In spite of government and professional recommendations in favor of VBAC, in 1988 almost 90 percent of women in the U.S. who had had a previous cesarean delivered their next child by cesarean.

Most problems with a uterine scar are not true ruptures but rather simple separations not requiring treatment. True rupture of a low-segment scar occurs in about 0.2 percent of births; most are not life-threatening emergencies. By contrast, the risks of other unexpected emergencies in labor, such as a prolapsed cord or placental separation, are 1 to 2 percent. Thus, a woman having a VBAC has no greater chance of needing an emergency cesarean than any other woman in labor. For this reason, any hospital capable of handling other childbirth emergencies can handle VBACs.

In the last 40 years not a single mother has been reported to have died due to the rupture of a cesarean scar. Although a few babies have died in connection with scar rupture, almost all involved the presence of other conditions such as vertical or unknown uterine scars, prematurity, or problems before labor. Some mothers and babies have died from the complications of elective (planned) cesareans, however.

The only factor known to increase the risk of rupture of a cesarean scar is a classical uterine scar. (The direction of the abdominal scar is not important.) A classical scar is somewhat more likely to give way (2 to 3 percent), but considerably more likely to be a severe emergency if it does. Most VBAC studies have excluded classical incisions, so a true comparison of the risks of labor with a classical scar, in a hospital able to perform an immediate cesarean, with the risks of a scheduled cesarean is not possible.

Although many other factors have been suggested, such as having had more than one cesarean, getting an infection after the cesarean, having twins, or having a breech baby, there is no evidence that any of them increase the risk of scar rupture. Whether a low vertical incision increases risk is uncertain.

Looking at many studies over the past 40 years, 75-80 percent of women attempting a VBAC have been successful. Although having had the prior cesarean for failure to progress or CPD slightly reduces the chances of a VBAC, one-third to one-half of women who have had a cesarean for CPD give birth to a baby larger than their first (supposedly too big) baby. Perhaps the most important factors in a successful VBAC are for the mother to be knowledgeable and committed to oneself, and to have strong support, especially from the physician or midwife.

A mother having a VBAC should be treated like any other laboring woman. Neither pain medication, epidural anesthesia, nor pitocin has been found to increase the risk of scar rupture. Since VBAC mothers have no higher chance of a sudden emergency than other mothers, they have no greater need for IVs or electronic monitoring, or to come to the hospital in early labor or give birth in a delivery room rather than a birthing room or center.

✱ BETH SHEARER

See also: Cesarean Birth: History and Legend; Cesarean Birth: Social and Political Aspects; Cesarean Birth: Trends in the United States

Resources

Cohen, Nancy Wainer & Estner, Lois J. (1983). *Silent Knife: Cesarean Prevention and Vaginal Birth after Cesarean.* New York: Bergin and Garvey.

Donovan, Bonnie. (1986). *The Cesarean Birth Experience.* Boston: Beacon.

Flamm, Bruce. (1990). *Birth after Cesarean: The Medical Facts.* Englewood Cliffs, NJ: Prentice-Hall.

Rosen, Mortimer & Thomas, Lillian. (1989). *The Cesarean Myth: Choosing the Best Way to Have Your Baby.* New York: Penguin.

Shearer, Beth & Cane, Aleta Feinsod. (Eds.) (1989). *Frankly Speaking: A Book for Cesarean Parents.* Framingham, MA: C/SEC Publications.

CESAREAN BIRTH: SOCIAL AND POLITICAL ASPECTS

Cesarean delivery refers to the surgical alternative to vaginal childbirth. The procedure is major surgery, entailing five layers of incision in order to penetrate the uterus and manually remove the newborn. To complete the procedure, each incision is sutured closed and the mother is prescribed a course of antibiotics and bedrest.

References to infants "untimely ripped from their mothers' wombs" can be found throughout Western literature, from Virgil's *Aenead* to Shakespeare's *Macbeth* to Anne Tyler's novel, *The Accidental Tourist.* Until recently, however, cesarean delivery was a rare event, considered too great a risk to the life of the mother. In cesarean deliveries clinically recorded in the 19th century, women usually died as a result of the procedure, with infection and hemorrhage the common causes of death. The modern technique of suturing the uterus was pioneered by the German physician Max Sanger, starting in 1882, depite the belief of many doctors at that time that the uterus should be left unsutured to heal itself. Sanger's commonsense innovation reduced the risks of hemorrhaging, but infection persisted as an acute problem in cesarean deliveries, as it was in vaginal deliveries.

It remained the main cause of cesarean maternal mortality rates which were between 70 and 80 percent in the first decades of the 20th century.

With general improvements in hospital sanitation and surgical procedures, the risks associated with cesarean delivery diminished, especially following the Second World War. The use of penicillin and sulfa drugs combatted infection. Improvements in anesthesia and transfusion techniques made major surgery less dangerous. Nonetheless, cesarean delivery remained a relatively rare procedure well into the 1960s, accounting for only 5 to 7 percent of births in the United States and Canada (where rates generally parallel those in the U.S.) and 3 to 5 percent in Europe.

The national rise in cesarean childbirth rates in the United States began toward the end of the 1960s and accelerated sharply over the next two decades. In 1978 the national rate reached 18 percent; by 1990, it had climbed to 25 percent. The National Center for Health Statistics in Washington has predicted a rate of 40 percent by the year 2000.

Professional Control. Many experts and a National Institutes of Health Task Force have attempted to explain exactly why cesarean deliveries have become increasingly frequent, more so in the United States and Canada than in other industrialized countries. The reasons are complex and involve changes in professional control of childbirth and in hospital organization, as well as a widespread social acceptance of surgical therapy. Since the end of the Second World War, general practitioners, who once delivered most newborns in the United States, have gradually lost professional turf to specialists. American obstetricians are now in charge of more than 80 percent of all deliveries. Since obstetricians are trained as surgeons, they are more apt to use surgical therapies when faced with labor-room crises. Surgical intervention is now often recommended for many medical indications, for example, breech presentation, twins, premature birth, first births, births to mothers over 35 or under 18 years of age, fetal distress, and dystocia, a general failure to progress in labor. All of these are conditions that many general practitioners, midwives, and even obstetricians trained in the 1950s approached successfully without radical surgical intervention.

There is also cross-national evidence demonstrating that healthy births are possible without surgical intervention. In Western Europe, cesarean rates have generally stayed under 10 percent, with good outcomes for parent and child. In the Netherlands today, in fact, 34 percent of births take place at home and many others at clinics with minimal technology. Midwives, strongly supported by the government, rely on hospital physicians for backup in predictably high-risk cases. Yet even in the hospital, a midwife may remain in charge of the delivery. The role of midwife or nurse-midwife in the United States is, in contrast, largely subservient to that of the physician.

When polled, obstetricians in the United States stated that they resort to cesareans as the best defense against malpractice claims. Parents may bring suit on behalf of injured children for as long as 21 years after birth, depending on state law. Although not necessarily in the best interests of all patients, the cesarean can be presented as evidence that the obstetrician did everything medically possible on behalf of the mother and infant.

More venal motivations ascribed to obstetricians—that they profit financially from cesareans or that they enjoy the convenience of a planned birth—cannot be substantiated and only distract from serious discussion of professional beliefs and behavior. Obstetricians are sued more than other medical specialists and many are leaving (or considering leaving) practice because of high malpractice insurance costs. This trend may increase the role of the midwives in and out of hospitals and, consequently, trends in medical intervention.

The Repeat Cesarean and VBAC. The greatest contributor to the rising cesarean rate appears to be physicians' reliance on the outdated rule, "once a cesarean, always a cesarean." Fifty and sixty years ago, some physicians performed cesareans using a vertical incision of the uterus that made its scar vulnerable to rupture the next time the woman went into labor. As early as the 1920s, many physicians had begun to use a low transverse incision (commonly called the Kerr technique after the physician who perfected it) that presents virtually no risk of scar rupture. Still, the tendency has been for women who have had cesareans once, for whatever reasons, to continue to have them.

Encouraged by a statement from the American College of Obstetricians and Gynecologists in 1988, medical centers have begun to promote vaginal birth after cesarean delivery. The VBAC, as it is called, has produced clinical results that are superior to those of cesarean births for both infants and mothers. If the choice for the VBAC increases, the current rate of cesarean deliveries might stabilize instead of increasing.

Institutional Forces. The institutional context for childbirth has also influenced the rise of cesarean deliveries. Since just after World War II, virtually all births in the United States have taken place in hospitals, but not in the high-technology environments available today. Small, local hospitals and obstetric wards in larger hospitals offered little compared with today's diagnostic and therapeutic options. The most common medical interventions were pain-killing drugs, episiotomies, and the use of forceps, relatively low technology when compared to cesareans. Most women spent a week or more in the hospital simply resting up from childbirth. In the last 20 years, however, increasing numbers of births have taken place in centralized hospital facilities. On a national level, many small hospitals with obstetric wards closed down entirely and local hospitals eliminated their obstetric units as unprofitable. In major medical centers, where the investment in surgical facilities, fetal monitoring, newborn intensive care, and other childbirth technologies is extensive, it is natural to expect that the number and degree of medical interventions is greater. The costs of childbirth are also higher and maternity beds are more profitable, provided the patients are fully insured.

In addition, physicians and nurses working in hospitals are under pressure to make maternity patients conform to the institutional schedule and rules. For example, labor that continues for 12 hours is often judged abnormal and, therefore, an indication for a cesarean. Since the failure of labor to progress ("dystocia") accounts for nearly one-third of all cesareans, the problem of institutional versus personal biological schedules is worth consideration. The onset and progress of labor is not well understood by medical science, yet it is known that, for many women, increased anxiety can inhibit and complicate its natural course. Once admitted to a hospital, a woman in labor must contend with the impersonal, organizationally efficient ways in which her particular labor and delivery will be handled. There are problems with women being left in isolation during labor, with women being required to remain immobile in their beds, with women automatically being given drugs to hasten labor, with mistakes in the use and interpretation of fetal monitoring, as well as with the physician's decision to perform the cesarean against the mother's wishes. While an extreme and rare occurrence, the court-ordered cesarean presents a serious dilemma, pitting medical authority against a woman's right to make decisions about her body.

Social Class Issues. Research on the rising cesarean rates shows that there are two categories of women most likely to have the procedure: (1) women of very low socioeconomic status and (2) well-educated, middle-class women. In the case of the former, poor maternal health and childbirth complications associated with poverty may be influencing the cesarean rate. Also, it is possible that women at the low end of the social spectrum have little control over delivery-room decisions and, in central teaching hospitals, serve as the patients on whom physicians in residence practice.

The more affluent group of educated mothers is medically at low risk yet appears to actively choose cesarean delivery. The procedure does seem to offer certain benefits. Interview studies suggest that educated women perceive cesarean delivery as less physically painful than vaginal birth and as more safe for their infants. The current use of local anesthesia during cesarean delivery makes it possible for a woman to be alert and relatively free of pain. Age is an additional factor. Women who delay having their first child until their mid-30s are also likely to choose cesarean delivery, on the premise that it is a safer procedure.

The Hazards of Cesarean Delivery. The hazards of cesarean versus vaginal delivery have only recently begun to be vigorously investigated by physicians. As women and their obstetricians become more aware of its risks, it is possible that cesarean delivery rates may decline. Historically, widespread, uncritical use of medical procedures is followed by a phase of professional criticism and rejection.

Risks to mothers undergoing cesarean delivery have been underestimated. Rates of maternal mortality (deaths related to childbirth) have been generally underreported, leading the Centers for Disease Control and the American College of Obstetricians and Gynecologists to establish in 1980 the Maternal Mortality Collaborative to improve reporting. Estimates of maternal mortality associated with cesarean childbirth used to represent it as little more than the 3 per 100,000 ratio associated with vaginal delivery. Based on new studies, the mortality rate associated with cesareans is estimated at from 2 to 26 times that of vaginal delivery. The old problems, hemorrhaging and infection, persist, along with stroke, injury to the urinary tract, and risks associated with anesthesia. Postpartum infection, or endometritis, reportedly follows 20 to 55 percent of cesarean deliveries and only 2 to 5 percent of vaginal births. Infection rates depend not only on the health of the mother but on the hospital environment.

If research showed that the cesarean delivery was clearly a medical benefit for newborns, then prospective mothers might in good faith assume the risks of surgery. However, medical benefits to infants delivered by cesarean are being questioned. The National Institutes of Health Task Force reported little difference in outcome for most infants. The claim of obstetricians that cesareans have contributed to decreased perinatal mortality rates, that is, stillbirths plus neonatal deaths, has recently been challenged by a longitudinal report from the National Maternity Hospital in Dublin, Ireland, which saw dramatic decreases in perinatal mortality rates without any increase in cesarean rates.

As for morbidity rates, infants born by VBACs appear to be in better clinical condition than infants of the same weight and gestational age delivered by cesarean. Physician skills have been shown to be significant determinants of cesarean case outcome. Physician miscalculation of fetal age, leading to a preterm delivery, was a major problem before the widespread use of ultrasound. Similarly, physician miscalculation of the size of a uterine incision in breech cases can entrap the fetus and result in serious injury to the nervous system. Thus, if the physician has been trained to deliver breech and twin infants only by cesarean, these infants are probably safer than if the physician attempted vaginal delivery.

✱ JEANNE HARLEY GUILLEMIN, Ph.D.

See also: Cesarean Birth: History and Legend; Cesarean Birth: Indications and Consequences; Cesarean Birth: Trends in the United States

Resources

Cohen, Nancy Wainer & Ester, Lois J. (1983). *Silent Knife, Cesarean Prevention and Vaginal Birth After Cesarean.* South Hadley, MA: Bergin & Garvey.

Guillemin, Jeanne. (1981, Jun). "Babies by Cesarean: Who Chooses, Who Controls?" *The Hastings Center Report 11* (3): 15-18.

Marieskind, Helen I. (1989, Dec). "Cesarean Section in the United States: Has It Changed Since 1979?" *Birth 16* (4): 200-201.

Placek, P.J., Taffel, S.M., & Liss, T. (1987, Sept). "The Cesarean Future." *American Demographics 12* (6): 46-47.

Rosen, M.G. (1981, Apr). "NIH Consensus Development Task Force Statement on Cesarean Childbirth." *American Journal of Obstetrics and Gynecology 57* (4): 537-545.

Sargent, Carolyn & Stark, Nancy. (1989, Mar). "Childbirth Education and Childbirth Models: Parental Perspectives on Control, Anesthesia, and Technological Intervention in the Birth Process." *Medical Anthropology Quarterly 3* (1): 36-51.

CESAREAN BIRTH: TRENDS IN THE UNITED STATES

The frequency of cesarean delivery in the United States has risen steadily in the last two decades. Since 1965, it has been possible to track national cesarean section rates from data collected in the National Hospital Discharge Survey (NHDS), conducted annually by the National Center for Health Statistics, Centers for Disease Control. Medical and demographic data entered on the face sheets of medical records are abstracted from a yearly sample of more than 200,000 inpatients discharged from approximately 400 nonfederal general and special short-stay hospitals that participated in the surveys. About 10 percent, or 20,000 of those sampled, are women discharged after giving birth (Graves, 1990).

The cesarean rate rose from 5.5 per 100 deliveries in 1970 to 16.5 in 1980 (Table 1), when the National Institutes of Health convened a Consensus Development Conference on Cesarean Childbirth (Department of Health and Human Services, 1981). The Conference recommended a number of approaches to reduce the rising cesarean rate, including the opportunity for women who have had a previous cesarean to undergo a trial of labor under certain conditions. These recommendations were published in two major obstetric journals shortly thereafter. In 1982, and again in 1985, the American College of Obstetricians and Gynecologists issued guidelines aimed at reducing the rate of repeat cesareans by promoting trial of labor (American College of Obstetricians and Gynecologists, 1982, 1985). However, despite these initiatives, the cesarean rate continued to rise, and reached 24.4 per 100 deliveries in 1987 (Taffel, 1989). But the U.S. cesarean rate appears to be stabilizing. The 1988 rate of 24.7 is not significantly higher than the rate of 24.4 observed in 1987, and the primary rate, the rate for first-time cesareans, of 17.5 in 1988 is almost identical to the rate of 17.4 observed in the two previous years (Taffel et al., 1990).

The number of cesarean deliveries for live births rose from 205,000 in 1970 to 966,000 in 1988, although the total number of births increased by only 5 percent in this period (Table 1). Repeat cesareans represent a growing share of total cesareans, increasing from 25.2 percent of all cesareans in 1970 to 36.3 percent in 1988. This increase reflects the very sharp rise in the primary cesarean rate for teenagers and women in their twenties. In 1988, the rates for these age groups were four to

Table 1. Cesarean Section Rates and Estimated Number of Live Births by Type of Delivery: United States, 1970-88

	Cesarean rate		Number of live births in thousands						Percent	
				Cesarean delivery[d]				Other	repeat	Percent
Year	Total[a]	Primary[b]	Total[c]	Total	Primary	Repeat	VBAC[d]	Vaginal	Cesarean	VBAC[f]
1988	24.7	17.5	3,910	966	615	351	50	2,894	36.3	12.6
1987	24.4	17.4	3,809	929	601	328	36	2,844	35.3	9.8
1986	24.1	17.4	3,757	905	595	310	29	2,823	34.3	8.5
1985	22.7	16.3	3,761	854	559	295	21	2,886	34.6	6.6
1984	21.1	15.0	3,669	774	509	265	16	2,879	34.2	5.7
1983	20.3	14.3	3,639	739	482	257	12	2,888	34.8	4.6
1982	18.5	13.3	3,681	681	462	219	11	2,989	32.2	4.8
1981	17.9	12.5	3,629	650	427	223	8*	2,971	34.3	3.6*
1980	16.5	12.1	3,612	596	418	178	6*	3,010	29.9	3.4*
1975	10.4	7.8	3,144	327	238	89	2*	2,815	27.1	2.0*
1970	5.5	4.2	3,731	205	153	52	1*	3,525	25.2	2.2*

a Number of cesarean deliveries per 100 total deliveries.

b Number of first cesareans per 100 deliveries for mothers who have not had a previous cesarean.

c Source: National vital registration data.

d Estimated by applying cesarean rates derived from the National Hospital Discharge Survey to the number of live births from national vital registration data.

e Proportion of all cesareans that are repeat cesareans.

f Number of women with a vaginal birth following a cesarean delivery per 100 women with a previous cesarean delivery.

* Figure does not meet standards of reliability of precision because the weighted numerator is less than 10,000 deliveries.

Source: National Hospital Discharge Survey of the National Center for Health Statistics, Centers for Disease Control.

five times as high as in 1970. Almost all of the subsequent births for these young women in the 1970-1988 period were repeat cesareans because of the low rate of vaginal birth following a previous cesarean (VBAC) during this time.

In 1970, only 2.2 percent of women who had a previous cesarean delivered vaginally. By 1988, VBAC had risen to 12.6 percent (Table 1), still well below what many practitioners believe is medically possible. According to a recent study, less than half of all hospitals offer a trial of labor to women who have had a previous cesarean, but the success rate for vaginal delivery following trial of labor in these hospitals is about 50 percent (Shiono et al., 1987). This suggests that VBAC rates are low, not because trial of labor fails, but because it is infrequently offered. In 1988 there were 50,000 VBAC deliveries (1.3 percent of all births), compared with 351,000 repeat cesareans (9.0 percent of all births).

Women most likely to have a cesarean delivery tend to be in the oldest years of childbearing. They are also more likely to deliver in a hospital located in the South, in a hospital that is not nonprofit or government owned, or in one that has more than 100 beds. In addition, they are more likely to have private insurance (Table 2).

Cesarean rates for common medical indications for 1988 compared with 1980 are shown in Table 3. In both years, almost all deliveries where feto-pelvic disproportion was diagnosed were by cesarean section. The cesarean rate for women who had a previous cesarean was 87.4 percent in 1988, down from 96.6 percent in 1980. These rates are the complements of the VBAC rates of 12.6 percent and 3.4 percent. The cesarean rate for breech presentation has been rising steadily. In 1988, it was 84.9 percent, up from 67.2 percent in 1980. The cesarean rate for a multiple birth doubled in this time period, rising from 32.7 percent to 64.8 percent.

In October 1988, the American College of Obstetricians and Gynecologists again issued revised guidelines for VBAC (American College of Obstetricians and Gynecologists Committee on Obstetrics, 1988). These guidelines emphasize the appropriateness of VBAC for women who have had a previous cesarean delivery with a low transverse incision, if there are no specific contraindications. The new guidelines stress that for such women VBAC may be safer than a repeat cesarean

Table 2. Cesarean Section Rates by Age of Mother, Region, Hospital Size and Ownership, and Expected Source of Hospital Payment: United States, 1988

(Cesarean rates are the number of cesarean deliveries per 100 total deliveries for specified category)

Total	24.7
Age	
Under 20 years	19.5
20-24 years	20.1
25-29 years	26.7
30-34 years	28.0
35 years and older	32.1
Region	
Northeast	23.5
Midwest	24.3
South	27.3
West	21.7
Bed size	
Less than 100 beds	22.3
100-299 beds	25.2
300-499 beds	25.9
500 beds or more	22.8
Ownership	
Nonprofit	25.0
State and local government	22.0
Proprietary	29.9
Expected source of payment	
Blue Cross	27.9
Other private insurance	26.8
Medicaid	22.8
Other government	24.4
Self pay	17.4
Other	20.9

Source: National Hospital Discharge Survey of the National Center for Health Statistics, Centers for Disease Control.

for both the mother and baby. The widespread adoption of these new VBAC guidelines, and a continued leveling off or reduction in the primary cesarean rate, will result in a decline in the overall cesarean rate in the United States.

✷ SELMA TAFFEL

See also: Cesarean Birth: History and Legend; Cesarean Birth: Indications and Consequences; Cesarean Birth: Social and Political Aspects

Resources

American College of Obstetricians and Gynecologists. (1982). "Guidelines for Vaginal Delivery after a Cesarean Childbirth." Statement of the Committee on Obstetrics: Maternal and Fetal Medicine. Washington, DC.

———. (1985). "New Guidelines to Reduce Repeat Cesareans." Statement by Dr. Luella Klein for VBAC News Conference, Washington, DC, January 25, 1985.

American College of Obstetricians and Gynecologists Committee on Obstetrics. (1988). Maternal and Fetal Medicine. "Guidelines for Vaginal Delivery after a Previous Cesarean Birth." Committee opinion No. 64, Washington, DC.

Department of Health and Human Services. (1981). "Cesarean Childbirth." Report of a Consensus Development Conference, sponsored by the National Institute of Child Health and Human Development. September 22-24, 1980. Bethesda, MD: National Institutes of Health, NIH Pub. No. 82-2067.

Graves, E.J. (1990). "1988 Summary: National Hospital Discharge Survey." Advance data from vital and health statistics 185. Hyattsville, MD: National Center for Health Statistics.

Shiono, P.H. et al. (1987). "Recent Trends in Cesarean Birth and Trial of Labor Rates in the United States." *JAMA 257* (4): 494-97.

Taffel, S.M. (1989). "Cesarean Section in America: Dramatic Trends, 1970 to 1987." *Statistical Bulletin* (70): 2-11.

Table 3. Cesarean Rates for Common Medical Indications: United States, 1980 and 1988

(Cesarean rates are the number of cesarean deliveries per 100 total deliveries for specified category)

ICD-9 CM Category		1988	1980
653.4	Fetopelvic disproportion	98.9	95.7
654.2	Previous cesarean delivery	87.4	96.6
652.2	Breech presentation	84.9	67.2
660	Obstructed labor	72.8	26.1
651	Multiple gestation	64.8	32.7
641	Antepartum hemorrhage	61.3	54.1
646.6	Genitourinary tract infections	52.2	49.8
661	Abnormal labor, uterine inertia	48.9	53.7
656.3	Fetal distress	48.0	66.9
642	Hypertension and eclampsia	41.5	38.1
647	Venereal and other infections	39.7	46.5
645	Prolonged pregnancy	36.7	34.0
648.2	Anemia	35.3	30.7
644	Early or threatened labor	31.8	25.2
662	Long labor	22.0	19.5

Source: National Hospital Discharge Survey of the National Center for Health Statistics, Centers for Disease Control.

Taffel S.M., Placek, P.J., & Moien, M. (1990). "1988 U.S. Cesarean Rate at 24.7: A Plateau?" *New England Journal of Medicine 323* (3): 199-200.

CHICKEN POX IN PREGNANCY

Chicken pox is relatively rare during pregnancy. Most women have had chicken pox during childhood and have become immune; only 2 percent of all cases of the disease occur in adults. The number of reported cases indicates an incidence of chicken pox of 1 to 5 per 10,000 pregnancies (Rosenfeld, 1989). Many obstetricians and midwives never have encountered chicken pox in the pregnant women they care for. However, when it does occur, chicken pox can present serious complications for the pregnant woman and the baby.

Maternal and Fetal Risks. Varicella pneumonitis occurs in about 14 percent of adults with chicken pox. The mortality rate is 30/100,000 for adults, whether or not they are pregnant. Several doctors recommend treatment with acyclovir (Zovirax) and aggressive use of a ventilator in adults with varicella pneumonitis (Rosenfeld, 1989).

Because of the low incidence of chicken pox during pregnancy and the corresponding low incidence of complications, it is difficult to ascertain the risk to the developing fetus. Proof that the syndrome exists is based on reports from around the world of infants with the same pattern of anomalies following maternal Varicella Zoster Virus syndrome (VZV) infection. Studies indicate that the earlier in pregnancy a woman acquires VZV, the greater the risk of congenital VZV. VZV syndrome consists of some combination of: (1) scarred, segmental, or dermatomal skin lesions; (2) limb deformities; and (3) central nervous system and/or ocular abnormalities (Fox and Strangarity, 1989).

Not all exposed infants will show signs of VZV. For example, one study indicated that only 2 of 27 fetuses of women with VZV in the first trimester were affected: one with a cataract and the other with microcephaly (Burrows and Ferris, 1988). In one study of 22 exposed infants with VZV, 38 percent were born prematurely and 39 percent were born small for gestational age. Several central nervous system abnormalities were seen in 77 percent; eye abnormalities were seen in 68 percent; and skin lesions were seen in 100 percent (Rosenfeld, 1989).

Perinatal Complications. Infants born to women in whom chicken pox occurs within five days before or after delivery are at high risk for severe neonatal disease; chicken pox develops in one-third of these infants. Mortality rates of 30 to 50 percent for infected infants have been reported. Complications include skin lesions, pneumonia, and uncontrolled bleeding. Studies have shown that the mortality rate and the severity of infection vary with onset of rash in the mother and the infant (Rosenfeld, 1989).

Treatment. Exposed neonates born during the high-risk period should receive varicella-zoster immune globulin (VZIG). There are reports of exposed infants who received acyclovir, in addition to VZIG, with good results. However, limited experience makes it difficult to conclude definitely that prophylactic acyclovir is effective and safe (Batik and Stevens, 1989).

Giving VZIG to a pregnant woman exposed to chicken pox may prevent her from developing clinically apparent varicella infection if given within 96 hours of exposure. However, there are no data about the effect of VZIG on fetal infection (Batik and Stevens, 1989). A live attenuated vaccine is being tested and may be available soon (Batik and Stevens, 1989; Fox and Strangarity, 1989).

✱ PAT DE LA FUENTE

See **Guide to Related Topics:** Pregnancy Complications

Resources

Batik, Odette & Stevens, Nancy. (1989). "Varicella in Pregnancy." *The Journal of Family Practice 28* (3): 315-21.

Burrows, Gerard N. & Ferris, Thomas F. (1988). "Varicella-Zoster Virus." In W.B. Saunders (Ed.) *Medical Complications During Pregnancy*. pp. 378-80.

Fox, Gary N. & Strangarity, Joseph W. (1989). "Varicella-Zoster Virus Infections in Pregnancy." *American Family Physician 39* (2): 89-98.

Rosenfeld, Jo Ann. (1989, Jun). "Chickenpox and Pregnancy: What Are the Risks?" *Postgraduate Medicine 85* (8): 297-300.

CHILDBEARING IN PRISON

Pregnancy and childbearing in prison must be understood against the backdrop of a profile of incarcerated women, the location and status of women's institutions, and the priority given to social control in the criminal justice system.

The majority of jailed and imprisoned women in the U.S. are young, undereducated, and under- or unemployed women of color. A large proportion of incarcerated women are likely to be drug abusers, and an increasingly larger number have acknowledged being physically and sexually abused. Property crimes and drug-related arrests represent the typical reasons for women's imprisonment; such crimes have registered gains in recent years as women's impoverishment has also increased.

The socially and economically marginal status of most imprisoned women who are pregnant means that they are not likely to have received adequate prenatal or reproductive health care prior to imprisonment. Many pregnant prisoners do not understand the physiological changes occurring within their bodies. Pregnant women with drug addictions pose additional medical needs. Yet, women's prisons typically fail to provide adequate reproductive health care or childbirth education classes for pregnant inmates. Although professional and advocacy groups have developed standards and guidelines for the care of pregnant prisoners, the level of available services varies significantly from community to community, state to state, and between local jails, state prisons, and federal institutions.

Generally inadequate health services result from a host of factors. One is the underfunding of prison programs, especially for women, whose small numbers in comparison to the male prison population make their needs seem less critical. Full-time doctors are not available, and physicians who conduct regular prison visits are not obstetricians or gynecologists. The often isolated location of women's penal institutions may even preclude the regular availability of appropriate medical personnel in the community to address pregnant women's needs. The philosophy of social control operating at any given prison will affect such critical issues as access to birth control (an especially important issue at coed prisons or institutions allowing conjugal visits), access to abortion (as a right of reproductive choice rather than a decision forced on a pregnant inmate by authorities or as an antidote to rape by prison staff), and the degree of freedom allowed during childbirth (e.g., with or without limbs shackled). Finally, negative attitudes of prison staff toward inmates affect the degree to which pregnant women's expressed needs will be viewed as legitimate and thus receive timely attention. Advocates report a startling number of cases in which pregnant women repeatedly requested medical attention to no avail until serious health consequences occurred. In short, whether neglect of pregnant inmates' needs and rights is intentional or unintentional, it is nevertheless an all too common feature of women's penal institutions.

Childbirth poses additional concerns. The imprisoned woman in labor is likely to be taken to a community hospital for delivery and returned to prison as soon as possible. If she has received inadequate prenatal care in prison, the likelihood of complications during childbirth and the birth of an unhealthy baby increases. The mother may be physically constrained during labor and afterward, a reminder of the prison's emphasis on inmate control. Upon her return to prison, the new mother may be subjected to routine vaginal searches and returned quickly to strenuous activity, without regard for her physical status.

In general, mothers see their babies for less than 72 hours before being returned to prison and separated from the infant. Policies regarding custody of prisoners' babies vary widely, from the unusual opportunity in a very few places to remain with a child in a prison alternative program to immediate custody hearings to determine the disposition of the newborn. Mothers typically rely on close female relatives to care for their children until their release.

Overall, the level of attention given pregnancy and childbirth for imprisoned women reflects the priority of social control within the U.S. criminal justice system. Recent efforts to prosecute pregnant drug users for child abuse signal the emergence of additional punitive stances toward pregnant women by legal institutions.

✱ PAULA DRESSEL, Ph.D., and
SANDRA BARNHILL, J.D.

See also: Pregnancy and Social Control; Pregnant Addicts, Treatment of; Violence against Pregnant Women

***See* Guide to Related Topics:** Pregnancy Complications

Resources

Baugh, Constance. (1985). *Women in Jail and Prison: A Training Manual for Volunteers and Advocates.* New York: National Council of Churches.

Holt, Karen E. (1982). "Nine Months to Life—The Law and the Pregnant Inmate." *Journal of Family Law 20:* 523-43.

New Directions for Women. (1990, Mar/Apr). *19* (2). Issue on Women in Prison.

Rafter, Nicole Hahn. (1990). *Partial Justice: Women, Prisons, and Social Control.* Second edition. New Brunswick, NJ: Transaction.

Richey Manns, Coramae. (1984). *Female Crime and Delinquency.* University, AL: University of Alabama Press, especially pp. 227-34.

CHILDBEARING IN SCIENCE FICTION

> "Don't ask me," snapped the imagination. "I could think up a dozen better arrangements before breakfast." (Le Guin, 1990, p. 236)

Frankenstein, widely regarded as the first science fiction story every written, is a cautionary tale of what can happen when men and science appropriate the process of creation. Since its publication, women writers have continued to imagine new reproductive technologies and to speculate on their effects on society and on women's lives. Some of the technologies they have imagined have been actualized. Most have not. But the real and immediate issues raised by the current medical simplicity of abortion, by surrogate mothers and test-tube conceptions and sperm banks have been anticipated and fought over in women's literature since the early 1900s.

Many of these stories are decidedly grim. They are written as warnings. In the time that has passed since Mary Shelley wrote *Frankenstein,* the experiences of women regarding new medical technologies have certainly been mixed. But many of these stories have imagined benefits to women in an altered reproductive process. Taken together, they constitute the efforts of women to think up "a dozen better arrangements."

Marge Piercy is one of several writers who has been both grim and hopeful. In her novel, *Woman on the Edge of Time,* Piercy's 20th-century protagonist, Connie, is introduced to Mattapoisett, a gentle community of the future. Children in Mattapoisett are birthed by machines. If pregnancy has been eliminated, motherhood has not, however. Each child has, in fact, three mothers, at least two of which nurse the child. All three mothers are volunteers. And any or all of the three mothers may be men.

At first, Connie is horrified by the sight of men altered with hormones so that they can lactate. She feels that the women of the future have thrown away the only area of power women had. Yet the community of Mattapoisett is set against the present-day sections of the book. In the real world where Connie lives, she has lost her only daughter in a custody case and undergone an unnecessary hysterectomy. There is nothing science-fictional about these experiences.

Mattapoisett is also set against a second possible future, an unnamed place glimpsed only briefly where women are differentiated and defined by sexual function. Some women are mothers. Some are contract prosititutes. When they cease to be useful in these functions, their body parts can be harvested for organ transplants. It is a high-tech, literal version of the religious dystopia Margaret Atwood imagines in *The Handmaid's Tale.*

Other dystopian visions include the Holdfast in Suzy McKee Charnas's *Walk to the End of the World,* where near-comatose women are raped in breeding rooms, and Kate Wilhelm's post-holocaust book, *Where Late the Sweet Birds Sang,* in which the protagonist is incarcerated and used as a host for clones. In both of these stories, motherhood is forced on women.

In Katherine Marcuse's short story "Twenty-first Century Mother," motherhood begins voluntarily but is stolen when the father surreptitiously turns his wife's pregnancy over to a machine. The artificial environment, he claims, is an improvement on nature. "It's got 300,000 valves . . . ," he says. "And that many can't go wrong!" (Marcuse, 1976, p. 23).

Other stories add technologically advanced reproductive methods to the concept of motherhood as a paid position. Artificial insemination and paid *mother-surrs* form the background to Connie Willis's "All My Darling Daughters." Nancy Freedman in *Joshua Son of None* imagines a cloned human created asexually into an enucleated egg, but carried in the womb of a young woman who is paid for her use. In Zoe Fairbairns' *Benefits,* motherhood is the only paying job available to women.

At the other extreme, women have imagined reproductive processes that women control absolutely. The title character of Joan Vinge's *Snow Queen* is a female genetic engineer who creates her own clone. Female cloning is also a feature of C.J. Cherryh's *Cyteen* and is the method of reproduction in the all-female future of James Tiptree Jr.'s (aka Alice Sheldon) "Houston, Houston, Do You Read?"

Artificial insemination offers another alternative for a reproductive process controlled entirely by women. In Carol Emshwiller's short story, "Abominable," women have disappeared and men speculate that the women are in hiding, impregnating themselves with the sperm of rock-and-roll stars. In Jody Scott's novel *I, Vampire,* the female vampire protagonist and her lover, an alien who appears in the form of Virginia Woolf, found the Company, an enterprise that sells famous men's sperm to women. "The basic pitch would be, 'Why have children by that miserable pauper, loser, and all-around grouch, your husband? Why not have John Travolta's glamorous baby instead? Think of it: yours to have and to hold—for only pennies a week.'" (Scott, 1984, p. 85). In time the Company will have the sperm of historical heroes for sale. In time the Company will offer all the benefits of unmixed genes—parthenogenesis—for the wealthy woman.

Parthenogenesis is imagined in several literary creations of all-women worlds. It appears as early as 1917 when Charlotte Perkins Gilman first published *Herland* and is refined in Joanne Russ's "When It Changed" and *The Female Man.* Russ explains the reproductive process in her all-female community Whileaway as follows:

> Whileawayans bear their children at about thirty . . . These children have as one genotypic parent the biological mother (the "body-mother") while the non-bearing parent contributes the other ovum ("other mother"). (Russ, 1975, p. 49)

Another all-female community is detailed in Suzy McKee Charnas's second novel, *Motherlines.* Having escaped from the Holdfast described above, the protagonist Alldera finds herself in the world of the Riding Women. Altered years ago in laboratories, these women are capable of reproducing daughters genetically identical to themselves. An infusion of sperm is required to initiate the birth process, and the Riding Women, therefore, mate ritually with their horses. Alldera is pregnant when she arrives and prized as someone who brings a potentially new genetic line. Like Connie in Piercy's book, Alldera finds a society in which, after the birth process itself, every child has many mothers. The daughters are raised by their blood mothers and four "share-mothers," among whom the "heartmother" holds those ties of particular tenderness. All mothers share in the nursing and help with the pregnancy and birth. No precedence is given in this arrangement to the woman who actually bears the child.

In other stories, as in Piercy's Mattapoisett, the process of childbearing, rather than being given to the exclusive control of the mother or the father, is imagined as shared more equitably between the two. In Vonda McIntyre's *Dreamsnake,* women and men are trained in "bio-control," a natural way of blocking conception. In Elizabeth A. Lynn's "The Man Who Was Pregnant," the pregnancy of the title character is mysterious and unexplained. But more often, equality involves technological alterations, taking some nips and tucks in male and female sexual differentiation. In *The Left Hand of Darkness,* Ursula Le Guin imagines the androgynous society of Winter. She postulates that the society was formed as an experiement in gender by an ancient race that populated the universe. The inhabitants of Winter are biologically neutral except during "kemmer," a kind of estrus that comes on them a few days every month. Based on the sexual stimulus they receive during kemmer, any inhabitant may become temporarily male or female. If intercourse results in pregnancy, the mother retains her femaleness through childbirth and lactation and then returns to a neutral state. *The Left Hand of Darkness* is, among other things, an exploration of the kind of society that might result if it were possible to be the father of several children and the mother of several more.

Stories such as Lynn's and Le Guin's might be argued to contain the most radical concept of all, the idea that through science or evolution or magic, somewhere, sometime, pregnancy might be something that could happen to *anyone.*

✱ KAREN JOY FOWLER

See **Guide to Related Topics:** Literature and the Arts

Resources

Anderson, Poul. (1970). *Virgin Planet.* New York: Paperback Library.

Atwood, Margaret. (1986). *The Handmaid's Tale.* Boston: Houghton Mifflin.

Bear, Greg. (1989). "Sisters." In *Tangents.* New York: Warner Books.

Berger, Thomas. (1973). *Regiment of Women.* New York: Simon and Schuster.

Bova, Ben. (1971). *THX 1138.* New York: Paperback Library.

Bryant, Dorothy. (1976). *The Kin of Ata Are Waiting for You.* Berkeley, CA: Moon Books.

Charnas, Suzy McKee. (1974). *Walk to the End of the World.* New York: Ballentine.

———. (1978). *Motherlines.* New York: Berkley.

Cherryh, C.J. (1988). *Cyteen.* New York: Warner Books.

Clear, Val et al. (Eds.) *Marriage and the Family through Science Fiction.* New York: St. Martin's Press.

Disch, Thomas. (1978). "Planet of the Rapes." In Douglas Hill (Ed.) *The Shape of Sex to Come.* London: Pan Books.

Emshwiller, Carol. (1980). "Abominable." In Damon Knight (Ed.) *Orbit 21.* New York: Harper and Row, Publishers.

Fairbairns, Zoe, (1979). *Benefits.* London: Virago.

Farmer, Philip Jose. (1960). "Father." In *Strange Relations.* New York: Avon Books.

Freedman, Nancy. (1973). *Joshua Son of None.* New York: Delacorte Press.

Gearhart, Sally Miller. (1978). *The Wanderground: Stories of the Hill Women.* Watertown, MA: Persephone Press.

Gilman, Charlotte Perkins. (1979). *Herland.* New York: Pantheon Books.

———. (1980). "The Yellow Wallpaper." In *The Charlotte Perkins Gilman Reader.* New York: Pantheon Books.

Godwin, Gail. (1983). *A Mother and Two Daughters.* London: Pan Books.

Huxley, Aldous. (1985). *Brave New World.* New York: Bantam Books.

Jorgensson, A.K. (1978). "Coming-of-Age Day" In Douglas Hill (Ed.) *The Shape of Sex to Come.* London: Pan Books.

Koontz, Dean. (1973). *The Demon Seed.* New York: Bantam Books.

Le Guin, Ursula. (1969). *The Left Hand of Darkness.* New York: Ace Books.

———. (1974). *The Dispossessed.* New York: Harper and Row.

———. (1976). "Nine Lives." In Pamela Sargent (Ed.) *Bio-Futures: Science Fiction Stories about Biological Metamorphosis.* New York: Vintage Books.

———. (1985). *Always Coming Home.* New York: Harper and Row.

———. (1990). *Dancing at the Edge of the World: Thoughts on Words, Women, Places.* New York: Harper and Row, Publishers.
Lynn, Elizabeth A. (1977). "The Man Who Was Pregnant." In *Chrysalis 1.* New York: Zebra.
Marcuse, Katherine. (1976). "Twenty-first Century Mother." In Val Clear et al. (Eds.) *Marriage and the Family through Science Fiction.* New York: St. Martin's Press.
McAllister, Bruce. (1988, May). "The Girl Who Loved Animals." In *Omni 10*: 100.
McIntyre, Vonda. (1978). *Dreamsnake.* New York: Dell.
———. (1979). *Fireflood and Other Stories.* Boston: Houghton Mifflin Company.
Piercy, Marge. (1976). *Woman on the Edge of Time.* New York: Random House.
Russ, Joanna. (1972). "When It Changed." In Harlan Ellison (Ed.) *Again Dangerous Visions.* Garden City, NY: Doubleday.
———. (1975). *The Female Man.* New York: Bantam Books.
Sargent, Pamela. (1976). *Cloned Lives.* Greenwich, CT: Random House.
Scott, Jody, (1984). *I, Vampire.* New York: Ace Books.
Shelley, Mary. (1965). *Frankenstein: Or, the Modern Prometheus.* New York: NAL.
Sturgeon, Theodore. (1960). *Venus + X.* New York: Dell.
Tepper, Sherry. (1988). *The Gate to Women's Country.* New York: Foundation Books.
Tiptree, James, Jr. (1976). "Houston, Houston, Do You Read?" In Vonda McIntyre and Susan Janice Anderson (Eds.) *Aurora, Beyond Equality.* New York: Random House.
Vinge, Joan. (1980). *The Snow Queen.* New York: Dell.
Werfel, Frantz. (1946). *Star of the Unborn.* New York: The Viking Press.
Wilhelm, Kate. (1974). *Where Late the Sweet Birds Sang.* New York: Pocket Books.
Willis, Connie. (1986). "All My Darling Daughters." In Terry Carr (Ed.) *Best of SF of the Year 15.* London: Victor Gollancz Ltd.
Wyndham, John. (1981). *Consider Her Ways and Others.* Middlesex, England: Penguin Books.

CHILDBED FEVER. *See instead* PUERPERAL FEVER

CHILDBIRTH PRACTICES IN AMERICAN HISTORY

Between 1650 and 1900, childbirth in America underwent a series of transformations. In the early period it was an event oriented toward family and community, dominated and defined by females, and occurring within the physical and emotional space of the home. By the end of the 19th century, childbirth was medically oriented and largely male-dominated, and though it still occurred mostly at home, it was directed by medical ideas rather than laywomen's everyday knowledge. During the 20th century, childbirth moved into the hospital where it became increasingly controlled and medicalized and where women's role, as birthing woman or as attendant, continued to diminish.

In early America, childbirth reflected age-old tradition as a woman-centered rite, a ritual attended, directed, and controlled by women. Based upon everyday domestic knowledge and experience passed down from one generation's women to the next, birth took place in the woman's home, where the expectant mother moved around at will and gave birth in one of a variety of positions: standing, sitting, kneeling, or even suspended from another's arms. Following birth, "the women" cleaned both baby and mother, who remained secluded for a period of time if someone was available to assume temporarily the new mother's household tasks. After a few days or weeks, visits by family and friends and sometimes a special ceremony for christening or naming the newborn would end this period of "lying-in."

Expectant mothers recognized the signs of impending labor and knew when to send for a midwife and what to expect in the hours ahead. In a place especially designed or prepared for birth, the expectant mother or "her women," as her attendants (midwives, friends, neighbors, family members) were called, would gather, bringing with them the benefit of generations of accumulated wisdom about ways to ease the trials of childbirth. They prepared soothing teas infused from amber, saffron, ground cumin seed, sage, or comfrey to ease her through the dilation stage of labor. As the labor and delivery progressed, attendants might offer other herbal preparations: myrrh to hasten the delivery, a mint syrup to quell

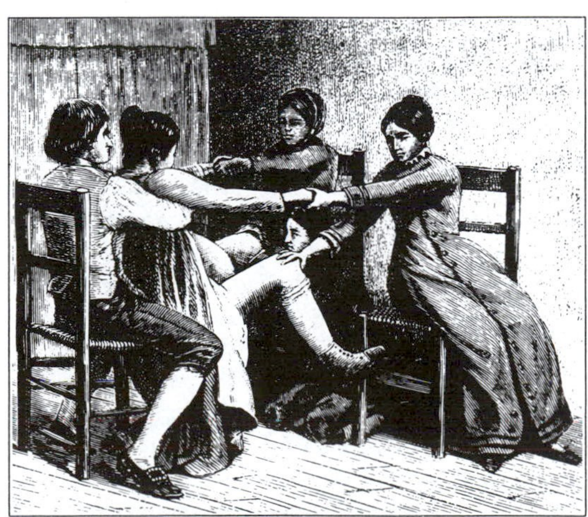

A pioneer birth in Virginia. Drawing after the work of George J. Englemann, 1882, courtesy of the National Library of Medicine. Illustration © by Janet Isaacs Ashford.

nausea, and fern paste to keep the perineum pliant during the delivery of the head and shoulders. To further ease passage of the fetus and to relieve pain, the expectant woman might sit atop a steaming pot of wild pennyroyal decoction. When she felt ready to deliver, she might do so on a birthing stool brought by the midwife or choose another position in which she felt comfortable. The midwife was in charge, and though well equipped to handle difficulties such as excessive pain, slow progress, and a poorly positioned fetus, most labors were normal and the women were used to waiting. After the baby's birth, the midwife might suggest a basil or rue decoction if the afterbirth was tardy, bayberry tea if the postbirth bleeding seemed excessive, or a betony root preparation as prophylactic against hysterics following the ordeal (Mather, 1972; Leighton 1966).

Specifics of women's childbirth experiences varied in early America as did particulars of practices surrounding the ritual. A 17th-century Fox Indian woman, for example, might give birth in a small isolated brush shelter with her mother, mother-in-law, and midwife present and assisting; she might kneel or lay supine on the ground during her labor while holding a strap suspended from the shelter roof on which she pulled whenever her contractions were intense; she might use special potions mixed and given her by the midwife, who would assist by giving herbal drinks to ease her pain, or by circling outside the shelter while singing special songs and chanting (Axtell, 1981).

Women held in slavery were often cultivated as breeders by owners in the latter 18th and 19th centuries, and so were encouraged in frequent pregnancies. Births took place in their quarters with friends, family, and neighbors helping out while the midwife oversaw the event. Though particular superstitions and beliefs about the best way to negotiate a pregnancy and birth might differ from their Northern sisters—their basis was in African heritage, after all—the childbirth itself did not. Midwives were usually the most skilled among the many women on a plantation who knew about birth, and they were regularly called upon to attend not only other bondswomen, but also the plantation owner's wife and other local white women (Norton, 1987; White, 1987).

After slavery, these "grannies," as lay midwives were usually called in the South, continued to serve as the main childbirth attendants for women of color and not infrequently for white women as well. As spiritual as well as medical advisors, these lay attendants helped to maintain the traditional nature of childbirth in African-American communities throughout the South (Holmes, 1986). Well into the 20th century—at first because they could not afford and/or did not with to have medical help at their births, and later because they were not permitted to enter white hospitals even if they might have chosen to do so—African-American women of the South continued to give birth in traditional ways and fared as well or better than their medically attended white sisters (Devitt, 1979).

Childbirth retained much of its tradition during the 19th and into the 20th century in many areas of the country. Utah's Mormon women, for example, relied upon midwives until the close of the 19th century when the Mormon Church began to sponsor women to attend women's medical colleges in the East (Rose, 1942; Arrington, 1976). Women traveling West worked to create a comfortable birthing situation for themselves that included whatever women were in the traveling group as well as any close enough to be called (Faragher, 1979). Both city and rural immigrant groups arranged childbirth in as traditional a way as they were able; custom—and not infrequently husbands—dictated female attendance at birth (Declerq, 1985; Ewen, 1985; Kobrin, 1966).

At first, physicians were called only as a last resort when a childbirth seemed hopeless, then "just in case" it became difficult, and then gradually in the 19th century, physicians handled all births, replacing the midwife as chief attendant. Called in because they were male, because they were "educated," because they claimed to be able to "do something" when women and midwives could not, men-midwives proceeded to redefine childbirth as disease, a pathology that called for medical attention and intervention.

The most dramatic intervention physicians held out was the forceps, a traditional instrument newly designed for use in saving both the birthing woman's *and* the infant's life under what would otherwise be hopeless conditions. Other interventions commonly practiced by late 18th- and early 19th-century physicians included venesection, or bloodletting, used to restart stalled contractions, or tobacco enemas if the bloodletting did not work. Ergot, a fungus that sometimes grows on rye grain and can be a potent oxytocic (substance used to speed up and intensify contractions), came into widespread use by physicians in the early 1800s after one Dr. John Stearns learned about it from a local midwife. He did not learn from her how best to prepare the ergot, however, and it alternately helped and harmed women and fetuses throughout the 19th century. Opium (in tincture form and known as laudanum) was used for pain relief, although it often slowed or even halted contractions. By mid-century, ether and chloroform were commonly used as anesthetics, sometimes given to accompany forceps use, sometimes given to erase pain or the memory of pain.

Interventions increased during the late 19th and early 20th centuries, often creating new childbirth problems which typically called for further interventions to address and manage. For example, anesthesia decreased contraction intensity but caused breathing difficulty for newborns. Instruments tore birth canal tissue and regularly introduced infection. Tissue tears were left torn. Why? Even though haphazard healing could result in chronic disability, suturing could create even worse problems. Solutions to problems created by interventive practices were usually developed, but hardly faster than new interventions arose and with them, new problems. This upward spiral has continued throughout the 20th century as childbirth practices have become ever more medically and technologically ordered.

✷ JANET CARLISLE BOGDAN, Ph.D.

See also: Midwifery: Overview; Midwives, Southern Black

***See* Guide to Related Topics:** Childbirth Practices and Locations

Resources

Arrington, Chris Rigby. (1976). "Pioneer Midwives." In Claudia Bushman (Ed.) *Mormon Sisters: Women in Early Utah.* Cambridge, MA: Emmaline Press, pp. 42-65.

Axtell, James. (1981). *The Indian Peoples of Eastern America: A Documentary History of the Sexes.* New York: Oxford University Press, pp. 28-29.

Bogdan, Janet. (1978). "Care or Cure?: Childbirth Practices in Nineteenth Century America." *Feminist Studies* 4: 92-99.

Declerq, Eugene. (1985). "The Nature and Style of Practice of Immigrant Midwives in Early Twentieth Century Massachusetts." *Journal of Social History* 19: 118.

Devitt, Neal. (1979, Spring). "The Statistical Case for the Elimination of the Midwife: Fact versus Prejudice, 1890-1935, (Part I)." *Women and Health* 2: 169-79.

Eakins, Pamela S. (Ed.) (1986). *The American Way of Birth.* Philadelphia: Temple University Press.

Ewen, Elizabeth. (1985). *Immigrant Women in the Land of Dollars: Life and Culture on the Lower East Side, 1890-1905.* New York: Monthly Review Press, p. 131.

Faragher, John Mack. (1979). *Women and Men on the Overland Trail.* New Haven, CT: Yale University Press, 139-40.

Holmes, Linda Janet. (1986). "African Midwives in the South." In Pamela S. Eakins (Ed.) *The American Way of Birth.* Philadelphia: Temple University Press, pp. 273-91.

Kobrin, Frances. (1966). "The American Midwife Controversy: A Crisis of Professionalization." *Bulletin of the History of Medicine* 40: 354.

Leavitt, Judith Walzer. (1986). *Brought to Bed: Childbearing in America, 1750-1950.* New York: Oxford University Press.

Leighton, Ann. (1966). *Early American Gardens 'For Meate or Medicine'.* Boston: Houghton Mifflin, pp. 237, 247, 263, 349, 382, 399.

Mather, Cotton. (1972). *The Angel of Bethesda (An Essay Upon the Common Maladies of Mankind).* Edited by Gordon W. Jones. Barre, MA: American Antiquarian Society and Barre Publishers, pp. 246-47. Katsi Cook, a lay midwife of the Mohawk Nation at Akwesasne, in a lecture on Native American midwifery, mentioned some of the same preparations Mather referred to as part of current Iroquois midwifery practice, e.g. fern paste (February 16, 1981, Syracuse, NY).

Norton, Mary Beth. (1980). *Liberty's Daughters: The Revolutionary Experiences of American Women, 1750-1800.* Boston: Little Brown, pp. 31, 78-84.

Rose, Blanche E. (1942). "Early Utah Medical Practice." *Utah Historical Quarterly* 10: 14-32.

Scholten, Catherine M. (1985). *Childbearing in American Society: 1650-1850.* New York: New York University Press.

Wertz, Richard W. & Wertz, Dorothy C. (1977). *Lying-In: A History of Childbirth in America.* New York: Free Press.

White, Deborah Gray. (1987). *Ar'n't I a Woman? Female Slaves in the Plantation South.* New York: W.W. Norton, pp. 67-69, 94-118.

CHILDKEEPING AND CHILDBEARING

Childkeeping refers to a unique decision-making process confronting pregnant families who choose prenatal diagnosis (see, for example, entries on amniocentesis, chorion biopsy, maternal serum alpha-feto protein screening, and ultrasound). With the advent of contraceptive and abortion technologies, families made childbearing decisions regarding conception (Fox, 1982) and/or continuation of a pregnancy (Luker, 1975). With the advent of prenatal diagnostic and fetal surgery technologies, families are faced with difficult, costly, and unique decisions that are called childkeeping decisions (Seals, 1989).

Regardless of family form, whether the family consists only of a pregnant woman, a wife and husband, or an extended set of relatives and friends, issues of childbearing and, to a large extent, childkeeping have been considered the domain of the legally recognized family unit within sociolegal limits (Arney, 1982; Medical Genetics Center, 1978). Childbearing decision making differs from that of childkeeping decision making in three important ways: (1) the context in which the decision is made; (2) the beliefs on which the decision is made; and (3) the interests in which the decision is made.

First, childbearing decisions are considered a matter to be handled within the family (Diamond and Orenstein, 1990; Fox, 1982). Even advice garnered from sources outside the family (doctors, midwives, etc.) is typically filtered through family preferences, prejudices, and experiences. Decisions to become pregnant or, if pregnant, to abort are based on practical considerations (such as the quality of living of the mother, the family, and the future child) and moral perspectives (such as attitudes toward abortion, birth defects, and life in general) (Fox, 1982; Seals, 1985).

Second, childbearing decisions are generally made with the presumption of a healthy newborn child (Lippman-Hand, 1977). That is, childbearing decisions are made with the belief that the child will be both healthy and without defect at birth. These worries aside, decisions regarding a potential or actual pregnancy are, in this context, primarily questions concerning the ability of the family to provide an acceptable quality of life to a well baby (Luker, 1985).

Third, it is the interests of the family that are of primary concern in childbearing decisions. The quality of life provided to a well baby is a function of family variables, including stability and economic, social, and psychological well-being. Childbearing decisions are made with an idealized image of the benefits to the family the child will bring (Lippman-Hand, 1977; Zelizar, 1985).

Childkeeping decisions stand in direct contrast to childbearing decisions. First, childkeeping decisions are made using information and advice provided by health care professionals to decide whether or not to keep a wanted pregnancy (Emery and Pullen, 1984). Although decisions regarding prenatal diagnostic techniques, selective abortion, and/or fetal treatments are deemed family decisions, health care professional and hospital preferences also are taken into consideration (Corea, 1985; Rothman, 1989; Scritchfield, 1987a). Families making childkeeping decisions may withhold knowledge of the pregnancy from their family and friends in order to guard against negative reactions to the decisions the family makes (Rothman, 1986; Kolker, 1989). In this isolated decision-making context, families attempt to make decisions based on information that is both definitive and probable (Ekwo et al., 1985). For example, a family may be told that a baby in utero has Down's syndrome but that the level of severity is not known and can be only roughly estimated (Emery and Pullen, 1984). Many fetal treatments are experimental and outcomes are uncertain (Rothman, 1989).

Second, based on the results of the prenatal testing, most families are reassured against certain defects, although fears of birth defects often resurface later in the pregnancy (Kolker, 1989). For the families who are told that their child has a birth defect, however, childkeeping decisions are made against the background of belief that the child will be unhealthy at birth and, in some cases, may not survive (Emery and Pullen, 1984). Families faced with this kind of information make their decisions comtemplating the worst possible case of the particular disorder (Lippman-Hand, 1977; Rothman, 1986, 1989). Instead of an idealized image of the benefits to the family, childkeeping decisions at this stage are made with an image of the financial, social, and personal costs to the family that the birth of a child with defects will create (Darling, 1979; Rothman, 1986; Seals, 1986).

Last, the interests of the family are no longer the primary concern in childkeeping decisions, particularly when a birth defect is diagnosed. Families who choose selective abortion face a difficult procedure and trauma at the loss of a wanted baby that may be similar to the experience of a miscarriage (Borg and Lasker, 1980; Rothman, 1986). The child's quality of life, if born, is not as dependent on family variables as are childbearing decisions. Families may be unable to assess what is best for the child when, for example, they must consider experimental treatments and chronic disabilities with a wide range of severity as is the case with many metabolic and chromosomal abnormalities (Emery and Pullen, 1984). Medical professionals may doubt whether or not families can objectively make decisions for the child; some health care professionals have suggested bringing fetal legal advocates into the decision-making process (Annas, 1984; Rothman, 1989). Here, the interests of the child are juxtaposed to the interests of the family (Overall, 1987).

As pregnancy is increasingly medicalized, that is, as more technologies and treatments are developed, even more families will be regarded as being at risk for having a child with birth defects, and more families will face both childbearing and childkeeping decisions (Corea, 1985; Blank, 1988; Rothman, 1989). With the expansion of prenatal diagnostic technologies, a wider range of known syndromes will be detectable, but the number of ambiguous diagnoses will also expand (Spallone, 1989). Beyond the medicalization of pregnancy decisions, childkeeping decisions may be even more difficult to make as the legality of selective abortion is questioned in many countries (Arditti et al., 1984; Hartman, 1987; Seals, 1991).

✱ BRENDA SEALS, Ph.D.

See also: Amniocentesis, History of; Prenatal Diagnosis: Overview; Selective Abortion

See **Guide to Related Topics:** Prenatal Diagnosis and Screening

Resources

Annas, George J. (1984, Aug). "Redefining Parenthood and Protecting Embryos: Why We Need New Laws." *Hastings Center Report*: 21-22.

Arditti, Rita et al. (1984). *Test-Tube Women: What Future for Motherhood.* Boston: Pandora Press.

Arney, William. (1982). *Power and the Profession of Obstetrics.* Chicago: The University of Chicago Press.

Blank, Robert H. (1988). "Making Babies: The State of the Art." In J. Gipson Wells (Ed.) *Current Issues in Marriage and the Family.* New York: MacMillan Publications, pp. 437-52.

Borg, Susan & Lasker, Judith. (1980). *When Pregnancy Fails.* Boston: Beacon Press.

Corea, Gena. (1985). *The Mother Machine: Reproductive Technologies from Artificial Insemination to Artificial Wombs.* New York: Harper and Row.

Darling, Rosalyn. (1979). *Families against Society: A Study of Reactions to Children with Birth Defects.* Volume 88. Sage Library of Social Research. Beverly Hills, CA: Sage Publications.

Diamond, Irene & Orenstein, Gloria. (1990). *Reweaving the World: The Emergence of Ecofeminism.* San Francisco, CA: Sierra Club Books.

Ekwo, E. et al. (1985). "Factors Influencing Maternal Estimates of Genetic Risk." *American Journal of Medical Genetics 20:* 491-504.

Emery, Alan E.H. & Pullen, Ian. (1984). *Psychological Aspects of Genetic Counseling.* New York: Academic Press.

Fox, Greer. (1982). *The Childbearing Decision: Fertility Attitudes and Behavior.* Beverly Hills, CA: Sage Publications.

Hartman, Betsy. (1987). *Reproductive Rights and Wrongs: The Global Politics of Population Control and Contraceptive Choice.* New York: Harper and Row.

Kolker, Aliza. (1989). "Advances in Prenatal Diagnosis." *International Journal of Technology Assessment in Health Care.* Cambridge: Cambridge University Press.

Lippman-Hand, Abby. (1977). "Genetic Counseling: Parents' Responses to Uncertainty." Unpublished thesis, McGill University, Montreal, Quebec, Canada.

Luker, Kristin. (1975). *Taking Chances: Abortion and the Decision Not to Contracept.* Berkeley, CA: University of California Press.

Massarik, Fred & Kaback, Michael. (1981). *Genetic Disease Control: A Social Psychological Approach.* Volume 116. Sage Library of Social Research. Beverly Hills, CA: Sage Publications.

Medical Genetics Center. (1978). "Father and Mother Know Best: Defining the Liability of Physicians for Inadequate Genetic Counseling." *Yale Law Journal 87*: 1488-515.

O'Brien, Mary. (1981). *The Politics of Reproduction.* Boston: Routledge & Kegan Paul Ltd.

Overall, Christine. (1987). *Ethics and Human Reproduction: A Feminist Analysis.* Boston: Allen & Unwin.

Rothman, Barbara. (1986). *The Tentative Pregnancy: Prenatal Diagnosis and the Future of Motherhood.* New York: Viking Penguin Inc.

———. (1989). *Recreating Motherhood: Ideology and Technology in a Patriarchial Society.* New York: W.W. Norton and Company.

Scritchfield, Shirley A. (1987a). "Becoming a Mother: Ambivalence and Oversight in the Feminist Perspective." Paper presented at the Annual Meetings of the Midwest Sociological Society, April, Chicago.

———. (1987b). "The Social Construction of Infertility: From Private Matter to Public Concern." Paper presented at the Society for the Study of Social Problems, August, New York.

Seals, Brenda. (1985). "Moral and Religious Influences on the Amniocentesis Decision." *Social Biology 32*: 13-30.

———. (1986). "Social Support, Well-Being and the Ease of Amniocentesis Decisions." Paper presented to the Society for the Study of Social Problems, August, New York.

———. (1989). *Families Who Must Decide: Amniocentesis and Childkeeping Decisions.* Unpublished dissertation, The University of Iowa, Iowa City, IA.

———. (1991). "Feminist Criticisms of Reproductive Technologies." Paper presented to the American Sociological Association, August, Cincinnati, OH.

Spallone, Patricia. (1989). *Beyond Conception.* North Hadley, MA: Bergin & Garvey Publishers.

Zelizar, Viviana A. (1985). *Pricing the Priceless Child.* New York: Basic Books.

CHIROPRACTIC CARE

An appreciation of the role of the chiropractic physician in the treatment of disease is predicated upon the understanding of the chiropractic vertebral misalignment as a perpetuating factor in disease. Chiropractors do not view disease as a static occurrence but as a process that manifests itself in certain signs, symptoms, and functional alterations. It is dependent upon irritants from the environment overcoming the innate resistance of an individual, with the nervous system acting as the mediating factor between. Chiropractic is concerned with prevention of these processes and the correction of existing structural lesions. The treatment, the chiropractic adjustment, is usually, although not always, a thrust administered by hand to the offending vertebrae in the plane that restores it to proper motion and function.

Obstetrics is a required course of study for all chiropractors, although they do not deliver babies. For many women, chiropractic is an important part of prenatal care. Chiropractic adjustments can correct the effects of spinal stress and postural distortions that may be causing unnecessary pain or discomfort during pregnancy. While some women are concerned about the safety of chiropractic adjustments during pregnancy, such adjustments can be modified to suit the patient's condition, and can be safely done at any time during pregnancy.

Adjustments are used to ensure that the pelvic bones are properly aligned in order to create an undistorted pelvic outlet, easing delivery. Pelvic bone adjustments have been found to stimulate past-due labors and nonprogressive labors that are due to pelvic outlet disproportion.

Low back, hip, and leg problems sometimes occur following the mechanical stress and trauma of pregnancy and delivery or due to pregnancy postural stress on the lumbar spine, sacrum, coccyx, and sacroiliac joints. Chiropractic adjustments can correct the insults to these joints following delivery. Regular chiropractic adjustments at recommended monthly intervals throughout the pregnancy will reduce the likelihood of symptoms.

Chiropractic care can also be important for the newborn to correct those spinal malpositions that are a result of birth trauma. Long, complicated labors where the infant's head was hyperextended or hyperflexed, causing a distortion of the cervical spine vertebrae or a shoulder dystocia that required a torquing effort by the birth attendant, or forcep delivery leading to a thoracic spine dysfunction, are situations where newborn chiropractic care can be helpful. These distortions in newborns, like adults, cause pain. This pain may be the foundation of infantile colic that is described as persistent, often violent crying for no apparent reason in otherwise healthy infants. It is different from normal crying because the distress does not stop when the infant's physiologic needs are met. A Danish study, published in 1989, showed a high incidence of cervical and thoracic spinal joint dysfunction in colicky infants. The spinal distortions can also inhibit normal function of the nerves associated with the vertebrae involved, inhibiting normal development.

Chiropractic adjustments are used to treat back pain associated with poor breastfeeding posture. Improper and tense posture by breastfeeding mothers strains mid-back musculature, leading to thoracic spinal dysfunction and pain. This tension-pain cycle leads to inhibited letdown reflex.

✷ TAMIE L. DIXON, D.C.

See also: Bodywork; Colic; Exercise Physiology in Pregnancy; Infant Movement

See **Guide to Related Topics:** Baby Care; Caregivers and Practitioners

Resources

Altman, Nathaniel. *The Chiropractic Alternative.* Los Angeles: P.J. Tarcher Inc., p. 33.

Fennison, Bernard E. (1981). *Low Back Pain.* Philadelphia: J.B. Lippincott Co., pp. 533-34.

Klougart, D.C., Nelsson, D.C. & Jacobson, D.C. (1989, Aug). "Infantile Colic Treated by Chiropractors: A Prospective Study of 316 Cases." *Journal of Manipulative Physiological Therapeutics 12:* 281-88.

Schafer, R.C. (1980). *Basic Chiropractic Procedural Manual.* Des Moines, IA: Associated Chiropractic Academic Press, p. I-1.

CHORIONIC VILLUS SAMPLING

Chorionic Villus Sampling (CVS) is a technique used for prenatal diagnosis of birth defects. CVS is done by inserting a catheter through the cervix or through the abdomen and suctioning some cells from the placenta. (The chorion is the membrane that surrounds the fetus early in the pregnancy and develops into the placenta; villi are hairlike projections from the membrane.) The procedure is performed under the guidance of ultrasound. Because the placenta has the same composition as fetal cells, the sample may be cultured in the laboratory and examined for chromosomal disorders, for example, the presence of an extra chromosome 21 (Down's syndrome). Biochemical disorders such as Tay Sachs may also be detected this way. However, neural tube defects, including spina bifida, cannot be diagnosed with CVS. A blood test, AFP (alpha-fetoprotein), may be done for this purpose.

The main advantage of CVS is that it is done earlier in the pregnancy than amniocentesis—at 9 to 12 weeks' gestational age. By comparison, amniocentesis cannot be done until the 12th to 16th week, with the results often taking another two weeks. If an abnormality is found and the parents decide on abortion, an early abortion is physically easier and safer. It should be remembered, however, that when the pregnancy is wanted, no abortion is easy. To the parents it represents the loss of a child, in some cases after years of difficulty in achieving or completing a pregnancy. Couples, their support networks, and health care providers should be aware that the emotional trauma cannot be avoided with CVS.

CVS is not risk-free. Studies have shown that the rate of combined pregnancy loss from all causes (including miscarriage, abortion of abnormal pregnancies, stillbirths, and neonatal deaths) is 7.2 percent after CVS, 5.7 percent after amniocentesis. Since most miscarriages occur in the first trimester, a miscarriage that follows CVS cannot be definitely attributed to the procedure; it may have been spontaneous. After adjustment for gestational age, researchers have determined that the CVS-related miscarriage rate exceeds that for amniocentesis by less than 1 percent. In centers with little experience in preforming CVS, the loss rate may be higher.

Beside making it possible to diagnose chromosomal disorders, CVS, like amniocentesis, can reveal the sex of the fetus. Knowing the baby's sex in advance may bring joy to some, disappointment to others. Some parents prefer not to be told. Some report that knowing the sex "personalizes" the baby and makes him or her more real, in addition to making it easier to shop for gender-stereotyped baby things. The disclosure of information on fetal sex also has a darker side. Because CVS is performed earlier in the pregnancy than amniocentesis, it may make it easier for a woman to abort a healthy baby just because it is of the "wrong" sex. There are no statistics on how many abortions are actually performed for this reason. In countries where a strong preference for male offspring is culturally ingrained, many famale fetuses are aborted, albeit illegally. This matter has raised a controversy among ethicists and health care providers.

Because of the risk associated with this invasive procedure, CVS is not recommended for all pregnant women. At present it is advised only for those who have had a history of genetic abnormalities or those aged 35 or older and hence faced with a somewhat higher-than-average chance of having a baby with chromosomal disorders. These women must decide what's right for them by weighing the information provided by genetic counselors together with their own feelings about genetic disorders, procedural risks, and abortion.

✷ ALIZA KOLKER, Ph.D.

See also: Amniocentesis, History of; Eugenics; Genetics; The Perfect Baby; Prenatal Diagnosis: Overview; Selective Abortion

See **Guide to Related Topics:** New Procreative Technologies; Prenatal Diagnosis and Screening

Resources

Green, Jeffrey E. et al. (1988, Feb). "Chorionic Villus Sampling: Experience with Initial 940 Cases." *Obstetrics and Gynecology 71* (2): 208-12.

Kolker, Aliza. (1989). "Advances in Prenatal Diagnosis." *International Journal of Technology Assessment in Health Care 5*: 601-17.

Kolker, Aliza, Burke, B. Meredith, & Phillips, Jane U. (1990, Fall). "Attitudes About Abortion of Women Who Undergo Prenatal Diagnosis." In Dorothy Wertz (Ed.) *Research in the Sociology of Health Care 9*: 49-73.

Rhoads, George G. et al. (1989, Mar 9). "The Safety and Efficacy of Chorionic Villus Sampling for Early Prenatal Diagnosis of Cytogenetic Abnormalitites." *The New England Journal of Medicine 320*: 609-17.

Wapner, Ronald J. & Jackson, Laird G. (1988, Jun). "Chorionic Villus Biopsy." *Clinical Obstetrics and Gynecology 31* (2): 328-43.

Wertz, Dorothy C. & Fletcher, John C. (Eds.) (1989). *Ethics and Human Genetics: A Cross-Cultural Perspective.* New York: Springer-Verlag.

CIRCUMCISION, FEMALE. *See instead* GENITAL MUTILATION, FEMALE

CIRCUMCISION, MALE

Circumcision is a surgical procedure in which the sleeve of skin that normally covers and protects the head of the penis is removed. As with any surgery, risks include surgical error, excessive bleeding, infection, and death.

Only in the United States will parents likely be asked to decide whether their newborn will be circumcised as a matter of routine. Children born in *any* European country, the former Soviet Union, Southeast Asia, China, Japan, or Latin America are rarely circumcised. The exceptions are that Jewish and Moslem children and those born in certain African countries and the Australian outback are usually circumcised.

Although the circumcision rate in the United States is declining, intense debate continues among physicians and also between parents, family members, and friends. In the late 1970s the U.S. circumcision rate was 85 percent; now it is less than 60 percent. If the decline continues at this rate, nonreligious circumcision may cease by the turn of the century. Yet, today, many prospective parents remain uninformed.

Beliefs about circumcision in the English-speaking countries—England, Canada, the United States, Australia, and New Zealand—have fluctuated. Circumcision was introduced about 100 years ago, during the Victorian era, in hopes of preventing masturbation and the many ills it was thought to cause—including asthma, epilepsy, alcoholism, and lunacy. Circumcision rates climbed rapidly until the 1940s. But today, nonreligious circumcision rates in England and New Zealand have dropped to zero; in Australia and Canada, they are about 25 percent and diminishing. Because beliefs about the preventive and curative powers of circumcision were never confirmed with research, the other English-speaking countries turned away from circumcision.

The United States remains the only country where a large proportion of male newborns are routinely circumcised for nonreligious reasons. Long after other countries abandoned routine newborn circumcision, American physicians continued to assert that the surgery provided health benefits. This was still true in 1979, even after the American Academy of Pediatrics, the American College of Obstetricians and Gynecologists, and the American Pediatric Urologic Society had all concluded that "there is no absolute medical indication for routine circumcision of the newborn." But, because circumcision is laden with social, cultural, religious, and sexual overtones, the debate goes on. Currently, unscientific, unsubstantiated assertions that circumcision prevents sexually transmitted diseases, including AIDS, are being made. The American Academy of Pediatrics neutralized its stand in 1989 by stating that "newborn circumcision has potential medical benefits and advantages as well as disadvantages and risks."

Today, almost all circumcisions in the United States are performed to prevent potentially and statistically unlikely future problems. Such thinking is reminiscent of the prophylactic tonsillectomies recommended for children a generation ago. When it became obvious that the risks exceeded the benefits, physicians rejected that procedure. As the public and the medical profession learn more about the risks and reputed benefits of routine nonreligious circumcision, it, too, may pass from the scene to join blood-letting and cupping in medical history. ✱ EDWARD WALLERSTEIN and MARILYN FAYRE MILOS, R.N.

See also: Circumcision Surgery; Genital Mutilation, Female

See **Guide to Related Topics:** Baby Care

Resources

"Report of the Ad Hoc Task Force on Circumcision." (1975). American Academy of Pediatrics. Washington, DC.

"Report of the Task Force on Circumcision." (1989). American Academy of Pediatrics. Washington, DC.

Wallerstein, Edward. (1980). *Circumcision: An American Health Fallacy.* New York: Springer Publishing Co.

———. (1980). "The Circumcision Decision." Seattle, WA: Pennypress, Inc. Pamphlet.

———. (1982). "When Your Baby Boy Is Not Circumcised." Seattle, WA: Pennypress, Inc. Pamphlet.

———. (1983). "Circumcision and Anti-Semitism: An Update." *Humanistic Judaism, XVI* (III): 43-46.

———. (1985). "Circumcision: The Uniquely American Medical Enigma." *Urologic Clinics of North America, 12* (1): 123-32.

———. (1986). "Circumcision: Information, Misinformation, Disinformation." San Anselmo, CA: National Organization of Circumcision Information Resource Centers.

CIRCUMCISION SURGERY

During a newborn circumcision, the infant is fastened spread-eagle to a plastic board with straps at the elbows and knees. A nurse scrubs his genitals with an antiseptic solution and covers the groin area with a surgical drape which has a hole in it to expose his penis. If a dorsal penile nerve block is used, two injections are given at the base of the penis. Although not always effective, the anesthetic reduces the stress response—if and while it is working. Once the effect has worn off, however, urination and defecation into the raw wound during the healing period cause obvious discomfort. Usually the surgery is done without anesthesia and is undeniably painful.

The foreskin of the newborn is normally attached to the glans (head of the penis) to provide protection from urine and feces during infancy. These two structures must be separated prior to circumcision. In order to perform this maneuver, two clamps are attached to the foreskin, a probe is inserted between the two, and the foreskin is torn from the glans. Another clamp is used to squeeze the foreskin lengthwise. This crushes blood vessels and prevents bleeding when the initial cut is made there. This cut enlarges the opening of the foreskin so the circumcision device can be inserted between the foreskin and the glans.

During the next stage of the surgery, the doctor clamps the foreskin against the circumcision instrument and then amputates it with a scalpel or scissors. One circumcision clamping device is removed immediately; another type remains tied in place for about a week while the remnant foreskin tissue dries up and falls off. Because of its prolonged attachment, this latter device is blamed for causing a higher incidence of postoperative infection.

As with any surgical procedure, circumcision has inherent risks, including hemorrhage, infection, mutilation, and even death. The potential benefits must be weighed against the potential risks. Since infant circumcision is very rarely necessary for therapeutic reasons, it is considered a prophylactic surgery. Specifically, how often is post-newborn circumcision necessary for therapeutic reasons? Wallerstein (1986) writes, "The Finnish National Board of Health in 1970 showed that 0.023% of males required hospitalization for foreskin problems (99.977% of Finnish males did not.) The U.S. rate is at least 50 times or 5,000% that of Finland . . . . The question is not foreskin problems, but the attitude of the American medical profession in pushing what most physicians throughout the world consider unnecessary surgery. Worldwide, foreskin problems are treated medically, rarely surgically."

Many Americans, having been subjected to other unnecessary surgeries—tonsillectomy, radical mastectomy, and hysterectomy—now question the need for circumcision. Many parents today believe that the foreskin is normal, healthy, functioning tissue; that circumcision serves no medical purpose and causes needless pain; that it leaves both physical and psychological scars; and that they do not have the right to make such a personal decision for their sons.

✷ MARILYN FAYRE MILOS, R.N.

See also: Circumcision, Male; Genital Mutilation, Female; Newborn Pain

See **Guide to Related Topics:** Baby Care

CLEFT LIP AND PALATE. *See instead* CENTRAL CLOSURE DEFECTS

CLITORIDECTOMY. *See instead* GENITAL MUTILATION, FEMALE

COLIC

Colic is an intermittent pattern of crying in a healthy, well-fed infant under three months of age that cannot be explained by any consistent theory or observation. Research has not produced an identifiable cause for this condition.

The proposed etiologies of colic are: gastrointestinal (GI) immaturity; central nervous system (CNS) immaturity; allergy; and infant temperamental factors that lead to parental anxiety and tension.

The gastrointestinal theory of etiology is supported by the observation that many young infants with intractable crying also show evidence of abdominal distention, flatulence, and irritability associated with feeding and bowel movements. This observation contributes to the choice of the term "colic" to describe this crying pattern. The work "colic" is derived from a form of the Greek work "kolikos," for colon. The GI theory of etiology indentifies swallowing air while feeding and inadequate burping as contributors to colic, and leads to recommendations for modifying feeding practices by feeding the baby slowly in an upright position and pausing frequently for burping. The infant whose colic is accompanied by gas and abdominal distention may, after careful physical examination rules out any abnormality, warrant prescription of antispasmodic medications as a method of decreasing GI irritability. Herbal remedies are used worldwide and include weak teas brewed from fennel, chamomile, anise, or comfrey. Despite the widespread belief that GI dysfunction is the cause of colic, there is little empirical data to support this theory.

Another proposed theory to explain colic is that the immature and developing central nervous system of a newborn baby may contribute to a lowered threshold to external stimulation. This lower threshold may cause the infant to cry in distress unless he or she is soothed in ways that override the stimulation of the ordinary environment. This theory is supported by observations that some newborn infants show an elevation in blood pressure and heart rate in response to environmental events such as sudden loud noises. Crying has been observed to decrease in some infants when they are swaddled or carried in a front pack, rocked, or exposed to continuous noise or vibrations, such as during car rides or when placed near a humming household appliance. Other interventions include encouraging the infant to suck on a thumb or pacifier, using a mechanical swing, massaging the infant, or going for walks outside. This neurological theory is also used as a rationale for the prescription of sedative medication for the colicky infant.

The theory that colic is caused by an allergic response is supported by studies that demonstrate symptom alleviation in some infants when cow's milk or other foods are removed from the diet of the breast-feeding mother, or cow's milk formula is replaced by a soy-based formula in the formula-fed infant. However, the majority of colicky infants do not improve with changes in diet, so this theory provides only a partial explanation and treatment plan.

The final theory of colic is that it is caused by temperamental characteristics of the infant. These characteristics include an innate lack of rhythmicity and predictability, a lower threshold of sensitivity to stimulation, and a high irritability and slower response to soothing, which makes it difficult for parents to read the infant's cues. The crying, irritable infant who cannot be soothed may cause the parents to become anxious as they try to respond to their infant's distress. Parents of colicky infants often express feelings of helplessness, frustration, anger, resentment, and rejection. These feelings are in conflict with the parents' desire to nurture the infant and can result in inconsistent responses to the baby's cues. Inconsistent parental responses may make it even harder for the colicky infant to settle down. This theory of infant colic supports interventions designed to alleviate parents' feelings of inadequacy or self-blame for the infant's behavior and to teach parents to read their baby's cues and respond consistently and calmly. Counseling by the health care provider, telephone contact, and parent support groups are effective interventions. Time away from caregiving responsibilities is essential, particularly for the mother. Knowledgeable professionals will recognize that although the infant's colic is self-limiting, the disruption of a family's transition to parenthood creates stresses that can persist beyond the newborn period.

Parents of newborn infants may confuse normal infant crying with colic. All newborn infants cry as a means of discharging tension and fatigue and as a precursor to other communication with caregivers. Crying behavior seems to peak between six to eight weeks of age and decline by 14 weeks. Interventions described to calm the colicky baby are appropriate for all infants. It is perhaps the success of these interventions with some babies and the lack of success with others that distinguishes true "colic" from normal newborn crying.

✱ MEG ZWEIBACK, R.N.

See also: Chiropractic Care; Swaddling
See **Guide to Related Topics:** Baby Care

Resources

Brazelton, T.B. (1962). "Crying in Infancy." *Pediatrics 29:* 579-88.
Carey, W.B. (1989). "Colic: Exasperating but Fascinating and Gratifying." *Pediatrics 84:* 568-69.
Levine, M. et al. (1983). *Developmental-Behavioral Pediatrics.* Philadelphia: W.B. Saunders Co., pp. 518-21.
Wessel, M.A. et al. (1954). "Paroxysmal Fussing in Infancy, Sometimes, Called Colic." *Pediatrics 14:* 421.

COMFORT OBJECTS

Parents either tolerate or struggle with young children over such behaviors as thumb-sucking, dragging a blanket or toy around, and needing a bottle into toddler years. The parent who reads childrearing books and articles may recognize that such attachments are "transition objects," which help the child move from union with the mother to a more "separate self" (Winnicott, 1987). On the popular TV show, "The Simpsons," the youngest child, Maggie, sucks a pacifier continually; some dolls available in stores suck their thumbs. Thus, the practice has become even more of an unquestioned norm. All of these behaviors may be cultural artifacts produced by attitudes toward mothering and child development.

Mothering in North America, when it includes nursing at all, does not tend to include nursing into toddlerhood. Lactation ends early (perhaps to six months), limiting the child's access to the mother body. Many youngsters (and bottle-fed youngsters from the start) turn to breast substitutes—objects or parts of their bodies, such as thumb and finger sucking and hair twirling—because they have species-specific biological and social needs for comfort contact (Cook, 1978). One child in a day care center, nursed for four years, answered a question differently from all others. When asked, "what do you hug when you are lonely?" children cited objects like "my blanket" and "my teddy bear." The nursed child said simply, "my mommy."

Much is lost by the use of comfort objects as substitutes for physical closeness with adult caregivers. When children are encouraged to develop an "automomous" self, they are discouraged from learning how to be, what Carol Gilligan (1983) calls, a "relational self." According to Jessica Benjamin (1988), a child can grow sovereign *within* a relationship to the mother, and this lesson carries over to all subsequent relationships. By encouraging a connection with the mother, rather than with a comfort object, cultural attitudes toward the maternal are no longer viewed as regressive, and children see that maturing does not mean having to settle for second best, or that satisfaction requires material objects.

✱ ROBBIE PFEUFER KAHN, Ph.D.

See also: Breastfeeding: Physiological and Cultural Aspects; Breastfeeding beyond Infancy
See **Guide to Related Topics:** Baby Care

Resources

Benjamin, Jessica. (1988). *The Bonds of Love: Psycholanalysis, Feminism, and the Problem of Domination.* New York: Pantheon Books.
Cook, Peter S. (1978). "Childrearing, Culture and Mental Health: Exploring an Ethological-Evolutionary Perspective in Child Psychiatry and Preventive Mental Health with Particular Reference to Two Contrasting Approaches to Early Childrearing." *The Medical Journal of Australia,* Special Supplement.
Gilligan, Carol. (1983). *In a Different Voice: Psychological Theory and Women's Development.* Cambridge, MA: Harvard University Press.
Winnicott, D.W. (1987). *The Child, the Family, and the Outside World.* Reading, MA: Addison Wesley.

COMMON COMPLAINTS OF PREGNANCY

Common complaints of pregnancy are basically normal side effects due to hormonal or physiological factors.

Nausea. Nausea is thought to be caused by high levels of estrogen and human chorionic gonadotrophin (HCG), which, while normal for pregnancy, require a period of maternal adjustment. Over 50 percent of women experience nausea to some degree. It usually abates by the 12th week. Relief may be found by (1) eating small amounts of food frequently, i.e., keep the stomach full; (2) increasing protein intake; (3) eating dry crackers or plain yogurt upon arising; (4) taking extra B-6—50 mg. at midday and 50 mg. at bedtime; (5) taking capsules of powdered ginger, three times a day; and (6) resting, relaxing, and slowing down.

Fatigue. Fatigue in early pregnancy is also due to high levels of estrogen and perhaps to a slowed metablic rate caused by progesterone. Plenty of rest is the obvious solution. Late in pregnancy, the sheer burden of carrying the baby and handling increased metabolic demands may lead to an increased need for sleep.

Headache. Headaches may be caused by circulatory distrubances, or as a reaction to hormone changes. Normal in early pregnancy, headaches may be a warning sign of pre-eclampsia in the latter half of pregnancy, especially if accompanied by swollen hands and face or visual disturbances. Simply lying down may help stimulate circulation and induce relaxation; cold cloths on the forehead and back of the neck may also help. Herbs like chamomile and skullcap may be taken, in consultation with a health care provider, in tea or tincture.

Frequent Urination. Frequent urination occurs in early pregnancy due to hormonally induced softening of the pelvic floor muscles, so that the enlarged uterus falls forward and impinges on the bladder. As the uterus grows and moves upward, the pressure is relieved, but at the end of pregnancy, the baby's head may press on the bladder as it enters the pelvis so that urination occurs more frequently again. It is fine to take more fluids early in the day and fewer in the evening, but limiting overall intake can be dangerous.

Dizziness and Fainting. Dizziness and fainting are due to circulatory disturbances caused by progesterone, which dilates major blood vessels so that blood tends to pool in the extremities, slowing return to the heart. Getting up slowly from resting positions, moving more slowly in general, and lying down when feeling faint are good common sense measures.

Constipation. Constipation in the first trimester is due to the softening of smooth muscle by progesterone; in later pregnancy, to the baby's head (or breech) compressing the intestines as it enters the pelvis. Fiber-rich foods such as bran cereals and raw vegetables, combined with two to three quarts of fluid daily, will usually help. Regular exercise stimulates the bowels and improves digestion. Over-the-counter laxatives, which may be harmful to the baby, should be avoided.

Hemorrhoids. Hemorrhoids are also caused by the softening action of progesterone, which causes blood vessels around the anus to dilate and prolapse downward. Later, the enlarged uterus may also put pressure on hemorrhoidal veins. Pregnant women should follow the guidelines for constipation, and avoid straining. Pelvic floor exercises (Kegels) may also help by stimulating circulation in the pelvic area. Pads of witch hazel may be applied to the area and are harmless (and are particularly soothing if kept chilled in the refrigerator).

Varicose Veins. Varicose veins are caused in the same way as hemorrhoids: Pressure of the baby in the pelvis late in pregnancy may hinder venous return from the legs, causing the veins to enlarge. Regular exercise is very important; swimming, in particular, is known to help. Clothes should not constrict the legs at any point (e.g., knee-highs or knee socks), but overall support with maternity support hose may help, as long as there is no constriction over the abdomen. Putting the feet up frequently during the day and wearing low-heeled shoes can make a difference. Many care providers recommend increased intake of vitamin E, up to 600 units daily.

Ankle Edema. Ankle edema is similar in origin to varicose veins, but more common. Nearly 40 percent of women experience some swelling of the ankles and feet towards the end of pregnancy. Often there is no lasting remedy until the baby is born, but putting the feet up periodically, changing positions throughout the day, and getting plenty of protein and fluid in the diet are useful measures. Pregnant women should strictly avoid diuretics, which seriously disrupt the metabolism and may cause harm to both mother and baby.

Leg Cramps. Leg cramps are also due to circulatory disturbances in the legs or pelvis. But they are mostly caused by pressure from the enlarged uterus on the nerves running through the pelivc area. They frequently occur in the night. It helps to straighten the affected leg, pulling toes towards the shin, or to quickly stand on a hard, cold surface (like the bathroom floor). Adequate intake of calcium, potassuim, and water are all important; calcium should be taken with vitamin C to aid absorption, and potassium can be found in bananas, oranges, and grapefruit.

Heartburn. Heartburn is caused by progesterone softening the valve that separates the stomach and esophagus, so that the acid contents of the stomach escape upward through the valve and cause a burning sensation. Heartburn is usually worse late in pregnancy when the baby puts pressure on the stomach, or when the mother is lying down and gravity cannot hold stomach acids in place. Small meals, plenty of fluids in small amounts, and sleeping/resting with head and shoulders elevated may be necessary. Some women find relief by taking digestive aids, such as papaya enzymes, with meals. But they should strictly avoid any bicarbonate of soda-based antacid, which can cause dangerous levels of fluid retention.

Shortness of Breath. Shortness of breath is caused primarily by the baby impinging on the diaphragm late in pregnancy, causing increased respiration. It helps to maintain good posture, to stretch with the arms over the head whenever feeling short of breath, and to breathe slowly and deeply.

Backache. Backaches are caused, once again, by progesterone, which softens the ligaments that support the growing uterus so that adjacent muscles are strained. Good posture is essential, as well as using the abdominal muscles to support the baby. Doing pelvic rocks (arching and straightening the back while on hands-and-knees) and wearing low-heeled shoes both help, as does adequate pillow support while sleeping.

✱ ELIZABETH DAVIS

See also: Bodywork; Herbal Treatments

See **Guide to Related Topics:** Pregnancy, Physical Aspects

Resources

Davis, Elizabeth. (1988). *Energetic Pregnancy.* San Francisco: Celestial Arts.

Jensen, Margaret & Bobak, Irene. (1985). *Maternity and Gynecological Care: The Nurse and the Family.* St. Louis, MO: C.V. Mosby Company.

Varney, Helen. (1988). *Nurse-Midwifery.* Boston: Blackwell Scientific Publications.

CONDOMS

The ordinary condom was not historically a contraceptive. The incentive for its development was the desire for protection against venereal disease. Many tropical peoples used coverings for the penis for a variety of reasons—sometimes for protection against tropical disease or insect bites, and sometimes as marks of rank, as amulets, or merely as decoration. Such a sheath was first publicized as a specifically antivenereal disease precaution by the Italian anatomist Fallopius (discover of the "Fallopian tubes"), an early authority on syphilis. In a book written in 1564 he suggested a linen cloth be made to fit the penis. By the 18th century the device had been transformed into something made of animal membrane, making it waterproof and effective as a contraceptive. By this time sheaths for the penis were widespread, were often given to men by prostitutes, and had acquired a wealth of charming nicknames and euphemisms: the English riding coat, assurance caps, the French letter, bladder policies, instruments of safety, condoms, cundums, and, of course, prophylactics. Through the mid-19th century books of home remedies gave instructions for making condoms.

Condoms were introduced to the American public in large part by World War I soldiers. Increased public consciousness about the possible spread of venereal disease from soldiers' and sailors' contacts broke through official prudery to force government action. By 1919 the Army alone was spending one million dollars a year on venereal disease prevention through sex education and prophylactics. Even fundamentalist Secretary of the Navy Josephus Daniels was forced, after initial oppositon, to authorize passing out condoms to sailors. A total of 4,791,172 men served in the U.S. armed forces in this war. This could only mean the introduction of condoms into public use on a mass scale. Strengthening that conclusion, comments from working-class Massachusetts and Rhode Island women interviewed in some small oral history projects suggest that many of them first learned about birth control from their husbands who had been in the service (Gordon, 1990). In the late 19th century the development of vulcanized rubber had made the manufacture of condoms easier and cheaper. Then after the First World War, latex made condoms thinner and cheaper yet, and their sales increased enormously.

Condoms—far more effective than chemical treatment in preventing veneral disease—had been available for centuries; rubber condoms since the mid-19th century. What made condoms objectionable to conservatives was that they had to be given out before the fact to be useful, possibly encouraging intercourse, and that they had a clear contraceptive capability. But the pressure to employ such effective devices was irresistible. The Navy had been distributing condoms before shore leave since early in the century.

It is surprising that the developers and popularizers of birth control did not pay more attention to the advantages of the lowly condom—cheap, disposable, easy, quick, and pocket-sized. The condom has a lower effectiveness rate than the properly used diaphragm but a much higher effectiveness rate than the improperly used diaphragm. Recent calculations of the effectiveness rates of contraceptives as actually used (thus excluding non-use, but including improper use) show a small difference between condom and diaphragm: the former producing 14.9 unwanted pregnancies per 100 women per year, and the latter 12.0 unwanted pregnancies.

One reason for the neglect of the condom was fear of licensing sexual immorality. The condom was well suited to be, as it indeed became, the chief contraceptive for "sinners." It was easy to get and required no doctors or special instructions.

Recently feminist health experts have argued for a greater emphasis on barrier methods of contraception, but there does not yet appear to be a major shift in focus. Since the mid-1960s there has been an increasingly successful movement, now further promoted by AIDS concerns, to relax or eliminate laws against advertising, displaying, and selling over-the-counter nonprescription contraceptives such as condoms, foams, and spermicidal creams or jellies. The proportion of unmarried people using condoms increased from 9 percent to 16 percent between 1982 and 1987, but among the married, condom use did not increase; the overall proportion of those using diaphragms declined in that period, while the pill experienced a revival.

The impact of AIDS on birth control is similar to the impact venereal disease had on birth control in the World War I era. Conservatives are finding themselves caught between two unpleasant choices—easing access to, or possibly even encouraging the use of, a form of birth control, or surrendering one of the only prophylactic devices against V.D. Condoms have been particularly objectionable to sexual conservatives because they are so distinctly nonmedical, and thereby unlicensed, without any intermediaries buffering popular access; on the other hand, it has been less acceptable to restrict condom availability because they are a man's device. The conservative "compromise" has been to try to keep condoms from certain captive populations. For example, in 1987 the Reagan administration moved to prevent provision of condoms in federal prisons on the grounds that doing so might contradict the regulation against homosexual sex. President Reagan himself several times insisted that the right approach to anti-AIDS work among teenagers is to promote sexual abstinence, not condom education or distribution. In fact there is widespread support for publicizing the availability of condoms. A 1987 Harris Poll showed approximately three-fourths of Americans, 85 percent of those aged 18 to 24, favorable to TV ads for condoms to help stop AIDS.

The most contested aspect of condom access, as previously mentioned, arises from proposals to make contraception and sex education available to teenagers, and to open birth-control clinics in schools. Even in New York City, which already operates eight health clinics in high schools and which has a high rate of AIDS, resistance had blocked, until recently, the provision of condoms in these clinics. The task is difficult even without opposition. It is more difficult to get boys rather than girls to take responsibility for birth control, and condoms require care in their use. A 1988 evaluation of the effectiveness of AIDS education for adolescents produced negative findings, for the same reason that programs against teenage pregnancy work poorly: the "just say no" to sex approach doesn't make sense to most teenagers.

There is not yet clear evidence about the impact of AIDS on heterosexual condom use. As noted, the proportion of unmarried people relying on condoms for their birth control has increased, but many men are still resistant to using condoms and women find it difficult to insist. AIDS is yet another reason why birth-control programs are being pushed to take a broad approach in considering all the circumstances of people's sexual lives. To be responsible to their clients, birth-control clinics must now consider disease prevention as well as birth control, recommending contraceptives that also protect against AIDS. Indeed, this should previously have been the policy in relation to other venereal diseases, but traditions of prudery and a narrow focus on contraceptive effectiveness as opposed to overall well-being prevented it. V.D. dangers constitute, of course, and additional argument against hormonal methods or IUDs and in favor of barrier methods. At the same time, birth-control clinics face another dilemma: they usually recommend combining condoms with an additional contraceptive, such as a spermicide, because condoms are not as effective as some other contraceptives, but they fear that this recommendation might actually deter condom use by making it too burdensome.

Condom distributors have reported sales increases of 20 to 25 percent and some drugstores report increases of up to 50 percent. Condom manufacturers have used the occasion to experiment with more aggressive advertising, some of it aimed at women. The breaking of taboos and silences about sex that the advertising necessitates seems likely to further the general cultural movement toward more explicitness about sex (a goal oddly called "desensitization"). "It's a way of talking about sex and having fun with it, to break down social fears against buying condoms"—this is not a family-planning advocate or an AIDS worker speaking, but an advertising executive.

✷ LINDA GORDON, Ph.D.

See **Guide to Related Topics:** Contraception

Resource

Gordon, Linda. (1990). *Woman's Body, Woman's Right: Birth Control in America.* Revised Edition. New York: Penguin Books.

CONTRACEPTION: DEFINING TERMS

All societies have provided ways of regulating fertility. In modern American society, while there is growing interest in treating and preventing infertility, most concern with fertility regulation has focused on avoiding births and limiting fertility. While obviously an issue of great personal and intimate concern, it is also an area of political concern. The language used to discuss approaches to limiting fertility—on both the individual and the societal levels—reflects a variety of perspectives. What follows are definitions of the most commonly used terms in the area of fertility limitation.

Birth Control. While sometimes used interchangeably with family planning and contraception, these terms do not mean exactly the same thing. Birth control is the most general and broadest of these terms, encompassing all means to limit fertility, including contraception, sterilization, and induced abortion. The birth control movement, which originated in England in the 1800s, promoted smaller families for the well-being of both society and the individual. In the United States, Margaret Sanger, founder of Planned Parenthood, first popularized the term "birth control."

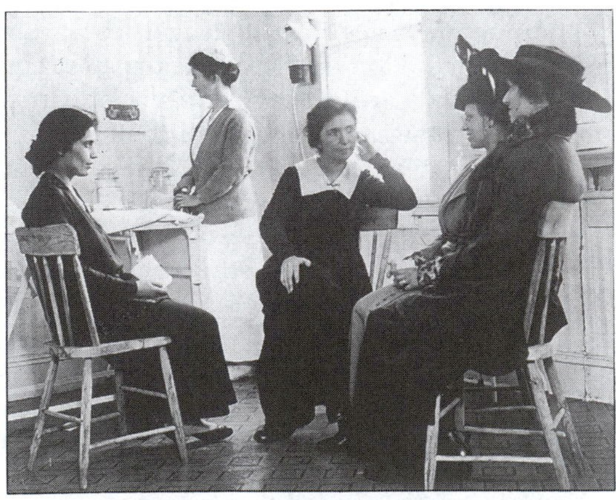

Margaret Sanger at the Brownsville Clinic in Brooklyn, New York, 1916. Photo courtesy of Planned Parenthood of New York City.

Family Planning. This is a more "user friendly" term than birth control. Advocates of family planning provide information and contraceptives to enable people to voluntarily regulate not only the number but also the spacing of their children. Family planning programs maintain that voluntary contraception is the best way to approach unwanted or unplanned pregnancies because it improves maternal and child health while contributing to effective personal freedom for couples.

Contraception. Contraception refers to conscious voluntary acts to prevent unintended pregnancy. There are reversible and permanent methods. Reversible methods of contraception include hormonal methods (oral contraceptive, injection, inplant, and vaginal ring), intrauterine devices (hormone or copper-releasing), barrier devices (diaphragm, condom, spermicide, foam, sponge, cervical cap), periodic abstinence (natural family planning, rhythm), and withdrawal (coitus interruptus—removal of the penis before ejaculation). Permanent or nonreversible methods of contraception, otherwise known as sterilization, are tubal ligation for women and vasectomy for men.

Abortion. Abortion can be spontaneous or induced. Spontaneous abortions (also called miscarriages) occur from natural causes; induced abortions are voluntary interruptions of pregnancy. Abortions can be induced either medically or surgically.

Abortion is termination of a pregnancy before the embryo or fetus is capable of independent life. The definition of abortion also relates to how one defines pregnancy. Abortion foes claim that pregnancy begins with fertilization, the union of egg and sperm, and label as abortifacients any contraceptive that might prevent implantation of that egg. Most scientists and physicians, on the other hand, believe that pregnancy begins when the fertilized egg is implanted in the lining of the uterus.

Population Control. This term is used by people who believe it desirable to use laws or government policies to curb or expand population growth to reach demographic goals. "Population control" is not found in dictionaries or encyclopedias of demographic or population terms, and it is not generally used by professionals who work in the population or family planning fields. People who believe in the importance of population control maintain that rapid population growth in the poorest countries is one of the world's most serious problems, to be solved through incentives, deterrents, or coercion, if necessary, for the good of society. On the other hand, some people believe that development alone will solve population growth problems and accuse population and family planning programs of a eugenics-inspired conspiracy to coerce couples into having fewer children. A third approach, that described under family planning, emphasizes information about and voluntary adoption of contraception.

✱ SANDRA WALDMAN, M.A., M.S.

See **Guide to Related Topics:** Contraception

Resources

Ehrlich, Paul R. (1968). *The Population Bomb.* New York: Ballantine Books.

Hartmann, Betsy. (1987). *Reproductive Rights and Wrong: The Global Politics of Population Control and Contraceptive Choice.* New York: Harper & Row.

Hatcher, Robert A. et al. (Eds.) (1989). *Contraceptive Technology: International Edition.* Atlanta, GA: Printed Matter, Inc.

Pressat, Roland (Ed.) (1985). *The Dictionary of Demography.* New York: Christopher Wilson, Basil Blackwell Inc.

Ross, John A. (Ed.) (1982). *International Encyclopedia of Population.* New York: The Free Press.

COUVADE: ANTHROPOLOGICAL ASPECTS

Originally regarded as male mimicry of the female role in childbirth, couvade has come to include a wide range of behavior associated with the father during pregnancy and birth. The biological irrelevance of couvade attracted the attention of early anthropologists as a classic example of the human potential for cultural divergence. In French the term "couvade" means "hatching," and is apparently drawn from the behavior of certain birds, such as mute swans, in which both parents participate in incubation. Indeed, any man whose wife was in labor in 17th-century France was called "Godard," the same name given to any individual swan. As applied to humans, couvade includes any restrictions in behavior and diet required of fathers, during pregnancy or following birth. In particular, couvade refers to the historically reported practice of Mediterranean-area fathers taking to bed for convalescence upon the birth of their child.

The earliest clear record of couvade comes from Marco Polo's 13th-century trip to the Upper Mekong area in China. "Then her husband goes to bed and takes the baby with him and lies in bed for forty days without leaving it except for necessary purposes. And all his friends and kinsmen come to see him and cheer him up and amuse him. This they do because they say that his wife has had her share of trouble in carrying the infant in her womb, so they do not want her to endure more . . ." (Polo, 1958). Before the demise of peasant communities in Europe, numerous accounts of couvade were collected in the Mediterranean area (Dawson, 1929). Common to all of these accounts is behavior required of the father but not directly involving the mother.

Turn-of-the-century reports appeared as remote parts of the Americas were explored. The most detailed accounts come from Im Thurn (1967) and Penard (see Roth, 1924) describing the highlands of the Guianas. As the mother returns to her duties after giving birth in the forest, the father takes to the hammock, refraining from his activities for several days, even weeks. In fact, the man has already prepared for impending fatherhood with dietary abstinences. Now, he limits his diet to cassava gruel and refrains from smoking or handling weapons. Meanwhile, women provide for his care.

It is assumed that any deviation will have a negative effect on the child. Although the mother is considered to have produced the child's body, the father is given credit for producing the child's soul. Moreover, the mystical connection of the father is not severed as early as the umbilical cord. Until the fontanelle at the back of the skull begins to harden, the child's spirit is considered capable of leaving the body and following the father. Therefore, the father must not hunt, since he would be unable to tell if the spirit-child was in the path of his arrows. If he must travel, the father must walk slowly and avoid thorns. In crossing a log or river, he would either place sticks or leave a floatable object to allow the spirit to follow his path.

Other restrictions were based on bodily correspondence, or connections between the father and the child. The father must not scratch himself vigorously nor eat foods difficult to digest. Another set of proscriptions was based on more arbitrarily imagined causal relationships. For example, certain meats ingested by the father were thought to cause spots on the child's skin.

This last set of restrictions was invoked during pregnancy as well as after delivery.

Three major theoretical approaches have attempted to account for the existence of couvade. Certain early evolutionists, rather innovatively saw couvade as a transitional practice allowing patrilineal kinship arrangements to overwhelm matrilineal forms. Couvade served as a device that allowed individual men to claim control over their offspring from birth forward (Tylor, 1889). The functionalist Malinowski (1953) found in couvade a socially acceptable way for the father to adjust to a new role and responsibilities. Some diffusionists claimed couvade as proof of the irrationality of culture and as evidence of a prehistoric "heliolithic" religion spread throughout world populations (Dawson, 1929).

The ethnographer Metraux (1948) pointed out that quite dissimilar practices had been improperly linked as forms of couvade. Chinese and Mediterranean men who took to bed were essentially convalescing in seclusion. However, Amazonian fathers took to their hammocks because all men of this area recline in their hammocks at times of inactivity. More important to the South American fathers were their restrictions from activities that would endanger a child, for it was believed that the child's spirit would follow him, being newly separated from the father.

Past confusion in the portrayal of couvade does not invalidate the relevance of further analysis in contemporary studies. Recent growth in the anthropology of gender may encourage a revival of interest. Such studies could examine the significant potential for manipulation of power stemming from couvade. Here Tylor's point is relevant: couvade strengthens the father's claim to the child. For the Macusi, couvade claims "a mysterious connection between the child and its father—far closer than that which exists between the child and its mother" (Im Thurn, 1967).

In analyzing relations of power inplicit in couvade, the future roles of the father, mother, and child must be recognized. What obligations are respectively incurred and what privileges are gained by each? How well are the child's paternal obligations balanced by the early acknowledgment of paternal responsibility? Analyses of egalitarian societies reveal a significant potential for manipulation of labor in a kin-ordered mode of production. Further studies of couvade may clarify its role in mobilizing labor, as a father incorporates children into a hunting or farming workforce, as well as the immediate reality of the father resting while the mother returns to a full workload. On the other hand, the slow, but extensive development of paternal commitment to the child may ensure that the mother is not alone in tending and provisioning the child, keeping the father in an active role in childcare. Lastly, the South American variety of couvade facilitates both a physical and emotional tenderness from the father to the child. Couvade may accord more social rights to the child at birth than would otherwise be issued. ✱ THOMAS BURGESS

See also: Couvade: Clinical Aspects

Resources

Dawson, Warren R. (1929). *The Custom of Couvade*. Manchester, England: Manchester University Press.

Im Thurn, Everard F. (1967). *Among the Indians of Guiana*. New York: Dover.

Malinowski, Bronislaw. (1953). *Sex and Repression in Savage Society*. London: Routledge and Kegan Paul.

Metraux, Alfred. (1948). *The Couvade: The Handbook of South American Indians*. Volume 5. Washington, DC: Smithsonian Institute.

Polo, Marco. (1958). The Travels of Marco Polo. Baltimore, MD: Penguin.

Roth, Walter E. (1924). "An Introductory Study of the Arts, Crafts, and Customs of the Guiana Indians." 38th Annual Report of the Bureau of American Ethnology. Washington, DC: Smithsonian Institute.

Tylor, E. B. (1889). "On a Method of Investigating the Development of Institutions Applied to Laws of Marriage and Descent." *Journal of the Royal Anthropological Institute 18*: 254-56.

COUVADE: CLINICAL ASPECTS

Couvade is derived from the French verb *couver*, which means "to brood or hatch." Ritual couvade, a magico-religious practice that has been observed among many primitive people, consists of deliberate actions performed by the husband of a childbearing women during pregnancy or the early postpartum (Frazer, 1910; Broude, 1988). Prior to or during the birth of the child, the expectant father takes to his bed and mimics the labor and delivery with expressions of pain, exhaustion, and other behaviors associated with childbirth. After delivery, the new father observes dietary restrictions, may not cut any objects, avoids the use of weapons, and does not hunt certain animals.

The couvade syndrome, in contrast, is the husband's *unintentional* acquisition of symptoms similar to those experienced by his wife during pregnancy and the postpartum (Trethowan and Conlon, 1965). The couvade syndrome may appear at any time during pregnancy or the early postpartum. Physical symptoms include indigestion, nausea and/or vomiting, bloating, changes in appetite, food cravings, increased urination, constipation, diarrhea, hemorrhoids, abdominal pain, backache, headache, elusive toothache, dyspnea, sensitivity to odors, skin rashes, itching, lassitude, leg cramps, unintentional weight gain, and syncope. Although discussions of the couvade syndrome emphasize physical symptoms, psychological symptoms have also been reported. These symptoms include body image changes and changes in mood, such as irritability, restlessness, insomnia, nervousness, inability to concentrate, anxiety, depression, or, conversely, and enhanced sense of well-being.

The couvade syndrome has been documented in several countries, including the United States, Canada, Great Britain, Sweden, British Honduras, and Kenya. The reported incidence of at least one couvade syndrome symptom ranges from 10 to 97 percent of husbands of childbearing women.

The couvade syndrome is thought to be a manifestation of the husband's identification with his pregnant wife (Trethowan, 1972), although research findings have failed to support this supposition (Drake, Verhulst, and Fawcett, 1988; Fawcett, 1977; Fawcett, Bliss-Holtz, Haas, Leventhal, and Rubin, 1986; Fawcett and York, 1987). Ambivalence about the pregnancy and unconscious envy of the woman's ability to create a child also are postulated to influence the development of the couvade syndrome, but these factors have not yet been substantiated through research. Factors that have been found to be associated with presence of symptoms of the couvade syndrome include ethnic minority status, working class social status, positive affective involvement in pregnancy, perceived economic stress, and health problems prior to the pregnancy (Clinton, 1986; Strickland, 1987; Twiggs, 1988). Absence of symptoms is associated with hostility and empathy (Strickland, 1987; Zelles, 1989). Furthermore, there is some evidence that the presence or absence of a symptom in the husband is directly related to the presence of absence of that symptom in his pregnant wife (Sullivan and Fawcett, 1991).

✷ JACQUELINE FAWCETT, Ph.D., R.N., FAAN

See also: Couvade: Anthropological Aspects

See **Guide to Related Topics:** Pregnancy, Psychological Aspects

Resources

Bogren, Lennart Y. (1986). "The Couvade Syndrome." *International Journal of Family Psychiatry 7*: 123-36.

Broude, Gwen J. (1988). "Rethinking the Couvade: Cross-cultural Evidence." *American Anthropologist 90*: 902-11.

Clinton, Jacqueline. (1986). "Expectant Fathers at Risk for Couvade." *Nursing Research 35*: 290-95.

Drake, Mary Louise, Verhulst, Dianna, & Fawcett, Jacqueline. (1988). "Physical and Psychological Symptoms Experienced by Canadian Women and Their Husbands During Pregnancy and the Postpartum." *Journal of Advanced Nursing 13*: 436-40.

Drake, Mary Louise, Verhulst, Dianna, Fawcett, Jacqueline, & Barger, Diane F. (1988). "Spouses' Body Image Changes during and after Pregnancy: A Replication in Canada." *Image: The Journal of Nursing Scholarship 20*: 88-92.

Fawcett, Jacqueline. (1977). "The Relationship between Identification and Patterns of Change in Spouses' Body Images during and after Pregnancy." *International Journal of Nursing Studies 14*: 199-213.

———. (1978). "Body Image and the Pregnant Couple." *American Journal of Maternal Child Nursing 3*: 227-33.

Fawcett, Jacqueline, Bliss-Holtz, Virginia Jane, Haas, Mary Beth, Leventhal, Marcia, & Rubin, Mary. (1986). "Spouses' Body Image Changes during and after Pregnancy: A Replication and Extension." *Nursing Research 35*: 220-23.

Fawcett, Jacqueline & York, Ruth. (1986). "Spouses' Physical and Psychological Symptoms during Pregnancy and the Postpartum." *Nursing Research 35*: 144-48.

———. (1987). "Spouses' Strength of Identification and Reports of Symptoms during Pregnancy and the Postpartum." *Florida Nursing Review 2*(2): 1-10.

Frazer, J. G. (1910). *Totemism and Exogamy*. Volume 4. London: Macmillam

Lipkin, Mack, Jr., & Lamb, Gerri S. (1982). "The Couvade Syndrome: An Epidemiologic Study." *Annals of Internal Medicine 96*: 509-11.

Munroe, Robert L. & Munroe, Ruth H. (1971). "Male Pregnancy Symptoms and Cross-sex Identity in Three Societies." *Journal of Social Psychology 84*: 11-25.

Strickland, Ora L. (1987). "The Occurrence of Symptoms in Expectant Fathers." *Nursing Research 36*: 184-89.

Sullivan, Jacqueline & Fawcett, Jacqueline. (1991). "The Measurement of Family Phenomena." In A.L. Whall & J. Fawcett (Eds.) *Family Theory Development in Nursing*. Philadelphia: F.A. Davis Company, pp.69-84.

Trethowan, W.H. (1972). "The Couvade Syndrome." In J.G. Howells (Ed.) *Modern Perspectives in Psycho-obstetrics*. New York: Brunner/Mazel, pp. 68-93.

Trethowan, W.H. & Conlon, M.F. (1965). "The Couvade Syndrome." *British Journal of Psychiatry 111*: 57-66.

Twiggs, Francis T. (1988). "Expectant Fathers: Couvade Syndrome and Stress." *Dissertation Abstracts International 48*: 2112B.

Zelles, Peter A. (1989). "Social Support and Empathy as Predictors of Couvade Syndrome in Male Partners of Abortion Patients." *Dissertation Abstracts International 49*: 2880B.

CREATION STORIES IN WESTERN CULTURE

Obstetricians use the term "birth from above" to signify cesarean section in contrast to "birth from below," where the mother gives birth by her own powers down and through her body. "Birth from above," associated with the male, has a long and distinguished heritage in creation stories of Western culture.

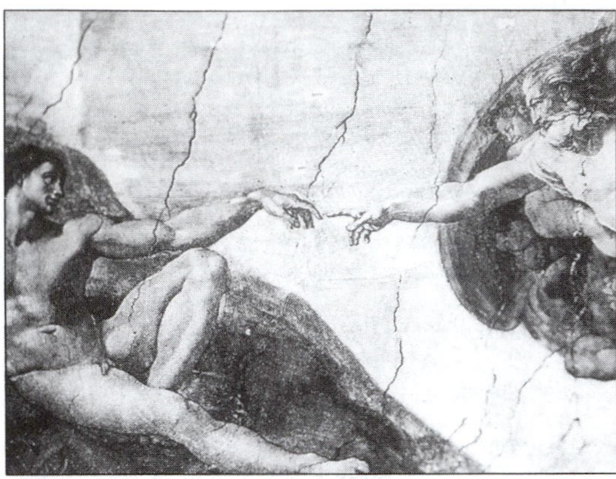

God creating man, Michelangelo's frescoes in the Sistine Chapel. Photo courtesy of Kip Kozlowski.

Because these stories of origin describe how order is established, they also are stories of power. In the Hebrew Bible, Yahweh creates solely through words, apart from matter; he is located above what he creates. "God's spirit hovered *over* the water. God *said* 'Let there be light,' and there was light" (Genesis 1:2-3)(emphasis added). In the Christian Gospel according to St. John, Jesus instructs that "unless a man is born from above/he cannot see the kingdom of God" (John 3:3). This second birth—the first is biological from the mother—is spiritual and ensures eternal life.

These two examples are from living religions of Western culture. In the Greek creation myth by Hesiod, the female creates but the male usurps her power (Hesiod, 1953). Mother Earth gives birth to all things out of her body; her grandson, the sky god Zeus, supersedes her. Zeus consolidates his power by giving birth to Athena from his head, who might otherwise, not under his control, have posed a threat to him. He couldn't accomplish this extraordinary birth, however, without first swallowing Athena's pregnant mother. Several centuries later, the Greek playwright, Aeschylus, depicts an Athena highly loyal to her father. Deciding a matter of social justice in favor of father right over mother right, Athena says, "I am always for the male with all my heart, and strongly on my father's side" (Aeschlyus, 1953).

As the Aeschylus example shows, transferring generativity from female to male erodes the mother/child bond. In the creation story by Hesiod, this bond threatened male power, for Mother Earth and her son Cronus conspire to castrate Father Sky. But their alliance came about because Father Sky, in fear of being overthrown by his offspring, pushed them back inside Mother Earth, undoing their birth. Father Sky's aggression became the reason for the formation of a mother/child bond hostile to the male.

These famous stories exert a lively influence on current attitudes toward childbirth. The foremost obstetrical text in the United States, *Williams Obstetrics*, provides a brief history of the procedure and the term "cesarean" (Hellman and Pritchard, 1971). After stating that cesareans did not become safe until the 20th century, the text associates cesarean birth historically with distinguished offspring, the powerful of the world like Pliny, Scipio Africanus, and Julius Caesar. The most telling geneological connection occurs in the following sentences:

> In Genesis (11:21) it is written: "And the Lord God caused a deep sleep to fall upon Adam, and he slept: and he took one of his ribs, and closed up the flesh instead thereof." Are we to conclude from this statement that general anesthesia and thoracic surgery were know in pre-Mosaic times? It would probably be just as logical to draw comparable conclusions about the beginnings of cesarean section from the myths and fantasies that have come down to us. (Hellman and Pritchard, 1971. pp. 1163-64)

Although the conscious intention in this example may be to distinguish myth from science, the unconscious result is just the opposite. Birth from above now is connected not only to figures of power in world history but to God himself. Far from being a case of thoracic surgery, Eve becomes the first recorded case of a cesarean section, as can be seen in early woodcuts showing her emerging from Adam's side; the obstetrician becomes the chief inheritor of birth from above.

Central texts of Western culture also can influence childbearing women who learn a cultural preference for birth from above brought about by the male, and absorb cultural ambivalence toward the mother/child bond. How can a six- to eight-week childbirth class undo cultural norms accumulated over a lifetime? For the effect of these texts is not confined to the classroom, or to those women and men fortunate enough to acquire a college education. Theologian Connie Buchanan explains that biblical accounts shape people's conceptions about the organization of the human world; these conceptions in turn affect their actions (Buchanan, 1987). Thus, central values of a culture may influence the actual social processes of reproduction. One woman on a public television show ruefully said, after an unwanted cesarean, that she had gotten her "miracle baby."

By contrast, what myths belong to the childbearing woman? Myths, according to Mircea

Eliade, quoted by Marta Weigle, "describe the various and sometimes dramatic breakthroughs of the sacred (or the 'supernatural') into the world" (Weigle, 1989). As a woman's body opens in birth and new life emerges, perhaps an aperture to what Carol Christ has called "powers of being and life," or the sacred, appears (Christ, 1980). A central text of Western culture, Dante's *Divine Comedy*, invites this perspective (Dante, 1939). At the end of the poem, when Dante comes before the creating source of all things, he first sees a simple light. Looking closer, a circle of three colors like a rainbow becomes visible, at the center of which is "our own likeness." What is this representation of the sacred if not a birth image? The circle with a human face in the center suggests the emerging baby's head ringed round by the mother's body. Without intending to, Dante dignifies birth from below because he cannot find any more powerful imagery for birth from above. But *actual* birth from below embodies the sacred in the world of "matter," a term that shares its root with the word "mother." Myths that confer prestige upon childbearing women help strengthen the belief in women's powers to give birth.

✱ ROBBIE PFEUFER KAHN, Ph.D.

See also: Art and Birth Metaphors: Nature-Culture Dichotomies; Goddess Imagery

See **Guide to Related Topics:** Literature and the Arts

Resources

Aeschylus. (1953). *Oresteia*. Translated by Richard Lattimore. Chicago: University of Chicago Press.

Buchanan, Constance H. (1987). "The Fall of Icarus: Gender, Religion, and the Aging Society." In Clarissa W. Atkinson, Constance H. Buchanan, & Margaret R. Miles (Eds.) *Shaping New Vision: Gender and Values in American Culture*. Ann Arbor, MI: UMI Research.

Christ, Carol. (1980). *Diving Deep and Surfacing: Women Writers on Spiritual Quest*. Boston: Beacon Press.

Dante, Alighieri. (1939). *The Divine Comedy*. Translated by John Sinclair. New York: Oxford University Press.

Hellman, Louis M. & Pritchard, Jack A. (Eds.) (1971). *Williams Obstetrics*. 14th edition. New York: Appleton-Century-Crofts.

Hesiod. (1953). *Theogony*. Translated by N.O. Brown. Indianapolis, IN: Bobbs-Merrill.

The Jerusalem Bible, Reader's Edition. (1966). Garden City, NY: Doubleday.

Kahn, Robbie Pfeufer. (1988). "Women and Time in Childbirth and during Lactation." In Freida Forman (Ed.) *Taking Our Time: Feminist Perspectives on Temporality*. New York: Pergamon Press.

———. (forthcoming) *The Language of Birth: Female Generativity in Western Tradition*. Chicago: University of Illinois Press.

Weigle, Marta. (1989). *Creation and Procreation: Feminist Reflections on Mythologies of Cosmogony and Parturition*. Philadelphia: University of Pennsylvania Press.

CUSTODY DETERMINATIONS: GENDER BIAS IN THE COURTS

Although 80 to 85 percent of custodial parents in North America are mothers, this does not mean that women always "win" custody of their children in a divorce; in many cases, mothers retain custody when fathers choose not to fight for it. In the last 15 to 20 years, when American fathers fought for custody, they won custody 63 to 70 percent of the time whether or not they were previously absent, distant, parentally uninvolved, or violent (Pascovitz, 1982; Polikoff, 1982, 1983; Weitzman, 1985; Chesler, 1991a; Takas, 1987). Similar trends have been documented in Canada (Lahey, 1989) and in Australia, France, Holland, Great Britain, Ireland, Norway, and Sweden (Smart and Sevenhuijsen, 1989; Chesler, 1991b). The data show that fathers do not win because mothers are unfit or because fathers have been participatory parents but because mothers are expected to meet more stringent standards of parenting. This double standard has been documented by ten 1989-1990 United States Supreme Court reports on "Gender Bias in the Courts," which confirm that there is one set of expectations for mothers and another, less demanding set for fathers. These reports have been published by the State Supreme Courts of Florida, Maryland, Massachusetts, Michigan, Minnesota, Nevada, New Jersey, New York, Rhode Island, and Washington. The reports explore the different ways in which both men and women are discriminated against in terms of custody. Although these studies demonstrate that some fathers are sometimes also discriminated against, it appears evident that women face greater custodial vulnerability.

In 62 countries surveyed worldwide, fathers were legally and automatically entitled to custody whether or not they fulfilled their paternal obligations (Chesler, 1991a). Mothers were obligated to care for and support their children without any reciprocal rights; most rose to the occasion heroically. Nevertheless, women had few rights as *individuals* and no rights as mothers over and against the rights that men have over women, that husbands have over wives, that fathers have over mothers, and that states have over citizens. In general, mothers everywhere are vulnerable to legalized father right. In custody battles, mothers are routinely punished for having a career or job or for staying home on welfare; for committing heterosexual adultery or for living with a man out-of-wedlock or for remarrying; or for failing to privide a male role model. Mental health experts tend to blame mothers, but not fathers, for any problems a child may have; to praise fathers, but not mothers, for the good they may do; and to have one set of expectations for mothers and another, lesser set for fathers (Caplan and Hall-McCorquodale, 1985a, 1985b). Experts also tend to label mothers diagnostically when they fall short of idealized expectations of motherhood (Caplan and Hall-McCorquodale, 1985a, Caplan, 1989a, 1989b; Surrey, 1990).

Divorcing fathers increasingly use the threat of a custody battle as an economic bargaining chip. When fathers persist, a high percentage win custody because judges tend to view the higher male income and the father-dominated family as in the "best interests of the child" (Polikoff, 1982, 1983). Many judges also assume that because the father who fights for custody is rare, he should therefore be rewarded for loving his children, or that something is wrong with the mother.

What may be "wrong" with the mother is that she and her children are being systematically impoverished, psychologically and legally harassed, and physically battered by the very father who is fighting for custody. However, mothers are often custodially punished for leaving a violent husband or, when the marriage does end, for staying. Some people, including psychiatrists, lawyers, and judges, deal with male domestic violence by concluding that women have either exaggerated it or have provoked it.

Today, more and more mothers, as well as the leadership of the shelter movement for battered women, are realizing that women risk losing custody of their child(ren) if they seek more (or sometimes any) child support or stability from fathers in terms of visitation. Mothers also risk losing custody if they accuse fathers of beating or sexually abusing them or their children—even or especially if these allegations are detailed and supported by experts (Pennington and Woods, 1991).

While neither mothers nor child advocates allege paternal incest more often during a custody battle than at other times, some father's rights activists, including lawyers and mental health experts, insist that the mothers or children are lying or misguided, and the media continue to cite an increase in "false" maternal allegations. Pearson and Thoennes (1988) and Paradise (1989) confirm that at least two-thirds of the maternal allegations about child molestation are true and that the remaining one-third may also be true but are difficult to substantiate. One-third of the allegations may therefore be considered "unfounded" but not necessarily "false."

Custodially embattled fathers kidnap children three times as often as mothers do (Chesler, 1991a). While some mothers or fathers may impede visitation, mothers rarely kidnap; when they have, it's almost never been to vindictively withhold a child from a loving father but to save a child from abuse.

Psychiatrists, psychologists, and social workers have tended to trust what a father tells them. They routinely minimize male violence and routinely pathologize the normal female response to violence. While at some level the evaluators do believe that these fathers have done something "wrong," they don't want to penalize them for their actions. Even when allegations of paternal violence are believed, the father is then exonerated by virtue of having a mental illness. Male mental illness is seen as either temporary or amenable to "therapeutic" intervention. Judges are reluctant to order a wife-batterer or child-abuser out of the house or into jail; based on such psychiatric evaluations, they can, instead, order violent fathers into therapy or mediation. Violent or mentally ill fathers rarely lose their rights to visitation or custody; mothers, however, do (Deed, 1991; Fineman, 1989; Crean, 1988).

✱ PHYLLIS CHESLER, Ph.D.

See also: Domestic Violence and Pregnancy
See **Guide to Related Topics:** Legal Issues

Resources

Caplan, P.J. (1989a). *Don't Blame Mother: Mending the Mother-Daughter Relationship.* New York: Harper & Row.

———. (1989b). *Assessing the Assessor: What You Need to Know.* Preliminary analysis of the Law Society of Upper Canada's quesionnaire survey of mental health professionals who conduct child custody assessment. Paper presented to the Law Society of Upper Canada, Toronto, December 1989.

Caplan, P.J. & Hall-McCorquodale, I. (1985a). "Mother Blaming in Major Clinical Journals." *American Journal of Orthopsychiatry* 55: 345-53.

———. (1985b). "The Scapegoating of Mothers: A Call for Change." *American Journal of Orthopsychiatry 55*: 610-13.

Chesler, P. (1976). *Women, Money and Power.* New York: William Morrow and Co.

———. (1989a). *Sacred Bond: The Legacy of Baby M.* New York: Vintage Books/Random House.

———. (1989b). *Women and Madness.* New York: Harcourt Brace Jovanovich.

———. (1990). *About Men.* New York: Harcourt Brace Jovanovich.

———. (1991a). *Mothers on Trial: The Battle for Children in Custody.* New York: Harcourt Brace Jovanovich.

———. (1991b, Feb). "Mothers on the Run and Other Atrocities in Sweden." *On the Issues,* p.1.

Crean, S. (1988). *In the Name of the Fathers: The Story Behind Child Custody.* Ontario: Amanita Enterprises.

Deed, M.L. (1991, Feb). "Court Ordered Child Custody Evaluations: Helping or Victimizing Vulnerable Families. *Psychotherapy*, pp. 19-91.

Fineman, M. (1989). "The Politics of Custody and Gender: Child Advocacy and the Transformation of Custody Decision Making in the U.S.A." In C. Smart and S. Sevenhuijsen (Eds.) *Child Custody and the Politics of Gender*. Sociology of Law and Crime Series. London, New York: Routledge.

Lahey, K.A. (Ed.) (1989). "Women and Custody." *The Canadian Journal of Women and the Law* 3 (1)

Paradise. J. (1989). "Substantiation of Sexual Abuse Charges When Parents Dispute Custody or Visitation." *Paediatrics 81*.

Pascovitz, P. (1982). *Absentee Mothers*. Totowa, NJ: Alanheld Universe.

Pearson, J. & Thoennes, N. (1988). "Summary of Findings from the Sexual Abuse Allegations Project." In E. Nocholson (Ed.) *Sexual Abuse Allegations in Custody and Visitation Cases: A Resource Book for Judges and Court Personnel*. Washington, DC: American Bar Association National Resource.

Pennington, H.J. & Woods, L. (1991). *Legal Issues and Legal Options in Civil Child Sexual Abuse Cases: Representing the Protective Parent*. New York: National Center on Women and Family Law.

Polikoff, N. (1982). "Why Mothers Are Losing: A Brief Analysis of Criteria Used in Child Custody Determinations." *Women's Rights Law Reporter* 7 (235).

———. (1983). "Gender and Child Custody Determinations: Exploding the Myths." In I. Diamond (Ed.) *Families, Politics and Public Policy: A Feminist Dialogue on Women and the State*. New York: Longman.

Smart, C. & Sevenhuijsen, S. (Eds.) (1989). *Child Custory and the Politics of Gender*. Sociology of Law and Crime Series. London, New York: Routledge.

Surrey, J.L. (1990). "Mother Blaming and Clinical Theory." *Women & Therapy* 10 (1/2): 83-97.

Takas, M. (1987). *Child Custody: A Complete Guide for Concerned Mothers*. New York: Harper & Row.

Weitzman, L.J. (1985). *The Divorce Revolution: The Unexpected Social and Economic Consequences for Women and Children in America*. New York: Macmillan

---

C.V.S. *See instead* CHORIONIC VILLUS SAMPLING

DAILY FETAL MOVEMENT COUNTING

As far back in written history as the Bible, fetal movement *in utero* has been recognized as a reassuring indication of a healthy pregnancy: "For behold, the moment that the sound of thy greeting came to my ears, the babe in my womb leapt for joy" (Luke 1:44-45) and "The children jostled each other within her . . . ." (Genesis 25:22). It is only recently that measurements of fetal movement have been used clinically to assess fetal well-being.

The use of Daily Fetal Movement Counting requires the pregnant woman to count and record the number of her baby's movements each day. Studies done over the last 20 years related to maternal perception of fetal activity and use of Daily Fetal Movement Counting charts (DFMC) indicate a correlation between fetal activity and fetal well-being (Pearson and Weaver, 1976; Sadovsky and Polishuk, 1977; Harper et al., 1981; Neldam, 1980; Rayburn, 1980; Rayburn et al., 1980; Leader, Baillie, and Van Schalkwyk, 1981; O'Leary and Andrinopoulos, 1981). Various researchers have reported maternal perception of fetal movements as being 75.7-90.3 percent accurate (Pearson and Weaver, 1976; Rabinowitz, Persitz, and Sadovsky, 1983).

DFMC is an inexpensive, uncomplicated, noninvasive, and clinically effective method of assessing fetal well-being in both low- and high-risk pregnancies. This is especially significant when one considers that, in a study conducted at the Hospital of the University of Pennsylvania between June 1, 1980, and May 31, 1981, Liston reported that 70 percent of all stillborns weighing greater that 1000g resulted from otherwise seemingly normal pregnancies (Liston et al., 1982; Davis, 1987).

The assessment of fetal movements may provide information regarding the status of the uteroplacental unit and the integrity of the fetal nervous system. Clinically, it is generally agreed that vigorous fetal activity demonstrates fetal well-being. A marked decrease or cessation of fetal movement may be indicative of intrauterine fetal compromise. Many health care providers are now using fetal movement information as one of several screening tools to help identify the fetus at possible risk. Though fetal activity varies with the individual fetus, many researchers agree that fewer than 10 movements within 12 hours constitutes an "alarm signal" requiring NST (nonstress test) follow-up (Pearson, 1977; Sadovsky and Polishuk, 1977). A change in the usual movement pattern of the fetus, and a sudden violent increase in movement followed by complete cessation of movement, or no movement within eight hours is almost invariably an indication of acute fetal distress and/or death. Immediate follow-up should be initiated by a health care provider.

Differing methods of counting fetal movements have been developed by various researchers. While there is, as yet, no universally accepted method of fetal movement counting, most research supports the fact that the use of DFMC has been shown to decrease fetal death (stillbirths) and poor fetal outcomes by providing the mother and health care provider with early warning signals that the fetus may be at risk.

* MARGARET R. PRIMEAU, R.N., M.B.A.

See also: Fetal Movement; Nonstress Tests

See **Guide to Related Topics:** Prenatal Diagnosis and Screening

Resources

Davis, L. (1987, Jan-Feb). "Daily Fetal Movement Counting. A Valuable Assessment Tool." *Journal Nurse-Midwifery 32* (1): 11-19.

Ehrstrom, C. (1979). "Fetal Movement Monitoring in Normal and High-Risk Pregnancy." *Acta Obstetricia et Gynecologica Scandinavica Supplement* (80): 1-32.

Harper, R.G. et al. (1981, Sept 1). "Fetal Movement, Biochemical and Biophysical Parameters, and the Outcome of Pregnancy." *American Journal of Obstetrics and Gynecology 141*(1): 39-42.

Leader, L.R., Baillie, P. & Van Schalkwyk, D.J. (1981, Apr). "Fetal Movements and Fetal Outcome: A Prospective Study." *Obstetrics and Gynecology 57* (4): 431-36.

Liston, R.M. et al. (1982, Oct). "Antepartum Fetal Evaluation by Maternal Perception of Fetal Movement." *Obstetrics and Gynecology 60* (4): 424-26.

Neldam, S. (1980, Jun 7). "Fetal Movements as an Indicator of Fetal Well-Being." *Lancet 1* (8180): 1222-24.

O'Leary J.A. & Andrinopoulos, B.C. (1981, Jan). "Correlation of Daily Fetal Movements and the Nonstress Test as Tools for Assessment of Fetal Welfare." *American Journal of Obstetrics and Gynecology 139* (1): 107-08.

Pearson, J.F. (1977, Apr 21). "Fetal Movements—A New Approach to Antenatal Care." *Nursing Mirror 144* (16): 49-51.

Pearson, J.F. & Weaver, J.B. (1976, May 29). "Fetal Activity and Fetal Well-Being: An Evaluation." *British Medical Journal 1* (6021): 1305-07.

Rabinowitz, R., Persitz, E. & Sadovsky, E. (1983, Jan). "The Relation Between Fetal Heart Rate Accelerations and Fetal Movements." *Obstetrics and Gynecology 61* (1): 16-18.

Rayburn, W.F. (1980, Sept 15). "Clinical Significance of Perceptible Fetal Motion." *American Journal of Obstetrics and Gynecology 138* (2): 210-12.

———. (1987, Dec). "Monitoring Fetal Body Movement." *Clinical Obstetrics and Gynecology 30* (4): 899-911.

Rayburn, W.F. et al. (1980, Sept 15). "An Alternative to Antepartum Fetal Heart Rate Testing." *American Journal of Obstetrics and Gynecology 138* (2): 223-26.

Sadovsky, E. & Polishuk, W.Z. (1977, Jul). "Fetal Movements in Utero: Nature, Assessment, Prognostic Value, Timing of Delivery." *Obstetrics and Gynecology 50* (1): 49-55.

DEAFNESS AND CHILDBEARING CONCERNS

The issues of prenatal care, labor, and birth are the same for the deaf woman as for any other woman. The only difference is that many deaf people depend on American Sign Language (ASL) as their sole method of communication, and in most hospitals, clinics, and doctor's offices, there is no one fluent in this language. The situation is identical to one in which a woman from France or Turkey would find herself if she went into a clinic in which none of the staff spoke French or Turkish.

It should not be assumed, however, that every deaf woman uses ASL; that needs to be determined, if possible, before the deaf woman arrives for her appointment. Some deaf people rely on lip reading and speech as their method of communication. A smaller number of deaf people prefer to communicate through writing. However, if the deaf woman in question is a signer, it is important for her to either be served by a medical professional who is fluent in ASL or else to hire an interpreter. If the deaf woman is sophisticated and comes from a middle-class background, she may have already arranged to have an interpreter with her. However, it is always best to ask the woman what method of communication she prefers and whether she will be bringing her own interpreter.

If the agency or doctor's office needs to hire an interpreter, that can be done through an interpreter referral agency. The National Registry of Interpreters for the Deaf in Silver Spring, Maryland, can act as a resource. Any interpreter hired should be certified by the Registry. The cost for the services of a certified interpreter ranges from $50 to $70 for the first two hours.

When using an interpreter, the health care consultant needs to remember these things:

1. He or she should sit next to the interpreter, and they should both face the deaf person so that she can watch both of them at the same time.
2. The health care consultant should talk directly to the deaf woman, not to the interpreter. For example, it is correct to say, "I understand, Mrs. Jones, that you are here for a pregnancy test." It is incorrect to say, "Ask Mrs. Jones if she is here for a pregnancy test."
3. The consultant should not make comments or ask questions of the interpreter that would be uncomfortable for the deaf person to hear.

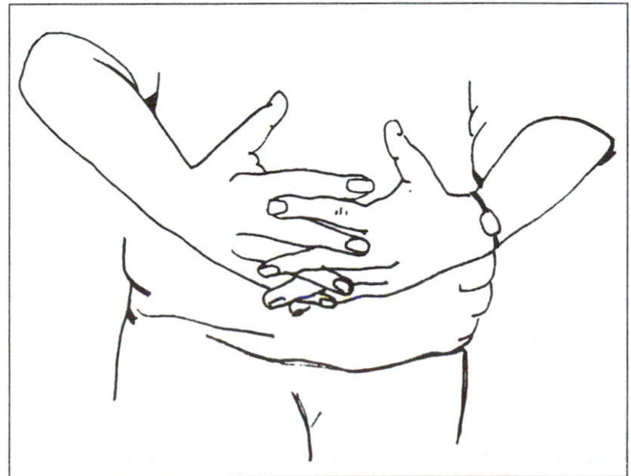

"Pregnant" in American Sign Language (ASL). Illustration courtesy of Meryl Weinman, Ph.D.

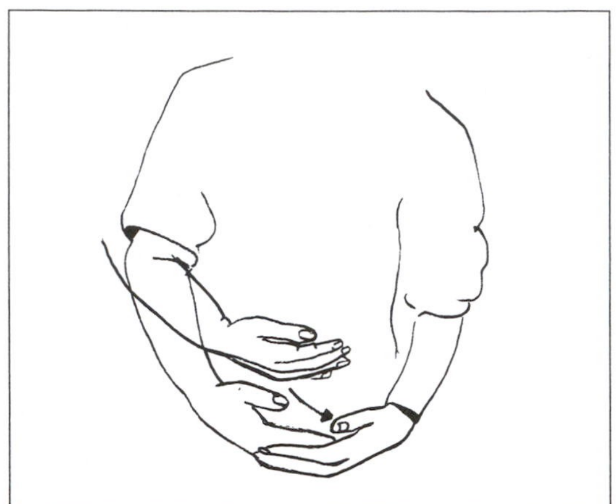

"Birth" in American Sign Language (ASL). Illustration courtesy of Meryl Weinman, Ph.D.

The interpreter will be signing everything said.

4. The consultant should not ask the interpreter for his or her opinion. The job of the interpreter is simply to facilitate communication between the health care provider and the deaf person.

If the deaf person is oral (communicates through speech and lip reading) an interpreter will not be necessary. The health care provider does need to keep in mind that he or she should look directly at the deaf person and make lip movements clear. It is not necessary or preferable to speak any louder than normal.

One issue that is unique to deaf women who seek medical attention for pregnancy will be their attitude regarding the likelihood of giving birth to a deaf child. If both parents of the unborn child are deaf and if the parents themselves come from families in which hereditary deafness is present, then it is very likely that the child will be born deaf. A genetic counselor will, no doubt, discuss this possibility with the deaf parents. All of the suggestions to facilitate communication with the deaf mother apply to the genetic counseling session as well.

Health care providers should not assume that the idea of having a deaf baby will be traumatic, upsetting, or even sad to the deaf parents. Many deaf couples state that they would prefer to have deaf children since then they will all communicate in the same language and become part of the deaf community. Other deaf people want very much to have a hearing child and will be upset upon being informed that their child is deaf. The first audiological exam is usually administered around three months; however, it is now possible to diagnose deafness at birth through a procedure known as the Auditory Brain Response (ABR). In families where hereditary deafness is present, the first exam is often given very early since these parents anticipate the possibility of deafness in their offspring. In these families, there are often several generations of deaf parents, grandparents, uncles, aunts, cousins, and siblings.

The deaf child who is born to deaf parents will grow up in an environment somewhat different from the deaf child born to hearing parents. As stated above, if the child is born to a family in which hereditary deafness is prevalent, he or she will grow up surrounded by deaf relatives and will become part of the deaf community at a young age. The most unifying factor of the deaf community is the fact that its members share a common language—American Sign Language or ASL. ASL is a language with its own syntax and grammar, different from English. It is not a universal language; for example, in France, the deaf community uses French Sign Language; in Israel the deaf community uses Israeli Sign Language. The deaf child who has deaf parents begins to learn ASL spontaneously in the first year of life by watching and imitating the signing of his or her parents. By two or three years of age, the deaf child is a fluent signer. Once the child reaches school age, many deaf parents opt to send their child to a school where he or she will learn to speak in order to become more integrated into the "hearing world."

When hearing parents are made aware that their child is deaf, they are presented with several different options as to how to facilitate their child's development and education. The two conflicting philosophies focus on whether the child should be raised with or without the use of sign language. Oralism is the name of the philosophy that advocates early introduction of the hearing aid, lip reading, and intensive training of residual hearing. The oral philosophy ascribes to the point of view that sign language should not be used, particularly in early childhood. Oralists propose that if the deafness is diagnosed early and the child receives the proper intensive training, he or she can learn to speak and will be able to function more like a hearing person. At the opposite extreme are those members of the deaf community who advocate early use of ASL and involvement in the deaf community, and even sometimes reject the use of the hearing aid. There are also several intermediate positions that propose the use of both sign language and lip reading. Hearing parents are faced with an assortment of conflicting philosophies regarding the best way to raise their deaf child. At the same time, one must keep in mind that hearing parents who have just found out their child is deaf are often in a state of desperation and mourning. The most valuable advice a health care professional can give such parents at this time is to encourage them to seek counseling and to explore all options thoroughly before making a decision that will influence the relationship they will form with their child, as well as set the course of their child's life.

✱ SUSAN KOLOD, Ph.D.

See also: Disability, Childbearing with; Disability, Parenting with

Resources

Meadow, K.P. (1980). *Deafness and Child Development*. Los Angeles: University of California Press.
Sacks, O. (1989). *Seeing Voices: A Journey into the World of the Deaf*. Los Angeles: University of California Press.
Walker, L.A. (1986). *A Loss for Words: The Story of Deafness in a Family*. New York: Harper and Row Publishers.

DECISION MAKING: NEWBORN CARE

Parents generally make decisions about health care for their children in cooperation with the health care professionals of their choice. However, the parents' right to make such decisions can be superseded by law; in the United States, all states have child neglect laws that permit officials to intervene on behalf of children and to provide medical care when the state decides that such care would best serve the child (Thomson, 1991).

In the past decade, judges and juries have heard hundreds of disputes in which parents fought for the right to use unconventional medical care, or to refuse care for their children, while doctors and hospitals insisted on treating the children with traditional medical methods. Almost always, courts have ruled against the parents and have granted governmental agencies the right to implement medical procedures. In some cases, the state has assumed custody of the child, and parents have been jailed (Thomson, 1991).

In the early 1980s, the "Baby Doe" regulations were promulgated, stating that no infant could be denied treatment solely on the basis of a disabling condition. These regulations could have required doctors and hospitals to provide maximum treatment to virtually all infants. However, in June of 1986, the U.S. Supreme Court ruled that the Baby Doe regulations were not authorized under Section 504 of the Rehabilitation Act of 1973. The Court agreed with the President's Commission on Medical Ethics that parents should be the primary decision makers for their children, but also emphasized that the state, not the federal government, has the authority to intervene under its existing laws if parents fail to act in the child's best interests (Scully and Scully, 1987).

Although most court cases have involved seriously ill children, their outcomes have ramifications for parents making decisions about health care for any child—for example, deciding whether or not to have a newborn child examined by a physician. In general, a physician or other health care worker is not legally permitted to care for a child without informed parental consent. Proposed treatments must be thoroughly explained, and all questions must be answered to the parents' satisfaction. However, the right to parental consent can be overruled in an emergency situation. In virtually all cases, it is the doctors, not the parents, who make the determination that there is a genuine emergency (Backus, n.d.).

Parents whose religious beliefs or personal preferences would lead them to choose alternative health therapies often think that they have lost their rights to make decisions about care for their children. Some believe that they have also lost the right to practice the tenets of their religion, such as refusing blood transfusions or using prayer instead of medical treatments. Although for many years proponents of prayer healing had managed to win considerable legal protection, a 1988 California Supreme Court ruling in the Walker case has left such rights in doubt. The court's written opinion stated that the state has a "compelling interest in assuring the provision of medical care to gravely ill children whose parents refuse such treatment on religious grounds . . . prayer treatment will be accommodated as an acceptable means of attending to the needs of a child only insofar as serious physical harm . . . is not at risk" (Thomson, 1991). In other words, prayer healing and, by implication, other forms of alternative treatment, will be allowed by the court so long as they never fail a standard of excellence that conventional medicine is not expected to meet. Nathan Talbot, a spokesperson for the Christian Science Church in Boston, estimates an overall death rate of Christian Science children between four days of age and 14 years to be 23 per 100,000 versus 51 per 100,000 in the general population. Children who do not receive blood transfusions lower their risk for acquiring hepatitis and HIV (AIDS) infections.

Parents may wish to spare their infants from painful, invasive procedures. To quote one doctor: "You can expect that virtually all doctors will treat an infant when there is doubt about the full nature of the child's condition or the possible benefits of treatment. . . . Typically, when faced with a life-or-death situation, most neonatologists treat the infant aggressively . . . You may be asked to give permission for a variety of tests and procedures, such as x-rays, blood tests, spinal tap, CAT scan, EEG . . . blood transfusions, inserting a chest tube, and possibly putting the infant on a respirator" (Scully and Scully, 1987).

Also at issue is payment for treatment. Can parents who refuse treatment for their children be forced to pay the doctors who insist on such care? If parents to not have adequate insurance coverage and financial resources, payments often will be made by Medicaid or Social Security; however, the choice of treatment options may thus be dictated by the source of payment rather than by the parents' wishes (Backus, n.d.).

At present, an unfortunate adversarial situation has been developing in which parents are pitted against doctors, with parents' rights viewed in opposition to children's rights. Parents who question the value of mainstream medical treatments need to be informed about state laws and about their rights. They need to be part of a community with similar beliefs, whether or not those beliefs are based on religion. Since the courts rarely intervene when parents and doctor agree, it is important to seek out doctors whose philosophy of care is compatible with their own. Many hospitals have set up infant bioethics committees for parents faced with making decisions about care for their newborn babies. If possible, parents should talk to other parents to find out how the committee operates, and what to expect when it meets (Scully and Scully, 1987).

✱ PAT DE LA FUENTE

See also: Vaccinations

See **Guide to Related Topics:** Legal Issues

Resources

Backus, Lois, (Ed.) (n.d.) "Your Child's Health: A Parents' Rights Guide." *People's Medical Society Health Bulletin*, 14 East Minor Street, Emmaus, PA 18049.

Scully, Thomas & Scully, Celia. (1987). *Playing God: The New World of Medical Choices*. New York: Simon and Schuster.

Thomson, Bill. (1991, Feb). "Treating Your Sick Child: Are Parents Free to Choose Alternative Therapies?" *East West: The Journal of Natural Health & Living*: 40-50.

DELAYED CHILDBEARING: SOCIAL FACTORS

Between 1970 and 1986, the number of women who delayed the birth of their first child until they were in their 30s quadrupled (Ventura, 1989). Effective and available contraception and other social changes made it possible for couples to postpone childbearing. While young women continue to give birth at high rates, the most significant demographic changes are occurring among older women having a first child.

During the 1970s the increases in first births were greatest among women between the ages of 30-34; during the 1980s, women between the ages of 35-40 showed the greatest increases in first births (Ventura, 1989, p. 1675). This suggests that women are continuing to delay the onset of parenthood and that they are also continuing to extend the age for first births. The number of first births to women ages 30-40 rose from 42,000 in 1970 to 182,000 by 1986; the number of first births to women between the ages of 35 and 39 rose from 12,000 in 1970 to 44,000 by 1986 (Exter, 1988, p. 63).

According to Stephanie Ventura (1989), there are four factors that account for this changing pattern of age at first birth, the first of which is a change in the timing of marriage. Since the 1960s, young people increasingly have postponed marriage by several years. In conjunction with delayed marriage, an increased divorce rate further delayed childbearing for many couples. Between 1970 and 1986, there was a 21 percent increase in women between the ages of 25 and 29 who were not married.

A second factor is the changing birthrate for women in their 20s, particularly among well-educated women. In the five years between 1970 and 1975, there was a one-third reduction of first births to women in their 20s and a 50 percent reduction among women who were college graduates. One consequence of these reductions in rates of first births is an increasingly large percentage of women in those age categories who are childless. In 1970, only 12 percent of women ages 30-34 were childless; by 1986, 25 percent of women in that age range were childless.

The third significant factor is that there are presently more women in these age categories than there were before. These are the women born in the post-World War II baby boom years; born in their own demographic bubble. Between 1970 and 1986, there was an 68 percent increase in the number of women between the ages of 25 and 39.

The fourth demographic trend that presaged the current pattern of delayed parenthood was that most women questioned in national surveys in the 1960s answered that they only wanted to have one child, and that 10 percent of the women in their early 30s planned to remain childless (Ventura, 1989, p. 1675).

While the demographic trends may have portended the current pattern of delayed first births among U.S. women, little else seems to prepare older first-time parents for their experience. "I feel like I need to be superwoman, constantly deflecting an array of potentially dangerous forces with my two small wrist bands"—35-year-old woman banker, mother of a one-year-old child (Whiteford, field notes). The same woman expressed the sentiments of many new mothers, but particularly those women who are older and already established in relatively powerful and high-stress jobs when she said: "I feel as though I'm an acrobat in the circus, spinning plates that go faster and faster. I don't know how long I can keep them all up in the air." Pressure at work, marital stress, and a highly dependent infant in combination with the lack of social supports often encountered by older new parents often cause severe disruptions in the early postpartum months (Whiteford and Sharinus, 1986). At the same time, these older first-time parents tend to be better educated, more financially secure, and more emotionally stable than younger couples. Based on their research and their analysis of others' research, Baldwin and Nord (1984, p. 32) suggest that many couples who delay childbearing find "the psychological impact of parenthood has been powerful and positive for these men and women and, in general, something they did not expect [the powerful effect] nor for which they were prepared" (Baldwin and Nord 1984, p. 30).

Whether babies born when parents are older cause disruptions in the carefully planned life—"Paradise Lost" (to paraphrase Dr. T.B. Brazleton paraphrasing Milton) or "Paradise Found" (by adding emotional depth to already established lives)—depends not only on the family, but also on how society responds to them. Good, affordable child care, and flexible working hours are two of the greatest needs expressed by new parents. Older working mothers are much less likely than younger working mothers to rely on relatives to provide child care. Forty-three percent of married mothers age 30 or over with a child under three and who held full-time jobs reported family child care arrangements, while their younger counterparts (women under 25) reported that, in 67 percent of the cases, family helped them care for their children (U.S. Bureau of the Census, p. 1987).

The trend toward delayed childbearing shows no diminution. Whether "Paradise Lost" or "Paradise Found," the demographics suggest that policymakers in the arenas of health care, child care, labor, and education need to pay careful attention to the reproductive trends of this generation of women; they presage the future.

✱ LINDA M. WHITEFORD, Ph.D., M.P.H.

See also: Delayed Childbearing: Trends in the United States

Resources

Anonymous. (1988). "Recent U.S. Fertility Patterns Continue: Birthrates Climb among Older Women, Childlessness Rises." *Family Planning Perspectives 20* (1): 44-45.

Baldwin, Wendy H. & Nord, Christina W. (1984). "Delayed Childbearing in the U.S.: Facts and Fictions." *Population Reference Bureau, 34* (4): 1-36.

Exter, Thomas. (1988, Dec). "Demographic Forecasts." *American Demographics 10* (12): 38-41.

U.S. Bureau of the Census. (1987). "Fertility of American Women: June 1986." *Current Population Reports*. Series P-20, no. 421. Washington, DC: U.S. Department of Commerce.

Ventura, Stephanie. (1989). "First Births to Older Mothers, 1970-86." *American Journal of Public Health 79* (12): 1675-77.

Whiteford, Linda M. & Sharnius, Michael. (1986). "Delayed Accomplishments: Family Formation among Older First-time Parents." In Karen Michaelson (Ed.) *Childbirth in America*. Hadley, MA: Bergin and Garvey Publishers, Inc.

DELAYED CHILDBEARING: TRENDS IN THE UNITED STATES

The rate of childbearing by women in their early 30s reached an 18-year high in 1988, at 74 births per 1,000 women aged 30-34, 41 percent higher than in 1975 (52 per 1,000) and just slightly above the previous high point in 1970 (73 per 1,000) (National Center for Health Statistics, 1990b). Generally, birth rates for women aged 30 and older have been rising since the mid 1970s, while rates for women in the peak childbearing ages (20-29 years) have been stable during this period. (See Figure 1.)

Of particular interest has been the dramatic increase in *first* births and *first* birth rates among women in their 30s. In 1988, about 1 in 6 women having their first child was 30 or older, compared with 1 in 25 in 1970 (Ventura, 1989; National Center for Health Statistics, 1990b). The number of first births per 1,000 for women 30 and older has more than doubled during the 1970-88 period; comparable rates for younger women have changed relatively little since the mid 1970s. (See Table 1.) The findings reported here are based on data drawn from the live birth certificates of all states and the District of Columbia, compiled and tabulated by the National Center for Health Statistics.

Figure 1.
Birth Rates for Women Aged 30-34 and 35-39 Years, All Births and First Births: United States, 1970-88

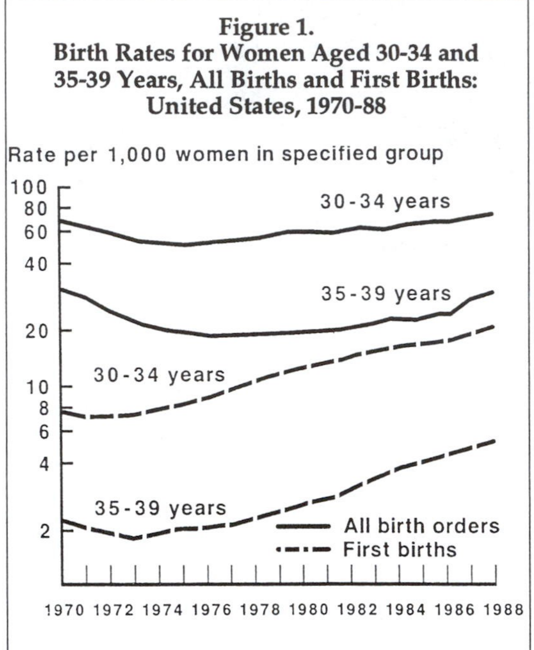

There are two important factors behind this shift in age at childbearing during the 1970s and 1980s. First, the number of women aged 30-44 increased 67 percent (from 17.7 to 29.5 million). Women aged 30-44 in 1988 are the baby boomers (born in the period after World War II through the early 1960s). In contrast, the number of women aged 15-29 increased only 16 percent (from 25.0 to 28.9 million) (U.S. Bureau of the Census, 1982, 1990), a reflection of the sharp drop in fertility during the 1960s and early 1970s. The other key factor is that the proportion of women reaching age 30 who are still childless increased from 15 percent in 1970 to 31 percent in 1988. National surveys show, however, that about half of these childless women intend to have at least one child (U.S. Bureau of the Census, 1989). The convergence of these factors resulted in the largest number of women aged 30-44 ever to be "at risk" of having a first child.

Older women having their first child in 1988 differ from younger first-time mothers in several important respects. For one thing, nearly half of them (48 percent) are college graduates, a level of educational attainment far higher than among mothers in their 20s (19 percent) and far higher than for women aged 30-44 in the general population (23 percent) (U.S. Bureau of the Census, forthcoming). Twelve percent were unmarried when their first child was born, compared with 23 percent of first-time mothers in their 20s. Nearly 9 out of 10 received prenatal care beginning in the first trimester. Of those who were college graduates, 94 percent began care in the first trimester. More than two-thirds were employed, a higher rate of labor force participation than younger first-time mothers, according to data from the June 1988 Current Population Survey (U.S. Bureau of the Census, 1989).

Clearly the socioeconomic status of these women is very high, creating a favorable impact on the health of their newborn infants. The best measure of pregnancy outcome is the proportion

Table 1. Number of First Births and First Birth Rates by Age of Mother: United States, 1970, 1980, 1985, and 1988
Age of Mother (years)

Year	15-44 years (1)	15-19 years	20-24 years	25-29 years	30-34 years	35-39 years	40-44 years
				Number			
1970	1,430,680	498,388	652,530	212,102	42,404	11,704	2,442
1980	1,545,604	425,676	605,183	371,859	112,964	18,241	1,964
1985	1,554,788	359,272	552,974	418,658	170,686	39,447	3,804
1988	1,595,587	364,073	505,975	447,219	206,649	54,531	6,745
				Rate (2)			
1970	34.2	53.7	78.2	31.2	7.3	2.1	0.4
1980	29.5	41.4	57.3	38.2	12.8	2.6	0.3
1985	27.6	39.7	53.0	38.8	16.9	4.4	0.5
1988	27.6	41.0	53.1	41.2	19.1	5.7	0.8

(1) Numbers include births to mothers under age 15 years and ages 45-49 years, which are not shown separately. Rates are computed by relating all births, regardless of age of mother, to women ages 15-44 years.

(2) First births per 1,000 women in specified group.

of babies weighing less than 5½ pounds (low birth weight). The most favorable ages in terms of low birth weight for first births are 20-29 years, with 6.1-6.6 percent of babies weighing less than 5½ pounds. Typically, first births to mothers in their 30s are at somewhat elevated risk of low birth weight (7.4-9.2 percent in 1988). However, when the data are further examined by educational attainment of the mother, the risk of a low weight outcome drops if the mother is a college graduate to 5.9 percent (mothers aged 30-34) and 8.0 percent (mothers aged 35-39). In addition to seeking early prenatal care, well-educated women are much more likely to have good diets, to gain adequate weight during pregnancy, and to be nonsmokers (Prager et al., 1984; Taffel, 1986; Mosher and Pratt, 1987).

Women who have delayed childbearing will likely continue to account for an increasing share of first births in future years. Data on childlessness by age do not suggest any reversal or halt in the recent trend. Two factors have tended to intensify the trend. The proportion of college graduates among women aged 30-34 years has increased from 16 percent in 1975 to 23 percent in 1988. Additionally, data from the vital registration system show that women are waiting longer to marry (National Center for Health Statistics, 1990a). Further intensifying the impact of these factors is the still growing number of women aged 30-44 years (U.S. Bureau of the Census, 1990). During the next several years, the population of women of childbearing age will have relatively more representation from those aged 30-44 than is now the case. Therefore, it can be anticipated that women in their 30s will probably account for more first births in future years.

✱ STEPHANIE J. VENTURA, A.M.

See also: Delayed Childbearing: Social Factors

Resources

Mosher, William & Pratt, William. (1987). "Fecundity, Infertility, and Reproductive Health in the United States, 1982." *Vital and Health Statistics.* Series 23, No. 14. Hyattsville, MD: National Center for Health Statistics.

National Center for Health Statistics. (1990a). "Advance Report of Final Marriage Statistics, 1987." *Monthly Vital Statistics Report 38* (12). Supplement. Hyattsville, MD: Public Health Service.

———. (1990b). "Advance Report of Final Natality Statistics, 1988." *Monthly Vital Statistics Report 39* (4). Supplement. Hyattsville, MD: Public Health Service.

Prager, Kate et al. (1984). "Smoking and Drinking Behavior before and during Pregnancy of Married Mothers of Live-born Infants and Stillborn Infants." *Public Health Reports 999* (2): 117-27.

Taffel, Selma. (1986). "Maternal Weight Gain and the Outcome of Pregnancy." *Vital and Health Statistics.* Series 21, No. 44. Hyattsville, MD: National Center for Health Statistics.

U.S. Bureau of the Census. (1982). "Preliminary Estimates of the Population of the United States, by Age, Sex, and Race: 1970 to 1981." *Current Population Reports.* Series P-25, No. 917. Washington, DC: U.S. Department of Commerce.

———. (1989). "Fertility of American Women: June 1988." *Current Population Reports.* Series P-20, No. 436. Washington, DC: U.S. Department of Commerce.

———. (1990). "U.S. Population Estimates by Age, Sex, Race, and Hispanic Origin: 1989." *Current Population Reports.* Series P-25, No. 1057. Washington, DC: U.S. Department of Commerce.

———. (Forthcoming). "Educational Attainment in the United States: March 1989 and 1988." *Current Population Reports.* Series P-20.

Ventura, Stephanie J. (1989). "Trends and Variations in First Births to Older Women, 1970-86." *Vital and Health Statistics.* Series 21, No. 47. Hyattsville, MD: National Center for Health Statistics.

DELEE, JOSEPH BOLIVAR

Joseph B. DeLee (1869-1942) was a caring, dedicated obstetrician. His practices, however, did much to dehumanize birth in the 20th century. His gentlemanly intentions were to protect women, not only from pain and danger, but from the birth process itself.

DeLee was a professor of obstetrics at Northwestern University and the University of Chicago, teaching many medical students, doctors, and nurses. He was the author of several obstetrical textbooks, a sought-after speaker, and the inventor or modifier of many obstetrical tools. Two of those tools, still in widespread use today, are the DeLee-Hillis head fetascope and the infant tracheal suction catheter.

Early in his career, DeLee became deeply concerned about high maternal and neonatal death rates. Investigation convinced him that infection carried by the attendant was one of the main causes of childbirth fever and death (*The National Cyclopedia of American Biography*, 1990). He began a vigorous campaign of cleanliness, which was revolutionary for the time. DeLee, however, went a step too far by negatively labeling childbirth itself as pathological, rather than pointing out the shortcomings of the caregiver or the surroundings.

DeLee had tremendous influence on obstetrical practice in the 20th century. His 1920 article and speech to fellow obstetricians noted that "labor is a pathological process," and that "few women escape without lasting injury." One of his solutions, among others, was to perform routine episiotomies and use prophylactic forceps at every birth. These emergency measures became standard practice in maternity hospitals throughout the country.

Why were these interventions so quickly accepted and used? Why would women submit to them? A brief background of the times may help explain.

Childbirth in the 19th and early 20th centuries did present many hazards to women. More pelvises were distorted by inadequate diets, tuberculosis was epidemic in some areas, and childbirth fever was not uncommon (Armstrong and Feldman, 1990). This was also the time when male doctors were fighting for autonomy and waging a relentless campaign to vilify midwives and their ways. Hospitals were emerging as scientific places for doctors to practice their ideas and to teach their students. So, many women, especially in urban areas, were willing to bypass traditional ways for new technology.

The dichotomous nature of DeLee's influence is exemplified by his founding in 1895, at his own expense, the Maxwell Street Lying-In Dispensary, which in 1932 became the Chicago Maternity Center. This was a home birth service for the very poor in the slums of Chicago. The Center's statistics were very good, compared to those of the hospitals at the time. It was run for over 40 years by Dr. Beatrice Tucker, the first woman resident accepted at the Maxwell Street Lying-In Dispensary.

The introduction of routine episiotomy and prophylactic forceps contributed strongly to dehumanizing childbirth and making it more technology-oriented. Because of this Joseph B. DeLee is viewed as a villain by many. DeLee himself revised his opinions about delivery, including his view of the preventive use of forceps "to protect the fetus from the crushing force of the pelvis." In a 1938 interview, he said, when asked about the issue, "I wish I hadn't done it" (Armstrong and Feldman, 1990). This dedicated, if somewhat misguided (by today's standards) obstetrician must be judged holistically, as a product of his times.

✱ MARY ANN M. SMITH, R.N., C.N.M.

Resources

Armstrong, Penny & Feldman, Sheryl. (1990). *A Wise Birth*. New York: William Morrow & Co.

Edwards, Margot & Waldorf, Mary. (1984). *Reclaiming Birth*. New York: The Crossing Press.

The National Cyclopedia of American Biography. (1990). Volume 31. Ann Arbor, MI: James T. White & Co., pp. 382-83.

Stewart, Lee & Stewart, David. (1978). *21st Century Obstetrics Now*. 2nd edition. Marble Hill, MO: NAPSAC Inc., Chapter 13.

DEPO-PROVERA

Depo-Provera is the brand name for depo-medroxyprogesterone acetate (DMPA), a long-acting injectable contraceptive administered usually every three months. Marketed by Upjohn Co. in about 90 countries around the world, Depo-Provera is approved by the U.S. Food and Drug Administration (FDA) only for the end-stage (palliative) treatment of uterine or renal cancer, *not* for contraceptive use. It nonetheless has been prescribed as a contraceptive for an estimated 15,000 U.S. women by physicians who believe it is a good birth control method. Many of these women received no information about its unapproved status or its possible negative effects.

DMPA, injected intramuscularly, is slowly released into the blood stream and acts primarily by inhibiting ovulation. In addition, it thickens cervical mucus and causes thinning of the endometrial lining, both of which interfere with fertilization and implantation. It is extremely effective (99 percent) and does not depend upon a woman's memory, as the birth control pill does, to be used properly.

In many respects the reproductive tract of a woman on DMPA resembles that of a menopausal woman. Cyclic hormonal surges stop and the endometrium stops proliferating, becoming thin and "atrophied" 20-30 days after injection.

DMPA may cause the following: disruption of menstrual bleeding patterns (most commonly, no bleeding, but sometimes heavy, prolonged bleeding); excessive weight gain; depression; hair loss; growth of facial hair; acne and skin rashes; blurred vision; joint pain and swelling of limbs; lowered glucose tolerance; changes in carbohydrate metabolism; and loss of sexual desire. There remains controversy about whether or not DMPA can cause cancer, but some data suggest strongly a relationship between DMPA and cervical cancer. DMPA has caused endometrial cancer in rhesus monkeys, a finding that has raised concern among some scientists.

Upjohn Co. has promoted Depo-Provera in other countries as the "ideal contraceptive for lactating mothers," although no long-term studies have established the safety of DMPA for breastfeeding infants. (The drug does appear in breast milk, as do many substances ingested by a nursing mother.)

One reason why some women who take Depo-Provera may have more severe reactions than with other long-acting progestin-based methods (e.g., injectable microspheres, and implantables like Norplant) is the fact that DMPA initially occurs in fairly high concentrations in the blood stream. Then, over time, blood levels taper off. In contrast, Norplant creates a relatively constant *lower* level of hormone, thus accounting for better toleration in some women.

In developing countries, where injections are often associated with effective cures for numerous conditions, some women have been given DMPA shots without understanding that it was for birth control purposes. This potential for abuse, coupled with its lack of individual control over the method, makes its use even more problematic in a setting where informed consent is unlikely.

In 1983, upon the request of Upjohn Co., the FDA held a special Board of Inquiry hearing to review once again whether DMPA should be approved for contraceptive use in the United States. The National Women's Health Network was the leading consumer organization presenting expert scientific witnesses arguing against approval. The special panel of physicians constituting the Board of Inquiry determined that the data presented were not adequate to demonstrate safety as required by the FDA and thus recommended denial of approval. Subsequently, Upjohn withdrew its request, indicating that it would resubmit an application for approval at some later date. As of 1992 no such request had been submitted.

✷ JUDY NORSIGIAN

See **Guide to Related Topics:** Contraception

Resources

Boston Women's Health Book Collective. (1989). Special packet of articles about Depo-Provera available for $10 from BWHBC, Box 192, West Somerville, MA 02144.

Branan, Karen & Turnley, Bill. (1985). "The Ultimate Test Animal." 45 min. color video about Depo-Provera. Available from The Cinema Guild, 1697 Broadway, New York, NY 10019.

Green, William. (1987). "The Odyssey of Depo-Provera: Contraceptives, Carcinogenic Drugs, and Risk-management Analyses." *Food Drug Cosmetic Law Journal 42* (4): 567-87.

Levine, Carol. (1979, Aug). "Depo-Provera and Contraceptive Risk: A Case Study of Values in Conflict." *Hastings Center Report 9* (8): 24-32.

Multinational Monitor. (1985). "The Case against Depo-Provera." *Multinational Monitor 6* (2 & 3). (A special issue on Depo-Provera, including articles and resource listings.)

Parsons, Claire. (1990). "Drugs, Science and Ethics: Lessons from the Depo-Provera Story." *Issues in Reproductive and Genetic Engineering 3* (2): 101-10.

Richard, B. & Lasagna, L. (1987). "Drug Regulation in the United States and the United Kingdom: The Depo-Provera Story." *Annals of Internal Medicine 30*: 886-91.

U.S. Food and Drug Administration. (1984). "Report of the Public Board of Inquiry of Depo-Provera" (Judith Weisz, Chair; Paul Stolley; Griff Ross). Available from Government Dockets, FDA, Parklawn Bldg., 5600 Fisher's Lane, Rockville, MD 20857.

DES: DIETHYLSTILBESTROL

The story of diethylstilbestrol (or DES) began with its synthesis in 1938 by Dr. Charles Dodd of the University of London. The first synthetic estrogen, DES was both inexpensive to produce and theorized to have many usages. It's first champions for use in pregnancy were Dr. George Smith and Dr. Olive Watkins Smith of Harvard Medical School who, in 1941, tested the drug on a group of women without the use of a placebo and decided that the drug was useful in preventing miscarriage. Drug manufacturers were not required by regulatory agencies to prove safety until 1962, so DES began to be commercially produced and the saga unfolded. At its zenith, DES was manufactured by as many as 200 pharmaceutical companies. Sadly, as Apfel and Fisher state, "With DES, the whole profession went awry. The DES case is an example of the inadequacies of research and communication, and of institutional hubris and the failure of regulation within the profession and the community" (Apfel and Fisher, 1984, p. 122).

Following the publication of the Smiths' research, DES was commonly administered to women who had a previous history of miscarriage or pregnancy complications. It was used for this purpose until 1971. About two million women were given DES, with the largest number receiving the drug in the 1950s, when it is estimated that as many as 10 percent of all pregnant women were taking it (Orenberg, 1981).

Criticism of the Smiths' research and scientific technique was extensive. As early as 1952, Dr. James Ferguson of Tulane University proved the drug's ineffectiveness in a study with a proper control group (Meyers, 1983). Using the "double blind" model in which neither the doctor nor the patient knows who is receiving the drug and who is receiving the placebo, Dr. William J. Dieckmann of Chicago Lying-in Hospital showed that those administered DES actually had a higher number of miscarriages. Other studies followed. Still, the drug's usage continued unchecked for 30 years.

In 1971, Dr. Arthur Herbst published a study in which DES was linked to a rare form of cancer called adenocarcinoma, which had been found in the vaginas and cervixes of a group of young women. In that year DES was banned by the FDA for use in pregnant women. Subsequently, Herbst established a registry of women afflicted with adenocarcinoma. In 1973, the National Cooperative Diethylstilbestrol Adenosis Project (DESAD) was begun by the National Cancer Institute. The four participating hospitals track children of mothers who took DES and continue to do so today.

What have been the effects of DES on mothers and their children? In daughters, 90 percent show evidence of an abnormal tissue growth called adenosis. This strawberry-colored, mucus-secreting glandular tissue mistakenly appears in the vagina or cervix (Orenberg, 1981). Virtually 100 percent of all daughters exposed to DES *in utero* at seven to eight weeks gestation develop adenosis, but among those exposed after the 19th week gestation, the number drops to less than five percent (Shapiro, 1983). The amount of DES taken by the mother appears to be inconsequential. Of those women who have adenosis, as many as one out of 700 will develop cancer, usually when they are 15 to 24 years old, with a peak incidence at 19. Those exposed *in utero* before the 10th week have the highest likelihood of developing cancer.

In addition, 16 percent of DES daughters, as compared to six percent of unexposed women, will develop genital abnormalities such as a "cocks comb" or hooded cervix, T-shaped uterus, or vaginal or cervical ridges (Herbst and Bern, 1981). These conditions cause a much higher incidence of infertility as they inhibit the movement of sperm or the implantation and growth of the egg. Ectopic pregnancies occur among six to seven percent of DES daughters' first pregnancies, about five times more frequently than among the unexposed. This is attributed to the more frequent evidence of small-diameter Fallopian tubes among this population. Miscarriage or premature dilation before the 37th week occurs much more frequently in DES daughters. It is theorized that an "incompetent cervix" may be the source of the problem and that the poor cervical musculature is a developmental abnormality attributed to DES.

What can be done to help these women? Treatment by a doctor familiar with DES is a must. Names of such doctors can be obtained from DES Action, a consumer group. The doctor will examine the woman's cervix and vagina for abnormalities by use of iodine staining to detect adenosis, do a palpitation and Pap smear, and conduct an internal examination with a colposcope, which can magnify and photograph abnormal tissue in the cervix and vagina. A biopsy may be taken. These procedures should be repeated every 6 to 12 months and are extremely expensive. Doctors may choose to treat the affected tissues by cryosurgery or freezing, or by conization, in which the tissue is cut away. Radical surgery for cancerous adenosis, called adenocarcinoma, might include a vaginectomy and vagina reconstruction. Careful monitoring of a DES daughter's pregnancy, which is considered "high risk," is essential. Cerclage, or the stitching shut of the uterus to prevent premature dilation, is sometimes used and bedrest is recommended.

Among DES mothers, there seems to be a somewhat higher tendency toward developing breast cancer, possibly as high as 44 percent higher than the general population (DES Action, 1984). It is theorized that this tendency may be dose related. Comparatively little research has been done on DES mothers.

In DES sons, as in their DES-exposed sisters, genital abnormalities have been found at much higher rates than in the general population. About one-third of those exposed may have abnormalities of the urinary tract, small penises, small or undescended testicles, epidymal cysts, or varicose veins in the testes (Orenberg, 1981). Some of these conditions contribute to sterility or at least poor sperm motility. DES sons have been spared of as high an incidence of DES-related structural abnormalities as their sisters because male genitalia form before the seventh week, and most DES therapy was started after that point in a woman's pregnancy. It is recommended that DES sons have complete examinations by urologists familiar with DES-related problems.

DES has been used for lactation suppression of mothers not intending to breastfeed, though the FDA in 1978 recommended that it not be used for this purpose (Seaman and Seaman, 1977). It has also been used as the "Morning After" pill, theoretically preventing egg implantation if taken within 72 hours of coitus. This usage has also been disapproved by the FDA. DES was given to cattle and chickens orally or as implantations as it made them meatier, though most of the increased density was fat and water. This usage was banned in 1979.

DES is still on the market. It is most often used to treat prostate cancer but, ironically, has been used to treat breast cancer as well. Its availability means that an uninformed physician could prescribe it for anything.

Several suits by DES daughters have been won against the drug companies that manufactured DES. These cases have added new concepts to the field of law. The landmark Bichler case was won on the grounds of joint-enterprise or industry-wide liability because manufacturers adhere to common standards. Additionally, market share liability, or the sharing of cost by the defendant drug companies according to their share of the DES market, has emerged as a result of DES prosecution (Orenberg, 1981). In 1986, New York State extended its statute of limitation on toxic substances, easing the way for DES prosecution (Helmrich, 1986). Most women do not discover they have been exposed to DES until many years after the exposure. The most successful cases have involved DES daughters with adenocarcinoma.

What we do know after 50 years of DES? No one knows the cumulative effects of hormones. For this reason, women exposed to DES should avoid other hormone use. No one knows yet if there will be a second wave of adenocarcinoma among DES daughters later in life. Benign adenosis does shrink spontaneously and may even disappear, being replaced by normal squamous epithelial tissue. It is theorized that contraceptive jellies may aid in this process (Seaman and Seaman, 1977). Eventually most DES daughters can have children. However, there have been instances of third-generation DES children injured during delivery due to their mother's malformed uterus, leaving these children with cerebral palsy.

The irony of the DES story is that the children of DES are among the most needy of reproductive technology, just as their mothers sought DES as a means of saving their pregnancies. It is hoped that the medical industry will never again make the terrible mistakes that it did with DES and cause such a sad legacy. ✷ DEIRDRE COLBY SATO, M.A.

See also: Research Issues in Childbirth; Thalidomide

See **Guide to Related Topics:** Pregnancy Complications

Resources

Apfel, Roberta J. & Fisher, Susan M. (1984). *To Do No Harm*. New Haven, CT: Yale University Press.

DES Action. (1984). *Fertility and Pregnancy Guide for DES Daughters and Sons*. New York: DES Action U.S.A.

Edelman, David A. (1986). *Diethylstilbestrol—New Perspectives*. Boston: MTP Press Limited.

Helmrich, Susan P. (1986, Fall). "Victory for the Victims in New York State." *DES Action Voice 30*: 1, 6.

Herbst, Arthur L. & Bern, Howard A. (1981). *Developmental Effects of Diethylstilbestrol (DES) in Pregnancy*. New York: Thieme-Stratton Inc.

Meyers, Robert. (1983). *D.E.S.: The Bitter Pill*. New York: Seaview/Putnam.

Orenberg, Cynthia Laitman. (1981). *DES: The Complete Story*. New York: St. Martin's Press.

Overall, Christine. (1989). *The Future of Human Reproduction*. Toronto: The Women's Press.

Seaman, Barbara & Seaman, Gideon. (1977). *Women and the Crisis in Sex Hormones*. New York: Bantam Books.

Shapiro, Howard T. (1983). *The Pregnancy Book for Today's Woman*. New York: Harper and Row.

DIABETES: CLINICAL AND GESTATIONAL

During the digestion of carbohydrates and sugars, enzymes convert the food into simple sugars, some of which are used immediately and some of which are stored for future use. Glucose, the most important sugar, enters the tissue cells, where it combines with oxygen to form carbon dioxide and water. The energy released by this chemical reaction is used for muscular work and for maintaining body temperature. Insulin, a hormone secreted by the pancreas, along with the insulin receptors on the cell wall, facilitates the transport of glucose across the cell wall.

Diabetes is more than simply a lack of insulin. The term "diabetes" can be applied to many different syndromes. The symptoms of diabetes mellitus, one of these syndromes, include the presence of sugar in the urine, excessive thirst, excessive urination, increased food intake, and an elevated plasma glucose (blood sugar) level. In an asymptomatic person, diagnosis of diabetes may also be made on the basis of test results alone if the fasting plasma glucose levels are persistently elevated.

The symptoms of diabetes mellitus are associated with one of three major physiological conditions, which in turn, have several root causes. (See Figure 1.) In addition, genetic factors can possibly predispose the body to *react* to any of these various influences (viruses, starvation, etc.) with symptoms of diabetes.

Gestational Diabetes. In gestational diabetes—also known as Class A, latent, chemical, or preclinical diabetes—a pregnant woman having no symptoms of diabetes has test results similar to those of nonpregnant clinical diabetes. By definition, this "diabetes" ceases once the pregnancy is over. Clinical diabetes that is diagnosed prenatally or persists beyond pregnancy is not properly called gestational diabetes.

Many birth attendants question the existence of gestational diabetes because it is usually diagnosed solely on the basis of a response to a test. Elevated blood sugars in an asymptomatic mother may only reflect the chemical gymnastics imposed by the test itself, since many glucose tests involve fasting followed by the consumption of concentrated glucose. Or blood sugar elevations during pregnancy can result from any of the root causes of clinical diabetes mentioned earlier. Or perhaps her body is registering a healthy response to the inherent dynamics of pregnancy. The pla-

Figure 1. Symptoms of Diabetes

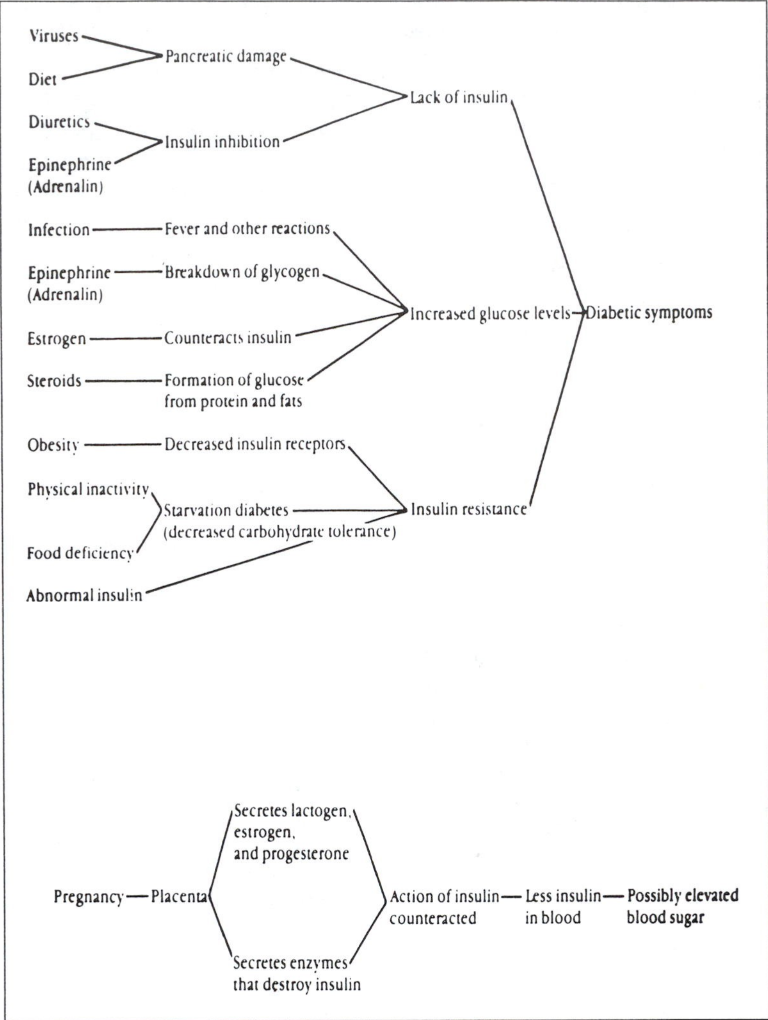

© 1990, Perinatal Support Services, 715 Monroe St., Evanston, IL 60202.

centa secretes lactogen, estrogen, and progesterone—hormones that counteract the function of insulin—as well as potent enzymes that destroy insulin. This placental function implies that the normal plasma glucose levels of the pregnant body are intentionally higher than those of the nonpregnant body.

One reason the pregnant body may need higher blood sugars is that "the continued demand for glucose and amino acids for fetal anabolism (tissue building) causes a state of 'accelerated starvation.' Lipolysis (fat break-down) to mobilize fat as metabolic fuel occurs more rapidly during pregnancy" (Burns, 1983). As a result of placental secretions, "instead of being rapidly converted to glycogen and stored in the liver for future use, the glucose remains for longer periods in the (woman's) bloodstream so that her developing baby has an easily available source of energy that can be used for growth and storage as fat (+glycogen)" (Inch, 1985).

Clinical Diabetes and Pregnancy. True clinical diabetes (different from gestational diabetes) can be diagnosed for the first time during pregnancy. A woman may have a latent diabetic condition that she is unaware of until pregnancy emphasizes the symptoms or until she discovers them in prenatal consultation with her birth attendant.

Some signs of undiagnosed clinical diabetes may come to light in the mother's history—for example, a family member with diabetes, a previous unexplained stillbirth, an unexplained premature labor, a previous baby with respiratory distress or tremors within a couple of hours after birth, or a previous baby weighing more than 10 pounds. However, none of these factors alone signifies diabetes. In conjunction with these signs, any of the following symptoms warrant further investigation: weakness, weight loss, increased thirst, increased urination, obesity at conception, polyhydramnios (excessive amniotic fluid), signs of pre-eclampsia, sugar persistently in the urine (every urination can be tested at home using a uristick), or plasma glucose levels higher than 200mg/100ml.

A pregnant woman with clinical diabetes needs to take extra measures to maintain good health. She can learn to test her own blood sugar level at home and adjust her insulin doses as necessary. She should eat "small frequent feedings of protein . . . as many as eight a day on a round-the-clock schedule." Recent research suggests that "diabetic mothers can eat the standard Brewer diet [2600 calories, 100-120g protein, salt to taste daily] plus enough extra protein so that she is getting 1 gram of protein per pound of body weight. Complex carbohydrates in quantity are essential, as are calories. Small, frequent meals will help to regulate the blood sugar. Exercise will help to utilize and normalize glucose levels. Weight gain and salt intake should NOT be restricted!" (Frye, 1985)

Glucose Screening Guidelines. Birth attendants (midwives and doctors) often recommend glucose screening tests for pregnant women. Several professional organizations have published testing guidelines. The American Diabetes Association recommends that all pregnant women take a one-hour glucose test. The Centers for Disease Control advise that preferably all pregnant women, but definitely those with diabetic risk factors or over the age of 25, take a one-hour glucose test. The American College of Obstetricians and Gynecologists recommends that women who have indications of diabetic risk or who are over the age of 30 have some kind of glucose screening. The American College of Nurse Midwives has not published any guidelines.

Glucose in the Urine. Sugar in the urine is not necessarily an indication of gestational diabetes. The kidneys filter 170 liters of filtrate out of the blood and reabsorb 168 liters daily. Some of the substances reabsorbed with the filtrate have a well-defined reabsorption limit, or a "renal threshold." Once that limit is reached, any more of that substance is "spilled" in the urine. The kidney's renal threshold for sugar is 160-180 mg/100ml in nonpregnancy, and 100mg/100ml in pregnancy. This change is due to the 40-60 percent increase in the blood volume of the well-nourished pregnant woman, and, with the increased load, a change in the kidney's reabsorption process. Consequently, in up to 50 percent of all normal pregnancies, women spill sugar in the urine (while maintaining normal blood sugar levels).

Newborn Care. Some health practitioners require 12 hours of hourly heel-pricks for blood glucose checks of babies born of mothers with gestational diabetes or babies who weigh more than a prescribed weight. Some require blood checks at ½-hour intervals, gradually increasing to 3-hour intervals, for 12 hours. Still others require only three hourly blood checks, and cancel the latter two checks if the first one is normal.

The purpose of this monitoring is to watch for the hypoglycemia (low blood sugar) that babies may show when they are born of poorly controlled clinical diabetics (different from well-controlled diabetics, and from gestational diabetics). These babies may have abnormally low blood sugar once they are removed from the presence of their mothers' abnormally high blood sugar levels. This hypoglycemia could lead to tremors, respiratory distress, listlessness, an abnormal cry, feeding difficulties, and convulsions.

Some pediatricians feel confident that they can tell by watching the baby whether he or she is experiencing hypoglycemia, and they require minimal or no testing. Others who do not believe the mother's glucose levels to be abnormally high require no testing of the baby. Some pediatricians also reason that infant hypoglycemia need not be a concern if the baby is nursing immediately at birth and frequently thereafter.

Testing Options. There are currently six tests that can be used to monitor blood sugar levels during pregnancy. Some of these tests require that the mother fast and then drink a concentrated glucose preparation, a metabolic stressor that is usually unrelated to the lifestyle of the individual mother and that may actually affect the accuracy of the test results.

The glucose tolerance test is often considered the most definitive procedure for determining whether or not glucose is being properly managed. However, this test is so inaccurate and prone to both false positive and false negative results that it has been described as "unhelpful in clinical practice although it may still have a place in research studies" (Foster, 1983).

Test Descriptions.

1. The GTT
   (a) Preparatory diet:
   250-300 g carbohydrate for 3 days before test
   (b) Fast 8-12 hours before test
   (c) Fasting blood sample
   (d) Drink 50-100 mg of concentrated glucose ("glucola")
   (e) Blood and urine samples at
   1 hour
   2 hours
   3 hours
   (f) Normal values for 3-hour GTT (if only plasma is tested; normal values are lower if whole blood is tested)
   fasting—<105 mg/100 ml
   ½ hour—<200 mg/100 ml (optional)
   1 hour—<190 mg/100 ml
   2 hours—<165 mg/100 ml
   3 hours—<145 mg/100 ml
2. The fasting blood sugar
   (a) Fast 8-12 hours
   (b) One blood sample
   (c) Normal values range from <150 mg/100 ml to <150 mg/100 ml, depending on the philosophy of the birth attendant
3. The 1-hour glucose
   (a) Fast 8-12 hours (sometimes not required)
   (b) Fasting blood sample
   (c) Drink 50 g of glucose ("glucola")
   (d) Blood sample 1 hour later
   (e) Normal values
   <140 mg/100 ml
4. The 2-hour postprandial blood sugar (two definitions)
   (a) First definition
   (1) No fasting
   (2) Mother eats a generous breakfast with a lot of carbohydrates, such as pancakes with syrup, sausages, and a large glass of orange juice
   (3) Blood sample is taken 2 hours after the meal
   (b) Second definition
   (1) No fasting
   (2) Mother drinks some concentrated glucose
   (3) Blood sample is taken 2 hours after the glucose
   (c) Normal values
   (1) Usual range—<120 to <140 mg/100 ml
   (2) Sometimes up to 170 mg/100 ml is acceptable
5. The random blood sugar
   (a) No fasting
   (b) Blood sample drawn at a random time of day and not within 2 hours after a meal (or it becomes a postprandial)
   (c) Normal values
   Upper range about 100-110 mg/100 ml
   On the Brewer Diet, normal range might be higher
6. The hemoglobin A1C
   (a) No fasting
   (b) One blood sample
   (c) Normal values
   (1) Usually <4-7 percent of total hemoglobin
   (2) Higher values seem generally associated with increasing rate of birth defects observed at birth

In 1979, the National Diabetes Data Group changed the commonly accepted standards for normal glucose levels in pregnancy. The accepted upper limit for the fasting glucose was lowered from 140 mg/100 ml to 105 mg/100 ml, and the accepted upper limit for the two-hour postprandial from 150 mg/100 ml to 120 mg/100 ml. Therefore, some pregnant women considered to have normal blood sugar levels before 1979 would now be described as gestational diabetics by those accepting the new standards.

✷ JOY M. JONES, R.N.

See **Guide to Related Topics:** Pregnancy Complications

Resources

American College of Obstetricians and Gynecologists. (1985). *Standards for Obstetric-Gynecological Services.* Washington, DC: American College of Obstetricians and Gynecologists.

American Diabetes Association. (1986, Jul-Aug). "Gestational Diabetes Mellitus." *Diabetes Care 9* (4): 430.

Brewer, Gail. (1983). *The Brewer Medical Diet for Normal and High Risk Pregnancy.* New York: Simon & Schuster.

Brewer, Tom. (1982). *Metabolic Toxemia of Late Pregnancy: A Disease of Malnutrition.* New Canaan, CT: Keats Publishing.

Burns, Evelyn. (1983). "Diabetes Mellitus and Pregnancy." *Nursing Clinics of North America 18* (4): 674.

Creasy, R. & Resnick, R. (1984). *Maternal Fetal Medicine Principles and Practice.* Philadelphia: W.B. Saunders.

"Diabetes Mellitus." (1977). In G.W. Thorne, et al. (Eds.) *Harrison's Principles of Internal Medicine.* 8th edition. New York: McGraw-Hill, pp. 568-83.

"Diabetes Testing." (1987, Winter). ("Staccato Briefs" section). *Midwifery Today 1* (1): 31.

Foster, Daniel. (1983). "Diabetes Mellitus." In G.W. Thorne et al. (Eds.) *Harrison's Principles of Internal*

Medicine. 10th edition. New York: McGraw-Hill, pp. 661-64.
Frye, Anne. (1985). *Understanding Lab Work in the Childbearing Year.* New Haven, CT: Informed Homebirth, Inc.
Garrey, Mathew M. et al. (1980). *Obstetrics Illustrated.* New York: Churchill Livingston.
"Homemade 'Glucola'." (1987, Winter). ("The Formalary" section). *Midwifery Today 1* (1): 11.
Hunter, David & Keirse, Marc. (1989). "Gestational Diabetes." In Murray Enkin et al. (Eds.) *A Guide to Effective Care in Pregnancy and Childbirth.* New York: Oxford University Press, pp. 41-43.
Inch, Sally. (1985). *Birthrights.* New York: Pantheon Books.
Jones, Joy. (1989). "Gestational Diabetes: Myth or Metabolism?" *Mothering* (50): 58-67.
———. (1991). "The Brewer Pregnancy Diet." Pamphlet. Evanston, IL: Perinatal Support Services.
National Diabetes Data Group. (1979, Dec). "Classification and Diagnosis of Diabetes Mellitus and Other Categories of Glucose Intolerance." *Diabetes 28*: 1039-57.
O'Brian, Mary Ellen & Gilson, George. (1987). "Detection and Management of Gestational Diabetes in an Out-of-Hospital Birth Center." *Journal of Nurse-Midwifery 32* (2): 79-84.
Pinckney, Edward. (1984). "The Accuracy of Medical Testing." In New Medical Foundation (Ed.) *Dissent in Medicine: Nine Doctors Speak Out.* Chicago: Contemporary Books, Inc., pp. 85-109.
Pritchard, J. & MacDonald, P. (1976). *William's Obstetrics.* 15th edition. New York: Appleton-Century-Crofts.
U.S. Department of Health and Human Services, Public Health Service, Centers for Disease Control, Center for Prevention Services, Division of Diabetes Control. (1986). *Public Health Guidelines for Enhancing Diabetes Control through Maternal and Child Health Programs.* Atlanta: Centers for Disease Control.

This article has been excerpted with permission from *Mothering*, Volume #50. Subscriptions: $22.00 per year (4 issues), from *Mothering*, P.O. Box 1690, Santa Fe, NM 87504. Back issues: $4.00. Vaccination and Circumcision Booklets: $12.00. All rights reserved.

DIAPERS: ENVIRONMENTAL CONCERNS

When disposable diapers were mass-marketed in 1961, they were hailed as an innovation that "made cloth diapers old-fashioned." Originally promoted as a convenience item to be used during travel, picnics, and the like, single-use diapers today account for 82 percent of all diaper changes in the United States.

The appeal of a diaper that could be tossed in the garbage was unquestionable. In recent years, however, shrinking landfill capacity and public health concerns have prompted a second look at where all those diapers are going. Over 18 billion are thrown away each year, enough to stretch to the moon and back seven times. Disposables constitute two percent of all solid waste (five million tons), more than any other single product except food and beverage containers and newspapers.

Composed of plastic, adhesives, and wood pulp fibers, single-use diapers can take up to 500 years to decompose in a landfill. Their durable plastics resist deterioration in the presence of ammonia and uric acid, making them difficult to degrade and potentially dangerous to burn.

Although most solid waste regulations prohibit the disposal of human excrement in residential garbage, 33 percent of the diapers contain fecal matter. Over 100 different enteric viruses, including polio and hepatitis, are known to be excreted in human feces, raising concerns about possible groundwater contamination and potential threats to the health of those who handle solid waste and to the public at large. Although labels on diaper packages advise the emptying of excrement into the toilet, few parents actually do so. Thus three million tons of untreated feces and urine end up

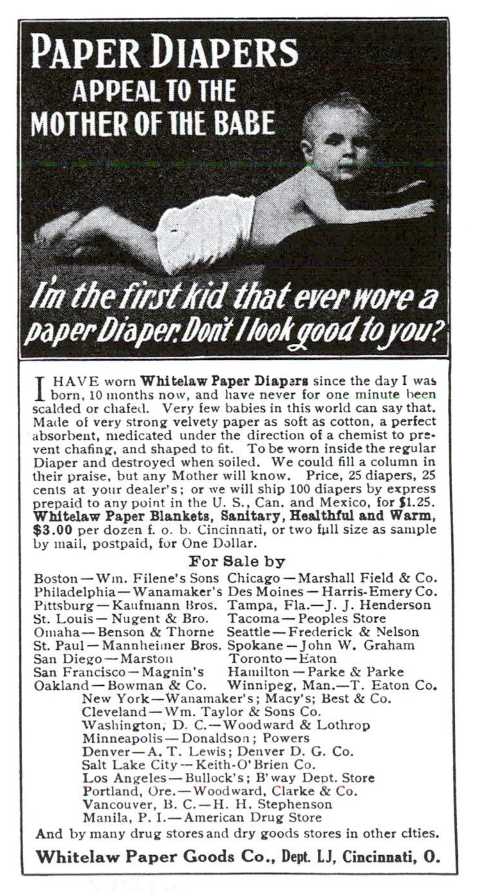

Advertisement appearing in *The Ladies Home Journal,* October 1, 1910. From the collection of Donna King.

in landfills rather than in the sewage system, a singular exception to the processing of human sewage through waste water treatment.

There is also some concern that the diapers may pose health hazards to the babies who wear them. The powerful chemicals used in synthetic, super-absorbent diapers can cause the skin to shrivel while absorbing the body's own protective fluids along with urine. Because the diaper seems dry, it remains on the baby for a long period of time. Synthetic diapers do not breathe and therefore raise the skin temperature, increasing the risk of infection. No long-term research has been conducted on the migration of super-absorbency chemicals and dioxins (present in bleached paper products) to the reproductive organs of babies who wear the diapers 24 hours a day for two to three years.

Numerous studies have compared the costs of various diapering options, and all find single-use diapers to be the most expensive, costing up to 50 percent more than reusable diapers laundered commercially and up to 66 percent more than those laundered at home. These figures do not account for the hidden costs of waste disposal and collection, which amount to three million dollars annually or about 10 cents for every dollar spent on disposables.

Despite growing awareness that single-use diapers are both costly and environmentally unsound, they are still chosen by most parents. An entire generation has grown up unacquainted with reusables, a generation for whom cotton diapers evoke an image of a harried mother with pins in mouth, frantically comforting a screaming baby underfoot while the soap kettle boils over. It is convenience, perceived or otherwise, that sells throwaways. Their sales are immensely profitable—over $4 billion in 1991. Major manufacturers spend hundreds of millions of dollars to advertise and promote diapers, including through hospital giveaways. One recent innovation is customized boy/girl diapers—pink for girls and blue for boys, with their respective packages depicting stereotypical male/female images. Manufacturers have also stepped up lobbying efforts in the face of legislation aimed at limiting the use of disposables. Twenty-two states had diaper legislation introduced or pending in 1990.

Many parents are switching to reusables, but many feel that doing so places a greater burden on already overworked mothers—for it is still mothers who chiefly care for and diaper their children. The issue demands a closer look. Marketing campaigns appeal directly to busy parents; some ads claim that disposables allow "more time with baby"—forgetting that time spent changing a diaper is time spent with baby. Underlying these ads is the promise of time saved, time that would otherwise be spent on a difficult and odious task. Some advertising even suggests that it is disposables that allow women to work outside the home.

In truth, no woman has to give up her job if she gives up disposables. Many families with working mothers use cloth diapers, including those with children in day care. Child care centers are increasingly required to accept children in cloth diapers, and many are beginning to encourage the use of cloth. By using diaper services, they no longer must contend with huge trash loads, feces in garbage, and the keeping track of individual throwaways.

Changing a cloth diaper is no more difficult or time-consuming than changing a disposable. Today's cloth diapers include such features as Velcro fasteners that eliminate the need for pins, custom-fitted diapers that eliminate the need for folding, and absorbent diaper covers. Use of a diaper service eliminates the need for home laundering. Four dozen diapers will last the entire two-and-a half to three years a child is in diapers and can be reused 80 to 100 times before going to the landfill, where they will decompose in six months. Babies using disposables exclusively will go through 7,000 to 10,000 of them, lugged home from the store every week at triple the cost of reusables and remaining in the landfill for five centuries.

Elimination of single-use diapers from the solid waste stream will require substantial changes in public policy. Asking parents to switch to reusable diapers is one part of a long-term solution that may require government and industry involvement as well as that of individuals. Proposed measures include consumer education programs designed to inform the public of the hazards of improper disposal of throwaways; active enforcement of health ordinances prohibiting the disposal of human excrement in garbage; education about ecologically sound diapering options; tax incentives for diaper services; incentives to institutions to switch to reusable diapers; and easing of import quotas on cotton that limit availability and threaten cost increases for cloth diapers. Suggested industry actions include the development of a single-use diaper with a flushable liner; stronger encouragement for customers to flush diaper contents; and research into composting techniques for diapers. The current "biodegradable" single-use diapers are not a viable option, since landfills lack the water and oxygen necessary for their rapid degradation. These diapers do nothing to reduce the volume of solid waste or to remove fecal matter from landfills.

✱ ELLEN BECKER, M.A.

See **Guide to Related Topics:** Baby Care

Resources

Becker, Ellen. (1991, Summer). "Are Single-Use Diapers Compostable?" *Mothering 60*: 53.

Braiman-Lipson, Judy. (1987, Spring). "Superabsorbent Disposable Diapers." *Mothering 43*: 36.

Center for Policy Alternatives. (1990). *Update on Diapers*. Washington, DC: Center for Policy Alternatives.

Henry, Sarah & Matthiessen, Connie. (1990, May). "The Diaper Dilemma." *Parenting*: 60-67.

Hollis, Robert W. (1989, Fall). "The Ethics of Diapering." *Mothering 53*: 29-35.

Lehrburger, Carl et al. (1991). *Diapers: Environmental Impacts and Lifecycle Analysis (Summary)*. Great Barrington, MA: Carl Lehrburger.

THE DIAPHRAGM

The diaphragm is a barrier method of contraception which has been in use since the 1800s throughout Europe. It was brought to the United States in the early 1900s by Margaret Sanger. She introduced the diaphragm and other barrier methods of contraception to the American people.

The diaphragm is a dome-shaped rubber cup with a flexible rim that is inserted into the vagina prior to intercourse. It is placed so that the anterior rim fits snugly behind the pubic bone and the posterior rim sits in the posterior fornix or aspect of the vagina (Hatcher et.al., 1990). It should completely cover the cervix at all times. The diaphragm is dome-shaped to promote effective covering of the cervix, as well as to serve as a reservoir for spermicidal jelly or cream. The spermicide must be used with the diaphragm for method effectiveness. The contraceptive effect of the diaphragm is twofold. The diaphragm itself acts as a barrier, keeping sperm from gaining access to the cervix. The spermicidal substance used with the diaphragm actually kills any sperm gaining access.

The diaphragm comes in three main types: (1) coil spring, in which the rim is a round, coiled metal wire; (2) flat spring, in which the rim is a flat, metal-banded ring; and (3) arching spring, in which the rim is a double metal spring, allowing the diaphragm to assume an "arching" shape when squeezed (Connell and Tatum, 1985). These different types allow for proper fitting for individual women, based on their pregnancy histories and musculature and pelvic architecture. Diaphragms also come in numerous sizes (55-105 millimeters in diameter), and a woman must be fit by a skilled practitioner. She is then taught the technique of insertion, checking for proper placement, removal, and care of the diaphragm. This promotes use effectiveness of the method. This method must be used prior to each act of intercourse, and the diaphragm must be left in place for a minimum of six to eight hours following the last act of intercourse. Women who have had Toxic Shock Syndrome should not use this method. Women suffering from chronic or repeated bouts of urinary tract infections (bladder infections or cystitis) are advised to choose another method of birth control.

Given correct use, the diaphragm can be an extremely reliable method of birth control. Various studies report a failure rate anywhere from 3 to 25 pregnancies per 100 woman years exposure (Varney, 1987). Barrier methods, in general, are quite effective for older women and careful users, and are less effective for younger women, for couples who have frequent intercourse, and for users who aren't diligent about careful use (Stewart et. al., 1987). Barriers have been shown to protect against certain sexually transmitted diseases, leading to increased protection against pelvic inflammatory disease. Additionally, the incidence of cervical cancer appears to be less in those women using barrier contraceptives.

Many women like the diaphragm method because it does not interfere with the body's hormones and does not have to be placed within the sterile cavity of the uterus. Women who are uncomfortable with touching their genitalia dislike the diaphragm because it requires manual manipulation for proper insertion, placement checking, and removal.

A woman who has been using the diaphragm should have the size rechecked if she has (1) had a baby or pregnancy termination or (2) gained or lost 10 pounds since the original fitting took place. Otherwise, the diaphragm needs to be replaced every two years.

✱ KAREN E. KATZ, C.N.M., M.S.

See **Guide to Related Topics:** Contraception

Resources

Connell, Elizabeth B. & Tatum, Howard J. (1985). *Barrier Methods of Contraception*. Durant, OK: Creative Infomatics, Inc.

Hatcher, Robert A. et al. (1990). *Contraceptive Technology 1990-92*. 15th edition. New York: Irvington Publishers, Inc.

Stewart, Felicia et al. (1987). *Understanding Your Body: Every Woman's Guide to Gynecology and Health*. New York: Bantam Books.

Varney, Helen, (1987). *Nurse-Midwifery*. 2nd edition. Boston: Blackwell Scientific Publications.

DIETHYLSTILBESTROL. *See instead* DES: DIETHYLSTILBESTROL

DISABILITY, CHILDBEARING WITH

Having a baby brings new joys and new challenges to all parents. For men and women who have a disability or chronic illness, the challenges are often greater.

General Public Attitudes. There are widespread misconceptions that people with disabilities cannot be adequate parents. Once they do become parents, they are all too often treated as if on trial and expected to conform to an ideal of parenthood that no one else must meet. There is also a tendency to treat all disabled people as the same; the hero/victim stereotypes focus on disability rather than ability and thus deny normalcy.

Health Professionals. The role of the health professional is to work with their client(s) to:

- provide accurate and appropriate family planning advice;
- build up a realistic picture of any risks to client and baby in advance of conception—if necessary, by referring the client(s) to genetic counselors and other specialists;
- provide appropriate prenatal care and advice that takes into account any potential effects of pregnancy on the disability and vice versa (including the effects of medication on fetus or via breastfeeding);
- seek out information relating to prenatal exercise, options in labor positions, use of medical forms of pain relief, and sources of nonmedical support;
- ensure accessibility of equipment and space in labor and postnatal wards;
- discuss childcare methods and adaptation of baby equipment as necessary;
- provide appropriate medical care as well as support and encouragement in labor and postnatally.

Problems often arise because health professionals lack general disability awareness and are often ill informed about the full nature of how a particular disability affects the individual in her day-to-day life; neither the disability nor the pregnancy is a purely medical issue but both are often treated as such. Prejudicial negative attitudes may encourage termination of pregnancy or paint an unnecessarily gloomy picture of the outcome so that the client feels guilty for wanting to have children. There is also a tendency in pregnancy, labor, and postnatal situations to overintervene or remove choices unnecessarily. This is often due to unfamiliarity and can be minimized by health professionals seeking out more information themselves and by prospective parents asking more questions to satisfy themselves of what the real options are.

Barriers. Prenatal classes, health clinics, hospital labor wards, and postnatal wards are often poorly equipped to welcome those clients who have a disability: for example, narrow doorways, staircases, high-sided baths that are inaccessible for those who use wheelchairs, beds that cannot be lowered for ease of transfer, baby cribs, and changing surfaces that cannot be reached. Apart from the lack of physical accessibility for those who have a mobility impairment, there are also barriers to information, e.g., inaccessibility of prenatal classes to those with a sight or hearing impairment. Through consultation with the client and other relevant agencies, such as occupational therapists, many of the barriers can be broken down by making adequate provision for the client to be accommodated or arranging alternatives that are accessible.

Personal Adjustment to Pregnancy and Parenthood. There may be anxiety on the part of potential parents due to lack of information and support as well as doubts about the long-term effects of the disability and, therefore, one's ability to cope. The changes of pregnancy may bring additional short-term or long-term physical problems. However it should be remembered that not all disabled people are ill and not all need major additional care. Disabled or not, childbearing can pose physical and emotional problems for any prospective parent, so the problems facing a woman with a disability should be kept in perspective.

Many people with disabilities are economically less well-off, so there may be additional financial stresses associated with pregnancy and parenthood. The attitudes of those close to them (family, neighbors, health professionals, teachers) are important in confidence building. Negative attitudes can undermine self-esteem and make it difficult to ask for help if it is needed.

Mobility may be further impaired with the arrival of the new baby because it may lead to isolation from other sources of support and shared experience. Finding or adapting equipment to suit the individual parent's needs can be a major factor in the ease, and therefore the satisfaction, of being a parent.

All of these factors may exacerbate the challenges that any parent faces in learning to look after a new baby. Most can be minimized by planning ahead and by support from professionals, family, and friends. ✷ MUKTI JAIN CAMPION

See also: Deafness and Childbearing Concerns; Disability, Parenting with

Resources

Asrael, W. (1983). "The Disabled Woman and Childbearing—The Nurse's Role." Nurses Association of American Obstetricians and Gynecologists (NAACOG) Update Series: USA

Campion, Mukti Jain. (1990). *The Baby Challenge—A Handbook on Pregnancy for Women with a Physical Disability* London; New York: Routledge.

National Childbirth Trust. (1984). *The Emotions and Experiences of Some Disabled Mothers.* London: National Childbirth Trust.

DISABILITY, PARENTING WITH

Parents who have a disability have a spectrum of needs just like any other parents: A few will need a lot of support most of the time, some will need help occasionally or with certain aspects of their day-to-day life, and many will manage perfectly well without any special outside help. Which sort of parent a person with a disability becomes may depend as much on the amount of planning ahead they do as on the nature of the disability. It should also be remembered that many of the needs of parents with disabilities may not arise from the disability itself—housing, employment, and relationships can produce challenges for all parents, though they may be exacerbated for those who are disabled.

To meet these challenges, it is important that disabled individuals have adequate information and support before deciding to start a family. Ideally, education should begin at school with appropriate advice about birth planning methods (since not all may be suitable) and positive adult role models. Thereafter, support and information may come from two principal sources other than friends and family: (1) health professionals and (2) self-help groups and disability organizations.

Health Professionals. Often a health professional is the first point of contact for people seeking medical information about parenting with a disability. It is therefore important that the information given be accurate, up-to-date, and based in reality without being unnecessarily negative. It is also vital that the information be intelligible (e.g., presented with due recognition of the client's disability, such as deafness) and that there is adequate opportunity for discussion of causes of concern to the client. The aim should be to create an atmosphere of trust and dialogue—for it is a major decision that will fundamentally affect the clients for the rest of their lives.

The vast majority of people with disabilities are physically able to become parents, but it is important that they be fully informed about any risks to either mother or baby, even though most such risks can be minimized with good prenatal care. All medical knowledge should be exchanged in a spirit of collaboration—the woman with a disability is usually very knowledgeable of her physical and emotional capabilities, and health professionals can learn from listening to her. While it is the responsibility of health professionals to discuss any potential problems, the final decision on whether to embark on parenthood should always remain with the client. Information about prenatal care, labor positions and pain relief, breastfeeding, and preparation for the baby's arrival should all be discussed well in advance.

Sources of postnatal support should be identified early on and be appropriate to the individual client and tailored as specifically to the individual (or couple or family) as possible. This requires empathetic consultation with the client. It is often helpful for the client to identify one professional who can coordinate the medical/social welfare services and support available. This care coordinator may have a better understanding of how, for example, medical referral processes work and may be better able to represent the client's needs within medical and social welfare departments. There should be detailed discussion of baby care methods, equipment, emotional adjustments of new parenthood, relaxation methods, and so on, particularly if the nature of the disability is such that it limits access to general sources of information (e.g., books, television, libraries).

Postnatal support should be planned ahead of the arrival of the baby and contact should be encouraged after the baby is born. In particularly stressed families, every effort should be made to provide support that enables families to stay together and function better rather than to take children into care.

Self-Help Groups and Disability Organizations (Local and National). The limited physical accessibility of so many public buildings can mean that many parents who are disabled miss out on the continuous exchange of information that takes place between parents at school gates, mother-and-baby groups, baby clinics, etc. This can result in isolation and additionally handicap a new parent. Awareness of this potential danger means parents can seek out activities that are accessible.

Not all people with disabilities want to be involved with other people just because they are also disabled. However, many disability organizations can provide valuable information, contacts, and sources of shared experience. Self-help networks serving those with a particular disabling condition can be especially useful for sharing tips and practical experiences—for a first-time parent, this can make a huge difference in day-to-day childcare strategies.

It is easy to focus on the problems that might face a parent who is disabled, but it is important to also highlight the fact that most veteran disabled parents report as normal a relationship with their children as any other parents. Because of the disability, many parents devote more time to their children, and it is often very noticeable that their children are more responsible and considerate of others at an early age. ✱ MUKTI JAIN CAMPION

See also: Disability, Childbearing with

Resources

Asrael W. & Kesselman, S. (1982). *Classes for the Disabled in Childbirth Educator.*

Campion, Mukti Jain. (1990). *The Baby Challenge—A Handbook on Pregnancy for Women with a Physical Disability.* London: Routledge.

Conine, T.A. & Carty, E.A. (1986, Nov). "Childbirth Education for Disabled Parents—Psychosocial Considerations." *International Journal of Childbirth Education.*

Nursing Mothers Association of Australia. (1982). *Where There's a Will There Is Usually a Way—A Guide to Breast Feeding Where the Mother Has a Disability.* Available from: Nursing Mothers Association of Australia, P.O. Box 231, Nunawading, Victoria 3131, Australia.

United States Department of Health and Social Services. (1981). *Family Planning Services for Disabled People—A Manual for Service Providers.* Washington, DC: United States Department of Health and Social Services.

DOMESTIC VIOLENCE AND PREGNANCY

One in 15 pregnant women are physically or sexually assaulted by their partners during the pregnancy, and battered women have twice as many miscarriages as pregnant women who are not battered.

These are shocking facts. Even more shocking is the conclusion of the Surgeon General that pregnancy increases a woman's risk of being beaten by her partner, in part shocking because the expectation of society is that pregnant women should receive special consideration, not abuse. Expecting "special treatment" for pregnant women, to a degree is based on perceiving pregnancy as a disability, akin to other temporary disabling conditions, such as a broken leg. But it also reflects cultural support for children, mothers, and mothering. Women in the later stages of their pregnancy, or with infants or small children in tow, could once count on courtesies from strangers, such as being given a seat on a crowded bus or train, or not having to wait in line at a store. In France, this practice is institutionalized: Pregnant women may sit in first-class train seats with second class tickets.

Since strangers were expected to offer such courtesies the expectation was that the family and friends of a pregnant woman would take even greater care of her. Some of this concern for her health was really aimed at protecting the fetus. Nevertheless, even if such courtesies are offered less frequently, most people still are deeply disturbed to learn that pregnancy not only does not protect women from physical abuse, but that it may itself be a risk factor. No one disputes that pregnant women are battered. The question is whether pregnancy increases a woman's risk of abuse.

Not insignificantly, the first awareness of pregnant women being beaten by partners came from service providers in battered women's programs. Physicians routinely in contact with pregnant women did not notice or report battering incidents and, for the most part, still do not. Advocates providing peer or clinical counseling to battered women found that a surprising number of women reported being beaten during their pregnancy. Some reported that the battery began during pregnancy and was itself focused on the pregnancy, with some women reporting being hit in the abdomen. That the pregnancy did not insulate women from such attacks surprised the victims and the counselors.

Subsequent studies of random households and of prenatal clinics confirmed both the regular incidence of abuse of pregnant women and the fact that some were indeed at special risk of being abused. Helton, McFarlane, and Anderson's clinic study (1987) confirmed that women who had been battered before were the most likely to be abused during their pregnancies. Eight percent received medical treatment for injuries, usually in an emergency room, from these assaults by their partners. Yet, the studies of abused pregnant women included one to three percent who had no previous history of being battered. For this much smaller group, abuse began with the pregnancy and, for some, focused on the pregnancy itself.

The prenatal clinic studies of battery were designed to calculate the incidence of battery during pregnancy and to make policy recommendations for health care providers and social workers in health care facilities. The several studies recommended that all pregnant women be screened for abuse, since the risks of violence from a partner were at least as common as such routinely screened risks in pregnancy as diabetes. As is common in nursing practice, evaluations of patients' social and medical needs were integrated. Prenatal clinic staff were encouraged to ask both the pregnant woman and her partner about their concerns related to the pregnancy and parenting so additional services could be offered as indicated.

Helton, McFarlane, and Anderson's (1987) studies of prenatal clinic patients confirms that at least seven to eight percent of pregnant women are beaten by partners. While 87.5 percent of those battered during pregnancy had been abused before, others reported that the assaults began during the pregnancy. That is, one percent of pregnant women, with no history of being battered, will be abused during pregnancy. This prenatal clinic study also verifies other work that shows that abuse is seriously underreported. In this sample, an additional 11 percent of those who denied being battered in the first interview showed symptoms of battery or reported abuse at the second meeting. Their study documents what others have found; that once trust has been established, additional reporting of abuse surfaces. This pattern indicates that most estimates of abuse from survey data should be considered conservative. Since poorer and younger women are less likely to receive prenatal care, and have greater risks of abuse, the studies based on private and public clinic patients would also underestimate the abuse experienced by pregnant women.

Explanations of the violence vary, but the most salient difference is whether they depict the pregnancy as directly connected to the partners' violence, or just coincidental. The kind of data one works from tends to shape the explanation offered. While Gelles (1988) accepted the prevalence of violence during pregnancy, he concluded that the age of the woman was critical to the violence, not her pregnancy. Using survey data, he found that women under 25 are both more likely to be beaten, and more likely to be pregnant, and concludes that the relationship between the pregnancy and the violence is a spurious one. However, some questions are begged by these data. Older men, whose battery rates are generally lower, have higher than expected rates of hitting their younger pregnant wives. Even this hypothesis that age of both the women and the men was the truly significant variable needs to be qualified. Gelles suspects that since pregnancy is significant to women, they are more likely to remember being hit during pregnancy and perhaps forget other abusive incidents that may have occurred.

Another clinic study of predominantly poor, urban, minority, women focused on substance abuse (Amaro et al., 1990). Battered pregnant women were more depressed and reported that they had less support from partners and other family members for the pregnancy. Several public health studies raised a concern that the depression often associated with a partner's abuse was being handled by the woman with alcohol, and by her physician with prescription drugs, placing the pregnant woman and the fetus at greater risk. Other studies have verified that women's drinking may be used to cope with a partner's violence. For men, drugs and alcohol are used to permit the violence, while escaping responsibility for it. The study also found that a pregnant woman's drinking and her partner's use of marijuana and/or cocaine were strongly tied to the risk of battery during the pregnancy. Substance use was a stronger predictor than race, age, or income, undermining popular stereotypes that spouse abuse is a problem limited to poorer, less educated families.

The correlations of unemployment, substance abuse, and social class with wife beating make them risk factors, too. Pregnancy, like some of the other risk factors, changes the family dynamic. Pregnancy also may exacerbate other problems. The number of American households without health insurance, and dependent on two incomes, means that the economic demands of the pregnancy and the fiscal and emotional demands of raising a child can be extremely difficult. Increasingly, women are expected to be in the paid labor force. The economic decline of a household in which a pregnant woman has had to leave work, or will leave work, is considerable.

Men who have learned that stress can be relieved by abusing others, with children and woman as the likely targets, are more likely to hit their pregnant wives. As well, pregnant women are more defenseless, more economically dependent. The most economically or socially dependent women endure a great deal of abuse because of their reduced options.

However, the dynamic between men and women who are intimate, is crucial to understanding this violence. Couples have specific expectations of one another that the culture supports. Many of these expectations are contradictory or are changing. In spite of the sharp disagreements among social scientists about the complexities of battered women's experiences, all agree that women's economic dependence and men's need for their subordination is at the root of the violence. The battery within dating relationships, and the special risks of battery for successful women married to less successful men, affirm that the abuse of women by their partners is based on a man's need to dominate or control "his" woman (Hornung, McCullough, and Taichi, 1981).

✱ EILEEN GEIL MORAN, Ph.D.

See also: Violence against Pregnant Women

See **Guide to Related Topics:** Pregnancy Complications

Resources

Amaro, Hortensia et al. (1990, May). "Violence during Pregnancy and Substance Use." *American Journal of Public Health 80* (5): 575-79.

Gelles, Richard. (1988, Aug). "Violence and Pregnancy: Are Pregnant Women at Greater Risk of Abuse?" *Journal of Marriage and the Family 50* (3): 841-47.

Helton, Anne. (1986). "Battery during Pregnancy." *American Journal of Nursing 86* (8): 910-12.

Helton, Anne S., McFarlane, Judith, & Anderson, Elizabeth T. (1987). "Battered and Pregnant: A Prevalence Study." *American Journal of Public Health 77*: 1337-39.

Hornung, Carlton A., McCullough, B. Claire, & Taichi, Sugimoto. (1981, Aug). "Status Relationships in Marriage: Risk Factors in Spouse Abuse." *Journal of Marriage and the Family 43* (3): 675-92.

Kantor, Glenda Kaufman & Straus, Murray A. (1987, Jun). "The Drunken Bum Theory of Wife Beating." *Social Problems 34* (3): 213-30.

DONOR INSEMINATION

Donor insemination (DI), the artificial introduction of semen into the female reproductive tract, has been practiced for over a century and is the most widely used method of assisted conception. The reasons why DI is performed include: primary male infertility, eugenics (20 percent of DI is done for genetic factors), immunological reasons (Rh incompatibility, "hostile" cervical mucus), vasectomy and remarriage, and lack of a male partner. Estimates of annual numbers of donor offspring in the United States range from 20,000 to 100,000, with 20,000 believed to exist in the state of California alone. The absence of records and statistics is a direct result of the secrecy that typically shrouds this procedure as well as the use of anonymous donors.

This process goes by many names: artificial insemination, AID insemination, donor insemination, alternative insemination, therapeutic insemination, heterologous insemination, abnormal insemination, non-spousal insemination, and vendor insemination. The mixed terminology reveals the social confusion that arises when the significance of biological ties is both denied and acknowledged in third-party conceptions. The donor is kept anonymous so that there can be a pretense to biological ties between the infertile husband and the offspring. Anonymity of the donor is also considered important by single women and lesbians, as well as married couples, to avoid a potential paternity claim. Different donors may be used in one cycle, or semen from different donors may be mixed (although that is less common nowadays) to make donor identity virtually impossible to trace. Openness is more likely when DI is done to avoid transmitting a hereditary disorder.

Donor sperm is usually procured by physicians from a semen bank for convenience and a wider choice of donors. Frozen semen is fast replacing fresh semen because cryopreservation permits quarantining and testing for HIV antibodies. Sperm banking has become a profitable commercial enterprise. While medical students made up the majority of donors in the past, sperm is now recruited from various sources and fees of up to $100 paid per ejaculate can yield many samples for insemination. The quality of donor screening and storage techniques is highly variable due to minimal or nonexistent state regulation. Guidelines have been drawn up by the Food and Drug Administration, the Centers for Disease Control, the American Association of Tissue Banks, and the American Fertility Society. However, these guidelines deal with public health issues and donor protection, not the rights of the unborn child, and are rarely enforceable due to absent or inadequate state legislation.

Matching of blood group and phenotype to the infertile husband are done primarily to deceive the child. The low-tech procedure of introducing sperm into the vagina (via syringe or cervical cap) facilitates secrecy; unlike adoption, DI leaves no legal trail. In such cases, the child will be raised up with the perilous "as if" factor created by deception. Secrecy reinforces the stigma and shame surrounding DI and creates a reluctance to reveal the fact even to family or close friends. Secrets result in lies and distortion; they generate anxiety, set up barriers, and create loyalty dynamics and co-conspiracy, affecting future generations too. Parental evasiveness with regard to sex, reproduction, and blood type arouses suspicion. "Leaking" and the temptation to gossip is ever present, and the most devastating consequence is the violation of trust when the deception is revealed, often during a family argument.

There is a dearth of information about how these families fare except for the testimonies of the few aware DI offspring who have spoken out, and experience with adoption and its reforms. A state of confusion results from no, uncertain, or partial knowledge of one's biological parents. This genealogical bewilderment has yet to be acknowledged in the case of the DI offspring who, like the adoptees of the past, are raised with the pretense of a biological connection.

Knowledge of and definite relationship to his or her complete genealogy is necessary for a child to build up a complete identity. When the fact of an anonymous donor conception becomes known, a host of other fears and feelings emerge as well. They include fear of unknown hereditary diseases, despair at not being able to find the identity of the donor because records are nonexistent or destroyed, lack of support from others in the same situation, and reluctant sharing of emotional burdens with family and community. Incest is another common fear. Donors can be used in small communities for a great number of births and some donate to several physicians and clinics.

It has been shown that where counseling is provided to parents, they are more likely to plan to inform the child of his or her DI status. However, the dilemma is that the identity of the donor is forever lost if the sperm broker, whether a semen bank or physician, keeps no records. The minimal standard would be to require permanent records to be available for the child at age of majority. Better still, the example of open and cooperative adoption could be followed.

✷ ELIZABETH NOBLE

See also: Adoption, Closed; Adoption, Open; In Vitro Fertilization for Male Infertility; Infertility: Cross-Cultural and Historical Aspects

See **Guide to Related Topics:** Infertility; New Procreative Technologies

Resources

Achilles, R. (1986). *The Social Meaning of Biological Ties: A Study of Participants in Artificial Insemination by Donor.* Ph.D. thesis, Department of Education, University of Toronto.

Baran, A. & Pannor, R. (1989). *Lethal Secrets: The Shocking Consequences and Unsolved Problems of Artificial Insemination.* New York: Warner.

Berger, D. (1986). "Psychological Patterns in Donor Insemination Couples." *Canadian Journal of Psychiatry 31*: 818.

Blizzard, J. (1977). *Blizzard and the Holy Ghost: Artificial Insemination—A Personal Account.* London: Peter Owen Ltd.

Bok, Sissela. (1978). *Lying: Moral Choice in Public and Private Life.* New York: Pantheon.

———. (1983). *Secrets: On the Ethics of Concealment and Revelation.* New York: Random House.

Lifton, B.J. (1987, Dec). "Brave New Babies in a Brave New World." *Women and Health.*

Noble, Elizabeth. (1987). *Having Your Baby by Donor Insemination.* Boston: Houghton Mifflin.

Rowland, R. (1983, Jun). "Attitudes and Opinions of Donors on an Artificial Insemination by Donor (AID) Programme." *Clinical Reproductive Fertility* 2: (249).

Sants, H.J. (1964). "Genealogical Bewilderment in Children with Substitute Parents." *British Journal of Medical Psychology 37*: 133.

DOULA

One of the shared characteristics of mammals is the appearance of support by others of the group during various periods in the life cycle. The stage of reproduction is just such a period. Very likely the supportive behavior among animals to protect females and their offspring was an adaptive response in the evolution of this species.

During the pregnancy/childbirth/early lactational stage in humans, one or more women, most often the mother's mother, assumes a supportive role. Though practically universal, this role had not been identified or studied until recently, when the term "Doula" was used to describe the person or persons whose role it is to care for the new mother (Raphael, 1973).

Several centuries B.C., this Greek word referred to a female slave. The present usage resulted from a casual remark of an elderly Greek woman. Listening carefully to a discussion between colleagues on the function of a supportive person around the new mother, she interjected, "Of course, that's a doula. It is the person who comes from across the road when a baby is born and helps the mother with the infant and the older children. They call her doula (auntie, grandmother). She bounces the fussing baby and gossips with the mother who needs her very much."

Frequently, the doula assists at the delivery, but it was the need for support during the postpartum period, when breastfeeding begins, that drew attention to the critical role the doula plays.

When this phenomenon was first studied, each of the 178 cultures examined revealed some sort of supportive, proscribed help around the mother as the ideal behavior (Raphael, 1966). This led to further study, revealing that without a doula, that is, without supportive help, women are usually unable to breastfeed. Without such assistance, someone to share the responsibility for the life of that child, the mother failed to eject the milk from the sinuses in the lobes within the breast, making it available for the infant to suck. Needless to say, in underdeveloped countries it is unlikely the child would survive without breastfeeding.

In traditional societies—India, China, and others—the preferred pattern is for a woman to return to her natal home during her last months of pregnancy. In that setting she is likely to feel safe, tendered and tended to by caring relatives. In India the "dai," or midwife, plays a very important role not only during delivery but postpartum as well. In this case, not only the mother's mother and other female relatives, but the dai share the role of doula—in this case a kind of "composite doula."

Human societies have developed a myriad of different patterns in response to the need for support, ranging from minimal support by the spouse to well-defined elaborate cultural mandates where different people—father and mother-in-law, mother's mother and father, even co-wives—have a culturally proscribed role in relation to the new mother. These mandates include performing special rites, tending the mother's garden, cooking for the family, or presenting the mother and babe with specific gifts.

The choice of who substitutes as doula if her own mother is not present is very complex. A woman may favor her aunt (mother's sister) as a substitute but finds she needs the consent of her own mother or her mother-in-law. During this century in England and the United States, maiden aunts, often "war widows," were expected to travel from one niece to another caring for the newborn.

In the United States it is unlikely that a "best friend" can be the doula. Frequently after marriage, miles, even continents, separate such friends, so this function is assumed by a newly acquainted "friend," one often in this close relationship for only a short time.

Such decisions may be influenced by the woman's economic and social position, as care is often a "statement" of familial responsibility with an underlying assumption that reciprocity is expected. Not surprising, women of high social status have more persons who will share the role of doula. Conversely, the presence of a doula and the amount of time she can spend with the mother is limited by the amount of food available to feed that helper. A new grandmother may come from the village to Mexico City to care for her daughter, but there must be adequate space for her and sufficient funds to pay for the additional food. If she lives in another part of the city, the duration of her participation may depend on whether or not she has the bus fare.

The amount of mothering the mother receives also depends on how much her child will enhance or stress resources of the family and the community. In China, where ideally each family is limited to one child, it becomes the responsibility not only of the family but the community to keep that infant alive. The common preference for male children is another factor influencing the quality and quantity of support given the mother.

An increasing body of research supports the thesis that such a relationship has a critical effect on postpartum behavior. In a pilot study conducted at the Social Security Hospital in Guatemala City, those women who, during labor, were assigned an untrained, unfamiliar woman—a doula—to provide reassurance and physical contact throughout labor and delivery, had a shorter labor and a lower rate of caesarean sections than did women who labored alone (Sosa et al., 1980). Twenty women who had the support of a doula experienced 8.7 hours of labor compared with 19.3 hours for the control group; the rate for caesarean sections was 6.5 percent among 200 women assigned a doula, compared with 18 percent among controls. Mothers with a doula also required less medication and were more likely than controls to remain awake after delivery and to interact more often with their babies.

As mentioned earlier the presence of support is intrinsic to many species of mammals. Hundreds of social mammals exhibit behaviors toward the female that appear to be very supportive, increasing the chances the young will survive (Raphael, Hale, and Breakstone, 1976; Raphael, 1981).

Patterns of grouping are extremely diverse: Sometimes they include one male and several females with their young, as in the silver-backed gorilla; a cluster of mothers and their young without a male (Kortland, 1962; Goodall, 1965); or female/female "families," as occur, for example, with the dolphin, elephant, and elk.

As human society changes, new forms of social arrangements for mother/infant care are invented. For example, in the 1950s in the United States, the La Leche League breastfeeding support group was created. The sole purpose was to support the primipara at a time when information about breastfeeding was minimal and when the preferred pattern was to feed infants with formula in bottles. These members shared their breastfeeding experiences with each other at monthly group meetings and acted as doulas in person or by telephone.

In the 1980s a new idea took hold. The generation of women who wanted to breastfeed also wanted immediate help on a one-to-one basis. Group meetings were no longer satisfying. In hospitals and pediatric practices, nurses were appointed to perform the role of doula. This lactation specialist was available, in person or by telephone, to answer the common, worrisome, and practical questions of breastfeeding mothers.

Another lactation specialist pattern emerged when leaders of breastfeeding support groups found they could no longer offer their service free. Small companies were formed, often with the word "doula" trademarked within the name of the organization. For a fee, these companies perform services for the new mother such as cooking, cleaning, and advising on breastfeeding problems. However, this work is labor-intensive and often not cost-effective. The role of doulaship is an extremely delicate one involving a form of mothering of the mother that does not easily lend itself to commercial practices. New ways of participating as doula are still being invented. An alternative "reciprocal doula" arrangement between two women with children of near ages is an effective option that, with careful and systematic planning, can be very effective (Raphael, 1973).

Recently, the doula relationship has taken on a broader context, becoming a term for anyone who helps another during some stressful state. A patient says his son became his doula when he had a coronary; a woman reports that her husband had tended to his mother's broken ankle, much like a doula.

"The need of mutual aid and support . . . always has been the chief leader towards further progress." Edward Wilson's tome *Sociobiology—The New Synthesis* (1975) provides new insight into altruism from a genetic standpoint—a form of supportive intelligence that becomes an instrument of natural selection—even in ants. The persistence of doula behavior in most mammals speaks to its intrinsic value, and the continuing invention of new responses in human beings attests to the ongoing value of this caring relationship.

✱ DANA RAPHAEL, Ph.D.

See also: Breastfeeding: Historical Aspects; Breastfeeding: Physiological and Cultural Aspects; Evolution of Human Birth; Labor Assistants

See **Guide to Related Topics:** Caregivers and Practitioners; Infant Feeding

Resources

Goodall, Jane. (1965). "Chimpanzees of the Gombe Stream Reserve." In Irven DeVore (Ed.) *Primate Behavior: Field Studies of Monkeys and Apes*. New York: Holt Rinehart & Winston, Inc., pp. 425-73.

Kortland, A. (1962). "Chimpanzees in the Wild. *Scientific American 2065* (5): 128-38.

Raphael, Dana. (1966). "The Lactation-Suckling Process within a Matrix of Supportive Behavior." Unpublished Ph.D. dissertation, Columbia University, New York, 1966. (Microfilm number 69-15,580).

———. (1973). *The Tender Gift: Breastfeeding*. Englewood Cliffs, NJ: Prentice Hall.

———. (1981). "Why Supportive Behavior in Human and Other Mammals?" *American Anthropologist 83* (3): 634-38.

Raphael, Dana, Hale, Lucinda & Breakstone, Amy. (1976, Oct 9). "Female/Young Groupings within Mammalian Social Organization." Animal Behavior Society Meeting, American Museum of Natural History, New York.

Sosa, Roberto et al. (1980). "The Effect of a Supportive Companion on Perinatal Problems, Length of Labor, and Mother-Infant Interaction." *New England Journal of Medicine 303* (11): 597-600.

Wilson, Edward O. (1975). *Sociobiology—The New Synthesis*. Cambridge, MA: Belknap/Harvard University Press.

Note: Doula™ is a registered trademark of the Human Lactation Center, Westport, CT 06880, Dr. Dana Raphael, director. Permission to use the term for commercial purposes may be obtained by writing to the Center.

DR. SPOCK. *See instead* SPOCK, DR. BENJAMIN

DREAMS DURING PREGNANCY

Researchers know a great deal about the frequency and content of the unusual dreams of pregnant women. These nightly visions are easily recalled, vivid, richly detailed, bizarre, and often nightmarish. Yet little has been said about the causes of these remarkable dreams, or how understanding them can shed light on the psychology of pregnancy.

Most psychologists (Krippner and Dillard, 1988) agree that dreams reflect our waking lives, so that analyses of dreams during pregnancy can provide clues to expectant mothers' innermost thoughts. Research (Maybruck, 1986, 1989, 1990) into thousands of pregnant women's dreams reveals that they are extremely anxious about six major concerns, as discussed below. Once identified and confronted, these typical, often needless fears can be resolved so that expectant mothers can experience a more relaxed, peaceful pregnancy and an easier, safer delivery.

Why Dreams during Pregnancy Are Different. Since 1968, there have been at least 14 major investigations of this phenomenon (Van de Castle and Kinder, 1968; Karacan et al., 1968, 1969; Cheek, 1969; Van de Castle, 1971; Winget and Kapp, 1972; Krippner et al., 1974; Ballou, 1978; Jones, 1978; Leifer, 1980; Maybruck, 1986, 1989; 1990; Garfield, 1988). All of these researchers found that pregnant women's dreams differ markedly from those of any other group.

Further, the themes and symbols of pregnant women's dreams appear to have similar meanings to most pregnant women regardless of age or background. For example, most women associate dreams of small animals, such as kittens, bunnies, or puppies, with the unborn child. Water images, such as overflowing tubs or toilets, storms at sea, and ocean waves, usually symbolize either the amniotic waters in which the fetus is suspended, the "waters breaking" at onset of labor, or the ebb and flow of labor contractions. Dreams about her mother may indicate the dreamer's concern about unresolved mother-daughter conflicts or her own mothering abilities. Themes of intruders, such as burglars or other threatening characters, often represent the dreamer's feelings that her body has been invaded, or her fears of a cesarean section.

There are several theories that attempt to explain these unusual dreams. One is that pregnancy's sudden increase in hormonal levels intensifies emotionalism and also affects both content and frequency of dreams. Another is that pregnant women sleep more so they are likely to have more dreams. A third explanation, based on Hartmann's investigations of nightmare sufferers (Hartmann, 1984), hypothesizes that, since everyone's dreams change dramatically during any transition or lifestyle change, it follows that pregnant women's dreams will reflect the concerns of approaching motherhood.

While all of these explanations appear to have some validity, Maybrock's research of thousands of pregnant women's dreams shows that the transition theory probably accounts for most of the unusual characteristics that are typical of this group. Moreover, contemporary mothers-to-be have more nightmares than ever before, indicating that pregnancy in these stressful times is often an emotionally difficult maturational phase of life-crisis proportions.

What Pregnant Women's Dreams Reveal. Hartmann found that only one in 200 nonpregnant people suffer from nightmares more than once a week. Yet more than 40 percent of pregnant volunteers reported nightmares from which they awoke feeling terrified. Moreover, another 30 percent had dreams containing fearful elements such as funerals, disasters, and threatening characters (Maybruck, 1989).

These statistics are alarmingly high, indicating that many expectant mothers are undergoing emotional upheaval that may adversely affect them and their babies' health as well as prevent them from achieving the deep relaxation necessary for a safe and normal childbirth. While many other factors undoubtedly affect duration and ease of labor, research has established (Winget and Kapp, 1972; Tapley et al., 1989) that relaxation between contractions greatly facilitates uterine motility, so that it becomes essential for women about to give birth to be free of stress and tension.

Upon analysis, anxiety-provoking dream themes revealed that these women experienced distress in six major areas: (1) fear of the baby being defective or dead; (2) fear of being an inadequate parent; (3) fear of the loss of the mate; (4) fear of losing control of the body and emotions; (5) fear of severe pain or death during delivery; and (6) fear of financial burdens (Maybruck, 1989). Investigation of the dreams and attitudes of literally hundreds of American and Canadian pregnant women indicates that most of the women studied experienced anxiety about two or more of these issues. Armed with this knowledge, both health professionals and pregnant women themselves can take positive steps to resolve these often needless fears.

Overcoming the Fears of Pregnancy. The pregnant woman's denial or repression of unpleasant emotions was noted by Deutsch more than four decades ago (Deutsch, 1945). Research shows that this response is even more typical today. Many women, striving to be self-sufficient, are reluctant to admit to any fears lest they be thought immature or inadequate as future mothers (Maybruck, 1989).

Careful examination of dream records will usually reveal the pregnant woman's true feelings, providing her and her caregiver the opportunity to uncover hidden anxiety. Once the fear has been identified, its reality and the choices available for preventing or minimizing it can be evaluated. As a final step in the resolution of each area of concern, expectant mothers can then be taught ways to integrate more positive attitudes within the unconscious.

High hormonal levels appear to enhance pregnant women's abilities to access skills associated with the brain's right hemisphere, so that they can achieve a semi-trance state more easily than they did before pregnancy. (This does not mean that they have no control over their waking state of consciousness; there is little need for concern about their driving or performing other tasks that require a more alert "left-brain" state of awareness.) This may be the reason relaxation and breathing techniques taught in prenatal classes are helpful during labor. In fact, teaching such techniques earlier in the pregnancy can help pregnant women overcome negative attitudes and a constant state of tension, which may otherwise be difficult to overcome at the onset of labor. Further, affirmations, guided imagery, and visualizations of a best-case scenario are especially effective in eliminating the often needless anxiety that causes stress. Pregnant women can also be taught to "incubate" or deliberately dream about topics they wish to explore. Dream incubation can help the dreamer resolve anxiety-provoking conflicts. Follow-up studies of 67 pregnant women showed that those who became assertive in dreams that once portrayed them as victims had an easier, shorter labor and delivery than those who made no attempts to defend themselves in such dreams (Maybruck, 1986, 1989).

Once their fears are released, those who suffer from nightmares will usually begin to have sweeter, more positive dreams that reflect their love for the child within and their joyous anticipation of motherhood. ✱ PATRICIA MAYBRUCK, Ph.D.

See also: Motherhood as Transformation

See **Guide to Related Topics:** Pregnancy, Psychological Aspects

Resources

Ballou, J. (1978). *The Psychology of Pregnancy.* Lexington, MA: Lexington Books.

Cheek, D. (1969). "Significance of Dreams in Initiating Premature Labor." *American Journal of Clinical Hypnosis 12*: 5-15.

Deutsch, H. (1945). *The Psychology of Women.* New York: Grune & Stratton.

Garfield, P. (1988). *Women's Bodies, Women's Dreams.* New York: Ballantine Books.

Hartmann, E. (1984). *The Nightmare.* New York: Basic Books.

Jones, C. (1978). "An Exploratory Study of Women's Manifest Dream Content during First Pregnancy." *Dissertation Abstracts International* (University Microfilms No. 76-199,359). Ann Arbor, MI: University Abstracts International.

Karacan, I. et al. (1968). "Characteristics of Sleep Patterns during Late Pregnancy and the Postpartum Periods." *American Journal of Obstetrics and Gynecology 101*:579-86.

Karacan, I. et al. (1969). "Some Implications of the Sleep Patterns of Pregnancy to Postpartum Emotional Disturbance." *British Journal of Psychiatry 115*: 929-35.

Krippner, S. & Dillard, J. (1988). *Dreamworking.* Buffalo, NY: Bearlike.

Krippner, S. et al. (1974). "An Investigation of Dream Content During Pregnancy." *Journal of the American Society of Psychosomatic Dentistry and Medicine 21*: 111-23.

Leifer, M. (1980). *Psychological Effects of Motherhood: A Study of First Pregnancy.* New York: Praeger.

Maybruck, P. (1986). "An Exploratory Study of the Dreams of Pregnant Women." *Dissertation Abstracts International* (University Microfilm No. 86-05,318). Ann Arbor, MI: University Abstracts International.

———. (1989). *Pregnancy and Dreams.* Los Angeles: Jeremy P. Tarcher, Inc.

———. (1990). "Pregnancy and Dream Content." In S. Krippner (Ed.) *Language of the Night.* Los Angeles: Jeremy P. Tarcher, Inc.

———. (1990, Jun 28). "Pregnant Women's Dreams: What They Reveal." Paper presented at the Seventh International Conference of the Association for the Study of Dreams, Chicago, IL.

Tapley, F. et al. (Eds.) (1989). *The Columbia University College of Physicians and Surgeons Complete Guide to Pregnancy.* New York: Crown Books.

Van de Castle, R.L. (1971). *The Psychology of Dreaming.* Morristown, NJ: General Learning Press.

Van de Castle, R.L. & Kinder, P. (1968). "Dream Content During Pregnancy." *Psychophysiology* 4: 375-80.

Winget, C. & Kapp, F.T. (1972). "The Relationship of the Manifest Content of Dreams to Duration of Childbirth in Primiparae." *Psychoanalytic Medicine 34*: 313-20.

This article is condensed from "Pregnancy and Dream Content" by Patricia Maybruck, Ph.D., in Stanley Krippner, Ph.D. (Ed.) *Language of the Night* (1990), Los Angeles: Jeremy P. Tarcher, Inc. and from *Pregnancy and Dreams* by Patricia Maybruck, Ph.D. (1989), Los Angeles: Jeremy P. Tarcher, Inc. with permission from the publishers.

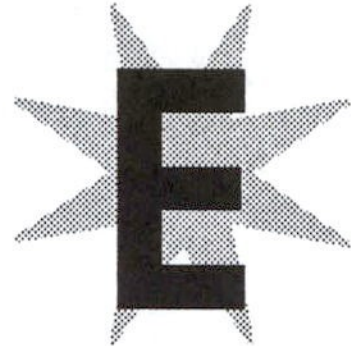

ECTOPIC PREGNANCY

The United States is in the midst of an epidemic of ectopic pregnancies. During the past decade, the number of reported ectopic pregnancies nearly tripled from about 17,800 in 1970 to about 52,200 in 1980 (Dorfman, 1984).

About 1 in 100 pregnancies begins to grow outside of the uterus. This is called an ectopic pregnancy, (meaning "out of place"). The most common site of ectopic pregnancy is in the Fallopian tube. There are also other sites where this can happen, such as the ovary or even the abdomen, but these cases are rare (American College of Obstetrics & Gynecology, 1983). In an ectopic pregnancy, the egg, which travels towards the uterus for eventual implantation during the first few days after fertilization, implants instead in the tube ("tubal pregnancy") or someplace outside of the uterus. In almost all cases, this means that the pregnancy is nonviable.

Some of the possible causes of ectopic pregnancy are believed to be: pelvic infections; infections following childbirth, abortion, previous surgery, or endometriosis, which can scar the tubes; and previous ectopic pregnancies. Ovarian tumors or cysts, pelvic adhesions, fibroids, or even on occasion urinary tract infections, plus previous use of the IUD or a tubal ligation are other possible causes of ectopic pregnancy (Dorfman, 1984).

Ectopic pregnancy is the leading cause of death in pregnant women. It also is a major factor in infertility or decreased fertility for those who have had one or more ectopic pregnancies. Delay in seeking care contributes to most of the deaths. Symptoms are often confusing and a fatal rupture can occur before the woman even knows she is pregnant.

Primary care physicians are being encouraged to "think ectopic": make the diagnosis promptly and act quickly. In years past, ectopic pregnancies often were not diagnosed until they ruptured, causing severe symptoms of lower abdominal pain on one side and dizziness, weakness, or fainting. Shoulder pain is also a symptom of a ruptured ectopic pregnancy, due to the irritation of the diaphragm by blood within the abdomen, which the body interprets as pain rising in the shoulder (Ilse, 1992).

What are the signs that might indicate an ectopic pregnancy? The usual ectopic pregnancy begins after an unexpectedly early, late, spotty, or missed menstrual period, and is often, but not always, accompanied by abdominal or pelvic pain, dull or stabbing, and irregular vaginal bleeding. However, many cases are confused with such other disorders as appendicitis, indigestion, kidney stones, bladder infections, or the stomach flu as well as normal pregnancy, threatened miscarriage, or the aftereffects of an induced abortion. If unusual abdominal or pelvic pain occurs after an irregular or missed period—with or without vaginal bleeding—it is important to see a gynecologist immediately because ectopic pregnancies are always a medical emergency (*Glamour*, 1987).

No single test can absolutely confirm the condition or rule it out and no two women have the exact symptoms. A pelvic exam, urine test, and the most common test—the Beta HCG—are used. The Beta HCG is a blood test that monitors the rise in levels of HCG. In a ectopic pregnancy the rise is slower than in a normal pregnancy. An ultrasound sonogram is used to detect whether there is an embryo in the uterus, the tube, or some other site. If an embryo is found in the uterus, an ectopic pregnancy is usually ruled out since it is rare to have both a normal pregnancy and ectopic pregnancy at the same time. If, however, the uterus appears empty, either another ultrasound will be scheduled or, depending upon the severity of the symptoms and test results, a culdocentesis (insertion of a needle through the vaginal wall to draw a sample of fluid) or laparoscopy (a small incision, usually at the naval where an instrument examines the tube and other organs for swelling or bleeding) will be performed. If, at this step, ectopic pregnancy is confirmed, surgery is usually required to remove the embryo and either repair the tube, if possible, or remove the tube when that is the site of pregnancy. The goal is to operate and remove the embryo before rupture occurs, thus reducing the risk of sudden hemorrhage. Many physicians use surgery to deal with every ectopic pregnancy, though there is some controversy whether this is always the only option.

Not very often do medical caregivers discuss the loss of a baby in this process, though surely there are some care providers who do. More often than not, they are concerned with the physical needs and impending emergency nature of the experience. Yet, for many families, there is a strong emotional response related to concern by the man for his partner and concern for the pregnancy and prospective baby by the woman (and occasionally the man). Some people feel a sense of failure and loss. Many people find themselves surprised at how disappointed, frustrated, sorrowful, and even angry they are. Families are encouraged to explore and discuss their emotional response after such an experience.

✱ SHEROKEE ILSE

See also: Miscarriage; Pregnancy after Pregnancy Loss; Pregnancy Loss: Family Response; Support Groups for Infant Loss

See **Guide to Related Topics:** Pregnancy Loss and Infant Mortality

Resources

American College of Obstetrics & Gynecology. (1983). Ectopic pregnancy pamphlet. Washington, DC.

Borg, Susan & Lasker, Judith. (1989). *When Pregnancy Fails: Families Coping with Miscarriage, Ectopic Pregnancy, Stillbirth and Infant Death.* New York: Bantam Books.

Devore, Nancy & Baldwin, Karen. (1987, Jun). "Ectopic Pregnancy on the Rise." *American Journal of Nursing*: 312.

Dorfman, Sally Faith. (1984). "Ectopic Pregnancy: 'Thinking Ectopic,' Key to Diagnosis." *Postgraduate Medicine 76* (12): 65-68.

———. (1986). "Ectopic Pregnancy." *The Female Patient 11.*

Glamour, Medical Report, April 1987.

Ilse, Sherokee. (1990). *Empty Arms: Coping with Miscarriage, Stillbirth and Infant Death.* Maple Plain, MN: Wintergreen Press.

———. (forthcoming). *Ectopic Pregnancy: An Epidemic on the Rise.* Maple Plain, MN: Wintergreen Press.

Limbo, Rana & Wheeler, Sara. (1984). "Ectopic Pregnancy." La Crosse, WI: Resolve Through Sharing.

EGG RETRIEVAL

Sophisticated procreative technologies, such as *in vitro* fertilization (IVF) or gamete intrafallopian transfer (GIFT) have been developed for the treatment of certain kinds of infertility. These technologies require that female eggs be available, either for fertilization by the sperm in the lab (IVF) or for transfer with the sperm into the Fallopian tube (GIFT). Because the eggs are embedded in the ovaries and are not easily accessible, egg retrieval involves either surgical procedures (such as laparoscopy) or ultrasound-directed approaches.

Egg retrieval is usually carried out after the ovaries have been stimulated by hormonal drugs to produce multiple eggs (Klein and Rowland, 1988). Ultrasound scanning of the ovaries is then carried out to follow the ovulation induction process, and blood samples are taken and analyzed for their hormonal levels. When the follicle attains a certain critical size (usually above 15 mm) and when blood estrogen levels reach a necessary value, hCG (human chorionic gonadotropin) is injected intramuscularly.

Egg retrieval is attempted 34 to 36 hours after the administration of hCG, around the 13th day of the menstrual cycle. Timing is an important factor in egg retrieval because the eggs need to be collected when they are mature but before they leave the follicles. Occasionally the ovaries may become quite enlarged and uncomfortable following the hCG injection.

The surgical procedure for egg retrieval is called "laparoscopy." A laparoscope (an optical device the size of a long ball-point pen) is inserted in the abdomen, allowing the physician to look at the organs within the abdomen. Though the laparoscopy is routinely described as a "minor surgical operation," it involves general anesthesia and two or three incisions in the abdomen of the woman. Carbon dioxide gas is pumped into the abdomen to separate the organs and make the manipulations easier. Through one of the incisions a needle is inserted and used to aspirate each ripe egg and its surrounding fluid. Three to four eggs are usually obtained through a laparoscopy, though in some cases up to 10-12 are found. At the end of the procedure, the gas pumped into the abdomen is removed. In some cases, however, adhesions in the women's pelvis prevent seeing the ovaries and no eggs can be obtained. There have been a number of deaths of women during laparoscopy, due mostly to errors by the anesthetists involved in the operation (Corea, 1988).

In the last few years, nonsurgical egg retrieval methods have begun to be developed, due in part to the fact that IVF success rates are very low and often women have to submit to egg retrieval procedures more than once.

The nonsurgical egg retrieval methods use ultrasound to guide the needle that will puncture the ovaries. Local anesthesia is usually used during these procedures. One method involves puncturing the bladder to empty it, then refilling it with saline solution (Wisanto et al., 1988). Another method introduces the needle through the back wall of the vagina (Dellenbach et al., 1985). When the needle transverses the bladder, blood in the urine is observed (Holmes, 1988).

Ultrasound-guided egg retrieval is less expensive, requires less anesthesia, and can be performed as an office procedure. However, it is also reported to be quite painful and women have suffered pelvic infection following transvaginal aspiration of eggs. This casual approach to sterile technique seems to be due to concern regarding the effect of prophylactic antibiotics on the oocytes. Other short-term possible risks of these procedures involve venipuncture, damage to the intestines or rectum requiring surgical repair, and reactions to sedatives and local anesthetics (Holmes, 1987). Practically nothing is known about the long-term risks of the procedure. Holmes also points out that because ultrasound-guided egg retrieval is now an office procedure, doctors are removed from the scrutiny of hospital ethical committees and "can try any variations at all that may happen to occur to them without justifying it to their peers; their methods of obtaining 'informed consent' are also not reviewed."

A feminist critique of reproductive technology is presented by Julie Murphy in her essay "Egg Farming and Women's Future" (Arditti, Duelli Klein, and Minden, 1984). In this article, Murphy contends that removing eggs from women's bodies is more aptly described as "egg farming" and that women are regarded as commodities with vital products to harvest: eggs. She makes the point that the scientific term "egg recovery" is a misnomer because, as she puts it: "Recovery implies prior attachment or ownership. One recovers something one once lost control of or misplaced. When eggs are taken out of women's bodies, however, women do not recover anything. Women lose something, namely, eggs."

Egg donation, in which women donate some of their eggs to women who cannot produce eggs themselves, relies on egg retrieval technology. A number of medical centers in the U.S. and abroad offer different forms of egg donation in spite of the fact that the many ethical and legal issues that this technique raises have not been adequately addressed.

✱ RITA ARDITTI

See also: In Vitro Fertilization for Male Infertility; Infertility: Overview; Preimplantation Diagnosis

See **Guide to Related Topics:** Infertility; New Procreative Technologies

Resources

Arditti, Rita, Duelli Klein, Renate, & Minden, Shelley. (1984). *Test-Tube Women—What Future for Motherhood?* Boston, London: Pandora Press.

Corea, Gena. (1988). *The Mother Machine—Reproductive Technologies from Artificial Insemination to Artificial Wombs*. London: The Women's Press.

Dellenbach, P. et al. (1985). "Transvaginally Sonographically Controlled Follicle Puncture for Oocyte Retrieval." *Fertility and Sterility 44* (5):656-62.

Edwards, Robert & Steptoe, Patrick. (1980). *A Matter of Life*. New York: William Morrow and Co., Inc.

Holmes, Helen Bequaert. (1988). "Risks of Infertility Diagnosis and Treatment." In *Infertility: Medical and Social Choices*. Contractor Documents. Volume IV: Social and Medical Concerns. Congress of the United States. Office of Technology Assessment.

Klein, Renate & Rowland, Robyn. (1988). "Hormonal Cocktails: Women as Test-sites for Fertility Drugs." *Reproductive and Genetic Engineering 1*(3): 251-74.

Wisanto A. et al. (1988). "Perurethral Ultrasound-Guided Ovum Pickup." *Journal of In Vitro Fertilization and Embryo Transfer 5*(2): 107-11.

ELECTRONIC FETAL MONITORING

Fetal assessment has gained more and more clinical importance in the last 25 years because of the rapidly expanding knowledge base regarding intrauterine fetal physiology and development.

Electronic fetal monitoring is one method of assessing fetal well-being *in utero*. The purpose of electronic fetal monitoring is to assess fetal oxygenation within the utero fetal-placental unit by recording contractions and fetal heart rate. Electronic fetal monitoring may be done externally or internally. Uterine contractions are detected either by an open-ended catheter inserted transcervically into the amniotic cavity and attached to a strain guage transducer or by an external device, called a tocodynamometer, that is placed on the maternal abdomen and recognizes the tightening of the maternal abdomen during a contraction.

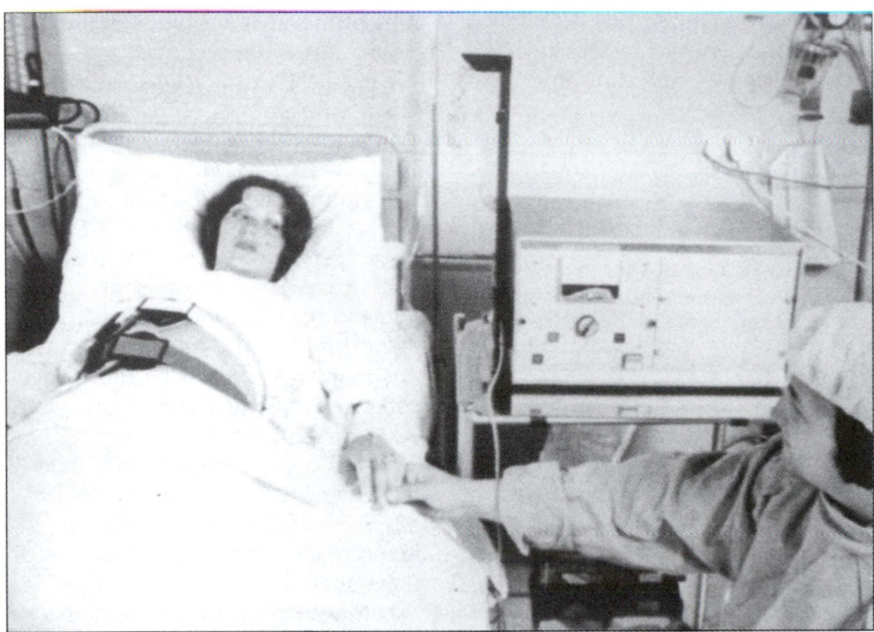

Laboring woman attached to an electronic fetal monitor. Photo courtesy of Kip Kozlowski.

The device identifies the fetal heart rate by using the R wave of the fetal electrocardiogram (EKG) complex, a signal generated by the movement of the cardiovascular structure and detected by a microphone pick-up using ultrasound and the Doppler principle or cardiac sounds. Internally, a fetal electrode is attached to the presenting part, usually the head, of the fetus to record the EKG complex. The peaks of the R wave are detected and the time interval between them is measured to give a baseline fetal heart rate (FHR) (Parer, 1983).

Several patterns of the fetal heart rate are used to help interpret the tracing. They are baseline changes and periodic changes. Baseline changes are defined as bradycardia (less than 110 beats per minute) and tachycardia (over 160 beats per minute). The rate must exist for over three to five minutes to be labeled as either a bradycardia or tachycardia.

Periodic changes are defined as changes in heart rate at specific intervals. These periodic changes may be grouped as accelerations or decelerations. Accelerations are defined as an increase in fetal heart rate in response to fetal movement or contractions of the uterus. Decelerations may be subgrouped into early, late, or variable decelerations. Early and late decelerations are a decrease in fetal heart rate in response to a contraction. Early and late terminology refers to when during the contraction the fetal heart rate begins to decrease. Variable decelerations are defined as sudden decreases in fetal heart rate with a quick return to baseline. These decelerations may or may not be related to a contraction of the uterus. Umbilical cord compression is a frequent reason for variable decelerations.

Not all baseline and/or periodic changes are defined as positive or negative. Many other variables must be considered before making a diagnosis of fetal well-being or stress/distress.

Electronic fetal monitoring is currently used as a means of antepartum assessment as well as intrapartum surveillance. All women with high-risk pregnancies should have antepartum and intrapartum fetal assessment. Some frequent indications for testing include diabetes, chronic hypertension, cardiac disease, or pregnancy-related conditions such as pregnancy-induced hypertension, growth-retarded fetuses, postdate pregnancies, or decreased fetal movement. During labor, meconium-stained fluid, abnormal presentations, or unusual labor patterns indicate the use of electronic fetal monitoring.

Much controversy over the increasing use of electronic fetal monitoring exists. Some of the concerns raised are the increasing cesarean birth rate, the increased risk of infection with invasive monitoring, the unknown risk of ultrasound exposure, the confinement of the mother during monitoring, and the skill level of personnel interpreting the monitoring strips.

✱ MARGARET MALNORY, M.S.N., R.N.

See also: Imaging Techniques

See **Guide to Related Topics:** Childbirth Practices and Locations; New Procreative Technologies; Prenatal Diagnosis and Screening

Resources

American College of Obstetricians and Gynecologists. (1983). *Electronic Fetal Monitoring*. (Patient Education Pamphlet).

Parer, Julian. (1983). *Handbook of Fetal Heart Rate Monitoring*. Philadelphia: W.B. Sanders Company.

Schifrin, B.S., Weissman, B.A., & Wiley, J. (1985). "Electronic Fetal Monitoring and Obstetrical Malpractice." *Law, Medicine and Health Care 13*(3): 100-04.

Tucker, Susan M. (1988). *Pocket Nurse Guide to Fetal Monitoring*. St. Louis, MO: C.V. Mosby Company.

EMOTIONAL RECOVERY FOLLOWING OBSTETRIC INTERVENTION

In this culture, it is expected that the majority of women will experience a period of upset and grieving following childbirth. The misunderstood and misused catch-all phrases "postpartum depression" and "baby blues" have been adopted as part of an authoritative childbirth vocabulary.

There are a number of cultures where postpartum depression is virtually unknown—celebrations and jubilation are the norm. These are predominantly cultures where birth is considered a truly natural process that takes place in the context of familial and social life (Jordan, 1981; Goldstein, 1984; Panuthos, 1984). At present, only a very small percentage of American women birth in a way that could be considered truly "natural," that is, without obstetric technological intervention; the vast majority of these women report feelings of satisfaction, pleasure, and empowerment. When a woman has had excellent nutrition, good prenatal care, and a smooth birth experience, her chances of "bouncing back" quickly are enhanced; the incidence of postpartum "blues" is greatly decreased.

While attention has been given for years to the physical and hormonal recovery after childbirth, until recently, little attention was given to the subject of emotional recovery. It became clear in the early 1970s, when cesarean support organizations such as C/SEC (Cesareans/Support, Education and Concern) were being developed, that the phrase "postpartum depression" did not explain the intense, negative feelings that were experienced by many women who had undergone cesareans; it did not express the frustration, confusion, rage, and sadness that many of them felt for extended periods of time after a surgical delivery. For example, it did not identify the feelings of loss that many women felt at being deprived, often unnecessarily, of the experience of giving birth, nor did it address a number of issues that seemed to be specifically related to the mode of delivery: the intense grief that occurred as a direct result of having their babies separated from them immediately after birth, and the difficulty of mothering a new child following major abdominal surgery. As the population of women experiencing cesarean sections grew, there arose a demand for more understanding and sensitivity toward this group. In the 1980s, a great deal of attention was focused on the special needs and concerns, including the emotional recovery, of cesarean mothers.

It has become evident over time that it is not only women who have had cesareans who are often enraged, confused, and depressed about the loss of the birth experience and separation from their newborns; many women who birth their babies vaginally are also extremely upset after their babies are born. They are often specifically disturbed by the myriad of interventions and interferences that are used at their deliveries, including analgesic drugs, labor-inducing and intensifying pitocin, fetal monitors, episiotomies, and anesthesia. Many American women report feeling abused, ignored, or deceived about their labor and birth. Some of the language used to express these feelings of violation is similar to that used by victims of rape. As information about unnecessary cesareans and other unnecessary, dangerous, and invasive interventions becomes more available, women who feel abused by the way that their births were managed exhibit emotional upset that does not fit into the category of "normal" postpartum depression. The issue of angry, sad, and depressed new mothers becomes extremely important when one considers the demands and dependencies of the newborn, and the significance of the mother's role during these first weeks, months, and years of the baby's life.

The depth and duration of emotional depression following birth is related to a number of factors, including expectations versus the reality of the experience; the extent to which the woman feels as if she was an active participant in the birth; the physical health and well-being of the mother and the baby; the degree or lack of support and respect granted the laboring and birthing woman; the circumstances and actual events of the particular birth; nutritional status; past experiences and losses; general coping abilities and personal philosophies; and present support systems.

A number of techniques are available for assisting women who are emotionally upset following a difficult, disappointing, or traumatic birth. These include active listening, visualization, creative and expressive outlets such as writing and painting, supportive readings, empowerment workshops, massage, and bioenergetics. It is important, however, to understand many of the personal, spiritual, and psychological aspects of pregnancy, labor, and birth, for herein lie many of the answers as to why so many women in the U.S. are unhappy following the births of their children. Prevention of emotional disturbance is preferable: it is an unnecessary tragedy that so many women in the United States experience negative feelings surrounding birth.

In sum, it may very well be that the frequency and intensity of depression and the need for emotional recovery so common after birth in this culture is a result of the obstetrical attitudes, philosophies, interventions, and methods accepted and practiced in the United States.

✱ NANCY WAINER COHEN

See also: Bonding; Matrescence and Patrescence; Postpartum Emotional Disorders; Social Science Research on American Childbirth Practices

See **Guide to Related Topics:** Pregnancy, Psychological Aspects

Resources

Cohen, Nancy Wainer. (1991). *Open Season: A Survival Guide for Natural Childbirth and VBAC in the 90's.* Westport, CT: Greenwood Publishing Group.

Cohen, Nancy Wainer & Estner, Lois. (1983). *Silent Knife: Cesarean Prevention and Vaginal Birth after Cesarean.* Westport, CT: Bergin & Garvey.

Demetrakopoulos, Stephanie. (1983). *Listening to Our Bodies: The Rebirth of Femine Wisdom.* Boston: Beacon Press.

Goldsmith, Judith. (1984). *Childbirth Wisdom from the World's Oldest Societies.* New York: Congdon and Weed.

Jordan, Brigitte. (1981). "Studying Childbirth: The Experience and Methods of a Woman Anthropologist." In Shelly Romalis (Ed.) *Childbirth: Alternatives to Medical Control.* Austin, TX: University of Texas Press.

Korte, Diana & Scaer, Roberta. (1990). *A Good Birth, A Safe Birth.* New York: Bantam Books.

Panuthos, Claudia. (1984). *Transformation through Birth.* Westport, CT: Bergin & Garvey.

Panuthos, Claudia & Romeo, Catherine. (1984). *Ended Beginnings: Healing Childbearing Loss.* Westport, CT: Bergin & Garvey.

Richards, Lynn. (1987). *The Vaginal Birth after Cesarean Experience.* Westport, CT: Bergin & Garvey.

ENDOMETRIOSIS

Endometriosis is a common gynecological disorder generally seen in women over the age of 30. It is a condition characterized by moderate to severe pelvic pain during menstrual periods, during sexual intercourse, and often with bowel movements or urination as well. This type of discomfort can also occur with infections; however, endometriosis is not an infective process at all. Many women experience no characteristic pain with this disease, and it is only diagnosed when they have unexplained difficulty becoming pregnant.

The cause of endometriosis stems from the growth of endometrial tissue (which lines the uterus) in other parts of the body. It is not cancerous or potentially dangerous. Essentially, it is normal tissue growing in places outside of its usual site. The pelvic region is the area where most endometriosis is found. The Fallopian tubes, the ovaries, the bladder, the lower bowel, and the ligaments that support these structures are often affected.

How this endometrial tissue got out of its normal site is widely speculated upon by experts. The most logical and popular explanation is that during menstruation, some blood and endometrial tissue, which normally flows down and out of the vagina, actually flows back up and out of the Fallopian tubes. This out-of-place tissue then implants itself on other pelvic structures and begins to grow.

There are several possible reasons that could explain exactly why this occurs in some women and not others. It seems to be hereditary. Some researchers think that there may be a malfunction in the immune system. Another theory proposes that the problem originates in the fetal stage. Unfortunately, funding for endometriosis research has been difficult to obtain. For years, doctors had written in medical literature that endometriosis is a "career woman's disease," describing its sufferers as "educated and egocentric." This sexist characterization has greatly impeded the raising of research dollars. But in recent years research efforts have improved and some current major studies have been performed to both establish clear diagnostic criterion and effective treatment plans.

Gynecological practitioners frequently suspect endometriosis on the strength of a symptom pattern for a woman and a pelvic examination. It usually requires a laparoscopy (a minor surgical procedure), however, to make a definite diagnosis. Once a diagnosis is established, a treatment plan can be formulated. This is a very individually tailored process. Age, location, and extent of the disease and desire for continued fertility are all significant factors.

Endometrial tissue responds strongly to changes in the female hormonal cycle. This is true if the tissue is in the uterus, where it naturally occurs, or if it is implanted in other sites. So, the first line of treatment is often the use of birth control pills to provide a low-dose, steady state of female hormones. Second-line-of-treatment drugs are also aimed at the manipulation of the female hormones to cause the ovary to be at rest, thereby not stimulating endometrial growth. However, these second-line hormonal medicines are slightly more complicated than birth control pills in that their side effects are often unacceptable. Many woman speak highly of treating their symptoms with such therapies as acupuncture, visualization, or homeopathy. Surgery for endometriosis is often the best remedy. It can vary from simply zapping the endometrial implants with a laser, to complete removal of the uterus, tubes, and ovaries.

As women age and the ovary ceases to function, the endometrial tissue no longer has any hormonal stimulus to which to respond. Menopause is thus the natural cure to this disorder.

✱ JOAN McTIGUE, R.N.

See also: Infertility: Diagnosis and Treatment
See **Guide to Related Topics:** Infertility

Resources

Boston Women's Health Book Collective. *Our Bodies, Ourselves.* New York: Simon and Schuster.
Novack, Edmund K. (1988). *Novack's Textbook of Gynecology.* 11th edition. Baltimore: Williams P. Wilkens Co.
Speroff, Leon et al. (1989). *Clinical Gynecologic Endocrinology and Infertility.* Baltimore: Williams and Wilkins Co.

ENGROSSMENT. *See instead* FATHERS AT BIRTH

EPIDURAL ANESTHESIA

Epidural anesthesia is an often used method of pharmaceutical pain relief for women in labor in the hospital. Epidural anesthesia is administered by injecting a numbing drug into the mid or lower back through a fine plastic tube (a cannula), which is left in place in case more anesthesia is needed.

Various studies reveal that epidurals are far and away the most effective form of obstetric analgesia. One report showed that pain relief was immediate, complete, and continued throughout labor and delivery for 74 percent of women (Doughty, 1975). In another study, 79 percent were satisfied with the pain relief they obtained; only 5 percent said the epidural did not help pain (Crawford, 1972).

Why Women Choose Epidurals. Women usually say they chose to have an epidural because they could not cope with the pain, and this is often the case when dilation is slow (Kitzinger, 1987a). Just under half of those who were asked why they had an epidural said they did so not only because pain was excessive, but because labor was very long. Other reasons given for having an epidural were induction, cesarean section, and breech birth.

But reasons for having an epidural are often more complex. The feeling of having lost control, or the fear of losing it, is a strong element in the majority of accounts of the events that led up to a woman choosing to have an epidural. Before they start labor, or in a very early phase of it, some women anticipate that they will lose control when in pain, and have an epidural to avoid embarrassment or the appearance of being "foolish." A women has in mind a model of how she should behave—calm, polite, cooperative. This model of conduct contrasts with the psychosexual reality of the experience of childbirth for most women. For, quite apart from the pain, childbirth can involve intense, urgent, and incredibly powerful physical sensations of pressure and opening and overwhelming emotions (Kitzinger, 1986, 1987b).

Some women asked for an epidural because they felt hustled through labor, subjected to uncoordinated management, or even abandoned. Being tethered to machines when already immobilized is also a very strong element in a woman's decision to have an epidural. Many women have an epidural because they feel helpless in a birth experience that can be highly medicalized. They may have tried to avoid interventions but find themselves "on the conveyer belt" and powerless to do anything about it. This powerlessness is frightening, and it destroys the laboring woman's self-confidence and increases her perception of pain. Choosing an epidural is the logical next step in trying to cope with a birth experience that is no longer a personal achievement, but a medical event.

Negative Experiences after Epidural. Many women have strong retrospective feelings about their experience of laboring and giving birth after having an epidural (Kitzinger, 1987a). Women were most likely to express regrets when they had felt under pressure to have an epidural, when an epidural failed to relieve pain effectively or had distressing side effects, and when they ended up with a forceps delivery. Almost half of the women reported a dominant feeling of being trapped and robbed of autonomy during labor (Kitzinger, 1987a).

One important element in a woman's retrospective assessment of an epidural is whether she felt coerced to have it or was able to make her decision freely. Pressure by hospital staff to have an epidural increases reports of regret. Pressure can range from gentle persuasion to obvious coercion. Occasionally, the woman has no chance to express her view, leaving her husband to make the decision, perhaps without opportunity to consult the woman first. Frequently "medical" reasons are used as a means of coercion. Women whose labors are induced are warned to expect long and painful labors. Such predictions increase the anxiety and tension and can actually contribute to a heightened perception of pain (Niven and Gijsbers, 1984).

It is often claimed that women who attend childbirth classes feel they have failed when they have an epidural, but this is rarely the case (Kitzinger, 1987a, p. 33). Even when women regretted having an epidural, they rarely talked about failure, but rather about uncaring attitudes, lack of information, or incompetence on the part of hospital staff. Those women who felt they had failed or that they had been "cheated" had usually experienced no sensation at all during delivery and had either a forceps delivery or cesarean section. Not only did they have little or no physical sensation at birth, but they were emotionally detached, as if watching the birth on a television screen.

Negative relationships with caregivers, difficulty or delay in obtaining an epidural once a woman decides to have one, lack of adequate information about the procedure, unskillful and painful administration by the anesthetist, and ineffective or insufficient results all contribute to dissatisfaction after having an epidural. Under these conditions, many women report disappointment and dissatisfaction with their birth experience.

When the Epidural Works Well. Those women for whom an epidural worked well expressed the most satisfaction with their experience. They reported tremendous relief from pain and a renewed sense of control. Many of these women had good relationships with their caregivers and were free of constraints either to have drugs or to manage without an epidural. All of the women who were entirely positive about their experience of birth with an epidural felt free from any pressure to have the epidural. They were far less likely than women whose experience was negative to have any other intervention—induction, for example—which led to staff advising an epidural. They were able to get the information they wanted and to share in the decision making. They all described instances where they had good emotional support, were able to rely on the continuing presence of a labor companion, and almost without exception gave birth in an unhurried, peaceful setting. Choosing to have an epidural was, for them, empowering rather than incapacitating.

In contrast, women who later regretted having an epidural had usually been under pressure to accept one, were out of touch with what was happening in their bodies at delivery, and were much more likely to have had a forceps delivery. They felt deprived of autonomy in childbirth.

Epidurals are sometimes given in the absence of strong emotional support, and pharmacological pain relief is offered in place of sensitive care. Many women have an epidural, not primarily because of pain, but because they feel trapped, helpless, and frightened. There are others who put off having an epidural, although they are in pain, because they feel they cannot trust their caregivers to respect their autonomy and they are concerned that a whole cascade of intervention will follow the epidural.

Much more work needs to be done to create an environment for birth in which each woman can handle pain in whatever way she chooses, without feeling that her autonomy is threatened, and can emerge from the experience with increased confidence and strength to face the new challenge of motherhood. Significant factors in obtaining a positive experience of birth with an epidural are not only being provided with pain relief, but being well informed about the procedure's risks and benefits, making one's own decision, and having the respect and consideration of caregivers and labor partners. ✱ SHEILA KITZINGER, LGSM

See also: Obstetric Drugs: Their Effects on Mother and Infant; Pain Relief in Labor: Nondrug Methods

See **Guide to Related Topics:** Childbirth Practices and Locations

Resources

Crawford, J.S. (1972). "The Second Thousand Epidural Blocks in an Obstetric Hospital Practice." *British Journal of Anaesthetics 44:* 1277-96.

Doughty, A. (1975). "Lumbar Epidural Analgesia—the Pursuit of Perfection with Special Reference to Midwife Participation." *Anaesthesia 30:* 741-51.

Kitzinger, Sheila. (1986). *Woman's Experience of Sex*. London: Penguin.

———. (1987a). *Some Women's Experiences of Epidurals: A Descriptive Study.* London: The National Childbirth Trust.

———. (1987b). *The Experience of Childbirth.* London: Penguin.

Niven, C. & Gijsbers, K. (1984). "Obstetric and Non-obstetric Factors Related to Labour Pain." *Journal of Reproductive and Infant Psychology* 2: 61-78.

EPISIOTOMY

Episiotomy is the most commonly performed surgery on women. Its use is so routine that people often seem to forget that it is a surgical procedure, with the attendant risks, complications, and consequences.

The episiotomy is a cut made in the perineum (the tissue and skin surrounding the vaginal opening and connecting to the rectum). It is generally made as the forthcoming fetal head pushes against the perineum, stretching it. The obstetrician or other birth attendant inserts a scissor and cuts either straight down (midline incision) or at an angle (pointing at "8:00," thinking of the birth outlet as a clock face—a mediolateral incision). North American obstetricians tend to favor the midline incision; those in the rest of the world, the mediolateral. More attention has been paid in the obstetric literature to which of these two types of incisions is preferable than to the more fundamental question of whether the episiotomy is itself a useful procedure.

Episiotomy developed with the medical management of birth. With the introduction of the lithotomy position for giving birth (flat on the back with legs in the air, strapped into stirrups), with routine forceps use, and with anesthesia, the woman's ability to slowly and effectively push her baby out while her perineum gradually stretched was severely compromised. Unconscious, strapped in, with metal forceps being inserted, tearing was common. The episiotomy substitutes a surgical incision for the tear; an incision surgeons found easier to repair. Obstetrical texts refer to the "straight, clean, surgical incision" in contrast to the "ragged laceration that otherwise frequently results" (Pritchard and MacDonald, 1980). Two questions are thus raised: Do women tear without episiotomies? Are episiotomies preferable to tears? The answers to these two questions do not support the routine use of episiotomies.

Under more natural conditions, women do not tear nearly as often as obstetricians seem to expect. Free to move around, to push as quickly or as slowly as feels appropriate, most women birth the baby over an intact perineum. Some birth attendants, particularly midwives, have worked to develop a variety of techniques to strengthen and support the perineum. More research is needed to determine whether these techniques are successful. But even without special support, massage, or other preparation and care, most women do not tear.

Nor does episiotomy prevent tearing: a very common tear is an extension, in which the surgical incision extends into a deeper tear. Some childbirth educators graphically demonstrate how this works: Take a regular 8½ by 11-inch sheet of typing paper and, holding both 8½-inch sides, pull at it, even snap it. Most paper will not tear. Now make a neat cut with a scissor into one of the 11-inch sides, hold the paper, and again pull apart the 8½-inch sides. The cut generally extends and the paper tears in half. A cut may weaken tissue and encourage tearing.

Episiotomies are painful, and more painful than comparable tears. A tear, in birth, is a separating of weakened tissue. It is less "neat" and less of a straight line to sew—but the body itself is not composed of straight lines. The pain of episiotomy is vastly underresearched. Sheila Kitzinger is one of the few people to have systematically asked women about their experiences with episiotomy. She reports that women are often shocked by the pain they experience (Kitzinger, 1987); though why wouldn't a surgical incision in the genitalia be painful? Studies of pain medication report moderate to severe pain in up to 60 percent of women with episiotomy and the need for pain relief for 85 percent of these women. Interestingly, these studies were done to compare pain relief techniques rather than to investigate the episiotomy per se. Episiotomy pain may persist for months. Nearly one-fourth of women with episiotomies in one study reported persistently painful sex after three months; another study reported 19 percent having painful intercourse for more than three months, compared to 11 percent of women with a tear (Thacker and Banta, 1983). Kitzinger (1987) reports that only 22 percent of episiotomy mothers said that intercourse was comfortable within the first month, compared with 39 percent of those with tears and 64 percent of those without injury to the perineum. No research has been done on the social, emotional, and psychological costs of this added stress on a woman and her partner at the time of early parenthood. A second, less common complication of episiotomy is infection, and there have even been reports of deaths from episiotomy infection.

✱ BARBARA KATZ ROTHMAN, Ph.D.

See also: Genital Mutilation, Female

See **Guide to Related Topics:** Childbirth Practices and Locations

Resources

Kitzinger, Sheila. (1987). *Your Baby, Your Way: Making Pregnancy Decisions and Birth Plans*. New York: Pantheon.

Kitzinger, Sheila & Simkin, Penny. (Eds.) (1986). *Episiotomy and the Second Stage of Labor*. 2nd edition. East Seattle, WA: Pennypress.

Kitzinger, Sheila & Walters, Rhiannon. (1981). *Some Women's Experience of Episiotomy*. London: National Childbirth Trust.

Pritchard, J.A. & MacDonald, P.C. (1980). *Williams Obstetrics*. 16th edition. New York: Appleton-Century-Crofts.

Thacker, S.B. & Banta, H.D. (1983). "Benefits and Risks of Episiotomy: An Interpretive Review of the English Language Literature, 1860-1980." *Obstetrical and Gynecological Surgery, 38*(6): 322-38.

ETHICS COMMITTEES

Ethics committees are multidisciplinary bodies in universities, hospitals, or other health care settings that participate in or oversee the resolution of ethically (and sometimes legally) difficult issues arising in health care.

Historically, biomedical committees with specifically ethical mandates (typically called "institutional review boards" or IRBs in the United States, but often termed "ethics committees" elsewhere) were initially developed to review proposals for biomedical and behavioral research to ensure the protection of human subjects. So-called "God Squads" were also briefly (and controversially) employed to assist with the allocation of scarce medical technologies, such as the artificial kidney machine, in the early 1960s (Alexander, 1962; Fox and Swazey, 1978). In the mid-1970s, the concept was borrowed and applied to decisions involving the withholding or withdrawal of life-sustaining treatments, most prominently in the well-known Karen Quinlan case (In re Quinlan, 1976; Teel, 1975; Veatch, 1977). Still more recently, and of special relevance to childbearing, ethics committees have become involved in the often tragic decisions concerning treatment of impaired newborns, brought out in the so-called "Baby Doe" cases. In contemporary American usage, the term "ethics committees" generally refers to committees involved in ethical aspects of treatment decisions.

There has been significant ongoing debate concerning the appropriate make-up, function, and role of ethics committees (Annas, 1984; Levine, 1984; Robertson, 1984; Fost and Cranford, 1985; Seay, 1985; Siegler, 1986; Lo, 1987; Moreno, 1988; Murray, 1988; Fleetwood, Arnold, and Baron, 1989). In the research setting, these issues are largely resolved through explicit federal regulations, which provide that IRBs should review the risks and benefits of proposed research and ensure appropriate informed consent by research subjects (45 *Code of Federal Regulations*, Part 46). IRBs may also play a role in supervising the criteria for selection of research subjects, where inclusion of women as research subjects has recently attracted needed attention (45 *Code of Federal Regulations*, §46.111(a)(3)).

In the context of withholding or withdrawing life-sustaining treatments, controversy has centered on whether ethics committees should confine themselves to general policy formulation and education functions or whether the committees should become actively involved in the resolution of individual cases. If the latter, should the committees focus solely on decision-making procedures, ensuring that the process is appropriate, or should they also become involved in the substance of the actual decisions, performing their own independent moral and legal analyses? Finally, should the committees' recommendations be purely advisory (to the patient and the patient's family, the physicians and other health care professionals, and/or the health care institution), or should the committees assume actual responsibility for making the decisions? Many scholarly commentators have encouraged committees to move beyond a purely educational mission to facilitate decision making on difficult cases and some have noted the tendency of committee recommendations to become *de facto* decisions in actual practice, but few have argued that committees should become the official decision makers (President's Commission, 1983; Fost, 1986; The Hastings Center, 1987).

Differing conceptions of the appropriate role of ethics committees came to broader public attention in the context of the federal government's response to the explosive "Baby Doe" cases in the mid-1980s. (*See* "Baby Doe.") The furor began with a series of decisions in which parents and physicians declined to perform corrective surgery on newborns with a variety of problems, many compatible with extended and happy lives. (One common situation involved children with Down's syndrome, a genetic condition formerly termed "mongolism" that is associated with highly variable mental retardation and certain physical anomalies.) These nontreatment decisions, which resulted in the (avoidable) deaths of several infants, were thought by many to reflect pernicious and unduly negative stereotypes of individuals with disabilities (Robertson and Fost, 1976; Fost, 1986), and resulted in a series of federal regulatory interventions and accompanying court challenges in the mid-1980s. The federal government's proposed regulations recommended, but did not require, use of so-called "infant care review committees," committees that are similar in format to ethics committees, that would specifically look at treatment decisions for impaired newborns (45 *Code of Federal Regulations*, §84.55(f)(1984). The federal proposal was widely criticized for limiting the scope of ethical considerations appropriate for such committees, for failing to require persons formally trained in ethics to be included in the committees' membership, and more generally, for envisioning committees primarily as enforcement agencies of the state (Fleischman and Murray, 1983; Annas, 1984; Murray, 1984; Weir, 1987; Mahowald, 1988; U.S. Commission on Civil Rights, 1989).

While there has been relatively little empirical research on the use of infant care committees (Leiken, 1987; University of Connecticut Health Center, 1987; Todres et al., 1988), reports from leading centers suggest that many hospitals have declined to follow the restrictive federal model and have conferred broader discretion on their institutional committees to consider a range of ethical concerns. These institutions have encouraged the committees to perform in an advisory, rather than primarily an enforcement, capacity (American Academy of Pediatrics, 1984; Fleischman, 1986, 1987, 1990; Kliegman, Mahowald, and Youngner, 1986; Shapiro and Barthel, 1986; U.S. Commission on Civil Rights, 1989). Recent controversies concerning real, potential, or perceived maternal-fetal or mother-infant conflicts, including forced cesarean sections, have elicited a tentative suggestion that ethics committees might play a constructive role in this domain as well (Chervenak and McCullough, 1990).

For patients or family members encountering difficulties with health care professionals or institutions, recourse to an ethics committee may provide a useful means of facilitating discussion or providing additional perspectives. In some settings, committees may prove more sensitive to patient and family wishes than individual health care professionals acting in isolation. Institutions and committees vary, however, in their willingness and ability to entertain such requests, to permit full participation by patients or family members in case review, and to ensure confidentiality of deliberations (Younger et al., 1983, 1984). At this time, only one state, Maryland, has enacted legislation governing such questions or other legal aspects of the status of hospital-based ethics committees (*Maryland, Health-General Code*, §§19-370-19-374), and many legal questions remain unresolved (Capron, 1986; Merritt, 1987, 1988).

Several books (Cranford and Doudera, 1984; Hosford, 1986; Ross et al., 1986; Macklin and Kupfer, 1988) and many articles address the range of practical and theoretical issues presented by ethics committees. The *Hastings Center Report* and a new journal, *HEC Forum*, are sources of continuing coverage, and recent bibliographic tools (McCarrick and Adams, 1989; Walters and Kahn, annual) provide useful guidance to the large and growing literature in the area.

✷ ALAN J. WEISBARD, J.D.

See also: Newborn Intensive Care

See **Guide to Related Topics:** Legal Issues; Special Needs Infants

Resources

Alexander, Shana. (1962, Nov 9). "They Decide Who Lives, Who Dies: Medical Miracle Puts Moral Burden on a Small Committee." *Life 53*: 102-03.

American Academy of Pediatrics Infant Bioethics Task Force. (1984, Aug). "Guidelines for Infant Bioethics Committees." *Pediatrics 74* (2): 306-10.

Annas, George J. (1984, Aug). "Ethics Committees in Neonatal Care: Substantive Protection or Procedural Diversion?" *American Journal of Public Health 74* (8): 843-45.

Capron, Alexander M. (1986). "Legal Perspectives on Institutional Ethics Committees." In Emily Friedman (Ed.) *Making Choices: Ethics Issues for Health Care Professionals*. Chicago: American Hospital Publishing, pp. 175-84.

Chervenak, Frank A. & McCullough, Laurence B. (1990, Feb). "Clinical Guides to Preventing Ethical Conflicts Between Pregnant Women and Their Physicians." *American Journal of Obstetrics and Gynecology 162* (2): 303-07.

Cranford, Ronald E. & Doudera, A. Edward (Eds.) (1984). *Institutional Ethics Committees and Health Care Decision Making*. Ann Arbor, MI: Health Administration Press.

Fleetwood, Janet E., Arnold, Robert M., & Baron, Richard J. (1989, Sept). "Giving Answers or Raising Questions: The Problematic Role of Institutional Ethics Committees." *Journal of Medical Ethics 15* (3): 137-42.

Fleischman, Alan R. (1986, Jun). "An Infant Bioethical Review Committee in an Urban Medical Center." *Hastings Center Report 16* (3): 16-18.

———. (1987, Jun). "Bioethical Review Committees in Perinatology." *Clinics in Perinatology 14* (2): 379-93.

———. (1990, Mar-Apr). "Parental Responsibility and the Infant Bioethics Committee." *Hastings Center Report 20* (2): 31-32.

Fleischman, Alan R. & Murray, Thomas H. (1983, Dec) "Ethics Committees for Infants Doe?" *Hastings Center Report 13* (6): 5-9.

Fost, Norman. (1986, Jan). "Treatment of Seriously Ill and Handicapped Newborns." *Critical Care Clinics* (1): 149-59.

Fost, Norman & Cranford, Ronald E. (1985, May 10). "Hospital Ethics Committees: Administrative Aspects." *Journal of the American Medical Association 253* (18): 2687-92.

Fox, Renee L. & Swazey, Judith P. (1978). *The Courage to Fail: A Social View of Organ Transplants and Dialysis.* 2nd revised edition. Chicago: University of Chicago Press.

Glasser, Gary, Zweibel, Nancy R., & Cassel, Christine K. (1988, Feb). "The Ethics Committee in the Nursing Home: Results of a National Survey." *Journal of the American Geriatrics Society 36* (2): 150-56.

The Hastings Center. (1987). *Guidelines on the Termination of Life-Sustaining Treatment and the Care of the Dying.* Briarcliff Manor, NY: The Hastings Center.

Hosford, Bowen. (1986). *Bioethics Committees: The Health Care Provider's Guide.* Rockville, MD: Aspen Systems.

Kliegman, Robert M., Mahowald, Mary B., & Youngner, Stuart J. (1986, Feb). "In Our Best Interests: Experience and Workings of an Ethics Review Committee." Journal of Pediatrics 108 (2): 178-88.

Leiken, Sanford. (1987, Sept). "Children's Hospital Ethics Committees: A First Estimate." American Journal of Diseases of Children 141 (9): 954-58.

Levine, Carol. (1984, Jun). "Questions and (Some Very Tentative) Answers about Hospital Ethics Committees." *Hastings Center Report 14* (3): 9-12.

Levine, Carol et al. (1986, Jun). "Ethics Committees: How Are They Doing?" *Hastings Center Report 16* (3): 9-24.

Lo, Bernard. (1987, Jul 2). "Behind Closed Doors: Promises and Pitfalls of Ethics Committees." *New England Journal of Medicine 317* (1): 46-50.

Macklin, Ruth & Kupfer, Robin B. (1988). *Hospital Ethics Committees: Manual for a Training Program.* New York: Albert Einstein College of Medicine.

Mahowald, Mary B. (1988, Dec). "Baby Doe Committees: A Critical Evaluation." *Clinics in Perinatology 15* (4): 789-800.

McCarrick, Pat Milmoe & Adams, Judith. (1989). "Scope Note: Ethics Committees in Hospitals." National Reference Center for Bioethics Literature. Washington, DC.

Merritt, Andrew L. (1987, Jul). "The Tort Liability of Hospital Ethics Committees." *Southern California Law Review 60* (5): 1239-97.

———. (1988, Feb-Mar). "Assessing the Risk of Legal Liability for Ethics Committees." *Hastings Center Report 18* (1): 13-14.

Moreno, Jonathan D. (1988, Nov). "Ethics by Committee: The Moral Authority of Consensus." *Journal of Medicine and Philosophy 13* (4): 411-32.

Murray, Thomas H. (1984, Feb). "At Last, Final Rules on Baby Doe." *Hastings Center Report 14* (1): 17.

———. (1988, Feb-Mar). "Where Are the Ethics in Ethics Committees?" *Hastings Center Report 18* (1): 12-13.

President's Commission for the Study of Ethical Problems in Medicine and Biomedical and Behavioral Research. (1983). *Deciding to Forego Life-Sustaining Treatment.* Washington, DC: U.S. Government Printing Office.

Robertson, John A. (1984, Jan). "Ethics Committees in Hospitals: Alternative Structures and Responsibilities." *QRB 10* (1): 6-10.

Robertson, John A. & Fost, Norman. (1976, May). "Passive Euthanasia of Defective Newborn Infants: Legal Considerations." *Journal of Pediatrics 88* (5): 883-89.

Ross, Judith Wilson et al. (1986). *Handbook for Hospital Ethics Committees.* Chicago: American Hospital Publishing.

Seay, J. David. (1985, Nov). "On Forming an Institutional Ethics Committee: The Doctor's Dilemma." *Bulletin of the New York Academy of Medicine 61* (9): 842-52.

Shapiro, Robyn S. & Barthel, Richard. (1986, May). "Infant Care Review Committees: An Effective Approach to the Baby Doe Dilemma?" *Hastings Law Journal 37* (5): 827-62.

Siegler, Mark. (1986, Jun). "Ethics Committees: Decisions by Bureaucracy." *Hastings Center Report 16* (3): 22-24.

Teel, Karen. (1975, Winter). "The Physician's Dilemma: A Doctor's View: What the Law Should Be." *Baylor Law Review 27* (1): 6-9.

Todres, I.D. et al. (1988, May). "Life-Saving Therapy for Newborns: A Questionnaire Survey in the State of Massachusetts." *Pediatrics 81* (5): 643-49.

EUGENICS

The word "eugenics" is derived from the Greek for "well-born" and was invented in 1883 by Francis Galton, a British mathematician and cousin of Charles Darwin. Galton wrote that he was looking for "a brief word to express the science of improving the stock, which . . . especially in the case of man [sic] takes cognizance of all the influences that tend . . . to give the most suitable races or strains of blood a better chance of prevailing speedily over the less suitable than they otherwise would have had." The political implications were there from the start. Galton realized that eugenics can take two forms: positive, which would involve getting the "better stocks" to have more children, and negative, which would involve restraining procreation among less desirable people. He was also quite specific about who fitted these categories. In the latter he included the "mentally ill" and "feeble-minded," as well as "habitual paupers" and "criminals."

Eugenics found immediate support among scientists and policymakers in Great Britain and the United States. Eugenics education fairs were instituted to inform people about the importance of judicious mating, and as late as 1941, the distinguished British biologist Julian Huxley wrote an article, entitled "The Vital Importance of Eugenics," in which he advocated selective prohibition of marriage, segregation in institutions and, where necessary, sterilization as ways to forestall "racial degeneration," and worried over "the absence of a eugenic sense in the public at large."

Early in this century, the United States developed two kinds of eugenic policies: compulsory sterilization laws at the state level and the Immigration Restriction Act of 1924 at the federal level.

The first compulsory sterilization law was enacted by Indiana in 1907, and by 1931, such laws existed in some 30 states. Although most of them were not enforced, by January 1935, some 20,000 people had been forcibly sterilized, nearly half of them in California, where the law remained on the books until 1980. Some states still have eugenic sterilization laws. The laws usually were aimed at the "insane" and "feeble-minded" and often included so-called sexual perverts, drug fiends, drunkards, epileptics, and other "diseased and degenerate persons.:

The Immigration Restriction Act of 1924 was intended to limit entry of people from southern and eastern Europe (immigration of people from Asia having been restricted earlier). The goal was to increase the predominance of persons of British and north European ancestry in the U.S. population.

Eugenics was introduced into Germany in 1895 by a physician, Alfred Plötz, who gave it the name "racial hygiene." From the start, eugenics in Germany was considered more a matter of public health than of social policy and was implemented by physicians and scientists.

The Nazis passed their first eugenic law in July 1933, barely six months after Hitler took over. It was a compulsory sterilization law and was, as in the United States, directed at people who were deemed feeble-minded or insane, or who exhibited other so-called hereditary defects (including "severe alcoholism").

The first racist eugenic measures, the Nürnberg anti-miscegenation laws, were passed in 1935. They forbade marriage or sexual relations between Jews and non-Jews and, for this purpose, provided a racial definition of who was a Jew. Included was a "Law for the Protection of the Genetic Health of the German People," which required premarital medical examinations to detect racial and other kinds of "damage."

The Nazis also instituted positive eugenic measures to encourage outstanding Aryan women to have many children, and they strictly enforced anti-abortion laws except for eugenic reasons. Later during the war, they went so far as to urge unmarried or widowed women of superior stock and SS men to produce children together as a sign of their dedication to the Führer.

The Nazi extermination programs, too, were initially developed to dispose of "defective" children and adult patients in mental hospitals and were extended only later to whole populations of Jews, gypsies, Poles and other east Europeans, and gay men and lesbians. In all of these cases, the intent was "hygienic": to improve the genetic health of the German *Volk* by "selecting and eradicating" inferior types.

While few people nowadays support the eugenic programs in use during the first half of this century, there is an uncomfortable link between them and the new tests that are being developed to detect so-called genetic defects. Some people argue that these tests are not eugenic because their aim is not to clean up the race, but to improve the lives of future parents and children. Furthermore, they say, as long as the measures are voluntary, they simply enhance people's procreative choices.

Yet, these choices readily translate into responsibilities. Once a test is available that foretells whether a future child may, or will, have some particular disability, the *choice* to bear that child implies the *responsibility* for whatever problems and pain may be associated with the disease in question. And the fact is that some scientists, physicians, and attorneys point to the "burdens" the choice to bear such a child imposes on society and question people's "right" to make it. But usually in today's liberal democracies, these practices are not frankly coercive.

Scientists and physicians have once again provided the ways to put societal prejudices about who should and should not be born into practice. Only now women are not forced to conform; they are merely expected to integrate these prejudices into their thought processes and "choose" to have appropriate tests and "elect" not to initiate, or to terminate, pregnancies whose outcome might meet with disapproval from society.

To a considerable extent, these choices may in fact be what women themselves want. But one reason they want (and perhaps need) these alternatives is because society takes little or no responsibility for children (and adults) who need protection, care, or perhaps just special opportunities.

✷ RUTH HUBBARD, Ph.D.

See also: Genetics; Genome Mapping; The Perfect Baby; Selective Abortion

See **Guide to Related Topics:** Prenatal Diagnosis and Screening

Resources

Duster, Troy. (1990). *Backdoor to Eugenics.* New York: Rutledge.

Nelkin, Dorothy & Tancredi, Lauence. (1989). *Dangerous Diagnostics: The Social Power of Biological Information.* New York: Basic Books.

Suzuki, David & Knudtson, Peter. (1988). *Genethics: The Ethics of Engineering Life.* Toronto: Stoddard.

EVOLUTION OF HUMAN BIRTH

Human biological evolution over the last five million years can be characterized by two major trends: bipedalism (upright stance) and encephalization (increasing brain size). Bipedalism results in a small pelvic opening whereas increasing brain size results in large-headed infants. These dimensions are in direct opposition to each other at the time of birth. In order to appreciate the impact of that opposition, it will be useful to compare birth in other primates to the way that birth is experienced by modern women.

Primates typically have high encephalization quotients, i.e., their brains are much larger, compared with their body size, than that of other mammalian species. Thus, for almost all primates, the birth process is challenging in that the fetal head size is close to or exceeds the size of the birth canal. Difficult birth, then, is characteristic of most primates, and has been part of the long evolutionary history of our ancestors. Beyond that, however, birth is even more of a challenge for human females because of the changes that have taken place in the pelvic basin as it has evolved for bipedal locomotion.

In quadrupedal primates, both the entrance and exit of the birth canal are longest in the front-to-back dimension as is the fetal head. Both the back of the birth canal (the sacrum) and the back of the fetal head (the occiput) are larger than the front of the canal and head. Thus, the fetus passes through the birth canal with the largest dimension of the head (occiput) against the largest dimension of the maternal pelvis (sacrum). That means that the monkey fetus enters the birth canal facing in the same direction as the mother, passes straight through, and emerges in that same direction.

In the human bipedal pelvis, the entrance to the birth canal is widest in the side-to-side dimension whereas the exit is widest in the front-to-back dimension. As with the fetal monkey, the human head is longest in the front-to-back dimension and the back of the head is the largest. Unlike the monkey pelvis, however, the human pelvis is largest in the front. Since fetal dimensions and maternal pelvic dimensions must be oriented in the same direction for successful birth, this means that the human infant must undergo rotation during birth. The human fetus enters the birth canal with its head in the diagonal or side-to-side dimension. It then must rotate so that the longest dimension of the fetal head is now oriented front-to-back in the longest dimension of the pelvic exit. The fetal occiput is against the front of the maternal pelvis, resulting in the infant being born facing away from the mother. Further rotation is necessary for the fetal shoulders to pass through the pelvic entrance and exit aligned in the correct position.

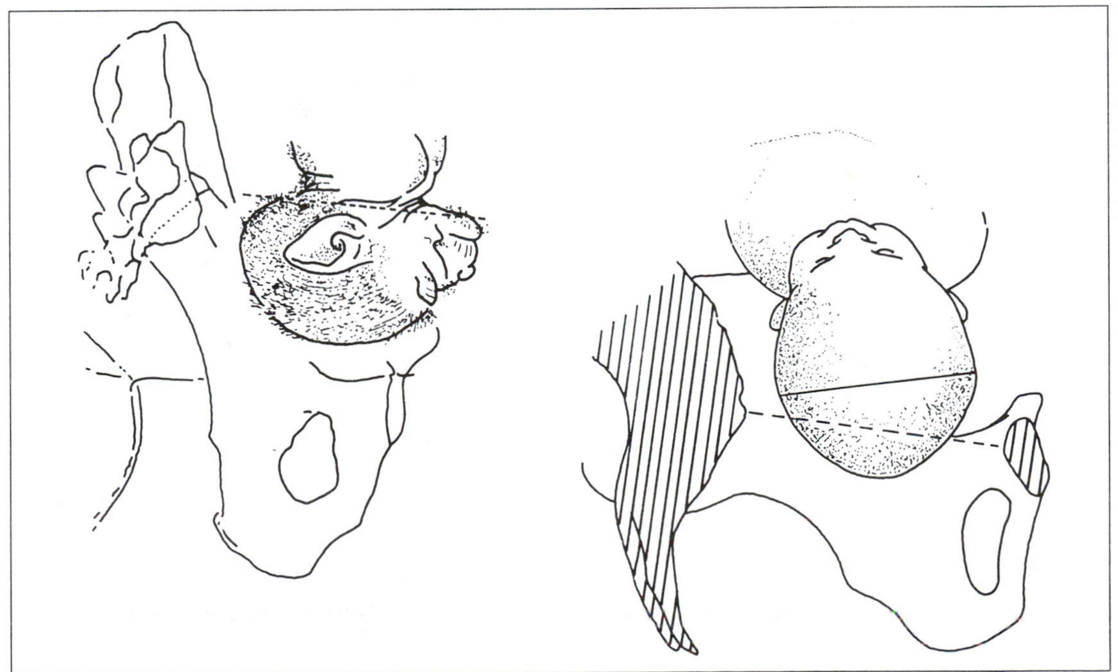

Primate and human fetal presentations. Illustration courtesy of Wenda R. Trevathan.

The human birth process presents additional challenges as a result of reorientation of the pelvis for bipedal locomotion. In a pelvis designed for quadrupedalism, the sacrum is high above the front (pubic portion) of the pelvis; thus, during birth the fetal head passes the sacrum before passing the bony portion of the pubis. In a pelvis designed for bipedalism, the sacrum and pubis are directly opposite each other; thus the infant's head must pass both bony portions of the pelvis at the same time, resulting in a much tighter squeeze.

The differences in orientation of the infant at birth have an impact on the mother's reaction as the child emerges from the birth canal. The monkey mother typically reaches down and pulls the infant toward her, along the normal flexion of its body. In some instances, the monkey infant is developed enough to assist in its own birth by pulling the rest of its body out of the birth canal once its head and arms have emerged. The mother is in a good position to wipe mucus from the infant's mouth and assist it in breathing.

For the human mother, the reception of her infant is more challenging, since it is typically born facing away from her. If she reaches down and pulls it against the normal flexion of its body, she risks damaging it, especially the nerves in the neck region. She is also hampered in her attempts to wipe mucus from the infant's mouth, in removing the umbilical cord if it is too tightly wrapped around the infant's neck, and in assisting the infant in breathing. These challenges are related to another major difference in nonhuman primate and human births: Nonhuman primates typically deliver alone with no assistance, whereas it is extremely rare for human females to deliver alone. It can be argued that human females began to seek assistance from others (probably other females) when they realized that having someone to help receive the infant increased survival rates of infants born facing away from them. Seeking assistance at birth may have thus been part of the human adaptation since the origin of bipedalism, more than four million years ago (Trevathan, 1987).

Brain size did not significantly increase in human ancestors until about two million years ago, with the appearance of the genus *Homo*. Birth was already a difficult process because of adaptation of the pelvis for bipedalism, as reviewed above. Neonatal brain growth could not proceed any further without compromising efficient bipedalism in the hominid female. The only other alternative was to have more of brain growth occur after birth, so that the infant could be born with a small enough head size to pass through the birth canal. The maximum brain size that can pass through a typical hominid pelvis is about 350 cubic centimeters. Most mammals, including most primates, give birth to infants with about 50 percent of their brain growth completed. *Homo habilis*, with adult cranial capacity of about 700 cc, was the last human ancestor to follow that pattern. As adult cranial capacity increased with *Homo erectus* and *Homo sapiens*, the only way that birth could continue to occur without compromising the ability to move efficiently was for more and more of the brain growth to occur after birth.

Today the human species has an adult cranial capacity of about 1400 cc, but females still give birth to infants with about 350 cc. Thus infants are born with approximately 25 percent of their adult brain size. Because of this, they are much less developed in motor skills and other systems at birth than are infants of our closest relatives, the Great Apes and monkeys. This evolution has been referred to as "secondary altriciality" because humans have most likely descended from species whose infants were much more developed at birth, more like those of other primates. Human mothers still produce milk that is more typical of primates who give birth to precocial infants who are able to cling to or follow their mothers at all times and thus can nurse at any time. Human milk is low in nutrients, requiring a high-frequency nursing pattern in order for sufficient food to be obtained. Thus, infants have to be in close contact with their mothers and, because they are so undeveloped in motor skills, maintaining that close contact is entirely up to the mothers for the first several months of life.

In addition to the requirement that infant brains be small enough so that the infant head can pass through the narrow maternal pelvis, it is probably advantageous that most of human brain growth occurs in the more stimulating environment outside the uterus. This is important for an animal as dependent on learning as we are, but as with maintaining contact, it also means that there is greater selective pressure on maternal caretaking ability since so much is dependent on the mothers of these very helpless infants.

In summary, selection for a narrow bipedal pelvis and larger adult brain size has led to the human pattern of giving birth to more helpless infants and to the behavior of seeking assistance at birth. Today the human species can be said to be characterized with "obligate midwifery" and "secondarily altricial" infants. Several million years of natural selection have been operating on human females to react to birth and their newborn infants in ways that increase their chances of survival. These behaviors and feelings that emerge at the time of birth are often in conflict with or are overridden by modern technologies and practices associated with birth. This can, in part, explain current dissatisfactions with the ways in which women and infants experience birth today in many industrialized nations.

✷ WENDA R. TREVATHAN, Ph.D.

See also: Doula; Midwifery: Overview; Social Science Research on American Childbirth Practices

See **Guide to Related Topics:** Caregivers and Practitioners

Resources

Berge, C., Organ-Segebarch, R., & Schmid, P. (1984). "Obstetrical Interpretation of the Australopithecine Pelvic Cavity." *Journal of Human Evolution 13*: 573-87.

Bowlby, J. (1969). *Attachment and Loss. Volume I: Attachment*. London: Hobarth Press.

Fisher, H. (1982). *The Sex Contract*. New York: William Morrow.

Freedman, D.G. (1974). *Human Infancy: An Evolutionary Perspective*. New York: John Wiley and Sons.

Gould, S.J. (1977). *Ontogeny and Phylogeny*. Cambridge, MA: Harvard University Press.

Klaus, M.H. & Kennell, J.H. (1976). *Parent-Infant Bonding*. St Louis: Mosby.

Leutennegger, W. (1981). "Encephalization and Obstetrics in Primates with Particular Reference to Human Evolution." In E. Armstrong and D. Falk (Eds.) *Primate Brain Evolution: Methods and Concepts*. New York: Plenum.

Lindburg, D.G. (1982). "Primate Obstetrics: The Biology of Birth." *American Journal of Primatology Supplement 1*: 193-99.

Rosenberg, K.R. (1988). "The Functional Significance of Neandertal Pubic Length." *Current Anthropology 29*: 595-617.

Stratton, P. (1982). *Psychobiology of the Human Newborn*. New York: John Wiley.

Trevathan, Wenda. (1987). *Human Birth: An Evolutionary Perspective*. Hawthorn, NY: Aldine deGruyter.

Trinkaus, E. (1984). "Neandertal Pubic Morphology and Gestation Length." *Current Anthropology 25*: 509-13.

EXERCISE PHYSIOLOGY IN PREGNANCY

Moderate exercise during pregnancy does not bring about and physiological changes that would be of concern to physiologists or physicians in a noncomplicated pregnancy. However, it is difficult to assess fetal responses to exercise. The two major areas of concern have been fetal oxygen supply and maternal/fetal temperature changes during strenuous exercise. In animals, the decrease in blood supply to the fetus that can occur during strenuous exercise is offset by mechanisms that increase the extraction of oxygen, resulting in no significant reduction in fetal oxygenation (Lotgering, 1988). The concern over fetal temperature regulation revolves around the fetus's inability to regulate temperature during the first trimester. Prolonged high maternal temperatures in animals during the first trimester of pregnancy are correlated highly with certain fetal abnormalities (Lotgering, 1988). In human populations this would translate to temperatures above 102 to 103 degrees Fahrenheit. Normal thermoregulation processes in humans would not cause these temperature increases during exercise. However, very hot, humid environments will reduce the amount of heat convected from the skin and dissipated from sweat, increasing the body's core temperature. Hence, pregnant women are cautioned to avoid becoming overheated.

The American College of Obstetricians and Gynecologists (1985) has published a series of recommendations for exercising pregnant women. These guidelines have been controversial and are deemed conservative by some professionals.

Moderate exercise during pregnancy has not yet been proven to be of any physiological benefit to mother or baby in terms of delivery, childbirth, or birth outcome. Neither has it been shown to be of any harm. Research on strenuous exercise during pregnancy suggests that highly trained women who continue to exercise strenuously throughout pregnancy may have lighter-weight offspring that nonexercising or moderately exercising cohorts (Clapp and Dickstein, 1984). Human studies have not shown significant changes in length of gestation, duration of labor, or measures of fetal outcome for pregnant women who participate in moderate programs of exercise (Collins, Curet, and Mullin, 1983; Lotgering, 1988).

✷ DIANE E. DEPKEN, Ed.D.

See also: Bodywork; Chiropractic Care; Pelvic Muscles

See **Guide to Related Topics:** Pregnancy, Physical Aspects

Resources

American College of Obstetricians and Gynecologists (ACOG). (1985). *Exercising during Pregnancy and the Postnatal Period*. Washington, DC: ACOG.

Clapp, J.F. & Dickstein, S. (1984). "Endurance Exercise and Pregnancy Outcome."*Medicine and Science in Sport and Exercise 16*: 556.

Collings, C.A., Curet, L.B., & Mullin, J.P. (1983). "Maternal and Fetal Responses to a Maternal Aerobic Exercise Program."*American Journal of Obstetrics and Gynecology 145*: 702-07.

Lotgering, F. (1988). "Pregnancy." In M. Shangold & G. Mirkin (Eds.) *Women and Exercise: Physiology and Sports Medicine*. Philadelphia: F.A. Davis Company, pp. 144-55.

EXTERNAL CEPHALIC VERSION

The popularity of External Cephalic Version (E.C.V), an age-old technique, has waxed and waned over the last century (Forunato et al., 1988). It may be best termed a "gentle art," whereby the health care provider places his or her hands on the skin of the mother's abdomen and, with carefully directed pressure and gentle manipulation, attempts to change the baby's position inside the uterus from a breech or transverse lie to a vertex or "head-first" position (Ranney, 1973), thus, attempting to avoid a cesarean section in favor of vaginal delivery.

During pregnancy, E.C.V. is used to convert a term breech singleton pregnancy to a head-down presentation. During labor, E.C.V. is used for vertex/breech twin gestations so as to enable the second twin to deliver vaginally as a vertex presentation (Chervenak et al., 1983, 1985). Also, E.C.V. has been advocated for use in labor when a previously undiagnosed breech has been discovered (Ferguson, 1985). E.C.V. has also been suggested for use either in pregnancy or during labor to convert a transverse lie to a vertex presentation (Phelan et al., 1986).

At term, the incidence of breech presentation is reported to be 3.5 percent, while E.C.V. can reduce the incidence to 1-2 percent (Savona-Ventura, 1986). Practitioners advise waiting until 37 weeks' gestation before attempting E.C.V. for a breech presentation for the following reasons: (1) prior to 37 weeks, a number of breech fetuses will spontaneously "turn" to a vertex position (Hofmeyer, 1983); (2) if complications occur secondary to E.C.V., a mature fetus can be delivered; and (3) while E.C.V. is less successful after 37 weeks, the fetus is less likely to revert back to a breech position (Morrison et al., 1986).

Contradictions to performing E.C.V. vary according to different authors, but most agree on the following as absolute contradictions: (1) bleeding during pregnancy; (2) placenta previa (the placenta blocking the birth outlet); (3) ruptured membranes; (4) fetal anomalies; (5) uteroplacental insufficiency (intrauterine growth retardation, abnormal fetal testing); (6) multiple gestation (except for planned E.C.V. of second twin after delivery of the first); and (7) cases where cesarean delivery would be required regardless of fetal presentation (Brocks et al., 1984).

Prior to attempting E.C.V., many practitioners believe the following criteria need to be met: (1) administration of an ultrasound to rule out fetal anomalies, document adequate amniotic fluid volume, confirm breech or transverse position and visualize placental location; (2) reassurance of fetal testing; (3) assurance of fetal lung maturity; (4) informed consent; and (5) in the case of unsensitized Rh-negative women, administration of Kleihauer-Betke tests (K.B.) drawn before and after attempted E.C.V. and administration of Rhogan after attempted E.C.V. (Stine et al., 1985). The K.B. test is an indicator of fetal-maternal bleeding.

Prior to performing E.C.V., the patient is given either tocolysis by injection or intravenous injection to ensure uterine relaxation. Anesthesia and analgesia are avoided. E.C.V. is stopped for maternal discomfort, fetal heart rate decelerations, and uterine contractions. The fetal heart rate is monitored during the E.C.V. Once E.C.V. is successful, the fetus is maintained in the new position for a few minutes and the fetal heart rate monitoring is reapplied. Reassuring fetal testing is obtained prior to discharging the patient home. (Most institutions allow the women to be discharged to home, with weekly follow-up rather than immediately inducing labor.) (Van Dorsten, 1982)

Fetal-maternal bleeding is reported as a consistent fetal risk of E.C.V.; incidence varies from 5 to 28 percent (Van Dorsten et al., 1981). The volume transfused is usually small, 0.1 to 6 ml, and the lowest incidences are reported by centers using ultrasound guidance and tocolysis, while avoiding anesthesia (Yeast, 1985).

✱ KATHERINE REESE, M.D.

See also: Fetal Presentations

Resources

Brocks, V. et al. (1984). "A Randomized Trial of External Cephalic Version with Tocolysis in Late Pregnancy." *British Journal of Obstetrics and Gynecology 91*: 653-56.

Chervenak, Frank et al. (1983). "Intrapartum External Version of Second Twin." *Obstetrics and Gynecology 62* (2): 160-65.

Chervenak, Frank et al. (1985). "Intrapartum Management of Twin Gestation." *Obstetrics and Gynecology 65* (1): 119-24.

Ferguson, James et al. (1985). "Intrapartum External Cephalic Version." *American Journal of Obstetrics and Gynecology 72* (1): 59-62.

Fortunato, Stephen et al. (1988). "External Cephalic Version with Tocolysis: Factors Associated with Success." *Obstetrics and Gynecology 72*(1): 59-62.

Hofmeyer, G.J. (1983). "Effect of External Cephalic Version in Late Pregnancy on Breech Presentation and Cesarean Section Rate: A Controlled Trial." *British Journal of Obstetrics and Gynecology 90*: 392-99.

Morrison, John et al. (1986). "External Cephalic Version of the Breech Presentation under Tocolysis." *American Journal of Obstetrics and Gynecology 154* (4): 900-03.

Phelan, Jeffrey et al. (1986). "The Nonlaboring Transverse Lie: A Management Dilemma." *Journal of Reproductive Medicine 31* (3): 184-86.

Ranney, Brooks. (1973). "The Gentle Art of External Cephalic Version." *American Journal of Obstetrics and Gynecology 116* (2): 239-51.

Saling, Erich et al. (1975). "External Cephalic Version under Tocolysis." *Journal of Perinatal Medicine 3*: 115-21.

Savona-Ventura, C. (1986). "The Role of External Cephalic Version in Modern Obstetrics." *Obstetrical and Gynecological Survey 41* (7): 393-400.

Stine, Lucille et al. (1985). "Update on External Cephalic Version Performed at Term." *Obstetrics and Gynecology 65* (5): 642-46.

Van Dorsten, J.P. et al. (1981, Oct). "Randomized Control Trial of External Cephalic Version with Tocolysis in Late Pregnancy." *American Journal of Obstetrics and Gynecology 141*: 417-21.

Van Dorsten, J.P. et al. (1982, Apr). "Safe and Effective External Cephalic Version with Tocolysis." *Contemporary Obstetrics and Gynecology 19*: 44-59.

Yeast, John et al. (1985, Mar). "External Cephalic Version for Breech Fetuses—A Neglected Alternative?" *Contemporary Obstetrics and Gynecology 25*: 45-52.

EYE PROPHYLAXIS

Administration of prophylactic agent to prevent the infectious conjunctivitis known as ophthalmia neonatorum in newborns is mandatory in most states. This preventative treatment, which originated in the 1880s when Karl Crede first proposed the use of silver nitrate to protect against newborn gonococcal eye infection, has been credited with saving the eyesight of countless babies worldwide. Conjunctivitis, an inflammation of the mucous membranes of the eye, is characterized by swelling of the eyelids and a sticky yellowish or watery discharge. If left untreated, ophthalmia neonatorum can lead to varying degrees of blindness (Avery, 1987). Although numerous agents can cause conjunctival inflammation, the most common are the sexually transmitted diseases chlamydia tracomatis and neisseria gonorrhea, which are currently on the rise in women (Avery, 1987). The newborn's eyes become infected during passage through the birth canal.

Although still widely used, silver nitrate 1 percent solution, the traditional drug of choice, is no longer recommended as a preventative agent since it is not effective against chlamydial infection, now considered the leading cause of conjunctival infection. Silver nitrate is also extremely irritating and produces a chemical conjunctivitis that will cause discomfort and interfere with the newborn's ability to focus his or her eyes (Schneider, 1984). The Centers for Disease Control (CDC), American Academy of Pediatrics, and National Society to Prevent Blindness (NSPB) agree that ophthalmic ointments containing 1 percent tetracycline or 0.5 percent erythromycin are acceptable and effective choices for prophylaxis of ophthalmia neonatorum. It is important to note that the CDC and the NSPB also consider a one to two hour delay in treatment safe and acceptable (Bobak et al., 1984). In most hospitals the treatment is administered in the delivery room, quite soon after birth. This interferes with eye-to-eye contact between parents and newborn, which has been identified as an important component of the bonding process. This first hour or so after birth is an emotionally sensitive period for both parents and newborns. Babies experience a quiet alert state that is extremely conducive to eye contact if postponement of prophylactic eye treatment can occur.

Several studies designed to evaluate the efficacy of prophylactic treatment have shown that a small but significant number of babies will develop conjunctival infection despite preventative treatment. Reasons postulated include improper instillation of ophthalmic ointment, nosocomial infection by hospital staff, and the potential for antimicrobial-resistant pathogens (Mooney, 1984; Hedberg et al., 1990). Prenatal screening and treatment for these sexually transmitted diseases is an

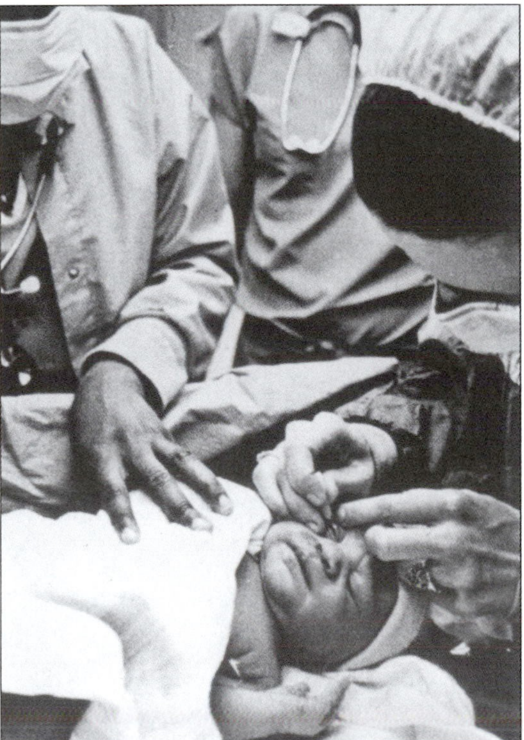

Prophylactic eye treatment of the newborn. Photo courtesy of Kip Kozlowski.

important component in the prevention of ophthalmia neonatorum. Parents should also be aware that the chemical conjunctivitis caused by prophylactic treatment is usually resolved within 24 hours after administration. Symptoms of conjunctivitis that appear after this period of time should not be attributed to the treatment and should be brought to the attention of a pediatrician for evaluation and treatment (Avery, 1987).

✱ KATHY ROSENBERG, C.N.M.

*See **also:*** Sexually Transmitted Diseases

See **Guide to Related Topics:** Baby Care

Resources

Avery, G. (1987). *Neonatology Pathophysiology and Management of the Newborn.* Philadelphia: J.B. Lippincott.

Bernstein, G.A. (1982). "Prophylaxis of Neonatal Conjunctivitis. An Analytic Review."*Clinical Pediatrics 21*(9): 545-50.

Black-Payne, C. (1989). "Failure of Erythromycin Ointment for Postnatal Ocular Prophylaxis of Chlamydial Conjunctivitis." *Pediatric Infectious Disease Journal 8* (8): 491-92.

Bobak, I. et al. (1984). *Essentials of Maternity Nursing.* St. Louis: C.V. Mosby Co.

Hedberg, K. et al. (1990). "Outbreak of Erythromycin-resistant Staphylococcal Conjunctivitis in a Newborn Nursery." *Pediatric Infectious Disease Journal 9* (4): 268-73.

Kitzinger, S. (1987). *Your Baby, Your Way.* New York: Pantheon Books.

Laga, M. et al. (1988). "Prophylaxis of Gonococcal and Chlamydial Ophthalmia Neonatorum. A Comparison of Silver Nitrate and Tetracycline." *New England Journal of Medicine 318* (11): 653-57.

Laga, M. et al. (1989). "Epidemiology and Control of Gonococcal Ophthalmia Neonatorum." *Bulletin of the World Health Organization 67* (5): 471-77.

Mooney, B.R. et al. (1984). "Non-gonococcal Ophthalmitis Associated with Erythromycin Ointment Prophylaxis of Gonococcal Ophthalmia Neonatorum." *Infection Control 5* (3): 138-40.

Schneider, G. (1984). "Silver Nitrate Prophylaxis." *Canadian Medical Association Journal 131* (3): 193-96.

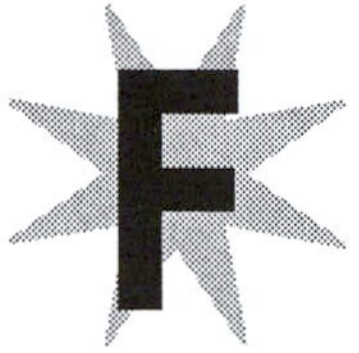

FAILURE TO THRIVE

"Failure to thrive" is a term used in pediatric medicine to describe a failure of physical growth in an infant or child. Such failure may be accompanied by delays in social, motor, and mental functioning. To make a diagnosis of failure to thrive, the physician must compare the child's physical development with standard growth charts, which measure average height and weight by percentile for specific ages. If the child's weight falls below a certain percentile compared with height, failure to thrive will be suspected. A typical standard used by physicians is weight that falls below the third percentile with height that is above the tenth percentile. Alternately, the physician may look for a rapid decline in a child's weight (for example, a drop from the 35th to the 10th percentile) (Chatoor and Egan, 1983).

The most significant distinction in the literature on failure to thrive is between organic and nonorganic failure to thrive. Organic failure to thrive is that which can be linked to physiological causes; nonorganic failure to thrive is linked to social-psychological causes. Historically, nonorganic failure to thrive has been defined as synonymous with maternal deprivation syndrome; it currently remains classified as the reactive disorder of attachment of infancy (Skuse, 1985).

The classic articulation of maternal deprivation syndrome describes a pattern of inadequate nurturance from a mother debilitated by her own psychological status; she may be acutely or chronically depressed, mentally ill, neurotic, or suffering from a personality disorder. Mothers are predisposed to deprivation because of their own experiences of inadequate nurture, and the child may represent a conflict that the mother is unable to resolve. The child is at risk when the mother's needs take precedence over those of the infant. The depriving mother may not be aware of her failure either because of mental disorganization or because she may have repressed her rejection of the child. Depriving mothers represent a continuum of psychosocial pathology, ranging from overt psychosis to subtle neuroticism; for this reason, such factors as normal appearance, articulateness, socioeconomic status, and appropriate demeanor may disguise pathogenic mothering (Kotelchuck, 1980).

Failure to thrive is the subject of much debate within the medical community. There is growing dissatisfaction with the way it has been conceptualized. Medical researchers complain of inadequate depiction of a causal sequence or etiology. In particular, they complain of a lack of research with adequate control groups for comparison (Kotelchuck, 1980).

A major criticism is that the diagnosis of nonorganic failure to thrive is made sheerly "on the basis of exclusion," that is, when organic factors cannot be found to explain the disease (Skuse, 1985). When the prevailing understanding of the nonorganic causes underlying the condition remains maternal deprivation, the result of this diagnosis "by exclusion" is an accusation of serious failure on the part of the mother. Overt maltreatment of the child is apparent in less than one-third of cases (Kotelchuck, 1980). Thus, the diagnosis of nonorganic failure to thrive is most commonly made in the absence of any positive indications of maternal neglect. Nevertheless, the maternal deprivation analysis remains salient because neglect can be understood as accomplished through subtle behavioral and emotionally communicated rejections of the child, for example, through unresponsiveness or inconsistency of response (Kotelchuck, 1980).

Of major concern to critics of maternal deprivation theory is the fact that psychological personality characteristics have not been shown to discriminate between mothers of failure to thrive children and control groups of mothers of healthy infants; other maternal factors that showed no significant differences between the two groups are demographic factors such as youth or first child, familial stressors such as unemployment, or pregnancy experiences (Kotelchuck, 1980). One maternal factor that has shown the ability to discriminate between healthy and nonhealthy outcomes is the degree of social isolation (Kotelchuck, 1980). One critic charges that clinicians have made use of "nebulous 'neglect' concepts," such as dysfunctional interaction or maternal bond failure, to cover cases where overt neglect is not observable (Kotelchuck, 1980).

There does exist an alternative tradition in the literature of failure to thrive—one that sees a need to attend to the heterogeneity of the failure-to-thrive population. In particular, there is a need to understand a variety of etiological sequences that may lead a child to fail to thrive. For example, researchers have distinguished between failure to thrive in the infant of less than six months, which is seen in classic terms of attachment disorder and maternal deprivation, and cases where the onset of the disease occurs in the second six months of life, which is seen as originating in the child's attempt to achieve autonomy and individuation from the mother through food refusal (Egan, Chatoor, and Rosen, 1980; Chatoor and Egan, 1983; Chatoor et al., 1984).

A more far-reaching criticism attempts to remove blame from the majority of mothers of infants who fail to thrive (Kotelchuck, 1980; Skuse, 1985). A first step has been to point out that the primary caretaker of the child may be the mother, father, or other relative (Skuse, 1985). An important reappraisal of the literature of nonorganic failure to thrive calls for an end to the emphasis on parental culpability in the absence of evidence of neglect (Skuse, 1985). Citing multiple possibilities for understanding the onset of failure to thrive, the problem becomes defined as one of undernutrition (Skuse, 1985). The specific etiology of emotional deprivation is seen as one possible diagnosis. Undernutrition, in this view, can stem from a variety of causes. It has been linked to ignorance of nutritional requirements on the part of the caregiver, as well as lack of financial resources needed to provide an adequate diet (Kotelchuck, 1980).

Of particular theoretical significance is a reinterpretation of dysfunctional parent-child interaction. An interactional model is proposed that presents a balanced view of the parent-child dyad, seeing the child as contributing to interactional functionality. The interactional approach replaces an oversimplified and universalized view of maternal deprivation as the precipitating factor with an image of parent and child as mutually influencing the nature of their interaction. Dysfunctionality can result from a mismatch of temperament or emerge from a self-perpetuating cycle of tension and anxiety (Kotelchuck, 1980; Skuse, 1985; Monahan, 1991). For example, a tense child who undereats could cause anxiety in the parental caregiver, who then adds to the tension of the child in the feeding process, leading to development of a dysfunctional interactional pattern. Or parent and child may have different hunger cycles, causing unsatisfactory feeding (Monahan, 1991). Treatment is centered on alerting the parent to the problem and increasing parental sensitivity (Skuse, 1985; Drotar, 1989; Monahan, 1991; Rostain, 1991).

The interactional view of nonorganic failure to thrive advocates the direct observation of the parent-child interactions, especially as they center around feeding behaviors. Behavioral patterns in instances of true neglect are characterized by fewer positive vocalizations and other attention-giving behaviors on the part of the caregiver, accompanied by an apathetic, nondemanding behavioral pattern on the part of the infant. The etiological question remains whether some characteristics of the child (lethargy, poor suck, sickliness) have had an interactional influence on parental neglect (Kotelchuck, 1980). Behavioral observations have revealed how differences in temperament affect feeding functionality (Skuse, 1985). They have also provided evidence that contingent factors such as familial distractions can interrupt the feeding routine (Kotelchuck, 1980). The importance of behavioral observation is emphasized in both diagnosis and treatment.

The interactional view has become increasingly acceptable to pediatricians (Monahan, 1991). Clinicians have also come to accept the interactional view that failure to thrive is a description of a condition of which there are many etiologies (Rostain, 1991). It is an empirical question as to what extent the emotional deprivation view continues to color the observation and treatment orientations of physicians and clinicians. If clinicians think of emotional neglect as the essential cause, then all cases of failure to thrive are subject to a diagnosis of relative psychopathology, and caretakers are guilty until proven innocent. Conceptually, what is needed is the formulation of discrete etiologies that can be distinguished from the genuine etiology of neglect.

✱ ALLISON CARTER

See **Guide to Related Topics:** Special Needs Infants

Resources

Barbero, Giulio J. & Shaheen, Eleanor. (1967). "Environmental Failure to Thrive: A Clinical View." *The Journal of Pediatrics 71* (5): 639-44.

Casey, Patrick H., Bradley, Robert, & Wortham, Betty. (1984). "Social and Nonsocial Home Environments of Infants with Nonorganic Failure-to-Thrive." *Pediatrics 73* (3): 348-53.

Chatoor, Irene & Egan, James. (1983). "Nonorganic Failure to Thrive and Dwarfism Due to Food Refusal: A Separation Disorder." *Journal of the American Academy of Child Psychiatry 22* (3): 294-301.

Chatoor, Irene et al. (1984). "Non-organic Failure to Thrive: A Developmental Perspective." *Pediatric Annals 13*: 829-43.

Drotar, Dennis. (1989). "Prevention of Emotional Disorders in Children with Nonorganic Failure to Thrive." In Stephen E. Goldston et al. *Preventing Mental Health Disturbances in Childhood*. Washington, DC: American Psychiatric Press, pp. 85-105.

Egan, James, Chatoor, Irene, & Rosen, Gerald. (1980). "Non-organic Failure to Thrive: Pathogenesis and Classification." *Clinical Proceedings, Children's Hospital National Medical Center XXXVI* (4): 173-82.

Kotelchuck, Milton. (1980). "Nonorganic Failure to Thrive: The Status of Interactional and Environmental Etiologic Theories." *Advances in Behavioral Pediatrics 1*: 29-51.

"The Maternal Deprivation Syndrome." (c. 1975). Author unknown: 56-61.

Monahan, Peggy. Children's Hospital of Philadelphia. Private communication, 1991.

Rostain, Anthony. Philadelphia Child Guidance Center. Private communication, 1991.

Skuse, D.H. (1985). "Non-organic Failure to Thrive: A Reappraisal." *Archives of Disease in Childhood 60*: 173-78.

Smith, Clement A. & Berenberg, William. (1970). "The Concept of Failure to Thrive." *Pediatrics 46* (5): 661-63.

FALSE LABOR. *See instead* BRAXTON HICKS CONTRACTIONS

THE FAMILY BED

"The family bed" refers to the practice of young children sleeping alongside their parents and/or siblings. The topic of where children should sleep has been much debated in American society. Doctors of great popularity, such as T. Berry Brazelton, are now beginning to admit that the concept of the family bed may not be so unhealthy after all. Brazelton, formerly adamantly against children sleeping with their parents, admits in his book *To Listen to a Child* (1984) that he has learned a great deal from parents who have happily reared children in a family bed. "Should we not re-evaluate our stance?" he asks. "Perhaps we should." At the same time, other forms of togetherness such as touching, increased communication, and the strengthening of interpersonal relationships are gaining force in American society. Breastfeeding and its related closeness is also making a comeback. Childbirth is becoming a family affair again. Parents are again being urged to pick up their babies whenever they cry. All of these changes in philosophy represent forms of closeness and togetherness, of which co-family sleeping is a part.

Children and babies have always slept next to or close to an adult, as they continue to do around the world. In a 1989 review article in the *New York Times Magazine*, Melvin Konner referred to research done at the University of Pittsburgh to determine where babies throughout the world sleep. Of the 173 cultures studied, not including Western culture, none kept the infant asleep in a separate room.

During the late 1800s, as families began to move away from the extended family to the big cities, young mothers turned to magazine articles and books to learn how to rear their children instead of learning from their own mothers. They began to read articles in which forced independence was sternly promoted. Parents were told that too much rocking, too much touching, too much nurturing, and sleeping together at night would lead to terrible psychological consequences, the least of which would be a very dependent child. While American parents obeyed these experts, the majority of the world continued to hold their babies, rock them, nurture them, and sleep with them. "What is an Oedipus complex?" people from other societies asked in amazement. "How does a mother get any sleep sleeping together with her infant in such a tiny crib?" "How come your babies cry so much?"

Over time, American doctors began to disagree with one another on the merits of the family bed. They wrote books and magazine articles stating their opinions of the precise method of rearing happy, independent children. Dr. Benjamin Spock came up with a technique for dealing with the pesky little tyke who insisted on climbing out of his or her crib to seek the mother: rig a netting over the crib (Spock, 1968). Some parents, wanting very much to follow doctors' advice that children should stay in their own isolated bed once they are put there, resorted to tying down the difficult-to-convince child.

The claim that co-family sleeping is detrimental to the child, that true independence is only learned through forced separation, is now being vigorously challenged. Dr. Peter S. Cook, a psychiatrist, writing in a special supplement to *The Medical Journal of Australia*, suggests that

> child rearing in English speaking societies is emerging from an era in which many widely held beliefs, values, attitudes and practices have been so out of harmony with the genetically influenced nature and needs of mothers and their developing children, that they have contributed to conflict, stress, and emotional and behavioral disturbance in the infant and developing child. An attitude of basic distrust towards the human biological "given" combined with a belief in coercion, have characterized this approach to child rearing. (1978)

But even though child authorities strongly advised against co-family sleeping, parents still, secretly, allowed their children in their bed, for either part of the night or all of the night. "This is a stubborn human characteristic well worth following up," commented Margaret Mead (Thevenin, 1987). The stubborn human characteristic has persisted through the years, despite expert advice against it, and now co-family sleeping, that age-old concept in child rearing, is again gaining acceptability. While in the early 1970s the subject was taboo, by the late 1980s the book *The Family Bed* had sold over 100,000 copies, was translated into two other languages, and was instrumental in reversing a 1988 Massachusetts criminal child abuse case. The subject has been discussed numerous times on television, on the radio, and in journals and magazines. Babies and children sleeping isolated from their parents is now understood not to be a natural human arrangement. No longer taboo, the acceptance of the family bed in America returns Western culture to practices prevalent in the rest of the world, where babies continue to sleep peacefully in proximity to their mothers.

✱ TINE THEVENIN

See also: Rooming-In

See **Guide to Related Topics:** Baby Care

Resources

Brazelton, T. Berry. (1984). *To Listen to a Child.* Reading, MA: Addison Wesley.

Cook, Peter S. (1978, Aug 12). "Childrearing, Culture and Mental Health." *The Medical Journal of Australia: Supplemental Issue*: 3-14.

Konner, Melvin. (1989, Jan 8). "Where Should Babies Sleep?" *New York Times Magazine.*

Spock, Benjamin. (1968). *Baby and Child Care.* New York: Pocket Books.

Thevenin, Tine. (1987). *The Family Bed.* Wayne, NJ: Avery Publishing.

FAMILY PLANNING. *See instead* CONTRACEPTION: DEFINING TERMS

FAMILY-CENTERED MATERNITY CARE

Family-centered maternity care (FCMC) is a philosophy and practice of care for the childbearing family that respects the needs of its individual members and fosters and supports the establishment of parent-newborn-family relationships. The term, introduced in the United States in the late 1950s (Stella, 1960; Engel, 1963), recognizes childbirth as a healthy life event for women and families. FCMC is designed for both healthy and high-risk women and combines the physical and psychosocial aspects of prenatal, intrapartum, and postpartum care. It emphasizes individualization of care and social interaction between mother, father, infant, family members, and chosen support persons.

Various organizations have defined and endorsed FCMC (International Childbirth Education Association, 1978; Interprofessional Task Force on Health Care of Women and Children, 1978; Canadian Paediatric Society, 1979; Canadian Institute of Child Health, 1980; McMaster University, 1981; American Academy of Pediatrics and American College of Obstetricians and Gynecologists, 1988), and components of a hospital FCMC program have been published (Stella, 1960; Haire and Haire, 1970; Bishop, 1980; Sumner and Phillips, 1981; Klaus and Kennell, 1982; Young, 1982; McKay and Phillips, 1984). Different physical designs for hospital FCMC units have been described (Fenwick and Dearing, 1981; Brans, 1983; Ross Planning Associates, 1988).

Changing from conventional maternity care to FCMC requires extensive planning and staff and

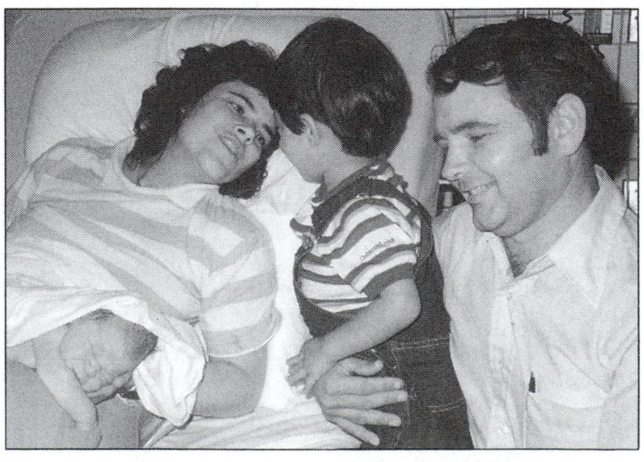

A new family rejoices. Photo courtesy of Paulina G. Perez.

public education. A recommended program includes a written philosophy, goals, and objectives for care; in-service staff education; orientation and tour of maternity facility; childbirth and parenting education; individualized care; informed consent for medical interventions; nurturing philosophy and attitudes of staff; partner presence for labor and birth; availability of midwives; trained labor companion (doula); Leboyer, or "gentle," birth; flexible protocols and practices; homelike birth environment; mother/baby nursing; rooming-in; breastfeeding promotion; early parent- and family-infant contact; flexible visiting hours; and an early discharge program.

In-hospital FCMC settings may include a diagnostic/admitting area; a waiting room or early-labor lounge; library area; conventional labor, delivery, and postpartum rooms; birthing or labor/delivery/recovery (LDR) room (Sumner and Phillips, 1981; Young, 1982; Brans, 1983; Ross Planning Associates, 1988); single-unit delivery system (Notelovitz, 1978; Fenwick and Dearing, 1981; Young, 1982; McKay and Phillips, 1984; Phillips, 1988) or combined labor/delivery/recovery/postpartum (LDRP) room (Ross Planning Associates, 1988); in-hospital birth center (Allgaier, 1978; American College of Obstetricians and Gynecologists, 1980; Young, 1982; McKay and Phillips, 1984); well-baby central nursery; newborn holding room (Fenwick and Dearing, 1981); special care and intensive care nurseries (Brimblecombe, Richards, and Roberton, 1978; Klaus and Kennell, 1982); and care-by-parent pediatric facilities (James and Wheeler, 1969; Klaus and Kennell, 1982; Ross Planning Associates, 1988). Free-standing (out-of-hospital) birth centers use FCMC principles and practices to care for healthy childbearing women and families (International Childbirth Education Association, 1978; National Association of Childbearing Centers, 1985; Lubic, 1980).

Advantages of FCMC to women, infants, and families are clinical safety; continuity and coordination of care; promotion of family attachment (bonding) and relationships; personal and family satisfaction; heightened maternal self-esteem, autonomy, and control; increased self-confidence in infant caregiving and parental adjustment; early and extended breastfeeding; active parent participation in health care decisions and childbearing process; fewer medical interventions; and elimination of room-to-room patient transfers.

Advantages of FCMC to maternity care providers are lower infection rates; personal job satisfaction; cost efficiency; better utilization of maternity staff; marketability; consumer popularity; improved provider-patient relations; improved community relations; elimination of duplication of services; and increased utilization of maternity services. ✱ DIONY YOUNG

See also: Birth Centers; Rooming-In; Social Science Research on American Childbirth Practices

See **Guide to Related Topics:** Childbirth Practices and Locations

Resources

Allgaier, A. (1978). "Alternative Birth Centers Offer Family-centered Care." *Hospitals* 52 (24): 97-112.

American Academy of Pediatrics & American College of Obstetricians and Gynecologists (AAP/ACOG). (1988). *Guidelines for Perinatal Care.* 2nd edition. Washington, DC: American Academy of Pediatrics/American College of Obstetricians and Gynecologists.

American College of Obstetricians and Gynecologists (ACOG). (1980). *Alternative Birthing Centers: A Survey and Bibliography.* Washington, DC: American College of Obstetricians and Gynecologists.

Bishop, J. (1980). *Family-centered Maternity Care: How to Achieve It.* Spokane, WA: The Cybele Society.

Brans, Y.W. (Ed.) (1983). "Symposium on Innovative Planning of Perinatal Centers." *Clinical Perinatology* 10 (1): 1-282.

Brimblecombe, F.S.W., Richards, M.P.M., & Roberton, N.R.C. (Eds.) (1978). *Separation and Special Care Baby Units.* Philadelphia: J.B. Lippincott Co.

Canadian Institute of Child Health (CICH). (1980). *Family-centered Maternity, Newborn, and Early Childhood Care in Canada.* Ottawa: Canadian Institute of Child Health.

Canadian Paediatric Society (CPS). (1979, Jun/Jul). "Family Centered Perinatal Care." *Canadian Paediatric Society News Bulletin Supplement* 10 (4): 1-2.

Engel, E.L. (1963). "Family-centered Hospital Maternity Care." *American Journal of Obstetrics and Gynecology* 85 (2): 260-66.

Fenwick, L. & Dearing, R.H. (1981). *The Cybele Cluster: A Single Room Maternity Care System for High- and Low-Risk Families.* Spokane, WA: The Cybele Society.

Haire, D. & Haire, J. (1970). *Implementing Family-Centered Maternity Care with a Central Nursery.* Minneapolis: International Childbirth Education Association.

International Childbirth Education Association (ICEA). (1978). Position Paper on Planning Comprehensive Maternal and Newborn Services. Minneapolis: International Childbirth Education Association.

Interprofessional Task Force on Health Care of Women and Children. (1978). Joint Position Statement on the Development of Family-centered Maternity/Newborn Care in Hospitals. Washington, DC: American College of Obstetricians and Gynecologists.

James, V.L. & Wheeler, W.E. (1969). "The Care-By-Parent Unit." *Pediatrics* 43: 488-94.

Klaus, M.H. & Kennell, J.H. (1982). *Parent-Infant Bonding.* 2nd edition. St Louis: The C.V. Mosby Co.

Lubic, R.W. (1980). *Evaluation of an Out-of-Hospital Maternity Center for Low-Risk Patients.* New York: Maternity Center Association.

McKay, S. & Phillips, C.R. (1984). *Family-Centered Maternity Care: Implementation Strategies.* Rockville, MD: Aspen Systems Corp.

McMaster University, Department of Obstetrics and Gynecology. (1981, Jun). "Family-centered Maternity Care." *Bulletin of the Society of Obstetrics Gynaecology of Canada 11* (3): 1-2.

National Association of Childbearing Centers (NACC). (1985). Standards for Freestanding Birth Centers. Perkiomenville, PA: National Association of Childbearing Centers.

Notelovitz, M. (1978). "The Single-unit Delivery System: A Safe Alternative to Home Deliveries." *American Journal of Obstetrics and Gynecology 132* (8): 889-94.

Phillips, C.R. (1988). "Single-room Maternity Care for Maximum Cost-efficiency." *Perinatology and Neonatology 12* (2): 22-24, 28-31.

Ross Planning Associates. (1988). *Perspectives in Perinatal and Pediatric Design*. Columbus, OH: Ross Laboratories.

Stella, Str. M. (1960). "Family-centered Maternity Care." *Hosp. Prog. 41*: (Mar) 92-94; *41*: (Apr) 70-72, 158.

Sumner, P.E. & Phillips, C.R. (1981). *Birthing Rooms: Concept and Reality*. St. Louis: The C.V. Mosby Co.

Young, D. (1982). *Changing Childbirth: Family Birth in the Hospital*. Rochester, NY: Childbirth Graphics, Ltd.

FATHERS AT BIRTH

What initial impact does a newborn have on its father? What does a father experience at his infant's birth? Animal studies indicate that newborns have considerable impact upon males within many vertebrate species. Studies of numerous cultures show that newborn infants have an intense early impact on their fathers, who may hold, cuddle, and show considerable enjoyment in their babies. Culture shapes both the amount of emotional commitment as well as who may show the greatest emotional commitment.

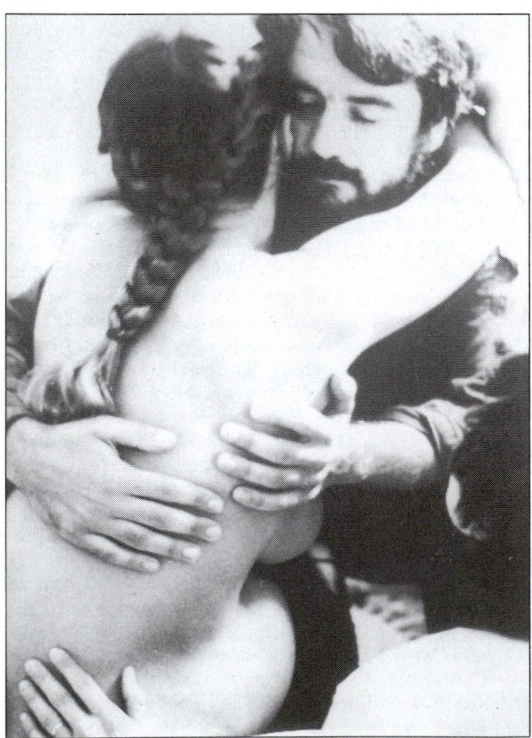

Loving support. Photo courtesy of Kip Kozlowski.

The extended family and other family support systems are seldom as readily available to most new parents as in the past. Early father attachment to the newborn is thus of greater significance today, especially in light of recent emphasis on the father's role in childrearing. Over the last two decades, fathers in contemporary Western society have become more involved in childbirth, assuming more nurturant roles. Approximately 80 percent of all American fathers now attend the birth of their children; it is now considered a given in American society that the father will be present at the birth. A father may be motivated to be present at the birth by many influences: his spouse or partner, friends, family, professionals, peers, his unborn child, and his desire for self-fulfillment.

Many men see childbirth as both awesome and fearful. Major concerns that a father usually keeps to himself may include fears of queasiness, expression of feelings, and loss of spouse or child, along with uneasiness about increased responsibility and obstetrical or gynecological matters. A review of nursing research on expectant fatherhood (Lemmer, 1987) revealed fathers' perceived needs and expectations during childbirth. Fathers want to know about labor and delivery and when to go to the hospital. They want frequent information on the mother-baby status, as well as a sense of control and a sense of being able to help their partners. Fathers expect an experienced birth attendant to be on hand at the birth and expect some idea of how to behave during childbirth. In addition, they want personal reassurance and care.

Popular readings, mass media presentations, and a variety of classes may help to determine fathers' beliefs about father-infant bonding. How a father feels and behaves toward his newborn is influenced both by internal factors brought into the situation as well as external factors that occur at the time. Internal factors include parental, family, and cultural values and practices; past attachment experiences; plus previous pregnancy and bonding experience. Other variables include financial stability and readiness and desire for the pregnancy. External factors include care received, attitudes and behaviors of attendants, newborn condition, infant responsiveness, and degree of separation between father and baby during the first hours or days of life.

Delivery is a slightly more positive experience for fathers than the emotional, sometimes stressful, and fatiguing labor. Following the birth, most fathers show an initial burst of behavior that occurs in sequence, beginning with hovering and visual contact, hands postured toward the infant, and continuing with face-to-face alignment followed by fingertip and palm contacts. The father may feel relief that the infant is healthy, that delivery is completed, and that his fears were suddenly released. He likely feels excited yet older, more mature, and has increased satisfaction when others see the newborn. He is filled with hope for the new life, and may feel overwhelmed. He knows he will always remember this day, and that he has accomplished a major goal. He has started a new experience that will continue to shape his life and that of his family.

Though research from the perspective of the father is relatively recent, many authorities have noted the powerful energy between newborn and father. Engrossment has been defined (Greenberg and Morris, 1974) as a father's sense of absorption, preoccupation, and interest in his infant. This sense initially unites father with newborn, and early contact with the infant is significant. Characteristics of engrossment include both visual and tactile awareness of the newborn, awareness of the baby's distinct characteristics, and perception of the infant as being perfect. A strong feeling of attraction focuses the father's attention on his infant. He experiences a "high" of extreme elation and feels an increase in self-esteem. The father may feel surprised at the degree of impact the newborn has on him. He is amazed at the infant's liveliness. Normal newborn movements and reflexes are perceived as communication and response of the infant to the father. The first hour of wakefulness and activity significantly reinforces and enhances the father's engrossment with the infant.

Many fathers report feeling drawn toward the baby as if by a magnet. They may have no control over this very powerful attraction, feeling stunned, surprised, ecstatic, dazed, relaxed, or as if dreaming. Some feel an intense, powerful, almost painful joy. Overwhelming love often begins with the first sight and touch of the newborn.

Much less research is available on how a father feels when his wife or partner does not experience an uncomplicated vaginal birth with a normal newborn. The more positive the birth experience, the greater the attachment to his newborn. Unfortunately, the greater his disappointment in the delivery not going as planned, the less responsive the father may be to his infant. A father at an unexpected cesarean birth may feel extreme terror, anxiety, a sense of loss and helplessness, complete emotional exhaustion, or alienation. Anger, disappointment, depression, and dissatisfaction may be mixed with acceptance and relief that the labor is over.

Not all fathers experience such adverse emotions, however. At planned or unplanned cesarean birth, some fathers feel relief that the long and difficult labor will soon be over, especially when a healthy newborn and mother emerge from surgery. If the newborn is critically ill, malformed, or stillborn, a father may experience rage, numbness, silence, or despair. Yet he also may feel great love, and a calmness at the wonder of birth, as well as death.

Do fathers at birth feel differently from fathers not present? Fathers who take an active role in the delivery of their own children often report a more satisfying experience than those who take a more passive role, yet not all men want to be present during labor and delivery.

A father witnessing his child's birth may have a profound spiritual experience and form an unusually close bond to his child. Presence at delivery seems to positively influence some father-infant attachment behaviors, especially inspection, verbalization, and many nonverbal behaviors. Almost all fathers, attending or not, report a sensation of elation that lasts two to three days. Involvement at delivery positively influences a father's perception of himself and his relationship with his mate. He is likely to show increased self-confidence and self-esteem plus an increased sense of self-growth and self-worth. His later parenting may be enhanced, and he may be remembered by his wife more positively for the emotional impact of having shared the birth event.

Attenders often remember a more positive experience than nonattenders. A father who attends birth is more likely than a nonattender to be quite certain that he can always identify his own newborn from other babies by how the infant looks. The attender is also likely to be more comfortable holding his baby during the immediate newborn period. On first sight of his newborn, a nonattender may feel surprised that the baby already moves around. Attenders likely will express certainty that the baby is theirs, while nonattenders do not mention the issue.

Fathers absent from their child's birth due to military, educational, or occupational obligations or sickness may notice their feelings of engrossment are less intense, or even absent. A critical period exists after which a father may have problems showing affection for his child. Fathers unable to attend the birth may experience guilt for longer than five months. Fathers not allowed with their wives at birth will likely be strongly concerned about the safety of mother and baby and the possibility of complications.

A father who is uncertain about attending the birth should be supported and encouraged but not pressured to do so, otherwise he will feel guilty if he does not attend or unhappy if he does. Once he sees the baby, it will not make much difference. Early newborn contact may be sufficient to help an ambivalent father establish engrossment. The reluctant father needs to know that whatever may happen at delivery, no one occurrence is singly necessary or sufficient to establish a positive, long-lasting relationship with his child.

Research into the father's experience of pregnancy and childbirth remains limited. More studies are needed relating to the feelings of unmarried, low-income, and poorly educated fathers as well as blue-collar, nonwhite, ethnic, and adoptive fathers at birth. Not enough is known about fathers at second or successive births or at planned or unplanned cesarean births. Further research would also be useful regarding fathers who do not attend childbirth education classes, fathers separated from their newborns for a long time, and fathers at the birth of a damaged or deformed child.

Fathers increasingly assist with the early physical and emotional care of their new infants, and more information is needed about the father-infant relationship. Though the expectant father's actions usually are viewed as supportive or secondary, he sees these actions as primary to his childbirth experience. Professional support of fathers before and during birth can give the father information, encourage questions, and facilitate engrossment. Encouraging the father's participation reinforces the concept that fathers do have a role in childbearing. Increasing his opportunity to become actively involved with the birth may strongly affect the father's involvement with his newborn, even to the enhancement of his future caretaking activities. Yet, although a man who has missed the moment of his child's birth has lost an experience no one can explain to him, building and maintaining the father-child relationship is a long-term, continuous process that extends far beyond the actual moment of birth.

✱ CATHRYN L. CALDWELL, R.N., B.S.N.

See also: Bonding

See **Guide to Related Topics:** Pregnancy, Psychological Aspects

Resources

Arms, S. (1975). *Immaculate Deception*. San Francisco: San Francisco Book Co./Houghton Mifflin.

Bowen, S.M. & Miller, B.C. (1980). "Paternal Attachment Behavior as Related to Presence at Delivery and Preparenthood Classes: A Pilot Study." *Nursing Research 29* (5): 307-11.

Brant, H. (1985). *Childbirth for Men*. Oxford, England: Oxford University.

Cronenwett, L.R. & Newmark, L.L. (1974). "Fathers' Responses to Childbirth." *Nursing Research 23* (3): 210-17.

Fein, R.A. (1976). "The First Weeks of Fathering: The Importance of Choices and Supports for New Parents." *Birth and the Family Journal 3* (2): 53-58.

Fortier, J.C. (1988). "The Relationship of Vaginal and Cesarean Births to Father-Infant Attachment." *Journal of Obstetrical, Gynecological and Neonatal Nursing 17* (2): 128-34.

Gaskin, I.M. (1978). *Spiritual Midwifery*. Summertown, TN: The Book Publishing Co.

Greenberg, M. & Morris, N. (1974). "Engrossment: The Newborn's Impact upon the Father." *American Journal of Orthopsychiatry 44* (4): 520-31.

Kitzinger, S. (1989). *Giving Birth: How It Really Feels*. New York: The Noonday Press/Farrar, Straus & Giroux.

Lemmer, C. (1987). "Becoming a Father: A Review of Nursing Research on Expectant Fatherhood." *Maternal-Child Nursing Journal 16* (3): 261-75.

Manion, J. (1977). "A Study of Fathers and Infant Caretaking." *Birth and the Family Journal 4* (4): 174-79.

McCall, R.B. (1987, Jan). "About Fathers: Father Bonding." *Parents*: 133.

———. (1989, Jan). "About Fathers: Present at Birth." *Parents*: 136.

McDonald, D.L. (1978). "Paternal Behavior at First Contact with the Newborn in a Birth Environment without Intrusions." *Birth and the Family Journal 5* (3): 123-32.

Merton, A. (1988, Dec). "My Son's Birth." *Glamour 86*: 126-32.

Palkovitz, R. (1987). "Fathers' Motives for Birth Attendance." *Maternal-Child Nursing Journal 16* (2): 123-29.

———. (1988). "Sources of Father-Infant Bonding Beliefs: Implications for Childbirth Educators." *Maternal-Child Nursing Journal 17* (2): 101-13.

Peterson, G. & Mehl, L. (1978, Oct). "Some Determinants of Maternal Attachment." *American Journal of Orthopsychiatry 135* (1).

Richards, L.B. (1987). *The Vaginal Birth after Cesarean (VBAC) Experience*. South Hadley, MA: Bergin & Garvey.

Shapiro, J.L. (1987, Jan). "The Expectant Father." *Psychology Today 21*: 36-39, 42.

Taylor, R. (1987, Mar 29). "A Fulfillment." *New York Times Magazine*: 67.

Varney, H. (1987). *Nurse-midwifery*. 2nd edition. Boston: Blackwell Scientific.

Wapner, J. (1976). "The Attitudes, Feelings, and Behaviors of Expectant Fathers Attending Lamaze Classes." *Birth and the Family Journal 3* (1): 5-13.

FEMINIST ANALYSES OF MOTHERHOOD

The meaning of motherhood to women has been a hotly debated subject in the West for about 200 years, or ever since Mary Wollstonecraft and other 18th-century European women tried to extend the principles of the French Revolution, the new Rights of Man, to women. Could women, defined by their duties to their families, be citizens, too? Was there a basic contradiction between the two identities, between public and private?

In the first mass wave of feminism in the 19th century, European and American women tended to make special claims for themselves as mothers: For example, many argued that they deserved the vote, not only because they were people, but because they were *special* people—more moral, nurturant, and peaceful. If women had the vote, some hoped the state would be more motherly.

For a number of reasons—the lack of consistently reliable birth control practices, the economic need for children, and the social meaning of the family—very few 19th-century feminists questioned motherhood as the central occupation of women. In the spirit of American Protestant individualism, the great 19th-century feminist thinker Elizabeth Cady Stanton spoke of women as ultimately independent, as souls who would meet their maker alone, but this ideal of self did not alter the fact that for most 19th-century women of all classes, motherhood was a social given, not a choice.

Some 19th-century women struggled to regulate their childbearing through a "cult of true womanhood," trying to establish an ideology that put women in control of the domestic sphere and of sexuality in marriage, but control and choice are subtly different. In the 19th century, the word "woman" and the word "mother" were one and the same, and it was only in the 20th-century wave of the women's liberation movement, beginning in the late 1960s, that women seriously considered separating these two identities in an effort to think of woman not only or primarily in her aspect as mother.

But if women are not mothers, who are they? Understandably, modern U.S. feminists have felt deeply ambivalent about just how far from "mother" women might want to go. How can the desire for liberation and the experience of motherhood combine?

For convenience, this ambivalence in modern feminism can be surveyed by simplifying the record into three general periods of contemporary feminist thought. From the beginning, feminists set out to break two taboos: the taboo on describing the complex and mixed experiences of actual mothers and the taboo on the celebration of a child-free life. But for reasons both inside and beyond the women's movement, feminists were better able in the long run to attend to mothers' voices than they were able to imagine a full and deeply meaningful life without motherhood, without children.

Period I: 1963-74. This period, which begins with the publication of Betty Friedan's book, *The Feminine Mystique*, might be called the era of the demon texts, books for which feminists have hastened to apologize, fearing that these early critiques of motherhood went too far. Friedan has herself denounced her first book in *The Second Stage* (1981), blaming her earlier work for being anti-family and for overemphasizing women as autonomous individuals. In fact, *The Feminine Mystique* is rather mild in making these points, but in her recantation, Friedan called her early radical feminism "strangely blind" about the real needs of women.

The most famous demon text is Shulamith Firestone's *The Dialectic of Sex: The Case for Feminist Revolution* (1970). This book is usually the starting point for discussions of how feminism has been "strangely blind" about motherhood. Certainly there are few of its sentences that Firestone would leave unmodified if she were writing with the same intent today. Her undertheorized enthusiasm for cybernetics, her self-hating disgust at the pregnant body ("Pregnancy is barbaric"), her picture of the female body as a prison from which a benign, nonpatriarchal science might provide release have all dated. Finally, though, it's her 1960s tone that seems strange—the atmosphere of freewheeling, shameless speculation. *The Dialectic of Sex* is an example of utopian writing, and part of the demonizing of this text arises out of a misreading of genre. Everyone colludes in calling it a mother-hating book. Search the pages. The evidence cannot be found, because the point of the book is always "smash patriarchy," not mothers.

Of course, there are real demon texts inside feminism, callow works like a few of the essays in the collection *Pronatalism: The Myth of Mom and Apple Pie* (1974), which reject childbearing in favor of having unsoiled white rugs and the extra cash to buy them. But such moments are rare. If one searches for early feminist mother-hating, what one usually finds is an absence. In major anthologies like *Sisterhood Is Powerful, Women in Sexist*

Society, and *Liberation Now!*, there are hardly any articles on any aspect of mothering. Nothing strange, really, about this blindness. Most of the writers were young, and many had been raised with the high expectations of the post-World War II generation, whose middle-class members were often promised a long period of self-development before marriage and motherhood. Hence a space opened for some relatively privileged women. Out of that space, and out of the kinetic social movements of that time, new questions emerged about the life trajectories of women.

The *Our Bodies/Ourselves* that was a newsprint booklet in 1971 reflects this new atmosphere. Under "Pregnancy," one finds such things as: "We, as women, grow up in a society that subtly leads us to believe that we will find our ultimate fulfillment by living out our reproductive function...." But soon, very soon, this criticism of pregnancy as destiny was misread as an attack on housewives. By the late 1970s, both mothers and nonmothers were on the defensive, a triumph of backlash.

Period II: 1976-80. With the publication of the glossy *Our Bodies/Ourselves* in 1978, women find themselves in a different feminist world. The book acknowledges that "until quite recently" having a baby wasn't really considered a decision, but then goes on to assume that now all that has changed, ending with this gee-whiz sentence: "Now almost 5 percent of the population has declared its intentions to remain child-free." Both people who have decided to have children and people who have decided against are quoted at some length, but the structural result is an aimless pluralism, a mere series of lifestyle questions with no recognition of the cultural asymmetry between the two choices.

If the 5 percent remained shadowy, nonetheless it was in Period II that feminism began the hard work of breaking that other taboo and speaking of the actual experiences of mothers. In these years, the feminist work of exploring motherhood took off: The year 1976 alone saw the publication of Adrienne Rich's *Of Woman Born*, Dorothy Dinnerstein's *The Mermaid and the Minotaur*, Jane Lazarre's *The Mother Knot*, and Linda Gordon's *Woman's Body, Woman's Right*. Also in that year, French feminism began to be a power in feminist academic thinking in the United States. *Signs* published Hélène Cixous's "The Laugh of the Medusa," which included these immediately controversial words: "There is always within [woman] at least a little of that good mother's milk. She writes in white ink."

In 1978, Nancy Chodorow's *The Reproduction of Mothering* and Michelle Wallace's *Black Macho and the Myth of the Super-Woman* were publishing events. The intellectual work of feminism has its renaissance in these years.

In her introduction to a brilliant special issue of *Feminist Studies* on motherhood in 1978, Rachel Blau DuPlessis honored what Rich was trying to do in *Of Woman Born*—to pry mothering away from the patriarchal institution: "motherhood." But then, DuPlessis went on to worry that Rich might be overreacting, overprivileging the body. "If, by the process of touching physicality," DuPlessis wrote, "Rich wants to find that essence beyond conflict, the place where all women necessarily meet, the essence of women, pure blood, I cannot follow there."

These discussions led to continuing feminist debates about the role of biology in women's situation. Feminists disagree about the extent to which motherhood is a socially constructed experience. DuPlessis asked the larger political question that nags throughout the period: Which construction of motherhood is productive for feminist work? If one takes Dorothy Dinnerstein at her word, men should become mothers. If one follows Rich, feminist energies move toward building a female culture capable of the support not only of women but also of their children.

Feminist theory is still far from sorting out the implications for activism, and right in the middle of this period, in 1977, the first Hyde Amendment was passed: Women lost Medicaid abortion. Abortion, the primal scene of this wave—won in 1973—was affordable for all classes for only four years before this right began slipping away.

Period III: 1980-90. The second period ends—and a third begins—with the brilliant threshold article by Sara Ruddick in 1980, "Maternal Thinking." Ruddick took seriously the question of what women actually do when they mother. She developed a rich description of what she called "maternal practice" and "maternal thinking," and her much reprinted article has been read, misread, and appropriated into a variety of arguments. Is motherhood really a separable practice? Are its special features capable of translation into women's public power?

Ruddick provides one of the best descriptions feminism has of why women are so deeply committed to the mothering experience, even under very oppressive conditions. Her work is a song to motherhood—multiphonic, without sugar—but still a song. "Maternal Thinking" is the fullest response since Adrienne Rich to the call to end the taboo on speaking the truth of mothers' lives. However, this work came at a time of retrenchment for feminism. During the Ronald Reagan presidency, talk of autonomous "women" disappeared into talk about "the family," though it is "women," not "families," who continue to do almost all domestic work.

On the whole the 1980s was a period of frustration and defeat for feminists, from the loss of the Equal Rights Amendment to new revelations about divorce, child support, rape, and incest. Many feminists lost heart about the more transformative goals of an earlier radical feminism and dug into more defensive political positions.

The year 1986—with Sue Miller's novel *The Good Mother* and Sylvia Ann Hewlett's *A Lesser Life*—was a peak year for backlash. Seeing that women are oppressed as mothers, Hewlett decided to demand special protections for them—a change from the demands for equality and shared child care that characterized earlier feminist work.

In spite of a political backlash against feminist thinking and action, women are in fact living out basically new story lines, making piecemeal changes in the balance they strike among work, childbearing, and relationships. While the U.S. birth rate declines (women had 3.7 children in 1956, 1.9 in 1990), feminists continue to debate the fundamental question of whether they want the identity "mother" to expand or contract.

If current experience is compared with that of the 19th century, it can be seen clearly that motherhood is a social institution that changes, a series of practices with a history. But inside an individual life, these changes are often invisible. Abortion has been a central demand of modern feminism, but it may be a long time before women's control of their reproductive capacity takes form as a basically different set of social relations between men and women. ✷ ANN SNITOW

See also: Feminist Analyses of Motherhood: Timeline

FEMINIST ANALYSES OF MOTHERHOOD: TIMELINE

Key: The items listed below are feminist or feminist-related. Relevant additional articles and events are denoted with an asterisk (*). Items in brackets are conferences.

1963

Friedan, Betty. *The Feminine Mystique*. New York: W.W. Norton & Co.

1964

Rossi, Alice. "Transition to Parenthood." *Journal of Marriage and the Family 1* (30).

1965

*Moynihan, Daniel Patrick. *"The Negro Family: The Case for National Action."*

1969

Pollard, Vicki. (Fall). "Producing Society's Babies." *Women: A Journal of Liberation.*

Willis, Ellen. (Sept). "Whatever Happened to Women? Nothing, That's the Trouble." *Mademoiselle.*

1970

Firestone, Shulamith. *The Dialectic of Sex: The Case for Feminist Revolution*. New York: William Morrow.

Tanner, Leslie. (Ed.) *Voices from Women's Liberation*. New York: Signet.

1971

Boston Women's Health Course Collective. *Our Bodies, Ourselves*. Boston: New England Free Press.

Peck, Ellen. *The Baby Trap*. New York: Pinnacle Books.

*Comprehensive Child Development Act passed by Congress, vetoed by Richard Nixon (Child care funds)

1973

Radl, Shirley. *Mother's Day Is Over*. New York: Charterhouse.

*Gilder, George. *Sexual Suicide*. New York: Quadrangle Books.

**Roe v. Wade*

1974

Bernerd, Jessie. *The Future of Motherhood*. New York: The Dial Press.

Mitchell, Juliet. *Psychoanalysis and Feminism: Freud, Reich, Laing, and Women*. New York: Pantheon Books.

Peck, Ellen & Senderowitz, Judith. Pronatalism: The Myth of Mom and Apple Pie. New York: Thomas Y. Crowell.

1975

Hammer, Signe. *Daughters and Mothers, Mothers and Daughters*. New York: Quadrangle Books.

Valeska, Lucia. (Winter). "If All Else Fails, I'm Still a Mother." *Quest 1* (3).

1976

Chodorow, Nancy & Cantratto, Susan. "The Fantasy of the Perfect Mother." *Social Problems 23* (2).

Cixous, Hélène. (Summer). "The Laugh of the Medusa." *Signs 1* (4): 875-93.

Dinnerstein, Dorothy. *The Mermaid and the Minotaur: Sexual Arrangements and Human Malaise*. New York: Harper & Row.

Gordon, Linda. *Woman's Body, Woman's Right: Birth Control in America*. Grossman Publishers.

Lazarre, Jane. *The Mother Knot*. New York: McGraw-Hill.

Rich, Adrienne. *Of Woman Born: Motherhood as Experience and Institution*. New York: W.W. Norton.

Russo, N.F. "The Motherhood Mandate." *Journal of Social Issues 32* (3).

1977

Friday, Nancy *My Mother/Myself: The Daughter's Search for Identity*. New York: Delacorte Press.

Joffe, Carole. *Friendly Intruders: Childcare Professionals and Family Life*. Berkeley: University of California Press.

Klepfisz, Irena. "Women without Children/Women without Families/Women Alone." Reprinted in *Dreams of an Insomniac: Jewish Feminist Essays Speeches, and Diatribes*. Eight Mountain Press, 1990.

Kristeva, Julie. (Winter). "Love's Heretical Ethics." *Tel Quel 74*: 39-49.

Rossi, Alice. "A Biosocial Perspective on Parenting." *Daedelus 106* (3).

*Hyde Amendment—no Medicaid abortions

*Lasch, Christopher. *Haven in a Heartless World*. New York: Basic Books.

1978

Boston's Women's Health Book Collective. *Ourselves and Our Children: A Book by and for Parents.* New York: Random House.

Chodorow, Nancy. *The Reproduction of Mothering: Psychoanalysis and the Sociology of Gender*. Berkeley: University of California Press.

Feminist Studies Special Issue. (Jun). "Toward a Feminist Theory of Motherhood." v.4, no.2

Hoffner, Elaine. *Mothering: The Emotional Experience of Motherhood after Freud and Feminism.* New York: Doubleday, Inc.

Wallace, Michelle. *Black Macho and the Myth of the Super-Woman.* New York: The Dial Press.

1979

Arcana, Judith. *Our Mothers' Daughters*. Berkeley: Shameless Hussy Press.

CARASA (Committee for Abortion Rights and Against Sterilization Abuse). *Women Under Attack: Abortion, Sterilization Abuse and Reproductive Freedom*. New York.

Chesler, Phyllis. *With Child: A Diary of Motherhood.* New York: Thomas Y. Crowell.

Feminist Studies Special Issue. (Summer). "Workers, Reproductive Hazards, and the Politics of Protection." no.5.

Friedan, Betty. "Feminism Takes a New Turn." *The New York Times*, Aug. 26.

Lorde, Audre. "Man Child: A Black Lesbian Feminist's Response." *Conditions 4.*

Willis, Ellen. (Sept 17). "The Family: Love It or Leave It." *The Village Voice XXIV* (38): 1, 29-35.

[Lerner, Michael. Friends of Families. Conference, c. 1979-1982]

[NOW, National Assembly on the Future of the Family, Conference, Hilton Hotel, Nov. 19]

[The Scholar and the Feminist VI: The Future of Difference. Conference, Barnard, April 29]

1980

Badinter, Elizabeth. *Mother Love: Myth and Reality.* New York: Macmillan.

Ehrensaft, Diane. (Summer). "When Men and Women Mother." *Socialist Review 10* (4): 49.

Eisenstein, Hester & Jardine, Alice. (Eds.) *The Future of Difference*. Boston: G.K. Hall & Co.

Marks, Elaine & de Courtivron, Isabelle. (Eds.) *New French Feminisms: An Anthology*. Amherst: University of Massachusetts Press.

Oakley, Ann. *Becoming a Mother*. New York: Schocken Books.

———. *Women Confused: Toward a Sociology of Childbirth.* New York: Schocken Books.

Ruddick, S. (Summer). "Maternal Thinking." *Feminist Studies 6* (2): 342-67.

Weisskopf, Susan Contratto. (Summer). "Maternal Sexuality and Asexual Motherhood." *Signs 5* (4).

1981

Bridenthal, Renate, Kelly, Joan, Swerdlow, Amy, & Vine, Phyllis. (Eds.) *Household and Kin: Families in Flux*. New York: The Feminist Press.

Brown, Carol. "Mothers, Fathers, and Children: From Private to Public Patriarchy." Reprinted in Lydia Sargent (Ed.) *Women and Revolution*. Boston: South End Press.

Dowrick, Stephanie & Grundberg, Sibyl. *Why Children?* New York: Harcourt Brace Jovanovich.

Friedan, Betty. *The Second Stage.* New York: Simon & Schuster.

Galinsky, Helen. *Parenthood.*

Hirsch, M. "Mothers and Daughters: A Review." *Signs 7* (1).

Lorber, J., Coser, R.L., Rossi, A.S., & Chodorow, N. "On *The Reproduction of Mothering*: A Methodological Debate." *Signs 7* (1).

O'Brien, Mary. *The Politics of Reproduction*. New York: Routledge.

*The Family Protection Act proposed.

1982

Barrett, Michele & McIntosh, Mary. *The Anti-Social Family*. London: Verso.

Gilbert, Lucy & Webster, Paula. *Bound by Love: The Sweet Trap of Daughterhood.* Boston: Beacon Press.

Gilligan, Carol. *In a Different Voice: Psychological Theory and Women's Development*. Cambridge and London: Harvard University Press.

Lerner, L. "Reproduction of Mothering: An Appraisal." *The Psychoanalytic Review 51* (1).

Rothman, Barbara Katz. *In Labor: Women and Power in the Birth Place.* New York: W.W. Norton.

Thorne, Barrie & Yalom, Marilyn. *Rethinking the Family: Some Feminist Questions*. New York and London: Longman.

*ERA defeated

1983

Dally, Ann. *Inventing Motherhood: The Consequences of an Ideal.* New York: Schocken Books.

Daniels, Pamela & Weingarten, Kathy. *Sooner or Later.* New York: W.W. Norton.

Diamond, Irene. (Ed.) *Families, Politics, and Public Policy: A Feminist Dialogue on the State.* New York: Longman.

Folbre, Nancy. (Summer). "Of Patriarchy Born: The Political Economy of Fertility Decisions." *Feminist Studies 9* (2).

Porter, Nancy reviewing "Mothering: Essays in Feminist Theory." *Women's Studies Quarterly*, v.VII (Winter).

Riley, Denise. *War in the Nursery: Theories of the Child and the Mother*. London: Virago.

1984

Alpert, J.L., Gerson, M., & Richardson, M.S. "Mothering: The View from Psychological Research." *Signs 9* (3).

Arditti, Rita, Klein, Renate Duelli, & Minden, Shelley. *Test-Tube Women: What Future for Motherhood?* London and Boston: Pandora Press.

Boston Women's Health Book Collective. *The New Our Bodies, Ourselves: A Book by and for Women.* New York: Touchstone/Simon & Schuster.

Delphy, Christine. *Close to Home: A Materialist Analysis of Women's Oppression*. Amherst: University of Massachusetts.

Gerson, Mary-Joan. (Sept). "Feminism and the Wish for a Child." *Sex Roles VII*.

Giddings, Paula. *When and Where I Enter: The Impact of Black Women on Race and Sex in America*. New York: William Morrow.

Greer, Germaine. *Sex and Destiny: The Politics of Human Fertility*. New York: Harper & Row.

Hooks, Bell. "Revolutionary Parenting." Reprinted in *From Margin to Center*. Boston: South End Press.

Luker, Kristen. *Abortion and the Politics of Motherhood*. Berkeley and London: University of California Press.

Petchesky, Rosalind. *Abortion and Women's Choice: The State, Sexuality, and Reproductive Freedom*. New York: Longman.

Rapp, Rayna. (Apr). "The Ethics of Choice: After My Amniocentesis, Mike and I Faced the Toughest Decision of Our Lives." *Ms*.

Sevenhuijsen, Selma & deVries, Petra. "The Women's Movement and Motherhood." Reprinted in *A Creative Tension: Key Issues of Socialist Feminism: An International Perspective from Activist Dutch Women, 9-25*. Boston: South End Press.

Simons, Margaret A. "Motherhood, Feminism, and Identity." *Women's Studies International Forum 7* (5): 349-59.

Trebilcot, Joyce. (Ed.) *Mothering: Essays in Feminist Theory*. Totowa, NJ: Rowman & Allanheld.

1985

Corea, Gena. *The Mother Machine: Reproductive Technologies from Artificial Insemination to Artificial Wombs*. New York: Harper & Row.

Folbre, Nancy. (Winter). "The Pauperization of Motherhood: Patriarchy and Public Policy in the United States." *Review of Radical Political Economics 16* (4).

Gerson, Katherine. *Hard Choices: How Women Decide about Work, Career, and Motherhood*. Berkeley and London: University of California Press.

Gittins, Diana. *The Family in Question*. London and New York: Macmillan.

Haraway, Donna. "A Manifesto for Cyborgs: Science Technology, and Socialist Feminism in the 1980s." *Socialist Review*: 80.

Pies, Cheri. *Considering Parenthood*. San Francisco: Spinsters Book Co.

Renvoize, Jean. *Going Solo: Single Mothers by Choice*. Boston: Routledge & Kegan Paul.

Schulenberg, Joy. *Gay Parenting: A Complete Guide...*

Weitzman, Lenore J. *The Divorce Revolution: The Unexpected Social and Economic Consequences for Women and Children in America*. New York: Free Press.

Zelizer, Viviana. *Pricing the Priceless Child: The Changing Social Value of Children*. New York: Basic Books.

1986

Allen, Jeffner. "Motherhood: The Annihilation of Women." In *Lesbian Philosophy: Explorations*. Palo Alto, CA: Institute of Lesbian Studies.

Atwood, Margaret. *The Handmaid's Tale*. Boston: Houghton Mifflin Co.

Barrett, Michele & Hamilton, Roberta. *The Politics of Diversity: Feminism, Marxism, and Nationalism*. London: Verso.

Chesler, Phyllis. *Mothers on Trial: The Battle for Children and Custody*. Seattle: Seal Press.

Gerson, Kathleen. "Emerging Social Divisions among Women: Implications for Welfare State Politics." *Politics and Society 15* (2): 213-24.

Heron, Liz. "Motherhood...to have or have not?" In *Changes of Heart: Reflections on Women's Independence* Boston: Pandora Press, pp. 177-218.

Hewlett, Sylvia Ann. *A Lesser Life: The Myth of Women's Liberation in America*. New York: William Morrow.

Hypatia Special Issue: "Motherhood and Sexuality." v.1, no.2 (Fall).

Kantrowitz, Barbara. (Sept 1). "Three's a Crowd." *Newsweek*: 68-76.

Mairs, Nancy. "On Being Raised by a Daughter." In *Plaintext*. Tucson: University of Arizona.

Miller, Sue. *The Good Mother*. New York: Harper & Row.

Ms. Special Issue: "When to Have Your Baby." (Dec.).

Omolade, Barbara. "It's a Family Affair: The Real Lives of Black Single Mothers." *Village Voice*.

Rothman, Barbara Katz. *The Tentative Pregnancy: Prenatal Diagnosis and the Future of Motherhood*. New York: Viking.

*McBroom, Patricia A. *The Third Sex: The New Professional Woman*. New York: William Morrow.

**New York Times Magazine*. "The American Wife." Oct. 26.

1987

Ehrensaft, Diane. Parenting Together. New York: Free Press.

Genevie, Louis E. & Margolies, Eva. *The Motherhood Report: How Women Feel About Being Mothers*. New York: Macmillan.

Gleve, Katherine. (Spring). "Rethinking Feminist Attitudes Towards Motherhood." *Feminist Review 25*.

Martin, Emily. *The Woman in the Body: A Cultural Analysis of Reproduction*. Boston: Beacon Press.

Petchesky, Rosalind. "Fetal Images." *Feminist Studies 13* (2).

Pollack, Sandra & Vaughan, Jeanne. (Eds.) *Politics of the Heart: A Lesbian Parenting Anthology*. Ithaca, NY: Firebrand Books.

Pruett, Kyle. *The Nurturing Father: Journeys toward the Complete Man*. New York: Warner Books.

Rosenfelt, Deborah & Stacey, Judith. "Second Thoughts on the Second Wave." *Feminist Studies 13* (2).

Segal, Lynne. "Back to the Nursery." *New Statesman*.

———. *Is the Future Female? Troubled Thoughts on Contemporary Feminism*. New York: Peter Bedrick Books.

Sojourner Special Issue. "Motherhood is Political: The Ideal vs. The Real."

Spallone, Patricia & Steinberg, Lynn. *Made to Order: The Myth of Reproductive and Genetic Progress*. New York: Pergamon Press.

Stanworth, Michelle. (Ed.) *Reproductive Technologies: Gender, Motherhood and Medicine*. Minneapolis: University of Minnesota Press.

*The Baby M Case in the news

**Time Magazine*. "Here Come the Dinks." April 20: 75.

*Wattenberg, Ben J. *The Birth Dearth*. Pharos Books.

1988

Aguero, Kathi & Gordett, Marea. (Jul). "Mothering and Writing: A Conversation." *Women's Review of Books*.

Benjamin, Jessica. *The Bonds of Love: Psychoanalysis, Feminism, and the Problem of Domination*. New York: Pantheon Books.

CARASA (Committee for Abortion Rights and Against Sterilization Abuse). *Women Under Attack: Victories,*

Backlash, and the Fight for Reproductive Freedom. Ed. by Susan E. Davis. Boston: South End Press, Pamphlet no.7 (The Athene Series).

Chesler, Phyllis. *Sacred Bond: The Legacy of Baby M*. New York: Times Books.

Eisenstein, Zillah R. *The Female Body and the Law*. Berkeley and London: University of California Press.

Epstein, Cynthia Fuchs. *Deceptive Distinctions: Sex, Gender, and the Social Order*. Boston: Yale University Press.

Grabucher, Marianne. *There's a Good Girl: Gender Stereotyping in the First Three Years of Life: A Diary*. Translated from the German by Wendy Philipson. London: The Women's Press Ltd.

Herman, Ellen. (Mar). "Desperately Seeking Motherhood." *Zeta*.

Quindlen, Anna. (Feb). "Mother's Choice." *Ms*.

Weideger, Paula. (Feb). "Womb Worship." *Ms*.

Weinberg, Joanna. "Shared Dreams: A Left Perspective on Disability Rights and Reproductive Rights." In Adrienne Asch & Michelle Fine (Eds.) *Women with Disabilities*. Temple.

*Family Support Act (workfare)

1989

Douglas, Susan J. (Sept). "Otherhood." *In These Times*: 12-13.

Edwards, Harriet. *How Could You? Mothers without Custody of Their Children*. The Crossing Press.

Ferguson, Ann. *Blood at the Root: Motherhood, Sexuality, and Male Dominance*. London: Pandora Press.

Gerson, Deborah. (Jul/Sept). "Infertility and the Construction of Desperation." *Socialist Review 19* (3).

Ginsburg, Faye D. *Contested Lives: The Abortion Debate in an American Community*. Berkeley and London: University of California Press.

Hirsch, Marianne. *The Mother-Daughter Plot: Narrative, Psychoanalysis, and Feminism*. Indiana University Press.

Hypatia Special Issue. "Ethics and Reproduction." v.4, no.3 (Fall).

Hochschild, Arlie. *The Second Shift*. London and New York: Viking Penguin.

Olivier, Christiane. *Jocastra's Children: The Imprint of the Mother*. New York: Routledge.

Rothman, Barbara Katz. *Recreating Motherhood: Ideology and Technology in a Patriarchal Society*. New York: W.W. Norton.

Ruddick, Sally. *Maternal Thinking: Towards a Politics of Peace*. Boston: Beacon.

Sevenhuijsen, S. & Smart, Carol. (Eds.) *Child Custody and the Politics of Gender*. New York: Routledge.

1990

Arnup, Katherine, Levesque, Andree, & Pierson, Ruth Roach. *Delivering Motherhood: Maternal Ideologies and Practices in the 19th and 20th Centuries*. New York: Routledge.

Chamberlayne, Prue. (Summer). "The Mother's Manifesto and Disputes over *'Mutterlichkeit,'*" *Feminist Review 35*: 9-23.

Cole, Ellen & Knowles, Jane Price. (Eds.) *Woman-Defined Motherhood*. Binghamton: Harrington Park Press.

Ehrensaft, Diane. "Feminists Fight (for) Fathers." *Socialist Review 4*: 57-80.

Finger, Anne. *Past Due: A Story of Disability, Pregnancy, and Birth*. Seattle: Seal Press.

Gordon, Tuula. *Feminist Mothers*. New York: New York University Press.

Kaminer, Wendy. *A Fearful Freedom: Women's Flight from Equality*. Addison-Wesley.

Morell, Carolyn MacKelcan. "Unwomanly Conduct: The Challenges of Intentional Childlessness." Dissertation, Bryn Mawr.

O'Barr, Jean et. al. (Eds.) *Ties that Bind: Essays on Mothering and Patriarchy*. Chicago and London: University of Chicago Press.

Rapping, Elayne. "The Future of Motherhood: Some Unfashionably Visionary Thoughts." In Karen V. Hanson & Ilene J. Philipson (Eds.) *Women, Class, and the Feminist Imagination*. Temple.

Sandelowski, Margarete. (Spring). "Fault Lines: Infertility and Imperiled Sisterhood." *Feminist Studies 16* (1): 33-51.

White, Evelyn C. (Ed.) *The Black Women's Health Book: Speaking for Ourselves*. Seattle: Seal Press.

Wilt, Judith. *Abortion, Choice, and Contemporary Fiction: The Armageddon of the Maternal Instinct*. Chicago and London: University of Chicago Press.

✱ ANN SNITOW and CAROLYN MORELL

See also: Feminist Analyses of Motherhood

FETAL ALCOHOL SYNDROME

Fetal Alcohol Syndrome (FAS) is a term invented in the 1970s to describe the potential effects of extreme, chronic alcohol intake by a pregnant woman on her developing fetus. Standards for diagnosing FAS were still being proposed as recently as 1980. Symptoms are usually listed to include three areas:

1. central nervous system damage, including mental retardation and/or behavioral disorders such as hyperactivity and poor impulse control;
2. impaired growth and/or failure to thrive, and;
3. a characteristic pattern of abnormal facial features, including a flattened mid-face region and thin upper lip.

In practice, the diagnosis of so-called "full-blown" FAS is often made when one or more of these symptoms is absent or extremely mild. Thus, making a distinction between FAS, its counterpart Fetal Alcohol Effects (FAE), also known as Alcohol Related Effects (ARE), and other confounding factors contributing to one or more of the above symptoms is ambiguous and problematic for epidemiological accuracy.

Although it has been described as "the leading cause of mental retardation in the Western world," and the only cause that is "totally preventable," (Abel and Sokol, 1987; Abel, 1990), there are still many unanswered questions about the prevalence of FAS, its target populations, and its basic causes. Reported incidence rates of FAS vary markedly according to researcher and population studied. According to Warren and Bast (1988) "the prevalence of FAS has never been determined using national probability methodology, so the U.S. incidence and prevalence is not precisely known."

Significantly, not every woman who is alcoholic and drinks excessively during pregnancy will produce a baby with FAS. Pregnancy outcomes for actively alcoholic women giving birth to an infant with FAS range dramatically from as many as 40.5 percent to as few as 2.7 percent, depending on the population studied (Bingol et al., 1987).

This remarkably wide range in percent of FAS babies born to alcoholic mothers suggests an array of critical confounding factors beyond alcohol intake as the primary and/or exclusive cause of FAS. Prominent among factors significantly associated with FAS is lower socioeconomic status and all of its attendant problems. These may include a genealogy of poor nutrition (when generations of mothers have been under- or poorly nourished), restricted access to prenatal care, and other life stressors associated with poverty and the hardship of marginal social existence.

The epidemiology of FAS along racial lines, clustering as it does in certain Native American tribes living on government reservations (May et al., 1983) and among the black urban poor, points to poverty and class as among the strongest predictors for FAS in the offspring of alcoholic women. Thus, any truly effective prevention strategy for FAS must widen its scope beyond the problem of alcoholism in pregnant women to confront the complex social context in which these women reside. ✱ DONNA LEE KING, M.A.

See also: Pregnancy and Social Control

See **Guide to Related Topics:** Special Needs Infants

Resources

Abel, E.L. (1990). *New Literature on Fetal Alcohol Exposure and Effects*. Westport, CT: Greenwood Press.

Abel, E.L. & Sokol, R.J. (1987). "Incidence of Fetal Alcohol Syndrome and Economic Impact of FAS-related Anomalies." *Drug and Alcohol Dependence 19* (1): 51-70.

Bingol, N. et al. (1987). "The Influence of Socioeconomic Factors on the Occurrence of Fetal Alcohol Syndrome." *Advances in Alcohol and Substance Abuse 6* (4): 105-08.

Cole, C. et al. (1987). "Prenatal Alcohol Exposure and Infant Behavior: Immediate Effects and Implications for Later Development." *Advances in Alcohol & Substance Abuse 6* (4): 87-104.

May, P.A. et al. (1983). "Epidemiology of Fetal Alcohol Syndrome among American Indians of the Southwest." *Social Biology 30* : 374-87.

National Institute on Alcohol Abuse and Alcoholism. (1985). "My Baby...Strong and Healthy." *Alcohol Health and Research World 10* (1).

U.S. Department of Health and Human Services. (1984). Fifth Special Report to the U.S. Congress on Alcohol and Health. DHHS Pub. No. (ADM) 84-1291. Washington, DC: Superintendent of Documents, U.S. Government Printing Office.

Warren, K.R. & Bast, R.J. (1988). "Alcohol-related Birth Defects: An Update." *Public Health Reports 103* (6): 638-42.

FETAL MOVEMENT

Historically, fetal movement has been considered to be the ultimate sign of fetal life and well-being. In the second half of the 20th century, people attempted to attribute these movements to various fetal physiological functions or patterns. It took the development of real-time ultrasonography to allow the visualization of the fetus within the uterus and the recording of the progression of fetal activity (motor function) that takes place in the uterine environment.

Studies of fetal movement can be generally divided into three major topic areas:

1. Fetal movement development and fetal movement cycles.
2. Correlations between fetal movement and fetal well-being and outcome.
3. Maternal perception of fetal movement and methods by which fetal movements can be counted and recorded.

Most pregnant women first become aware of fetal movement (quickening) between 16 and 20 weeks' gestational life. Researchers now know that fetal movements take place much earlier than this. The fetal heart has been observed, on ultrasound, to beat as early as the sixth week of gestation. Studies on the development of fetal movement and fetal movement cycles describe "jerky" or "sporadic" fetal head and neck movements as early as the seventh gestational week, and some studies have reported fetal respiratory movement at 10 weeks' gestation (Jouippila and Piiroimen, 1975; Birnholz, Stephens, and Faris, 1978; Sadovsky, Weinstein, and Polishuk, 1978; deVries, Visser, and Prechtl, 1984).

Fetal movements vary according to gestational age. Separate movement patterns have been identified in normal pregnancy—Birnholz identified nine characteristic patterns that he associated with various musculoskeletal movements (Birnholz, Stephens, and Faris, 1978; Cintas, 1987). Timor-Tritsch categorized fetal movement patterns as rolling, simple (jab, startle, or kick), high frequency (hiccough, weak kick, or flutter), and respiratory (Timor-Tritsch et al., 1976). As the neuromuscular systems develop, the complexity of fetal movements increases (Cintas, 1987). This developmental progression of muscular activity occurs first from the head and then downward to include the trunk and finally the limbs (Lehman and Estok, 1987). When fetal compromise occurs, movements will generally be lost in the reverse order of their development—fetal heart rate accelerations being the first to go, followed by breathing movements, body movements, and finally muscle tone (Vintzileos et al., 1983; Johnson, Besinger, and Thomas, 1988). The fetal heartbeat may still be audible.

As pregnancy progresses, movements become stronger and more frequent. Some studies indicate a general increase in fetal movements starting at about 18 weeks' gestation until a maximum is reached between weeks 29 to 38. Movements then decrease slightly until delivery (Sadovsky and Yaffe, 1973). Although the reasons for this decrease in movement are not fully understood, it may be directly related to the decreased amount of space and amniotic fluid left within the uterus, or to the increasing maturation of the neonatal central nervous system (Mathews, 1978; Baskett and Liston, 1989). It should be noted that a reduction in the number of daily movements without a change in the distribution of types of movements is not necessarily an indicator of fetal distress (Coleman, 1981).

A great deal of interest, in the last 15 to 20 years, has been focused on maternal perception of fetal movement and Daily Fetal Movement Counting (DFMC). Introduced in the early 1970s, DFMC is being used as one tool for evaluating fetal well-being and identifying the fetus at risk for complications or death. Different methods by which maternally perceived fetal movements can be counted and recorded have been developed.

Studies have not indicated a significance in an absolute number of fetal movements per day, except for very low rates with a definite trend toward decreasing motion (Sadovsky and Polishuk, 1977; Sadovsky, 1985). Each fetus demonstrates individuality in rhythm or (sleep/wake) cycle. Fetal movements may also be affected by other variables, both internal and external, such as light, touch, sound, temperature changes, vibrations, maternal activity levels and stress, smoking, maternal drug use, fetal anomalies, intrauterine growth retardation (IUGR), Rh isoimmunization, ultrasound, and intrauterine hypoxia caused by diminished uteroplacental blood flow.

Fetal movements are an indicator of central nervous system integrity and function. By studying fetal movements, through maternal perception, real-time ultrasonography, and with electromechanical devices (i.e., fetal heart rate monitors and nonstress testing), it is possible to obtain state of the art information regarding fetal well-being (Rayburn, 1987).

✱ MARGARET R. PRIMEAU, R.N., M.B.A.

See also: Daily Fetal Movement Counting; Nonstress Tests

See **Guide to Related Topics:** Prenatal Diagnosis and Screening

Resources

Baskett, T.F. & Liston, R.M. (1989, Sept). "Fetal Movement Monitoring: Clinical Application." *Clinics in Perinatology 16* (3): 613-25.

Birnholz, J.C., Stephens, J.C., & Faris, M. (1978, Mar). "Fetal Movement Patterns: A Possible Means of Defining Neurologic Developmental Milestones In Utero." *American Journal of Roentgenology 130* (3): 537-40.

Cintas, H.M. (1987, Fall). "Fetal Movements: An Overview." *Physical and Occupational Therapy in Pediatrics 7* (3): 1-15 (80 ref) Haworth Press.

Coleman, C.A. (1981, Jan/Feb). "Fetal Movement Counts—An Assessment Tool." *Journal of Nurse Midwifery 26* (1): 15-23.

deVries, J.I., Visser, G.H., & Prechtl, H.F. (1984). "Fetal Motility in the First Half of Pregnancy." In H.F. Prechtl (Ed.) *Continuity of Neural Functions from Prenatal to Postnatal Life. Clinics in Developmental Medicine, 94.* Philadelphia: JB Lippincott, pp. 46-64.

Johnson, T.R.B., Besinger, R.E., & Thomas, R.L. (1988, May). "New Clues to Fetal Behavior and Wellbeing." *Contemporary OB/GYN*: 108-23.

Jouippila, P. & Piiroimen, O. (1975, Nov). "Ultrasonic Diagnosis of Fetal Life in Early Pregnancy." *Obstetrics & Gynecology 46* (5): 616-20.

Lehman, A.E. & Estok, P.J. (1987, Jan). "Screening Tool for Daily Fetal Movement." *Nurse Practitioner 12* (1): 40-42, 44.

Mathews, D.D. (1978). "Fetal Wellbeing in Gravidas with Diminished Fetal Activity at Term." *Obstetrics and Gynecology 51* (3): 281-83.

Rayburn, W.F. (1987, Dec). "Monitoring Fetal Body Movement." *Clinical Obstetrics and Gynecology 3* (4): 899-911.

Sadovsky, E. (1985, Apr). "Monitoring Fetal Movement: A Useful Screening Test." Reprinted from *Contemporary OB/GYN.*

Sadovsky, E. & Polishuk, W. (1977, Jul). "Fetal Movement in Utero." *Obstetrics and Gynecology 50* (1): 49-55.

Sadovsky, E., Weinstein, D., & Polishuk, W.Z. (1978). "Timing of Delivery in High Risk Pregnancy by Monitoring of Fetal Movements." *Journal of Perinatal Medicine 6* (3): 160-64.

Sadovsky, E. & Yaffe, H. (1973). "Daily Fetal Movement Recording and Fetal Prognosis." *Obstetrics and Gynecology 41* (6): 845-50.

Timor-Tritsch, I. et al. (1976, Sept). "Classification of Human Fetal Movement." *American Journal Obstetrics and Gynecology 126* (1): 70-77.

Vintzileos, A.M. et al. (1983). "The Fetal Biophysical Profile and Its Predictive Values." *Obstetrics and Gynecology 62* (3): 271-78.

FETAL PRESENTATIONS

Fetal presentation is determined by the anatomical landmarks of the fetus in relation to the maternal pelvis. Fetal lie, attitude, and position are also determined in this manner. These descriptive terms provide a common language for the health care practitioner in assessing essential information. Fetal presentation and position describe how the fetus and mother's pelvis may accommodate each other in the birth process. Hence, anticipatory plans can be made to prepare for the birth.

The first portion of the fetus to enter the pelvic inlet is called the presenting part. Presentation is defined by the presenting part. Approximately 96 percent of babies born are in the cephalic, or head down, presentation. Approximately 3.5 percent are in the breech, or feet first, position. The fetal lie is the relationship of the long axis of the fetus to the long axis of the mother. In both cephalic and breech presentations, the lie is longitudinal. In the very rare (.04 percent) case of a persistent transverse lie (the fetus is "sideways") or shoulder presentation, a vaginal birth is not possible, and a cesarean section becomes life-saving.

The fetal attitude is the relation of the fetal parts to each other, or the fetus's basic posture of flexion or extension. The most common is one of flexion, with the head bent in front of the chest, arms and legs folded, and the back curved slightly.

The fetal position gives the most complete information and includes in its definition the presentation, lie, and the relationship of the fetal presenting part to the front, back, or side of the mother's pelvis. (See Figure 1.) The most common position at term is known as left occiput anterior, or LOA. This term denotes the occiput of the fetal skull facing towards the left and front of the maternal pelvis. The combination of both the decreased amniotic fluid at term and the roomier uterine fundus, which provides more space for the bulkier fetal parts, probably explains the predominance of this position.

Presentation may be determined by abdominal exam and/or digital vaginal exam in labor. Diagnostic ultrasound may confirm clinical diagnosis. Once the cervix has begun to dilate, fetal suture lines, fontanels, and portions of the face and fetal body can be felt. The practitioner must be well versed in the anatomical landmarks of the fetus, and especially of the fetal skull, in order to determine vaginally a more definitive diagnosis of presentation. ✱ LAURA ZEIDENSTEIN, C.N.M., M.S.N.

See also: External Cephalic Version

See **Guide to Related Topics:** Pregnancy, Physical Aspects

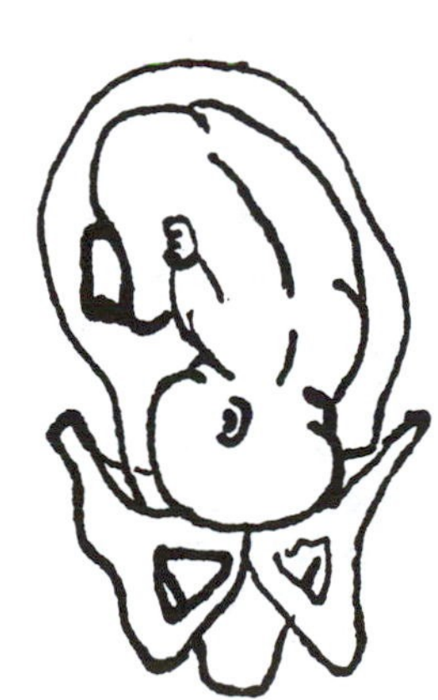

LOA: left occiput anterior
LIE: longitudinal
PRESENTATION: vertex
ATTITUDE: well-flexed

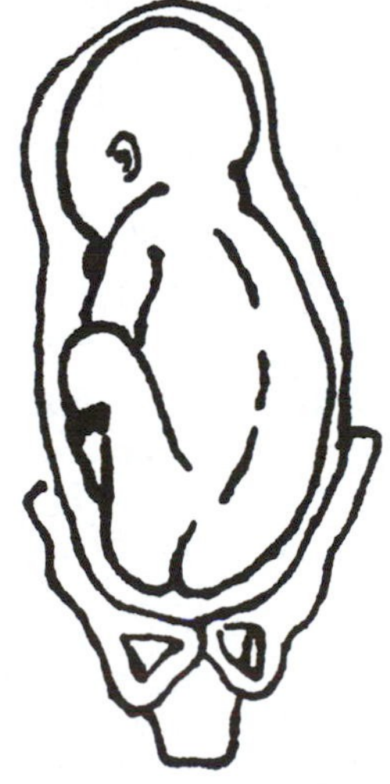

LSA: left sacrum anterior

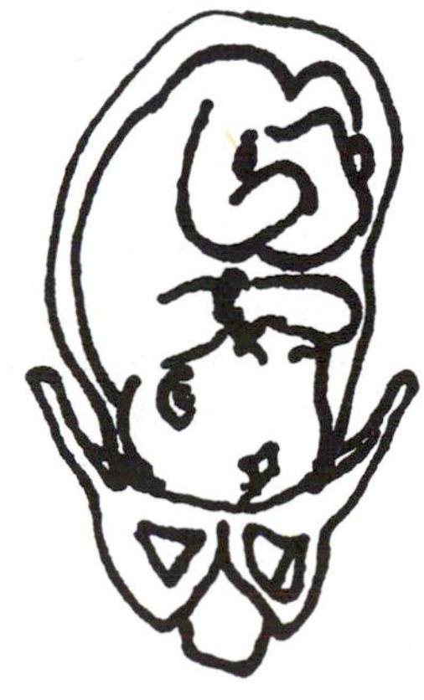

ROP: right occiput posterior

Illustrations courtesy of Laura Zeidenstein, C.N.M.

Resources

Cunningham, F. Gary et al. (1989). *Williams Obstetrics.* 18th edition. Norwalk, CT: Appleton and Lange.

Davis, Elizabeth. (1987). *Hearts and Hands: A Midwife's Guide to Pregnancy and Birth.* 2nd edition. Berkeley, CA: Celestial Arts.

Gaskin, Ina May. (1978). *Spiritual Midwifery.* Revised edition. Summertown, TN: The Book Publishing Co.

Myles, Margaret F. (1981). *Textbook for Midwives.* 9th edition. Edinburgh, Scotland: Churchill Livingstone.

Oxorn. (1986). *Oxorn-Foote Human Labor and Birth.* 5th edition. Norwalk, CT: Appleton-Century-Crofts.

Scott et al. (1990). *Danforth's Obstetrics and Gynecology.* 6th edition. Philadelphia: J.B. Lippincott Co.

Varney, Helen. (1987). *Nurse-Midwifery.* 2nd edition. Boston: Blackwell Scientific Publications.

Whitley, Nancy. (1985). *A Manual of Clinical Obstetrics.* Philadelphia: J.B. Lippincott Co.

FETUS, MATERNAL EXPERIENCE OF

The experience of carrying a fetus within one's body is unique to pregnancy. How does one experience being tied to another, a very dependent being, in such an intimate, deep way? Women talk about this experience of the embodied "presence" of the fetus-becoming-child, as they learn to become "present" for the fetus/child as a mother (Bergum, 1989). The exceptional intimacy of the woman-fetus interaction, this interrelationship, has been described by Rabuzzi (1988) as a "kind of interactive, two-in-one-self," where the selfhood of the woman becomes "motherselfhood" (pp. 43, 52). Does not the pregnancy experience, as a primordial experience, tie people together in the many-leveled commitments to relationship, to family, to community, and to the environment? The woman-fetus relationship—transient, undefinable, powerful, trustworthy—is the foundation of the strongest connection between human beings, and the basis for all others (Sarah, 1987). As women begin to recognize the reality of the Other, the fetus/child, they also become more attentive to the Self. In pregnancy, this experience is not a detached sense of Self as one responds to an Other; rather, it is an understanding of Self within relationship to the Other. Women, during pregnancy, talk about the changing understanding of Self from "Who am I?" to "Who are you?" (Bergum, 1990).

This Is My Body: The Idea of Baby. On first recognition of pregnancy, the sense of the Other, the baby, is distant. Of course, women say, "I am going to have a baby," but that baby is just an idea, perhaps even a secret for a while, something that a woman may hold close to her heart. Later she shares her "going to have a baby" news with others, such as husband, family, and friends. Women experience the baby as an idea or as an abstraction as they wait for inner signs of movement or heartbeat or outer signs, such as the ultrasound picture or the tight skirts, to make them realize that there indeed is a fetus/child present.

With the baby an idea rather than a reality, the woman focuses on the Self, on bodily changes that are often uncomfortable, on a growing body that many feel just fat, or on emotional changes, such as increased vulnerability about being faced with overwhelming tasks, and on the fear that the Self will be lost in the process and will no longer have control of her life. This early experience of pregnancy is primarily focused on the Self: "How am I feeling? How can I handle this new experience? I need friends and family to care for me. I fear losing myself. I fear losing control and becoming dependent on others." The idea of the baby is found in the words "Is there really a baby in there?" since the woman has not yet begun, in a bodily way, to recognize the Other.

This Is My Body and My Baby. The first encounter with the living Other, the fetus/child, is through hearing the heartbeat, seeing the ultrasound, feeling a movement. These first encounters bring women to a place of sensing someone other than themselves. It is real, that is, pregnancy is real, and the abstract baby is "really" there, not yet as an individual, a separate being, but rather as an extension of oneself. During this time there is talk about planning for the baby and planning on fixing a space for the baby (but not necessarily doing anything). There is also discussion with the partner about how this coming baby will change their relationship. In talking with others, some women talk about being let into a "secret" club, a club that consists of women who are already mothers. This theorizing about the baby and what being a mother will be like is part of the recognition that pregnancy is preparation for an actual child, and preparation for becoming attentive to an Other.

This Is My Body: This Is My Baby. Women start to see the beginnings of the fetus/child as an individual when they guess about what the movements of the fetus/child mean and imagine his or her characteristics. They find satisfaction in making sense of this behavior. The encounters with the fetus remind the woman that "before it was me, but it's not anymore; this is my baby, I really feel *somebody*." The coming to know the *individual* child continues to develop through play, through the characteristic movements that the mother gives to this child, toward a more distinct recognition that this fetus/baby is a separate/separating being. Here we see the beginning attention to the Self *and* the Other—that is, attention to both the needs of the Self (woman) and the needs of the Other (fetus/child).

Talking to the baby, shifting to make room (e.g., "He reminds me to sit up.") is recognition that this "presence" is someone who is strong and vigorous, and someone who can "make up its own mind." Now the baby is one that women hold in their arms, or whose foot they touch when it is pushing too hard, or with whom they play and talk. The give and take between woman and fetus begins before birth and leads the woman to talk about the separation itself, to the meeting of the independent child. As the fetus/baby gets bigger, the woman can imagine pushing the baby out and begins to prepare for that separation. Some expect pain as a necessary part of this separation, a recognition that the pain will help the woman to accept the separation of this close intimacy that the "presence" of the fetus/child had begun. When the child leaves the woman's body, the woman comes, through the pain, to see the child face to face. The inner intimacy opens to outer commitment. ✱ VANGIE BERGUM, R.N., Ph.D.

See also: Motherhood as Transformation

See **Guide to Related Topics:** Pregnancy, Psychological Aspects

Resources

Bergum, Vangie. (1989). *Woman to Mother: A Transformation*. N. Hampton, MA: Bergin & Garvey Publishers.

———. (1990). "Abortion Revisited: Toward an Understanding of the Nature of the Woman-Fetus Relationship." *Phenomenology & Pedagogy* 8: 17-26.

Rabuzzi, K.A. (1988). *Motherself: A Mythic Analysis of Motherhood*. Bloomington, IN: Indiana University Press.

Sarah, R. (1987). "Power, Certainty, and the Fear of Death." *Women & Health* 33 (2-3): 59-72.

FORMULA MARKETING

The marketing of commercially manufactured breastmilk substitutes and other foods promoted for infant consumption is not a unique problem for the so-called "Third World," but is a global issue. The marketing and promotion of infant foods is damaging to the practice of breastfeeding in rich as well as in poor countries. The infiltration of health facilities and information channels by the baby food companies has led to the assumption that artificial feeding is a "normal" and therefore acceptable process for large numbers of infants. The results are a question of scale; not to be breastfed increases the risk of infection for infants in industrialized countries, but widely available health services can treat illnesses early enough to minimize the risk of death. For example, a study in Scotland showed a threefold risk of gastrointestinal illness in bottle-fed infants regardless of socioeconomic conditions (Howie et al., 1990). However, in a developing country, there is a fourteenfold increase in death from gastrointestinal illness if a child is not breastfed (Victora et al., 1987). The United Nations Children's Fund calculates that, in poor conditions, a bottle-fed child is 25 times more likely to die than a breastfed one (UNICEF/WHO/UNESCO/IBFAN, 1989).

Biologically, lactation is a successful survival strategy. Breastfeeding failure is virtually unknown among traditional societies, such as gatherers/hunters, and is mainly caused by cultural, iatrogenic, and commercial factors. The medicalization of childbirth and infant feeding during the 19th and 20th centuries has led to a misunderstanding of breastfeeding. Medically prescribed "management" of breastfeeding continues to undermine the process and, worldwide, the more contact women have with health services, the more rapid the decline in incidence and duration of breastfeeding. This applies to both industrialized and nonindustrialized countries. The development of damaging practices, such as restricted feeding, incorrect positioning, and the use of supplementary bottle feeding, grew from 18th- and 19th-century theories developed by influential doctors (mostly male) both in Europe and the United States. Traditional breastfeeding knowledge was ignored because it lay with uneducated women.

This trend toward bottle feeding and away from breastfeeding could not have endured if its establishment had not coincided with changes in dairy technology that led to cows' milk surpluses and the development of the artificial baby milk market. Both doctors and milk companies gained financially through breastfeeding failure (as they still do), for the baby whose mother's milk had been sabotaged by mistaken management was dependent on a human-made product for survival. Until the 19th century, orphans and the infants of mothers who did not breastfeed were foster-nursed by other women; the life-saving properties of breastmilk were appreciated, and wet nursing was a respected practice whether carried out for financial gain or from goodwill. The development of the artificial baby food market led to the demise of the wet nurse, though the practice of suckling other women's infants survives to this day.

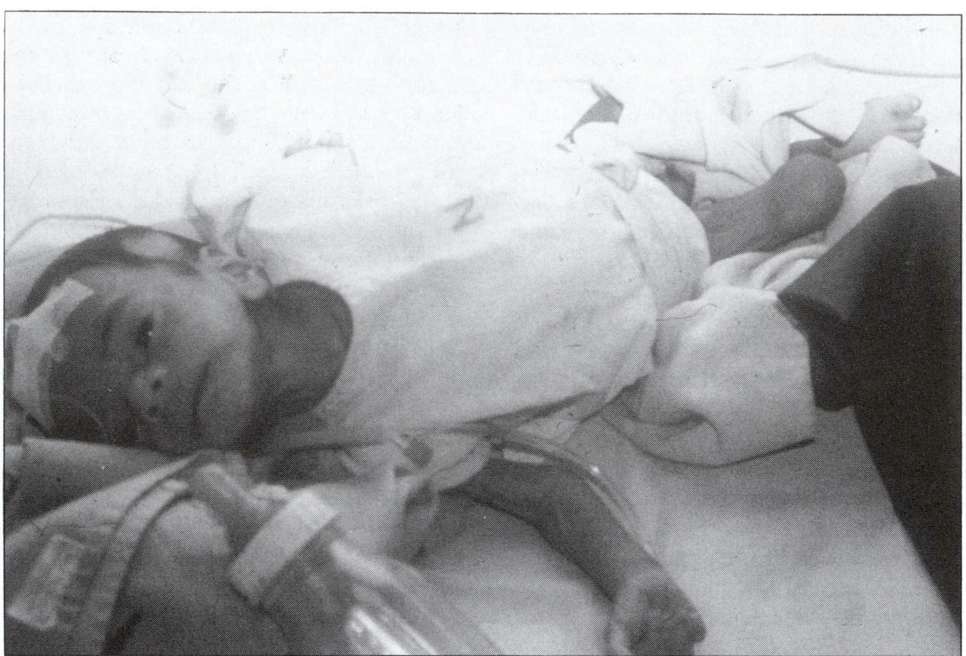

A malnourished, bottle-fed Filipino baby. Photo courtesy of Baby Milk Action, Cambridge, U.K.

The expansion of 20th-century industrialized capitalism facilitated the mass marketing of infant foods. Public advertising, promotion through health services, and a symbiotic relationship with the medical profession were well established by the 1920s and persist to this day all over the world. Research and study design are influenced by the baby food industry, which gives grants and awards, financially supports medical associations, and maintains close relationships with governmental health bodies. Companies distribute misleading infant feeding information that is echoed in pediatric text books. Company employees may even teach infant nutrition as part of medical, midwifery, and nursing courses.

The Swiss company Nestlé (the market leader) was already promoting infant foods in Europe, the U.S., and tropical countries in the 19th century. The marketing and availability of these products undermine breastfeeding wherever they occur. At the turn of this century, rising morbidity and mortality, particularly from diarrhea, was noted by contemporary doctors to be related to a lack of breastfeeding. A common reaction was either to blame the mother for allegedly "refusing to breastfeed" or to accept lactation failure as an unresolvable fault of nature. Acknowledgment of the roles of industry and the medical profession was rare, although there were exceptions. The high prevalence of infant infection, malnutrition, and death that is now associated with Third World conditions existed in turn-of-the-century Europe and the United States. Poverty and urbanization were key factors, but uncontrolled promotion of commercial infant foods and indifference and/or collusion by doctors played a significant part as well.

Although concerned individuals, such as Dr. Cicily Williams in 1939, made strong public statements, the harm of infant food promotion in poor countries was not an issue of public awareness until the 1970s when information was published in popular media. The magazine *New Internationalist*, the British charity "War on Want," and citizens' groups took up the issue. Publicity was heightened by a libel suit brought by Nestlé in 1974 against the Berne Third World Action Group for translating the "War on Want" document "The Baby Killer" into the German equivalent of "Nestlé Kills Babies." Nestlé won on a technicality, and the Berne group was fined a nominal sum, but the case evolved into a public exposé of the company's promotional practices. In 1977 a boycott against Nestlé was launched in the U.S. and spread to Canada, New Zealand, and Europe. This action, together with lobbying by concerned groups and individuals, led to meetings at the United Nations level. The result was the drafting and adoption by the World Health Assembly (WHA) in 1981 of the WHO/UNICEF International Code of Marketing of Breastmilk Substitutes, which gives clear guidelines for the ethical marketing of baby foods and feeding utensils. This Code was adopted by 118 member states, with 3 abstentions and a single "no" vote from the United States.

Nestlé, though stating publicly in 1981 that it would follow the WHO/UNICEF Code, continued to violate its principles despite some changes in marketing practices. However, by 1983 the company appeared to be making real changes, and the boycott ended in 1984 when Nestlé signed a written agreement with the International Nestlé Boycott Committee (INBC) promising to adhere to the International Code. Other baby food companies, including Abbott-Ross (U.S.); Mead-Johnson/Bristol-Myers (U.S.); Wyeth/AHP (U.S.); Milupa (West Germany); Nutricia (Netherlands) and its UK subsidiary Cow and Gate; Boots/Farley (UK); Meiji (Japan); Amul (India); and other smaller companies all violate the International Code. Nestlé is still (1990) the baby food leader with a 50 percent market share, which far exceeds that of any of the other large infant food companies. Nestlé is a founder member of the International Association of Infant Food Manufacturers, whose stated purpose is "to develop common industry policy" and "to promote high ethical standards."

In 1988, a new Nestlé boycott was launched in the United States and West Germany by the groups Action for Corporate Accountability (ACTION) and Actionsgruppe Babynahrung (AGB), both members of the International Baby Food Action Network (IBFAN). This boycott was triggered by Nestlé's breaking of the agreement that ended the first boycott, expressed by its refusal to abide by a 1986 WHA Resolution (39/28) that clarified an article in the WHO Code regarding the provision of free or low-cost supplies of baby milk. Nestlé and other companies use the free supply tactic as a marketing strategy, which is against the WHO Code. This second Nestlé boycott has spread to Australia, Canada, Mauritius, Mexico, the Philippines, and eight European countries (Baby Milk Action, August 1990).

✷ GABRIELLE PALMER

See also: Breastfeeding: Historical Aspects; Nipples, Artificial; Weaning Food

See **Guide to Related Topics:** Infant Feeding

Resources

Baby Milk Action (BMAC), 6 Regent Terrace, Cambridge CB1 4AP, UK.

Chetley, Andrew. (1986). *The Politics of Baby Foods*. London: Frances Pinter.

Howie, P. et al. (1990). "Protective Effect of Breastfeeding against Infection." *British Medical Journal 300*: 11-16.

Minchin, Maureen. (1985). *Breastfeeding Matters*. Sydney, Australia: Alma Publications/George Allen and Unwin.

Palmer, Gabrielle. (1988). *The Politics of Breastfeeding*. London: Pandora Press.

UNICEF/WHO/UNESCO/IBFAN. (1989). "Facts for Life: A Communication Challenge." Geneva.

Van Esterick, Penny. (1989). *Beyond the Breast-Bottle Controversy*. New Brunswick, NJ: Rutgers University Press. (Published in the U.K. by Zed Press under the title *Mother Power Infant Feeding*.)

Victora, G. Cesar et al. (1987, Aug 8). "Evidence for Protection by Breastfeeding against Infant Deaths from Infectious Diseases in Brazil." *Lancet*: 319-22.

WHO/UNICEF. (1981). "The WHO/UNICEF Code of Marketing of Breast-milk Substitutes." Geneva.

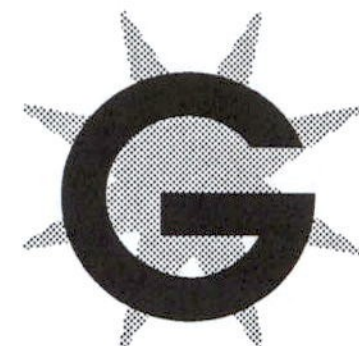

GENETIC COUNSELING

Genetic counseling is a communication process that translates genetic knowledge into practical information for individuals and families. It is concerned with the occurrence and the risk of recurrence of genetic disorders within a family. It involves establishing a diagnosis, explaining inheritance patterns, and discussing options available to at-risk individuals and/or couples (Ince, 1987).

Frequently, genetic counseling occurs *retrospectively*, that is, after the birth of a child with a birth defect or genetic disease. At this time, genetic counseling can provide important information as well as emotional support and understanding. If there are decisions to be made about the care of a child, about having more children, and about the ability of the familyto cope, parents can make more informed decisions with the facts at hand.

However, more and more couples are seeking *prospective* genetic counseling prior to a family because either one member of the couple is affected with a disorder or there are questionable genetic problems on one or both sides of the family (Scott, 1988). Genetic counseling is appropriate for:

- Persons who themselves have or are concerned they might have an inherited disorder or birth defect.
- Women who are pregnant or planning pregnancies in their 30s or 40s.
- Couples who have a child with mental retardation, an inherited disorder, or a birth defect.
- Couples whose infant has a genetic disease diagnosed by routine newborn screening.
- Women who have had two or more miscarriages or early infant deaths.
- Persons concerned that their jobs, lifestyles, or past medical history may pose a risk to pregnancy (including exposure to radiation, medications, chemicals, infections, drugs, or known cancer-causing substances).
- Couples who would like testing or information about genetic defects that occur more frequently in their ethnic group.
- Couples who are first cousins or other close blood relatives.
- Pregnant women who, based on a blood alphafetoprotein test or ultrasound, have been told their pregnancy may be at increased risk for complications or birth defects.

Before a family can be counseled, the nature of the birth defect or disease in question must be precisely established. The correct diagnosis is crucial—some environmentally produced birth defects (which are unlikely to occur again) can look very much like genetic disorders. Similar medical conditions may follow different inheritance patterns, and a hereditary illness can sometimes affect two family members in quite different ways.

To establish the diagnosis, the affected individual and sometimes others in the family may be examined or given laboratory tests. If a family member is unavailable, valuable information often can be gathered from medical records, autopsy reports, or old photographs. A family health history, or pedigree, is taken by the genetic counselor. Questions may be asked about current family members as well as past generations to gain information on babies who died early, the age and cause of death of a relative, and ancestors' country of origin. Prior to counseling, it is often possible to supplement family health information through discussion with relatives (Balkite, 1986).

Genetic conditions are caused in whole or in part by an alteration in one or more genes or in the amount of chromosomal material. Conditions are classified into the following categories: chromosome disorders, single-gene or Mendelian disorders, and polygenic or multifactorial disorders. On the basis of the way they are transmitted, single-gene defects are further divided into these categories: autosomal dominant, autosomal recessive, and X-linked conditions. All have characteristic inheritance patterns and risks, ranging from little or no risk of recurrence to 50 percent or more (Scott, 1988). Once a diagnosis is established, the inheritance pattern, recurrence risks, tests for the disorder, and options available can be discussed. Options discussed may include one or more of the following: (1) having children without any further testing; (2) electing not to have children; (3) having prenatal testing of a pregnancy either by chorionic villus sampling (CVS), amniocentesis, or ultrasound; (4) using artificial insemination by donor sperm; (5) investigating surrogate motherhood or embryo transfer; and (6) adopting (Gelehrter and Collins, 1990). The risks, benefits, limitations, and various outcomes of each option must also be discussed.

How the counseling information is viewed depends not only on the risk, but on the burden conferred by the disorder. For example, 2 percent of a severely disabling disorder (e.g., spina bifida) may be considered more significant to couples than a 50 percent risk of a minor problem such as extra toes. Counselees' perceptions for the risk/burden relationship depend on their own philosophic and religious beliefs, educational background, lifestyle, and prior experience, as well as the counseling information (Emery and Pullen, 1984). Genetic counseling is informational and a source of support. Counselors do not prescribe a particular course of action but help families reach the right decision for them, respecting individual values and choices (Balkite, 1986).

The genetic counselor should be a doctor or nurse with expertise in genetics, or a specially trained genetic counselor. A family can seek genetic counseling directly or be referred by a physician. More than 200 comprehensive genetic centers are available in the United States, usually located within obstetric or pediatric departments at large medical centers or teaching hospitals. Persons who think they could benefit from genetic counseling can call their nearest hospital or medical center, ask their health care provider, or contact the National Society of Genetic Counselors, 233 Canterbury Drive, Wallingford, PA (215) 872-7608 for the genetic counseling center nearest to them.

✱ ELIZABETH BALKITE, M.S.

See also: Eugenics; Genetics; Genome Mapping; Prenatal Diagnosis: Overview; Selective Abortion; Wrongful Birth and Wrongful Life

See **Guide to Related Topics:** Prenatal Diagnosis and Screening

Resources

Balkite, Elizabeth. (1986). "Genetic Counseling Prior to Amniocentesis." *Hospimedica* 4 (4): 51-55.

Emery, Alan & Pullen, Ian. (1984). *Psychological Aspects of Genetic Counseling.* New York: Academic Press.

Gelehrter, Thomas D. & Collins, Francis S. (1990). *Principles of Medical Genetics.* Baltimore: Williams & Wilkins.

Ince, Susan. (1987). *Genetic Counseling.* New York: March of Dimes.

Scott, Joan. (1988). "The Role of Genetic Counseling." In *Genetic Applications: A Health Perspective.* Lawrence, KS: Learner Managed Designs.

GENETICS

Genetics is the scientific description of hereditary mechanisms. An important impetus behind this effort has been the hope that a better understanding of genetics will explain the ways socially significant traits are passed from one generation to the next, so that this knowledge can be used for purposes of social and genetic engineering.

In his classic paper in 1865, Gregor Mendel, the "father" of genetics, enunciated the formal rules that describe the conditions under which specific traits in pea plants, such as flower color or seed shape, are transmitted to successive generations and suggested that such traits might be correlated with hypothetical "factors" inside the organisms. Later, scientists assumed these "factors" to be particles, carried on the chromosomes inside cells, and called them genes. In the late 1940s and early 1950s, the genes became molecules of DNA, the "double helix." But as was true of Mendel's "factors," specific genes can only specify differences between specific, simple traits: whether a pea plant has white or red flowers; whether someone has blue or brown eyes. More complex traits are generated by the participation of many genes and other metabolites in processes that take place within and outside of cells and organisms.

The fact that the pattern of inheritance of certain specific differences between two individuals of a species can be described by Mendel's laws has led scientists to assume that such differences are mediated by different forms of the same gene, called "alleles." But this in no way implies that any of the allelic forms of a gene can program or control that trait, only that the gene is one of the many components required for the trait to exist.

For example, hemoglobin, the protein that gives blood its red color and helps transport oxygen around the body, has two forms (normal and sickle cell). These forms constitute a pair of "traits" whose inheritance follows Mendel's laws. They differ in a specifiable way that is mediated by a relatively simple difference in the gene involved in hemoglobin synthesis. It is correct to say that, all other things being equal (which they never are outside of controlled laboratory experiments), the difference in the two forms of the gene exerts a decisive influence during the synthesis of the two forms of hemoglobin. It is *not* correct to say that either form of the gene *causes* the corresponding form of hemoglobin to be synthesized. That process involves a battery of additional reactants (including other genes) and energy sources that must be available at appropriate times and under the appropriate conditions.

All observable traits are produced by many interacting, and often mutually regulating, processes that involve many substances, including genes. But unfortunately the concept of the gene is used loosely by scientists and their public. Genes are invoked to explain the origin of specific traits as well as of major structures and functions of organisms. They are said to program the orderly transformations that take place while organisms develop and age, and they are said to be decisive for the slow, cumulative changes thought to have occurred during evolution and species formation. Much of this conjecture rests on assertions that are not based on observations or experiments.

Genes (DNA) contain four different, but related, chemical building blocks and differ from one another by virtue of differences in the sequence of these building blocks. These differences introduce specificity into the way genes interact with other molecules. Genes mediate the synthesis of proteins, and because of their structural differences, different genes mediate the synthesis of different proteins. As far as is known, that is all they do.

One of the most interesting features of the double-helical structure of DNA is that one strand of the helix can serve as a template for the synthesis of the other. This is how genes are duplicated when a cell divides and gives rise to two identical cells that constitute the next generation. This process is often described by saying that genes "replicate themselves." But in fact even their own duplication only happens as part of the metabolism of living cells in which many other molecules and processes participate.

The mistaken belief that genes cause or program a wide range of traits that are of personal and social significance recently has led scientists to undertake the gigantic project of trying to determine the composition and sequence of all of the DNA (the genes) located in the nuclei of human cells. They hope that once they know the complete DNA sequence, they will be able to understand the molecular basis of a wide range of diseases and disabilities and therefore to diagnose, treat, and eventually cure them. But genes affect only very few diseases in a direct and readily traceable way, and even for these, identifying the gene has rarely yielded treatments, much less cures. The best example is sickle cell anemia. The fact that the specific genetic and metabolic defects responsible for this disease have been known for several decades has been of little practical benefit.

Identifying a gene that is linked to a disease may indeed enable scientists to develop better diagnostic tests, but without therapies or cures, diagnoses are of questionable benefit. On the other hand, the increased focus on genes will increase the mythic importance our culture attributes to genetics and genes, so that people's complex physical and psychosocial characteristics will be explained in excessively individualistic, genetic terms that can be used to blame the victims. ✱ RUTH HUBBARD, Ph.D.

See also: Eugenics; Genome Mapping; The Perfect Baby

See **Guide to Related Topics:** Prenatal Diagnosis and Screening

Resources

Duster, Troy. (1990). *Backdoor to Eugenics.* New York: Routledge.

Nelkin, Dorothy & Laurence, Tancredi. (1989). *Dangerous Diagnostics: The Social Power of Biological Information.* New York: Basic Books.

Suzuki, David & Knudtson, Peter. (1988). *Genethics: The Ethics of Engineering Life.* Toronto: Stoddard.

GENITAL MUTILATION, FEMALE

Female genital mutilation, also known as female circumcision, is still widely practiced in a major part of present-day Africa and, to some extent, on the Arab Peninsula. The number of affected women has been estimated to be well over 80 million (Lightfoot-Klein, 1989a). The procedures involve extensive damage and irreversible mutilation of healthy external female genitalia.

Ritual circumcision, as it is performed in Africa, has as its intent the sexual desensitization of females and the attenuation of their sexual desire (Lightfoot-Klein, 1989b). Mutilations in varying degrees of severity are routinely inflicted on girls or young women, depending on the customs of the tribe and geographical area involved, with or without their consent and most often by force.

Excision of the clitoris and part or all of the labia minora is performed on females in most of sub-Saharan Africa. These parts of the female genitalia are generally believed to be unclean and are often feared as dangerous to the manhood of the husband and lethal to newborns. Excision is regarded as an essential purification rite (Lightfoot-Klein, 1989c). The severest and most profoundly damaging circumcision practices are found among Arabic-Islamic peoples along the Horn of Africa, in an area encompassing Southern Egypt, Northern and Central Sudan, parts of Ethiopia and Kenya, Somalia, Djibouti, and Mali in Western Africa. In these areas infibulation, as well as excision, is practiced (Hosken, 1982). This drastic procedure is known as Pharaonic Circumcision.

Infibulation involves the scraping out of the fleshy, inner layers of the labia majora, the remaining outer edges of which are then brought together so that when the wound has healed, they are fused to leave only a pinhole-sized opening, barely adequate for urination and menstruation. This infibulation is, in effect, an artificially created chastity belt of thick, fibrous scar tissue. At marriage the genitals are subjected to further trauma when the bridegroom either tears or cuts this infibulation to make sexual penetration possible and then prevents the wound from healing shut once more by repeated intercourse. Yet more trauma occurs at each birth, when the infibulation must be incised anteriorally to permit the expulsion of the baby, after which it is sewn shut once more.

Most commonly genital mutilation is performed on small girls and adolescents. The age at which the girl is subjected to circumcision may vary, however, from early infancy to after the birth of the first child, depending on custom. Throughout Africa there is now a tendency to perform the surgery at ever younger ages, since "a small girl is more easily managed."

Female circumcisions have traditionally been performed by medically untrained midwives, with no knowledge of antiseptic procedure or anatomy, on an unanesthetized child, kept from struggling by several women who hold her immobile. The instruments used are razor blades, kitchen knives, scissors, or pieces of glass. Within recent years some medical training has been made available to these practitioners, and in many African cities circumcisions are now performed in a rudimentary clinic-like setting, under what passes for sterile conditions, with the use of local anesthesia and antibiotics.

While these improved techniques tend to reduce the fatalities and immediate complications following circumcision, such as hemorrhage, infection, fever, and shock from pain, the long-term effects, particularly when there is infibulation, are much the same. These most frequently take the form of chronic infections, due to a build-up of urinary and menstrual debris behind the infibulation—infections that may eventually spread to the entire reproductive and renal systems. Childbirth is made exceedingly hazardous to both mother and infant by the fact that massive and often keloidal scarring of the infibulation obstructs and prevents dilation (Koso-Thomas, 1987; Sami, 1986; Dareer et al., 1982; Verzin, 1975).

Despite increased levels of education and exposure to Western influence, no significant decrease in female genital mutilation has been observed in any part of Africa; in fact, female circumcision practices are spreading into areas where they had previously been unknown (Lightfoot-Klein, 1989a). The reasons for this are manifold. Traditionally, female circumcision has been associated in most African societies with premarital chastity and, therefore, has been a prerequisite for marriage. Even today an uncircumcised woman simply will not find a man who is willing to marry her, and few if any options other than marriage and motherhood have ever been open to the African woman. In some societies, such as Sudan and Egypt, custom requires female circumcision as a guarantee of family honor, as increasing the chances of obtaining a high bride price for a daughter, and as a sign of prominent social status within the community. It has served through the ages to differentiate the "decent" circumcised and infibulated woman from prostitutes and slaves, who are uncircumcised and considered common property, unprotected by any male and his family or clan, and subject to rape and abduction.

Women in Africa traditionally have been regarded as property and are just now becoming aware of their human rights. Since circumcision practices are ubiquitous within the circumcised woman's limited sphere, she is not able to compare her condition with that of uncircumcised women. Therefore, within the boundaries of her own experience, she accepts the long-term health consequences that go with being circumcised as simply "a woman's lot."

It is of some importance to recognize that while the woman in Africa is still under familial and tribal influence, her circumcision is a source of pride and community acceptance to her. Whatever painful and traumatic consequences she may have suffered as an adult woman are generally not related in her mind to the procedure inflicted on her in childhood, especially if she was very small at the time it was performed and she does not remember the event clearly. Until she is exposed to an explanation of a causal relationship, she has no reason to question the necessity or essential rightness of her own circumcision, or indeed the one she will inflict on her own daughter.

Nurses and midwives are much respected by women in African societies since they are their primary source of medical services, and therefore they have the power of life and death. The role of the nurse as a potential educator is a particularly important and poignant one, because a clear understanding of the harmful effects of circumcision and infibulation on a woman's health is necessary before the family can make an educated choice on whether or not their daughters should be circumcised (Lightfoot-Klein, 1989a).

✷ HANNY LIGHTFOOT-KLEIN, M.A.

See also: Circumcision, Male; Circumcision Surgery

See **Guide to Related Topics:** Baby Care

Resources

Dareer, A. et al. (1982). *Woman, Why Do You Weep?* London: Zed Books.

Hosken, F. (1981). *The Universal Childbirth Picture Book.* Lexington, MA: Women's International Network.

———. (1982). "Female Circumcision in the World Today: A Global Review." In *WHO/EMRO Technical Publication: Seminar on Traditional Practices Affecting the Health of Women and Children in Africa.* Geneva: WHO.

Koso-Thomas, O. (1987). *The Circumcision of Women: A Strategy for Eradication.* London: Zed Books.

Lightfoot-Klein, Hanny. (1989a). *Prisoners of Ritual: An Odyssey into Female Genital Circumcision in Africa.* New York: Haworth Press.

———. (1989b). "The Sexual Experience and Marital Adjustment of Genitally Circumcised and Infibulated Females in an Afro-Islamic Society (Sudan)." *Journal of Sex Research* 26 (3): 375-92.

———. (1989c). "Rites of Purification and Their Effects: Some Psychological Aspects of Female Genital Circumcision and Infibulation (Pharaonic Circumcision) in an Afro-Islamic Society (Sudan)." *Journal of Psychology and Human Sexuality* 2 (2): 79-91.

Lightfoot-Klein, H. & Shaw, E. (1991). "Special Needs of Ritually Circumcised Woman Patients." *Journal of Obstetrics, Gynecology and Neo-natal Nursing* 20 (2): 102-07.

Sami, I.R. (1986). "Female Circumcision with Special Reference to Sudan." *Annals of Tropical Paediatrics,* 6: 99-115.

Shaw, E. (1985a). "Female Circumcision: Perception of Clients and Caregivers." *American Journal of College Health* 33: 193-97.

———. (1985b, Jun). "Female Circumcision: What Kind of Maternity Care Do Circumcised Women Need and Can United States Caregivers Provide It?" *American Journal of Nursing*: 684-87.

Verzin, J.A. (1975). "Sequelae of Female Circumcision." *Tropical Doctor* 5: 163-69.

GENOME MAPPING

Projects are underway in the United States and elsewhere to map and sequence the human genome. The genome represents all of the genetic material in the chromosomes of an organism; the goal of mapping is to locate the 50,000 to 100,000 human genes (the exact number is not known for certain) on the 23 pairs of chromosomes. So far, about 2,000 genes have been mapped. With changing techniques increasing the mapping rate (currently about 12 additional genes are located per week), a human gene map may be completed as predicted by the year 2005.

Sequencing, a distinct but interrelated activity, aims to identify the specific order of the approximately three billion pairs of nucleotide bases that make up the DNA molecules encoding the genetic material passed from parent to offspring. Its end product, a complete catalog of the genetic material of humans, will take longer to achieve.

While the size and scope of the recently initiated human genome projects are new, mapping and sequencing have been underway for many years. In fact, photographs showing the alternating dark and light bands of chromosomes that frequently illustrate media reports about medical genetics depict one version of the genome map. This map is akin to a picture of the earth's continents taken from a high-flying airplane. Maps generated by targeted genome projects will refine these "views," yielding close-up pictures with fine details of the entire genetic terrain—the contents of cabinets in houses on the continents previously photographed, as it were.

What is the purpose of these mapping and sequencing activities? Most often, advocates present them as approaches for the relief of human suffering and the improvement of human reproduction, claiming they will greatly increase physicians' ability to diagnose and treat genetic disease. In this perspective, then, they would not appear problematic. But, is this the full picture?

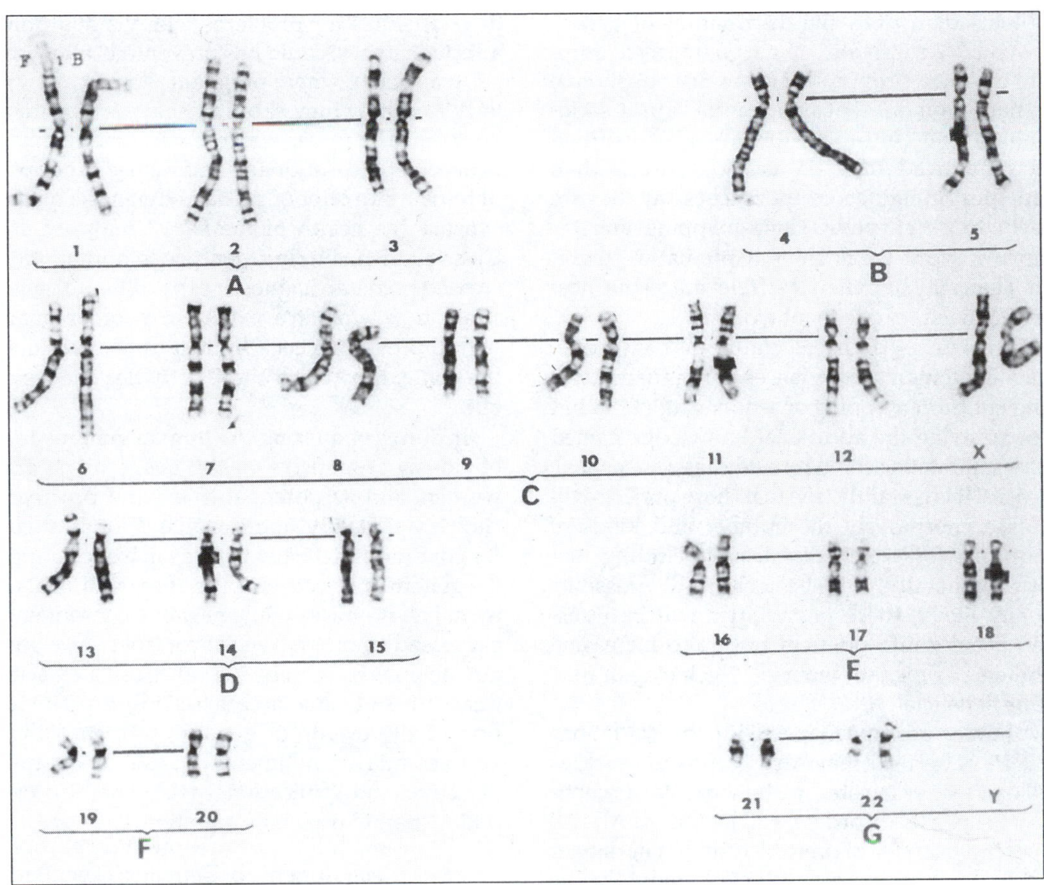

A human genotype. Photo courtesy of Dr. M. Vekemans, Cytogenetics Service, Montreal Children's Hospital.

The "usefulness" of a map of the human genome depends in large part on what genes can do. Here, the reality is quite discordant with the hyperbolic statements appearing in professional and popular magazines. Identification of the exact location of a gene, even complete knowledge of the DNA sequences it comprises, allows one only to determine its presence in a specific person. It does not—and cannot—predict what will happen to that person, what that person will be like. Even if the gene is associated with some disease or disorder, knowing where it is will neither foretell the severity of the condition nor solve the health problem(s) that affect those with the gene. Genes do not function independently or in isolation. Thus, knowing whether a specific gene is present or absent, even having a complete "genetic profile" of an individual, is not like having a blueprint that reveals how the person will turn out.

This fact becomes apparent in considering sickle cell anemia, a disorder associated with a change in a single gene pair. The exact DNA alteration associated with sickle cell anemia was identified over 20 years ago. Nevertheless, predicting beforehand how severe the condition will be in any particular person is still impossible—and a cure remains elusive. There is little reason to expect mapping will be any more "useful" for far more prevalent physical and mental conditions (e.g., high blood pressure, Alzheimer's disease, schizophrenia) where a genetic component, if any, is likely to be quite complex.

In North America, the major causes of perinatal morbidity and mortality continue to be low birth weight and prematurity. Whether or not genes contribute to these problems, the social and economic inequalities of women with which these risks are associated are already well "mapped." The "location" of women who are at increased risk is known; the sequences of events that lead to their excessively and unnecessarily high rates have been well described. Even if genes were shown to be related to these problems, how would knowledge of their location and sequence be useful when the distribution of wealth probably explains more of the variation in pregnancy-related health problems than does the distribution of genes? Low-tech "treatments" (e.g., guaranteed minimum incomes; provision of necessary nutrition to pregnant women) that remove the causal socioeconomic and cultural factors already identified and sequenced may be less glamorous than biomedically engineered approaches, but they are known to be effective. Gene mapping and sequencing efforts are not merely premature, therefore. They may be generally irrelevant to the most pressing needs of pregnant women.

However, supporters claim that improvements in women's experiences of pregnancy will come not from mapping or sequencing per se but from applying the additional knowledge gained of the genome to screen for and diagnose genetic diseases. It is certainly true that those projects will increase enormously the number and kinds of conditions for which diagnosis, including that made prenatally, will be technically possible. Equally likely, these possibilities will be translated rapidly into offers of testing to increasing numbers of pregnant women, which may or may not be beneficial.

A human genome map will identify variations in DNA patterns. Genes that "cause" disease, as well as those associated with increased susceptibility to specific disorders, will be found. All will be potential targets of prenatal testing. The danger may be to those who will have hemophilia, be color-blind, be susceptible to schizophrenia, for instance, and be identified before birth. Women have always been the principal health care providers for their families and they lack real options for using information obtained through prenatal diagnosis. If a problem—or the potential for one—is diagnosed, the absence of public facilities and social supports for families with a disabled child, as well as the generally negative societal attitudes that unnecessarily preclude the participation of the disabled, may make termination of pregnancy seem, at least to health professionals, the "logical" outcome. Moreover, because the gap between diagnostic capabilities and effective treatments and cures is widening, not narrowing, as the number of mapped genes increases, abortion of fetuses thought to carry the genes sought after becomes less the temporary alternative it is said to be than a necessary sequela of having prenatal diagnosis. This process is accelerated by insurance companies that threaten to withdraw coverage to women who choose to give birth to children they know in advance might at some time have the health problem diagnosed during pregnancy and by commercial forces that may make it seem inefficient to develop cures for problems that, via abortion of affected fetuses, could be "prevented" altogether.

In a society where pregnant women are regularly told how they should behave to ensure the health of the fetus, where those who smoke or drink elicit accusations of "fetal abuse," the option of refusing an offer of prenatal diagnosis made to "ensure the health of the baby" may not exist. Clearly, then, linking genome mapping to increased prenatal diagnostic capabilities to demonstrate how women's experiences of pregnancy will improve reflects a limited understanding of the context in which these activities are carried out.

In sum, conquering the human genome is not obviously responsive to the needs of pregnant women, and its potential to expand procreative choice is certainly questionable. Promised cures for conditions detected before birth elicit support for genome projects, but the cures will likely remain just promises while negative consequences, expressed as external social control over women, are no longer merely hypothetical. Legislating guarantees of equal access to and proper regulation of the results of genome projects will not address more fundamental questions about the objectives and applications of the genome projects that demand immediate attention.

✱ ABBY LIPPMAN, Ph.D.

See also: Eugenics; Genetics; The Perfect Baby; Prenatal Diagnosis: Overview

See **Guide to Related Topics:** Prenatal Diagnosis and Screening

Resources

Botstein, D. et al. (1980). "Construction of a Genetic Linkage Map in Man Using Restriction Fragment Length Polymorphisms." *American Journal of Human Genetics 32*: 314-31.

Donis-Keller, H. et al. (1987). "A Genetic Linkage Map of the Human Genome." *Cell 51*: 319-37.

Friedmann, T. (1990). "Opinion: The Human Genome Project—Some Implications of Extensive 'Reverse Genetic' Medicine." *American Journal of Human Genetics 46*: 407-14.

Holtsman, N.A. (1989). *Proceed with Caution*. Baltimore: Johns Hopkins University Press.

Macklin, R. (1985). "Mapping the Human Genome: Problems of Privacy and Free Choice." In A. Milunsky & G.J. Annas (Eds.) *Genetics and the Law III*. New York: Plenum Press, pp. 107-14.

National Research Council. (1988). *Mapping and Sequencing the Human Genome*. Washington, DC: National Academic Press.

Nelkin, D. & Tancredi, L. (1989). *Dangerous Diagnostics: The Social Power of Biological Information*. New York: Basic Books.

Rose, S., Kamin, L.J., & Lewontin, R.C. (1984). *Not in Our Genes: Biology, Ideology and Human Nature*. Middlesex, England: Penguin Books.

Stephens, J.C. et al. (1990). "Mapping the Human Genome: Current Status." *Science 250*: 237-44.

U.S. Congress, Office of Technology Assessment. (1988). *Mapping Our Genes—the Genome Projects: How Big, How Fast*. Washington, DC: U.S. Government Printing Office.

White, R. & Lalovel, J.M. (1988). "Chromosomes Mapping with DNA Markers." *Scientific American 258*: 40-48.

White, R. et al. (1985). "Construction of Linkage Maps with DNA Markers for Human Chromosomes." *Nature 313*: 101-05.

Wilfond, B.S. & Fost, N. (1990). "The Cystic Fibrosis Gene: Medical and Social Implications of Heterozygote Detection." *Journal of American Medical Association 263* (20): 2777-83.

GERMAN MEASLES. *See instead* TORCH SYNDROME

GERMANY

Though women have always had children, the circumstances under which they have had them have frequently been determined by politics. Today's trust in progress has pushed traditional midwives aside. Fortunately, some of their accounts from German-speaking areas have recently been published. Practicing mostly in remote areas, they assisted birthing women whenever and wherever needed.

Under Hitler, midwives were often coerced into obeying Nazi ideology. In 1935, they received, along with their midwife certificates, instructions to disregard the special needs of weak or disabled newborns. Sometimes, against regulations, they assisted pregnant Polish or Russian foreign workers—who were not supposed to have babies. Nevertheless, in teaching hospitals these pregnant women served as objects of study and training, even for demonstrations of nontreatment. They had to return to work the day after delivery, and their babies were taken from them, often for "special treatment."

In the 1950s and 1960s, the midwives' comprehensive care for women's physical, mental, and spiritual well-being was replaced by the medical care of usually male doctors in the cold atmosphere and isolation of clinics—where the social and spiritual side of giving birth was ignored. People do not know that German midwives may manage birth independently. Today, feminist criticism of the medicalization of pregnancy has resulted in a hospital environment that appears more humanized. Consequently, most babies are still born in hospitals, although home births are increasing in number. While some of the traditional social components of having children have been regained, much remains to be done to restore the birth process to the more humanistic level on which it once existed.

American and German women's birthing experiences have historically been similar, differing only in degree: Because German doctors have tended to be slower in accepting medical "progress," fewer German women have had "programmed births," cesarean sections, etc. But being pregnant in Germany is different than being pregnant in the United States.

The German Constitution states: Men and women shall have equal rights. Maternity legislation is not considered discriminatory against men but merely a special issue. Maternity protection is accepted as a societal responsibility, a tradition that dates back to the 19th century. It covers most employed women. Following are some of its provisions:

- A pregnant woman's job is guaranteed until four months after birth.
- Her work may not endanger her health or that of the growing child.
- Particular kinds of work are forbidden.
- The employer has to compensate her for financial losses incurred by the above restrictions.
- Maternity leave continues from six weeks prior to eight weeks after delivery.
- During maternity leave, women receive payments equal to their former net income.
- Pregnancy regulations apply to nursing mothers.
- Mother and child are fully covered by health insurance; if the mother is without work or other income, medical expenses are paid by welfare.

Once the child is born, the mother or father can take parental leave for up to 18 months. Up to the sixth month, a fixed allowance is paid; subsequent allowances depend on family income. During parental leave the job is guaranteed. In 1989, 1.5 percent of the fathers were house husbands.

Recent improvements in maternity and child care provisions are in part a reaction to dropping birth rates. What about abortion in such a pronatalist atmosphere? In 1974, after a long struggle against section 218 of the 1871 criminal code, which prohibited abortion, a coalition of Social Democrats and Liberals legalized abortion during the first three months of pregnancy. A few months later, a court appeal by Christian Democrats resulted in the present "indication rule," which provides abortion under some circumstances, with physicians' letters stating the indication for abortion.

At this point, Catholic church influence on German politics (where there is no clear separation of church and state) becomes obvious. Christian Democrats do not want to oppose Catholic fundamentalist interests for fear of losing power (many church officials are party members). They consider even the "indication rule" too liberal. Consequently, in German states with a Catholic and/or conservative majority, the "indication rule" has been undermined, making legal abortion for poor women tremendously difficult.

A recent "witch hunt" in Bavaria added fuel to the abortion issue: Prosecution of a gynecologist who had assisted women without the obligatory "indication letter" made abortion a criminal offense. On the basis of evidence from his confidential records, he was convicted, imprisoned, and his career destroyed. Two hundred of his patients were fined.

The unification of Germany in October 1990 renewed the abortion debate because East German law gave women freedom of choice. In light of this, government attempts to enforce West German law nationwide met with fierce resistance from a few women politicians (pro-choice men buckled under party discipline). An interim solution permitting abortion was achieved that may lead to new legislation that would give German women the right to choose.

Abortions based on prenatal testing like amniocentesis or chorionic villus sampling are rarely discussed publicly. German feminists, sensitized by Third Reich history, see a continuity between eugenics, euthanasia, and today's selective abortions for eugenic—usually called medical—reasons. Just as in the U.S., the public perceives prenatal testing as a medical advancement that offers women more control over their lives. The horrible choices women face in case of a bad test result can (in an atmosphere of subtle social pressure toward abortion) be publicly ignored because they are viewed as isolated occurrences and are kept private. Therefore, the underlying issue of eugenic population control remains hidden.

Some German doctors also have become sensitized to the social and psychological issues, resulting in a more careful approach to prenatal diagnosis. For example, although many American doctors check the alpha-fetoprotein in pregnant women's blood routinely without asking, German doctors are advised to perform this test only after genetic counseling and informed consent from the pregnant woman. Some data indicate that in Germany counseling leads to the rejection of prenatal diagnosis more often than in the U.S. Moreover, only women above age 35 or with a special indication are considered for testing in Germany. This reflects on another issue: German doctors feel less threatened by insurance claims, since suits are much less common than in the U.S.

One area where Germans reject American practices is that of surrogacy: Largely to avoid the commodification of life, surrogacy is not allowed. A woman giving birth to a child is considered its mother, regardless of the source of the genetic "material." ✷ JULIETTE LIESENFELD, M.A.

See **Guide to Related Topics:** Cross-Cultural Perspectives

Resources

Allen, Ann Taylor. (1985, Spring). "Mothers of the New Generation: Adele Schreiber, Helene Stöcker, and the Evolution of a German Idea of Motherhood, 1900-1914." *Signs 10*: 418-38

Blatt, Robin J.R. (1988). *Prenatal Tests*. New York: Vintage.

Bridenthal, Renate et al. (Eds.) (1984). *When Biology Became Destiny: Women in Weimar and Nazi Germany*. New York: Monthly Review Press.

Grabrucker, Marianne. (1989). *Vom Abenteuer der Geburt. Die letzten Landhebammen erzählen. [The Adventure of Birth: The Last Rural Midwives Tell Their Stories.]* Frankfurt/Main: Fischer.

Hubbard, Ruth. (1990). *The Politics of Women's Biology*. New Brunswick, NJ: Rutgers University Press.

Rothman, Barbara Katz. (1986). *The Tentative Pregnancy*. New York: Viking Press.

Schindele, Eva. (1990). *Gläserne Gebär-Mutter. [The Transparent and Birthing Mother/Uterus.]* Frankfurt/Main: Fischer.

Schroeder-Kurth, Traute M. (Ed.) (1989). *Medizinische Genetik in der Bundesrepublik Deutschland. [Medical Genetics in the Republic of Germany.]* Frankfurt/Main: J. Schweitzer Verlag.

Zimmermann, Susan. (1989). "Weibliches Selbstbestimmungsrecht und auf 'Qualität' abzielende Bevölkerungspolitik." ["Women's Right to Self-Determination and a Quality-Oriented Population Policy."] *Beiträge 21/22*: 53-71.

G.I.F.T. *See instead* INFERTILITY: OVERVIEW

GODDESS IMAGERY

It all began during the early 1960s in Turkey with excavations at Catal Huyuk by archeologist James Mellaart and his team. The remarkable and hitherto unthinkable living refinements and art production of this Neolithic culture astonished scholars, preceding by over 3,000 years the ad-

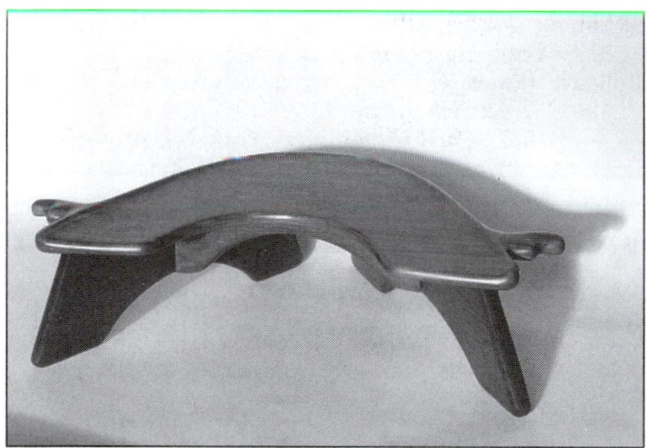

A modern birth stool, walnut, designed by Mark Parrish, 1980. Photo courtesy of Mark Parrish.

vanced civilizations of Mesopotamia and Egypt. What is really significant about this culture is its reverence for the Mother. "Sweeter than honey and date wine was the ancient Mother, for it was She who made all life ....," wrote the ancient Mesopotamians (Stone, 1990). Yet in an even more distant past, people living in Catal Huyuk actually made images honoring the Mother giving birth (Mellaart, 1967).

So who is this old mother who is so intoxicating because she's fertile? Who has statues and poems made in her honor for doing what is natural? Behind the images and the words is a deeper meaning. She is no ordinary mother. She is the Goddess.

In viewing these images, it is first necessary to strip away the conceits of culture that suggest that what is different is marked by intellectual and moral deficiencies of the highest order. This is especially necessary in the matter of religion. Sacred birth imagery at Catal Huyuk is brutally frank, its makers unmoved by today's notions of holy. A primal force of existence is apprehended, based on spiritual dimensions seemingly in tune with the shifting stresses of nature (Frankfort, 1956).

Plaster wall reliefs decorating shrines are the basic form of birthing representation found at Catal Huyuk. They depict the Goddess as a generalized, upright, human figure who has given birth to the head of a bull or ram. The juxtaposition of head and pubis, accentuated by widespread legs, shows plainly what has occurred. The meaning seems clear: The Goddess has borne a male deity (Mellaart, 1967).

An exception to this format is the clay statuette discovered in a grain-and-vegetable bin located next to a shrine. Its style is unique. This work of art is a naturalistic portrayal of the Mother as a seated woman in the process of giving birth. An infant's head is just visible between her thighs. Her full maternal body, characteristic of pregnancy, is perhaps symbolic of generative power. It is suggested on the basis of other figurines unearthed at Catal Huyuk that the seated Goddess also gives birth to a male principle.

The clay statuette embodies the rich diversity of Goddess worship documented at Catal Huyuk. Although the inhabitants left no written record, evidence found in shrines reveals complex religious concepts centering around a female deity that developed approximately 8,000 years ago in this early farming community. Symbols of life and death—states that appear to conflict—converge in this clay image; states that appear to conflict. Remember that this image was found in a grain bin, stressing a connection between the fertility of the Mother and crops (Mellaart, 1963). Embracing all aspects of life, including the animal kingdom and death, the Goddess gives birth in a chair, supported on either side by a feline, while her right foot likely rests on a skull. It is in this contrariness, refuting an either/or mentality, that the essence of what the Goddess may have meant most clearly emerges (Gimbutas, 1989).

It is generally assumed that the feline chair of the clay Goddess is a throne. The roots of this assumption are based partially on comparisons to genuine examples of feline thrones seen in art of later cultures, but also on the patriarchal-conditioned association of divinity and domination (Eisler, 1988). It is worth noting that the concept of rulership implicit in the idea of throne was virtually unknown at Catal Huyuk; social hierarchies suggested by burial gifts and building sizes were not dramatic there (Mellaart, 1967).

If one looks beyond the conceptual barrier to what is actually portrayed, the image becomes what it is—a chair for delivery and birth (Diskerud, 1988). It is conjecture but consistent with a cultural and religious outlook that Mellaart showed was highly respectful of women, procreation, and life. The art, sex ratio, burial practices, and room designs support this conclusion (Angel, 1971). With a record of a high level of technology at Catal Huyuk, it can well be imagined that the women of this village had a practical method of confinement that was eventually translated into a pictorial symbol system. It would be sobering to discover that feline thrones of the ancient Near East were derivations of the birthing chair of the Goddess, knowing what that spelled for the civilizing influence of the Mother. ✷ MARY DONAHUE

See also: Art and Birth Metaphors: Nature-Culture Dichotomies; The Birth Symbol; Creation Stories in Western Culture

See **Guide to Related Topics:** Literature and the Arts

Resources

Angel, Lawrence J. (1971). "Early Neolithic Skeletons from Catal Huyuk: Demography and Pathology." *Anatolian Studies 21*: 77-99.
Diskerud, Louise. (1988). Personal communication.
Eisler, Riane. (1988). *The Chalice and the Blade*. New York: Harper & Row.
Frankfort, Henri. (1956). *The Intellectual Adventure of the Ancient Man*. Chicago: University of Chicago Press.
Gimbutas, Marija. (1989). *The Language of the Goddess*. New York: Harper & Row.
Mellaart, James. (1963). "Excavations at Catal Huyak, 1962." *Anatolian Studies 13*: 43-105.
———. (1967). *Catal Huyuk*. New York: McGraw-Hill.
Stone, Merlin. (1990). *Ancient Mirrors of Womanhood*. Boston: Beacon Press.

GRANNY MIDWIVES. *See instead* MIDWIVES, SOUTHERN BLACK

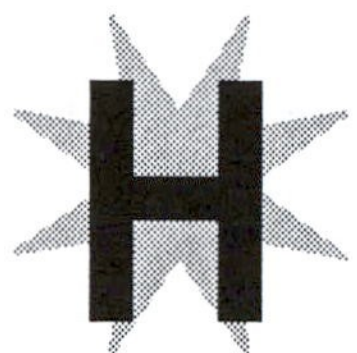

HERBAL TREATMENTS

Many modern mothers and midwives continue to use herbal treatments as an alternative to drugs during pregnancy and childbirth. Herbal medicine has been used by women from the beginning of time, and much of the knowledge on its use has been passed down over hundreds of years. Methods of using plants in North America commonly include drinking teas and ingesting powdered herbs in gelatin capsules or drops of tincture. A tincture is made by steeping fresh or dried plant material in 100 proof (or grain) alcohol in a tightly closed jar. This mixture is shaken daily and stored for several weeks. The liquid is then poured off into amber glass dropper bottles. The advantages of tinctures over teas are that: (a) they are much more concentrated, so even unpleasant-tasting herbs are easy to take; (b) they travel easily and keep potency for several years; and (c) because of the alcohol base, they enter the blood stream quickly.

Herbs are also used topically in salves, powders, compresses, and baths. Aromatherapy uses the essential oils of plants. Herbs are also used to make many homeopathic preparations.

Though certainly not all-inclusive, the following is a brief summary of some of the most commonly used herbs employed by North American midwives at present.

Angelica Root (Angelica Archangelica): Used in tincture for retained placenta.

Arnica (Arnica Montana): Used topically as a salve, in infusion as a compress, or internally in homeopathic pellets for aching, bruised, sore feeling from prolonged pushing or trauma to muscle tissues.

Blessed Thistle (Cnicus Benedictus): Used as a tea postpartum to increase milk supply.

Blue and Black Cohosh (Caulophylum Thalictroides and Cimicifuga Racemosa): Used in tea or tincture as an oxytocic action to stimulate or regulate contractions or "ripen" cervix.

Chamomile (Matricaria Chamomila): Used as a tea, for baby's colic and to calm the mother.

Echinacea (Echiniacea Augustifolia) Tincture: Known as the "herbal antibiotic"; used for all types of systemic infections, flus, breast infections, and as a prophylactic to infection.

Fennel (Foeniculum Vulgare): Used in tea to treat gas and colic, and to stimulate milk production.

Ginger Root (Zingiber Officinale): Used in capsules or tea to treat nausea and vomiting in the first trimester.

Red Raspberry Leaf (Rubus Indicus): Used as a tea; used by pregnant women worldwide during pregnancy to tone the uterus, nourish, and "prepare for an easier birth."

Shephard's Purse (Capsela Bursa Pastoris): Used as a tincture or tea to control or prevent hemorrhage postpartum.

Skullcap (Scuteleria Lateriflora): Used as a tincture or in tea; used as a sedative, pain reliever.

Wild Yam Root (Dioscorea Villosa): Used, powdered (in capsules), during pregnancy for nausea or threatened miscarriage. * ALISON PARRA

See **Guide to Related Topics:** Pregnancy, Physical Aspects

Resources

Gardner, Joy. (1982). *Healing the Family: Pregnancy, Birth and Childrens Ailments Vol. I.* New York: Bantam Books (out of print). Currently available by same author on similar vein: *Healing Yourself During Pregnancy.* (1989).

Koehler, Nan. (1985). *Artemis Speaks: VBAC Stories and Natural Childbirth Information*. Occidental, CA: Jerald Brown Inc.
Milinaire, Catherine. (1978). *Birth*. New York: Harmony Books.
Parvati, Jeannine. (1978). *Hygieia: A Woman's Herbal*. Provo, UT: Freestone Collective.
Weed, Susan. (1986). *Wise Woman Herbal for the Childbearing Year*. Woodstock, NY: Ash Tree Publishing.

HERPES. *See instead* TORCH SYNDROME

HISPANICS: UNITED STATES

Comprehensive information on the fertility of Hispanic women in the United States has been available since 1978. That was the first year that a number of states added a question to the birth certificate to determine if the parents were of Hispanic origin.

Prior to 1978, scattered studies were available that differentiated the Hispanic population by Spanish surname, native language, or place of birth. While all these identifiers can be useful, they do not have the advantage of individual self-identification. People several generations removed from their country of origin and with Anglo surnames may or may not identify themselves as Hispanic. In 1978, 17 states, which accounted for about 60 percent of U.S. Hispanic births, reported this information to the National Center for Health Statistics (NCHS) (Ventura and Heuser, 1981). By 1980, the number of reporting states had increased to 22, and for the years 1983 to 1987, the reporting area included 23 states and the District of Columbia, representing at least 90 percent of U.S. Hispanic births. The reporting area in 1988, the latest year for which detailed birth certificate information is available, included 30 states and the District of Columbia, representing an estimated 95 percent of the U.S. Hispanic population (U.S. Bureau of the Census, 1989). Beginning in 1989, all but three states have reported the Hispanic origin of the parents on the birth certificates. Since this information first became available from the birth certificate, the National Center for Health Statistics has shown data for Hispanics in five major categories—Mexican, Puerto Rican, Cuban, Central and South American, and other and unknown Hispanic.

Nearly 450,000 babies were born to Hispanic mothers in 1988 in the reporting states. If this figure is inflated to estimate the number of Hispanic births in the other states, the likely total is about 475,000 for the U.S. as a whole. To put it another way, about one in every eight babies born in this country is to a Hispanic mother.

Birth and fertility rates for the Hispanic population have been relatively stable over the past several years, but both rates increased 3 to 4 percent in 1988 (Ventura, 1982, 1983, 1984, 1985, 1987; National Center for Health Statistics, 1989, 1990). The birth rate per 1,000 population was 24.1 in 1988, compared with 23.3 in 1987. The fertility rate per 1,000 women aged 15 to 44 years was 96.4 in 1988, compared with 93.0 in 1987. (Rates for 1988 are shown in Table 1.) These rates were 54 and 47 percent higher than rates for the non-Hispanic population (15.7 and 65.7, respectively). The differential in rates between the Hispanic and non-Hispanic populations has changed little since 1978, when the rates were first computed.

About 1 in 6 Hispanic-origin births was to a teenaged mother in 1988, compared with 1 in 10 white non-Hispanic births and nearly 1 in 4 black non-Hispanic births. In 1988, teenagers accounted for 17 percent of births to Mexican Americans and 21 percent of Puerto Rican births but only 6 percent of Cuban births. (See Table 2.)

Because Hispanic mothers, except for Cubans, tend to start childbearing at relatively young ages,

Table 1. Birth and Fertility Rates, by Hispanic Origin of Mother: Total of 11 Reporting States, 1988

	Origin of mother						
		Hispanic					
Measure	All origins	Total	Mexican	Puerto Rican	Cuban	Other Hispanic[1]	Non-Hispanic[2]
Birth rate[3]	16.9	24.1	23.2	19.6	9.8	34.2	15.7
Fertility rate[4]	70.5	96.4	98.0	67.9	47.7	118.6	65.7

[1] Includes Central and South American and Other and Unknown Hispanic origin.
[2] Includes origin not stated.
[3] Rate per 1,000 total population.
[4] Rate per 1,000 women aged 15-44 years.

Note: The 11 states are Arizona, California, Colorado, Florida, Illinois, Indiana, New Jersey, New Mexico, New York, Ohio, and Texas.

Table 2. Percent of Births with Selected Characteristics, by Hispanic Origin of Mother and by Race of Child for Mothers of non-Hispanic Origin: Total of 30 Reporting States and the District of Columbia, 1988

	Origin of mother									
		Hispanic						Non-Hispanic		
Characteristic	All origins[1]	Total	Mexican	Puerto Rican	Cuban	Central and South American	Other and unknown Hispanic	Total[2]	White	Black
Mothers under age 20 years	12.7	16.4	17.3	21.4	6.1	8.1	18.4	12.2	9.7	22.9
Fourth and higher order births	10.2	15.6	18.1	12.3	5.8	11.7	12.1	9.2	7.6	14.1
Births to unmarried mothers	26.2	34.0	30.6	53.3	16.3	36.4	35.5	24.9	14.9	63.7
Mothers completing 12 years or more of school[3]	78.4	57.5	43.1	54.8	81.9	68.2	65.9	79.8	83.4	68.5
Mothers born in the United States	83.4	43.0	40.9	53.4	16.9	3.9	83.7	91.1	95.4	92.1
Mothers who began prenatal care in first trimester	75.0	61.3	58.3	63.2	83.4	62.8	67.3	77.3	82.0	60.8
Mothers who had late or no prenatal care	6.5	12.1	13.9	10.2	3.6	9.9	8.8	5.6	4.1	10.9
Births of low birth weight[4]	7.0	6.2	5.6	9.4	5.9	5.6	6.8	7.2	5.6	13.1
Preterm births[5]	10.4	10.8	10.6	13.3	9.0	10.1	10.8	10.4	8.2	18.5
1-minute Apgar score less than 7[6]	8.5	7.3	7.8	6.8	4.9	6.0	9.3	8.7	8.0	11.2
5-minute Apgar score less than 7[6]	1.6	1.4	1.3	1.6	1.0	1.2	1.6	1.6	1.3	2.9

1 Includes origin not stated.

2 Includes races other than white and black.

3 Excludes data for California, New York State (exclusive of New York City), Texas, and Washington, which did not require reporting of educational attainment of mother.

4 Birth weight of less than 2,500 grams (5 lb. 8 oz.).

5 Born prior to 37 completed weeks of gestation.

6 Excludes data for California and Texas, which did not require reporting of either 1- or 5-minute Apgar score.

they also tend to have large families. Mexican mothers are more likely than any other Hispanic or non-Hispanic group to have at least four children. The larger completed family size for Mexican women is due in part to the relatively large fraction (one-fourth in 1988) of Mexican teens who give birth to two or more children.

Although nonmarital childbearing is relatively common among most ethnic groups, most researchers assume that it is an additional risk factor for childbirth (Berkov and Sklar, 1976; Ventura, 1988; Centers for Disease Control, 1990). In addition to being younger, unmarried mothers generally are less educated, have lower incomes, and possibly have less emotional and other support than would accompany childbearing in a two-parent family. Childbearing by unmarried mothers has been increasing for Hispanic and non-Hispanic women alike. In 1988, one-third of Hispanic mothers were unmarried. There were wide variations among the various Hispanic and non-Hispanic groups, as shown in Table 2.

Except for Cuban women, Hispanic mothers are much less likely than non-Hispanic mothers to have completed high school. In 1988, 58 percent of all Hispanic women giving birth were high school graduates compared with 83 percent of white non-Hispanic mothers and 69 percent of black non-Hispanic mothers. Educational attainment varies considerably among the individual Hispanic groups: 43 percent of Mexican mothers, 55 percent of Puerto Rican mothers, 68 percent of Central and South American mothers, and 82 percent of Cuban mothers were high school graduates. Some of the differences in educational attainment may be attributed to the fact that a very high proportion of Hispanic mothers were born outside of the United States (57 percent in 1988). Presumably many foreign-born Hispanic mothers have not been exposed to a universal education system. Important differentials have been observed between the childbearing characteristics of U.S.- and foreign-born Hispanic mothers (Ventura and Taffel, 1985).

Consistent with their limited educational attainment and economic status, Hispanic mothers, except Cubans, are substantially less likely to begin prenatal care in the critical first trimester of pregnancy than are white non-Hispanic mothers. Comprehensive prenatal care is particularly important for those without the economic and other resources to care for themselves adequately during pregnancy and is especially important in the prevention of low birth weight. In 1988, 58 percent of Mexican mothers began prenatal care in the first trimester compared with 82 to 83 percent of Cuban and white non-Hispanic mothers. Teenagers, who are particularly vulnerable to health problems and complications during pregnancy and could benefit from guidance on nutrition and other matters during pregnancy, are even less likely to begin prenatal care early.

One in eight Hispanic mothers and one in nine black non-Hispanic mothers received late prenatal care (beginning in the third trimester) or no care at all, compared with just 1 in 25 white non-Hispanic mothers. Teenagers are particularly at risk of having delayed or no prenatal care. Among Puerto Rican teen mothers, more than one in five women had late or no prenatal care in 1988, a higher level than for any other group.

A critically important measure of birth outcome is the incidence of low birth weight. Babies weighing less than 2,500 grams or 5½ pounds have a greatly elevated risk of infant mortality, congenital malformations, mental retardation, and other physical and neurological impairments. As a measure of pregnancy outcome, low birth weight has the advantage of being accurately and completely reported directly on the birth certificate. One of the most inexplicable findings over the years has been the consistently low level of low birth weight among Mexican American babies. Because of their mothers' limited educational attainment and use of prenatal care, babies born to Mexican mothers would be expected to have a relatively high rate of low birth weight; this is the pattern that has been observed for Puerto Rican and black non-Hispanic babies. However, just 5.6 percent of Mexican babies weighed less than 5½ pounds, about the same as for Cuban and white non-Hispanic babies, but consistently below the level for Puerto Rican and black non-Hispanic infants. These levels have been the same since this information was first reported in 1978. Furthermore, data by nativity of the mother show that Mexican mothers born in Mexico are even less likely to have a low birth-weight infant than their counterparts born in the United States, 5.0 percent compared with 6.7 percent.

Finally, even when the incidence of low birth weight by trimester that prenatal care began is examined, it is clear that Mexican babies fare relatively well compared with other Hispanic or non-Hispanic babies, regardless of how late care began. Even babies born to Mexican mothers whose care did not begin until the third trimester or who had no care at all were at a relatively favorable risk of low birth weight, 7.2 percent.

To account for the relatively favorable levels of low birth weight among Mexican babies, data on related topics have been examined. For example, Hispanic women are much less likely to smoke than non-Hispanic women. Unpublished data from the 1980 National Natality Survey conducted by NCHS showed that only 10 percent of Mexican women, compared with 27 percent of white non-Hispanic women, smoked during pregnancy. The data further suggested that foreign-born Mexican women were less likely to be smokers than their U.S.-born counterparts. Another smaller-scale study confirmed this pattern for teens, and also found that Mexican teens tend to gain more weight during pregnancy than their white and black peers (Felice et al., 1986).

✱ STEPHANIE J. VENTURA, A.M.

See **Guide to Related Topics:** Cross-Cultural Perspectives

Resources

Berkov, Beth & Sklar, June. (1976). "Does Illegitimacy Make a Difference? The Life Chances of Illegitimate Children in California." *Population and Development Review* 2: 201-17.

Centers for Disease Control. (1990). "Infant Mortality by Marital States of Mother—United States, 1983." *Morbidity and Mortality Weekly Report 39* (30): 521-23. Atlanta: Public Health Service.

Felice, Marianne E. et al. (1986). "Clinical Observations of Mexican-American, Caucasian, and Black Pregnant Teenagers." *Journal of Adolescent Health Care* 7: 305-10.

National Center for Health Statistics. (1989). "Advance Report of Final Natality Statistics, 1987." *Monthly Vital Statistics Report 38,* (3) supplement. Hyattsville, MD: Public Health Service.

———. (1990). "Advance Report of Final Natality Statistics, 1988." *Monthly Vital Statistics Report 39,* (4) supplement. Hyattsville, MD: Public Health Service.

U.S. Bureau of the Census. (1989). "The Hispanic Population in the United States, March 1988." *Current Population Reports,* Series P-20, No. 438. Washington, DC: U.S. Department of Commerce.

Ventura, Stephanie J. (1982). "Births of Hispanic Parentage, 1979." *Monthly Vital Statistics Report 31,* (2) supplement. Hyattsville, MD: National Center for Health Statistics.

———. (1983). "Births of Hispanic Parentage, 1980." *Monthly Vital Statistics Report 32,* (6) supplement. Hyattsville, MD: National Center for Health Statistics.

———. (1984). "Births of Hispanic Parentage, 1981." *Monthly Vital Statistics Report 33,* (8) supplement. Hyattsville, MD: National Center for Health Statistics.

———. (1985). "Births of Hispanic Parentage, 1982." *Monthly Vital Statistics Report 34,* (4) supplement. Hyattsville, MD: National Center for Health Statistics.

———. (1987). "Births of Hispanic Parentage, 1983 and 1984." *Monthly Vital Statistics Report 36,* (4) supplement. Hyattsville, MD: National Center for Health Statistics.

———. (1988). "Births of Hispanic Parentage, 1985." *Monthly Vital Statistics Report 36*, (11) supplement. Hyattsville, MD: National Center for Health Statistics.

Ventura, Stephanie J.,& Heuser, Robert L. (1981). "Births of Hispanic Parentage, 1978." *Monthly Vital Statistics Report 29*, (12) supplement. Hyattsville, MD: National Center for Health Statistics.

Ventura, Stephanie J. & Taffel, Selma M. (1985). "Childbearing Characteristics of U.S.- and Foreign-born Hispanic Mothers." *Public Health Reports 100* (6): 647-52.

HIV AND PREGNANCY

Knowledge of the effects of HIV infection on pregnancy is limited, due to the preliminary and inconsistent nature of current studies and incomplete data. Some studies indicate an acceleration of the disease in pregnant women, and others show no effect on pregnancy or neonatal outcome (Selwyn et al., 1989). An American prospective controlled study of 125 pregnancies in IV drug users indicated no increase in the frequency of spontaneous or elective abortion, ectopic pregnancy, preterm delivery, stillbirth, or low birthweight births in 39 births to HIV-positive women (Selwyn et al., 1989). Infected women were more likely to be hospitalized for bacterial pneumonia during pregnancy and had an increased tendency for breech presentation (Selwyn et al., 1989). In studies of HIV-infected women who tended to be sicker on enrollment, some clinical progression during pregnancy was noted, with an increase in prematurity and a relatively high rate of neonatal deaths (Minkoff et al., 1987).

Of the total AIDS population in the United States, 6.9 percent is female, most of whom are of childbearing age (Weber and Alger, 1988). The disease is not distributed evenly among ethnic groups. Fifty-four percent of women affected are black, 24 percent are Hispanic, and 21 percent are white (Selik et al., 1988). These figures reflect the poverty-based barriers to education and intervention that disproportionately affect minorities. Many women are diagnosed as being HIV-positive as a result of voluntary testing offered at their prenatal care clinic (Rich, 1989).

Research shows that the fetus can become infected while *in utero*, but it is possible that infection can also occur during the birth process (Wofsy et al., 1986). Performing a cesarean-section, however, has not proven to be protective, since the virus can be introduced to the uterine cavity in this procedure. Amniocentesis is contraindicated for similar reasons (Weber and Alger, 1988).

Perinatal transmission is the cause of more than 75 percent of pediatric AIDS cases (Weber and Alger, 1988). It is not possible to predict which women will transmit HIV to their babies and the reasons why. Studies have revealed rates of transmission from 30 to 50 percent (Holman et al., 1989). Some women have infected more than one child, but babies born following an infected sibling may be uninfected. There are also cases of twin births where only one of the infants is infected (Scott, 1989).

There have been a few reports of women who were infected with HIV immediately postpartum and transmitted the HIV infection by breastfeeding (Hauer and Dattel, 1989), but the presence of the virus in breastmilk is not proven to be sufficient to infect. HIV-positive women have breastfed for up to seven months without infecting their babies (Scott, 1989). Breastfeeding could be beneficial for the infant, possibly inactivating the HIV. However, current public health service recommendations discourage breastfeeding by HIV-positive women (Senturia et al., 1987). Incubation in newborns varies. The majority of infected newborns appear normal at birth but within 24 months have clinical illness. A small number remain asymptomatic for as long as eight years (Blanche, 1986).

Testing a newborn for HIV antibodies can give accurate information only about the mother. This is because all newborn babies receive antibodies against infection, including HIV, from their mothers while in the womb. They retain these maternal antibodies for several months after birth. Even though the babies of HIV-infected women test positive, most have not acquired the virus itself and therefore are not truly infected.

✱ PAT RICHTER, M.P.A.

See also: HIV Testing during Pregnancy

See **Guide to Related Topics:** Pregnancy Complications

Resources

Blanche, S. (1986). "Longitudinal Study of 18 Children with Perinatal LAV/HIV III Infection: Attempt at Prognostic Evaluation." *Journal of Pediatrics 109*: 965-70.

Hauer, Laurie B. & Dattel, Bonnie J. (1989). "Management of the Pregnant Woman Infected with the Human Immunodeficiency Virus." *Journal of Perinatology VIII* (3): 258-62.

Holman, Susan et al. (1989, Feb). "Women Infected with Human Immunodeficiency Virus: Counseling and Testing during Pregnancy." *Seminars in Perinatology 13* (1): 7-15.

Minkoff, H. et al. (1987). "Pregnancies Resulting in Infants with Acquired IDS or ARC: Follow-up of Moth-

ers, Children, and Subsequently Born Infants." *Obstetrics and Gynecology 69*: 288-91.
Rich, K.C. (1989). "Maternal AIDS: Effects on Mother and Infant." *Annals New York Academy of Sciences 562*: 243.
Scott, Gwendolyn B. (1989, Sept). "Perinatal HIV-I Infection: Diagnosis and Management." *Clinical Obstetrics and Gynecology 32* (3): 477-84.
Selik, R.M. et al. (1988, Dec). "Racial/Ethnic Differences in the Risk of AIDS in the U.S." *American Journal of Public Health 78*: 1539.
Selwyn, Peter et al. (1989, Mar 3). "Prospective Study of Human Immunodeficiency Virus Infection and Pregnancy Outcomes in Intravenous Drug Users." *JAMA 261* (12): 1289-94.
Senturia, Y.D. et al. (1987). "Breastfeeding the HIV Infection." *Lancet 2*: 400.
Weber, Anne & Alger, Lindsey S. (1988, Sept). "HIV in Women and Their Pregnancies." *MMJ 37* (9): 717-24.
Wofsy, C.B. et al. (1986). "Insolation of AIDS: Associated Retrovirus from Genital Secretions of Women with Antibodies to the Virus." *Lancet 1*: 527-29.

HIV TESTING DURING PREGNANCY

In 1987, the Centers for Disease Control (CDC) expanded their guidelines for HIV testing of women in their childbearing years, defining women at risk as follows: intravenous drug users; prostitutes; women known to have had infected, bisexual, IV drug-using, or hemophiliac sexual partners; residents of communities or immigrants from countries with a known or suspected high prevalence of infection; and those who received a blood transfusion between 1978 and 1985 (Holman et al., 1989).

The CDC emphasized the importance of voluntary testing with informed consent. However, if testing is offered only to women who fit risk criteria, as many as half of those infected could be missed (Landesman et al., 1987). Because of this, some policymakers recommend routine testing with specific informed consent in high-risk communities, regardless of personal histories. Others believe that offering screening to all women would avoid stigmatization of poor, black, and Hispanic women.

Debate continues on possible hidden agendas of public policy concerning HIV testing of women. Is it to empower women to make informed choices regarding continuation of a pregnancy according to her own personal values, or is it to serve a communal public health interest of preventing the birth of infected newborns? There is potential for compromising the parental right to bear children at the expense of children who would be born uninfected should the latter of these opinions prevail. The director of the CDC's AIDS program has stated, "There's no reason that the number of cases . . . shouldn't decline. Someone who understands the disease and is logical will not want to be pregnant and will consider the test results when making family planning decisions" (Centers for Disease Control, 1988). However, research shows that infected women do not choose to postpone pregnancy (Bayer, 1989).

In recent years, public health officials almost never urged women to avoid pregnancy because of the possibility that a congenital disorder might be transmitted. The principle of nondirective counseling has become officially accepted by the medical establishment and genetic counselors. There is a close analogy between HIV disease and genetic disorders as they apply to reproductive choices. Yet some health professionals support a directive approach in conveying the importance of protecting sexual and needle-sharing partners, even though they do not support it for reproductive decisions. Others feel that explicit discouragement of pregnancy is in order. A policy designed to prevent the birth of HIV-infected children runs the risk of tacitly condoning directive counseling. It seems likely that time will reveal that no mode of individual counseling is more effective than another in influencing the reproductive choices of women. Overall, HIV-infected women seem to make choices about pregnancy for the same reasons that uninfected women do (Sunderland et al., 1988).

Many women choose not to share their test results with health care providers because they fear discrimination. Many women share their test results with their sexual partners but report physical or emotional intimidation when attempting to introduce safer sex into the relationship. The most important issue is that identification of this disease in a child simultaneously diagnoses the mother, who may have been unaware of her own illness. Revealing her diagnosis may expose her to discriminatory and possibly catastrophic experiences at work and in her community.

✱ PAT RICHTER, M.P.A.

See also: HIV and Pregnancy; Prenatal Diagnosis: Overview

See **Guide to Related Topics:** Prenatal Diagnosis and Screening

Resources

Bayer, Ronald. (1989). "Perinatal Transmission of HIV Infection: The Ethics of Prevention." *Clinical Obstetrics and Gynecology 32* (3): 497-505.
Centers for Disease Control. (1988, Oct). "Curran Supports Testing, Counseling for Pregnant Women. *CDC AIDS Weekly*: page 2.
Holman, Susan et al. (1989, Feb). "Women Infected with Human Immunodeficiency Virus: Counseling and

Testing during Pregnancy." *Seminars in Perinatology 13* (1): 7-15.

Landesman, S. et al. (1987). "Serosurvey of Human Immunodeficiency Virus Infection in Parturients." *JAMA 258*: 2701-03.

Sunderland, A. et al. (1988). "Influence of HIV Infection on Pregnancy Decisions." IV International Conference on AIDS, Stockholm, Abstract #6607.

HOME BIRTH

Since a time predating recorded history, women have helped other women give birth at home. (*See* "Evolution of Human Birth.") Around 150 years ago, however, there began a slow evolution of birth from a woman-dominated, family experience in the home to a male-dominated, medical experience in the hospital. In the mid-1800s, a process began that drew childbirth under the umbrella of sickness, medicine, and hospitalization. As more hospitals were built, they were used for procedures that used to be performed in the home. It cost more to have the procedure done in the hospital, but that simply added to its appeal as a status symbol. At the same time, doctors realized that obstetrics and gynecology were becoming lucrative fields. A doctor's time could be spent more efficiently if a woman gave birth in the hospital. He could attend to several medical tasks and receive assistance from nurses and orderlies during the time it would take to sit at one woman's bedside for a home birth.

Women also played their part in following doctors to hospitals to have their babies. According to social historian Judith Walzer Leavitt (1986), there has always been a female determination to overcome the obstacles of childbirth, and a major obstacle to overcome before the 20th century was the fear of dying or being permanently injured. Leavitt maintains that fear of death or debility led women away from traditional birthing patterns to a long search for safer and less painful childbirth. Drugs and instruments, women believed, could provide relief and successful birth outcomes.

The switch of birth place from home to hospital, much more than the switch of birth attendant from midwife to physician, is what changed childbirth for Western women. Leavitt states that "for the entire home birth period, until women moved to the hospital to deliver their babies in the 20th century, women friends, neighbors and relatives continued to offer birthing women psychological support and practical help . . . these female-centered activities dominated most American births, whether or not they were attended by male physicians." Once birth switched to the hospital, the female relatives, friends, and neighbors were excluded. Now the laboring woman was denied not only their emotional support and sips of soup from their kitchens, but also their protection. Leavitt points to documented instances when women helpers would ask the physician to leave the home if they didn't like what he was doing.

By 1960, when most births took place in the hospital, women were alone and unsupported in their birth experience, feeling obliged to accept whatever the large institution prescribed for them. This could range from being forced to wear an impersonal and revealing hospital gown to being strapped by her hands and feet to a delivery table. In recent years, many hospitals have begun changing some of the old rules, and most allow one support person (usually the woman's husband) to stay with the woman during labor. But even with these changes, more women are going back to choosing home birth.

More and more women see the advantages of home birth as not only emotional well-being and comfort, but as an effective way to avoid procedures they would feel forced to accept in the hospital. Many women view these procedures as not just uncomfortable or unnecessary but potentially dangerous.

Electronic fetal monitoring is just one example. In almost every hospital in the United States, a woman in labor is hooked up to a machine that records the baby's heart rate. It records that rate either by a belt around the mother's waist, which sends the heart rate to the machine by ultrasound, or by screwing an electrode into the baby's scalp when it is still inside her, with wires from the scalp electrodes that are then attached to the machine. With ultrasound, women wonder what the effect of the waves on the baby will be. With the electrode, they wonder about reports of hemorrhage and infection entering at the site on the baby's scalp. And with either way of monitoring the baby's heart, the woman has to stay in bed, which slows down her labor and may interfere with the baby's blood and oxygen supply if the mother lies on her back. A recent study of almost 35,000 pregnancies showed that there is no greater benefit to the mother or baby of using this type of monitoring as opposed to the fetoscope, the kind of stethoscope used at most home births (Levano et al., 1986). But most hospitals continue to use the electronic fetal monitor on all women having babies.

The long-range effects of some of the current hospital procedures, such as electronic fetal monitoring, are not yet known, because they have not been in use long enough. However, consumers have seen in retrospect how some procedures may not be in their best interests. The use of forceps is an example of a procedure introduced to save babies that, when first widely used, caused many injuries or death due to overuse and improper use.

"Hospitals have never been proven to be the safest place to have a baby," says David Stewart, Ph.D., executive director of the International Association of Parents and Professionals for Safe Alternatives in Childbirth (Stewart and Stewart, 1983). When births first took place in hospitals, many women died of a disease called puerperal fever. Physicians moved from touching cadavers to examining laboring women without washing their hands properly. Although antiseptic technique is now followed, infection control is still a major problem in hospitals.

Other hospital procedures women currently are questioning, in addition to electronic monitoring, include shaving the pubic hair, giving enemas, limiting the number of support people, encouraging the use of drugs, refusing to permit the consumption of food, being examined by numerous personnel, starting an intravenous line, and being put to bed. At a home birth, a woman can do simple things like walking, eating, going to the bathroom—things that a person normally does at home—that also expedite labor.

Most women choosing home birth state they want control over what they do during labor. At home, women can control not only who is in the room with them but what procedures are used on them. In the hospital, it is harder to have this control, as the institutional needs of the hospital often preclude concern for the woman giving birth. Hospital staff members report that, in teaching hospitals, a procedure might be done because a doctor needs practice in doing it, or a drug to

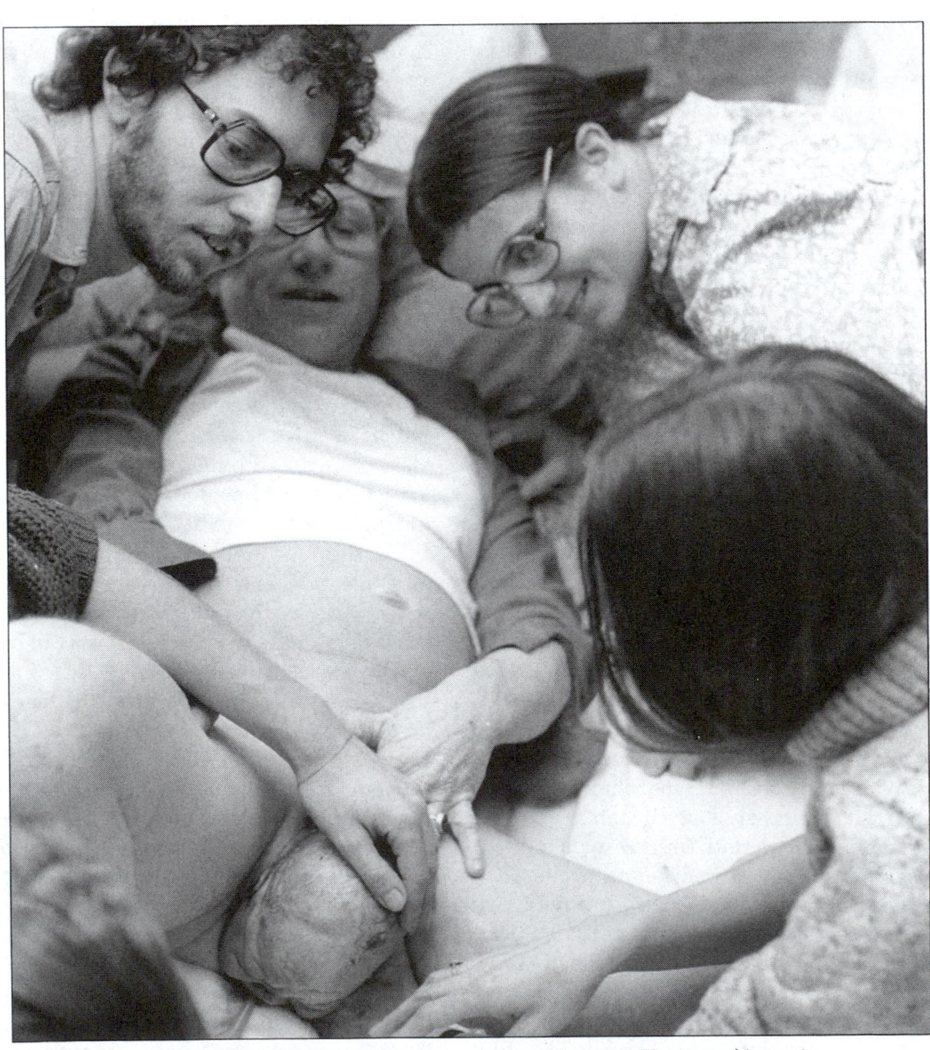

A family sharing the moment of birth. Photo courtesy of Harriette Hartigan/Artemis.

speed up labor may be given because there are so many women waiting to give birth.

Over the past 10 years, studies have begun to appear in the medical literature that support the safety of home birth, and home birth procedures and practitioners (Burnett et al., 1980; Sullivan and Beeman, 1983; Hinds et al., 1985). In spite of these research studies and the increasing desire of women to have available home birth programs, a few families and home birth midwives have been targets of legal action, although home birth itself is not illegal. Doctors may initiate lawsuits against midwives for practicing without a license (although some home birth supporters believe the real complaint is losing money).

While more than 90 percent of babies are born in hospitals under the American birth system, the United States continues to rank poorer and poorer in United Nations-published statistics of infant mortality among industrialized nations. Such findings have given support to the idea that the American way of birth needs to be reviewed and alternative methods explored.

A typical home birth today is not unlike those births that took place before hospitalization became the norm. The laboring woman walks around, finishing up her activities while she is in early labor. When her labor contractions increase, she calls the midwife, who comes over and examines her and the fetus periodically. When labor gets difficult, the mother can lean on a friend, or take a bath, or drink some special tea, or change her position many times. She can say and do whatever she wants because she is at home. Most home births are attended by midwives who are there to make suggestions and help, but not to take control of the birth process away from the mother.

Any time a laboring woman could benefit from being in a hospital, the midwife takes her there. Most midwives require that the woman have back-up arrangements with a doctor or hospital should they become necessary. Women preparing for home birth are generally carefully screened for risk well before labor and delivery begin. Last-minute complications requiring hospital equipment or procedures are generally uncommon in women who have received adequate prenatal care.

After the birth, the midwife gives the baby a newborn checkup and treats the mother if she has a complication, such as excessive bleeding. Hemorrhage is actually a rare occurrence after home birth for mothers who nurse their newborns, because frequent breastfeeding causes the uterus to firm up quickly. Most midwives bring medications and suturing materials with them in case they are needed.

There are some women who have their babies at home without any midwife or doctor present. They just give birth to the baby on the bed and tie off the umbilical cord with dental floss, clean themselves and the baby, and rest a bit. Or the baby's father may help the woman. Since labor and birth are normal functions of a woman's body, usually nothing goes wrong with this way of having a home birth. But most women choosing home birth prefer to have an experienced midwife present.

More than 90 percent of pregnant women in the United States continue to have their babies in hospitals, many without thinking there is another way. Most mothers choosing home birth have done a lot of reading and thinking about the advantages and disadvantages of home versus hospital birth, and then conclude, like Ashley Montagu, "Where else . . . if not in the home?" (Ward and Ward, 1976). ✱ ALICE GILGOFF

See also: Hospital Birth: An Anthropological Analysis of Ritual and Practice; Labor: Overview; Midwifery: Overview; The Netherlands; Social Science Research on American Childbirth Practices

See **Guide to Related Topics:** Childbirth Practices and Locations

Resources

Annas, G. (1975). *The Rights of Hospital Patients.* New York: Avon Books.

Arms, S. (1975). *Immaculate Deception.* Granby, MA: Bergin & Garvey.

Bean, C. (1977). *Labor & Delivery: An Observer's Diary.* Garden City, NY: Doubleday.

Burnett, C. et al. (1980). "Home Delivery and Neonatal Mortality in North Carolina." *Journal of the American Medical Association 244*: 2741-45.

Gaskin, I.M. (1975). *Spiritual Midwifery.* Summertown, TN: The Book Publishing Co.

Gilgoff, A. (1978). *Home Birth.* New York: Coward, McCann & Geoghegan.

———. (1989). *Home Birth: An Invitation and a Guide.* Granby, MA: Bergin & Garvey.

Hinds, M. et al. (1985). "Neonatal Outcome in Planned vs. Unplanned Out-of-Hospital Births in Kentucky." *Journal of the American Medical Association 253*: 1578-82.

Korte, D. & Scaer, R. (1990). *A Good Birth, A Safe Birth.* New York: Bantam Books.

Leavitt, J. (1986). *Brought to Bed: Childbearing in America 1750-1950.* New York: Oxford University Press

Levano, K. et al. (1986). "A Prospective Comparison of Selective and Universal Electronic Fetal Monitoring in 34,955 Pregnancies." *New England Journal of Medicine 315*: 615-19.

Sousa, M. (1976). *Childbirth at Home.* Englewood Cliffs, NJ: Prentice-Hall.

Stewart, D. & Stewart, L. (Eds.) (1983). *The Childbirth Activist's Handbook.* Marble Hill, MO: NAPSAC Reproductions.

Sullivan, D. & Beeman, R. (1983). "Four Years' Experience with Home Birth by Licensed Midwives in Arizona." *Journal of the American Public Health Association* 73: 641-45.

Ward, C. & Ward, F. (1976). *The Home Birth Book.* Washington, DC: Inscape.

HOSPITAL BIRTH: AN ANTHROPOLOGICAL ANALYSIS OF RITUAL AND PRACTICE

All known human societies channel the physiological process of being born into pathways—better known as rites of passage—imprinted with their cultural world view. It is commonly held that the de-ritualization of birth—its liberation from ancient superstition and taboo—accompanied its movement into the hospital. But, in fact, this movement into the hospital resulted in the most elaborate proliferation of birth rituals yet seen in the human cultural world.

A ritual is a patterned, repetitive, symbolic, and transformative enactment of a cultural belief or value; its primary purpose is the alignment of the belief system of the individual with that of society. A rite of passage is a series of rituals through which individuals are conveyed from one social status to another (for example, from girlhood to womanhood, boyhood to manhood), thereby transforming both society's definition of the individual and the individual's self-perception. The most important feature of most rites of passage is that they place their participants in a transitional realm that has few of the attributes of the past or coming state (Turner, 1979). Existing in such a nonordinary realm facilitates the gradual psychological opening of the initiates to profound interior change. In many initiation rites involving major transitions into new social roles (e.g., military basic training), this openness is achieved through a ritualized combination of physical and mental hardships that serve to break down the initiates' belief systems—the internal mental structure of concepts and categories through which the initiates perceive and interpret the world. Such breakdown leaves the initiates profoundly open to new learning and the construction of new categories. The rite of passage then restructures their belief systems in accordance with the dominant belief and value system of the society or group into which they are being initiated.

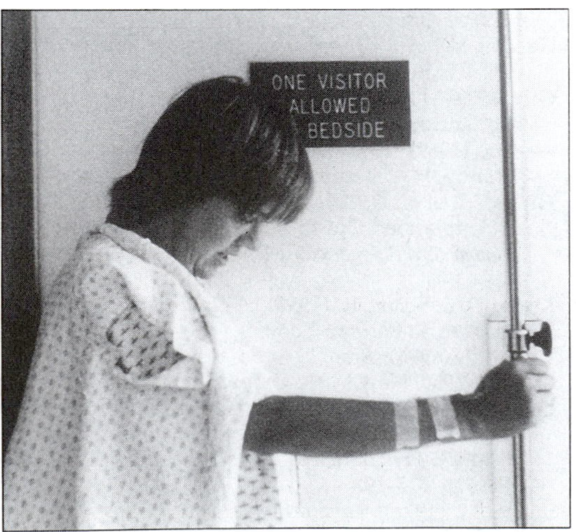

Laboring woman in a hospital. Photo courtesy of Kip Kozlowski.

By making the naturally transformative process of birth a cultural rite of passage for the mother, a society can ensure that its basic values will be transmitted, as the mother is generally the one primarily responsible for instilling these values in the minds of her children—society's newest members and the guarantors of its future. The core value and belief system of American society centers around science and technology and the institutions that control and disseminate them. Ritual is the most powerful communication tool available for perpetuating these—or any society's—values. Its effectiveness results from some of its primary characteristics, which are discussed here as springboards for understanding ritual's role in hospital birth.

Symbolism. Ritual sends its messages through symbols. (A symbol, most simply, is an object, idea, or action loaded with cultural meaning.) Unlike symbols, straightforward verbal messages are intellectually analyzed by the left hemisphere of the human brain, enabling the recipient to accept or reject their content. Symbols, in contrast, are received through the right hemisphere of the brain as a gestalt. They are felt in the body and the emotions; their meanings are often internalized without conscious awareness.

Hospitals are replete with symbols. Routine obstetrical procedures—the rituals of hospital birth—manipulate such symbols to convey messages to birthing women (and their partners, and the hospital personnel who attend them). For example, to be seated in a wheelchair, as many laboring women are, is to receive through their bodies the symbolic message that they are disabled; to be put to bed is to receive the symbolic message that they are sick. The intravenous drips commonly attached to the hands and arms of birthing women may be viewed as making an especially powerful symbolic statement: They are umbilical cords to the hospital. The long cord connecting the woman's body to the fluid-filled bottle places the woman in the same relation to the hospital as the baby in her womb is to her. By making her seem dependent on the institution for her life, the IV conveys to her one of the most profound messages of her initiation experience: Everyone is dependent on institutions for life.

A Cognitive Matrix. Rituals are not arbitrary; they come from within the belief system of a group. Their primary purpose is to enact and transmit that belief system into the emotions, minds, and bodies of their participants. The belief system enacted by the rituals of hospital birth is the technological model of reality (Davis-Floyd, 1987a, 1992) that forms the philosophical basis of both Western medicine and American society. This model, originally developed in the 1600s by Descartes, Bacon, Hobbes, and others, assumes a mechanistic universe available for exploitation by those who can figure out its laws through science and manipulate them through technology (Merchant, 1983). Under this model, the human body came to be viewed as a machine that can be taken apart and put back together. The male body was held to be the prototype of the properly functioning body-machine, while the female body, insofar as it deviated from the male, was regarded as inherently defective—a metaphor that eventually formed the philosophical basis of modern obstetrics (Rothman, 1982) and led to the development of tools and technologies for the manipulation and improvement of the inherently defective mechanical process of birth.

Repetition and Redundancy. For maximum effectiveness, a ritual concentrates on sending one set of messages over and over again in different forms. Many obstetrical procedures (such as electronic monitoring, frequent cervical exams, the administration of pitocin to speed labor) convey in different forms the same basic messages of the defectiveness of the woman's birthing machine and her dependence on the institution and its technology. The additional and powerful message of such rituals is that technologically obtained information and institutional schedules are much more important than the woman's internal rhythms and personal experience of labor.

Cognitive Destructuring. The initiate's belief system must be broken down before it can be restructured. In rites of passage, this cognitive breakdown is accomplished through techniques of hazing, strange-making (making the commonplace appear strange by juxtaposing it with the unfamiliar) (Abrahams, 1973), and symbolic inversion (turning things upside down and inside out) (Abrahams, 1973; Babcock, 1978). Birthing women are made to feel strange to themselves through exposing hospital gowns, ID bracelets, and the shaving of their pubic hair. They are sometimes hazed by frequent and painful cervical checks, during which their most private and intimate parts are symbolically converted into institutional property.

Cognitive Stabilization. When humans are subjected to extremes of stress and pain, they may move past the cognitive destructuring desirable in rites of passage into a dysfunctional panic condition in which learning cannot take place (McManus, 1979). Here, ritual plays a critical role, for it can stabilize individuals under stress by giving them a conceptual handhold. The rhythmic breathing taught in many childbirth education classes serves this purpose, as do pain-relieving obstetric drugs and fear-relieving obstetric technologies.

Order, Formality, and a Sense of Inevitability. Its exaggerated and precise order and formality set ritual apart from other modes of social interaction, enabling ritual to establish an atmosphere that feels both inevitable and inviolate (Moore and Myerhoff, 1977). To perform a series of rituals is to feel oneself locking onto a set of "cosmic gears" that will safely crank the individual right on through a perceived danger to safety on the other side. Just as the Trobriand sea fisherman performs an elaborate series of rituals in precise order because he hopes that, if he does his part, the gods of the sea will do their part to bring him safely home, so the obstetrician hopes that, if he or she precisely follows procedure, a healthy baby will result. In both cases, the rituals provide a sense of control that gives individuals the courage to act in the face of the challenge and caprice of nature. (Once these gears have been set in motion, though, there is often no stopping them: One obstetrical procedure often appears to necessitate the next, and the next—a process often referred to as the "cascade of interventions.")

Cognitive Transformation. The goal of most initiatory rites of passage is cognitive transformation. It occurs when the belief system enacted in the rite and the belief system of the initiate become one. Such transformation must usually be preceded by the cognitive destructuring described above. For nascent mothers, this process of conceptual fusion is usually gradual. Routine obstetrical procedures cumulatively work to map the technological model of birth onto the birthing woman's perceptions of her labor experience; if these rituals are successful in a cognitive sense, the pregnant woman will begin to experience her own body as a defective machine incapable of birthing without science, technology, and the institution. One woman experienced it this way:

> As soon as I got hooked up to the monitor, all everyone did was stare at it. The nurses didn't even look at me anymore when they came into the room—they went straight to the monitor. I got the weirdest feeling that *it* was having the baby, not me.

Drama and Intensification. Belief tends to follow emotion. Behavioral psychology has shown that people are far more likely to remember and internalize the messages of events that carry an emotional charge. Ritual's ability to generate strong emotions is enhanced by the fact that it is set apart from everyday life, by its high stylization, by the self-conscious acting often required of its participants, and by the repetitious bombardment of the participants with symbolic messages, which often intensifies toward a climax.

As the moment of physical transformation approaches, the number of ritual procedures performed upon the woman intensifies toward the climax of birth. These procedures work to heighten the emotional effect that the birth itself has, and to focus the attention of the ritual actors on the physician as protagonist and the woman's body as the stage upon which he or she performs the drama of birth.

Preservation of the Status Quo. Through explicit enactment of a culture's belief system, ritual works both to preserve and to transmit that belief system and so becomes an important force in the preservation of the status quo in any society. Wherever this stabilizing characteristic of ritual is paramount, those in positions of power tend to have unique control over its performance.

In spite of tremendous advances in equality for women, the U.S. is still a patriarchy. Nowhere is this more evident than in the continued use of the physiologically disadvantageous lithotomy position for birth. This position completes the ritual process of symbolic inversion that has been in motion since the woman put on the backward hospital gown. Her legs are in the air, her buttocks at the table's edge, her vagina totally exposed. As the ultimate symbolic inversion, it is ritually appropriate that this position be reserved for the peak transformational moments of the initiation experience—the birth itself. The official representative of society and its core values of science, technology, patriarchy, and institutions stands, in control, at the mother's bottom, where the baby's head is beginning to emerge. American culture views "up" as good, "down" as bad. To enact these values, the babes born of science and technology must be born "up" toward the positively valued cultural world of men, in opposition to the natural force of gravity, instead of "down" (as they would in the physiologically efficacious squatting position) toward the negatively valued natural world of women. The overthrow of the initiate's category system is now complete: This position marks and reinforces her now total openness to the new messages she is about to receive, and itself constitutes one of those messages, as it speaks so eloquently to her of her powerlessness and the power of society at the supreme moment of her own individual transformation.

The episiotomy performed by the physician just before birth symbolically enacts the high cultural value technological society places on one of its basic organizing features—the straight line. Through episiotomies, physicians (society's representatives to the human body-machine) can deconstruct the vagina (and its symbolic representations of the power of female sexuality and creativity), then reconstruct it (and its representations) in accord with technological values.

The more a society's dominant model of reality differs from actual reality, the more rituals that society must employ to bolster its paradigm. In reality, women's bodies are not defective machines, and birth is not a mechanical process. Thus, obstetrics has had to develop an enormous number of rituals to fulfill one of its primary cultural roles—making the technological myth about how society is reproduced appear to be true.

An Agent of Social Change. Paradoxically, with all its insistence on continuity and order, ritual can be an important factor not only in individual transformation but also in social change (Turner, 1974). New belief and value systems are most effectively spread through new rituals designed to enact and transmit them; entrenched belief and value systems are most effectively altered through alterations in the rituals that enact them. In the cultural arena of birth, some of society's most visible battles over core values are being waged. Medical personnel, pressured by the threat of malpractice suits, are working to develop increasing control over the birth process and place ever greater reliance on technology, while many women are demanding more options in birth and seek greater autonomy and self-responsibility.

A small percentage of American women choose not to participate in the technological socialization of women and instead give birth at home. These women often adopt an alternative paradigm—the wholistic model. Based on systems theory, this model stresses the organic integrity and inherent trustworthiness of the female body; communication and oneness between mother and child—and mother and midwife; the integrity and self-sufficiency of the family; and self-responsibility. Home birthers enact this model and send its messages to themselves and their families and friends through rituals such as singing, visualizations, traditional Native American Blessing Way ceremonies, and the preparation of special foods. The persecution that home birth mothers and midwives occasionally experience from physicians and police is a reflection of the degree to which their alternative reality model differs from and challenges the hegemony of the dominant technological model.

How Effective Is Ritual? Every society in the world attempts to socialize its citizens into conformity with its norms; successfully socialized citizens derive many benefits from wholehearted participation in their society. As has been seen, hospital birth is an intensive process of ritual socialization into the dominant values of American society. Yet human beings are not automatons, and the extent to which such socialization succeeds depends to a great extent on the individual involved. Many American women actively choose technological births precisely because they wish to fully participate in American society's dominant belief and value system and to achieve status and success within that system, on its terms; their induced labors and scheduled cesareans reflect beliefs they already hold. Others take a middle road between the technological and wholistic extremes, attempting to avoid conceptual fusion with the technological model without rejecting it altogether, by substituting some self-empowering rituals that enact aspects of the wholistic model for some obstetrical procedures (e.g., eating their own food instead of having an IV, walking the halls instead of going to bed). Some succeed in achieving their goal of "natural childbirth" and emerge from the hospital unsuccessfully socialized, from society's point of view. Others succumb to the force of the socialization process, internalizing messages of dependency, mechanics, and defectiveness. Those whose pre-birth beliefs are in greatest conflict with their ritual socialization will often experience long-term psychological trauma. In contrast, those women who already hold values in accord with the technological model will not experience hospital rituals as traumatic, but as reassuring and affirming of their own value and importance in the larger society.

✱ ROBBIE DAVIS-FLOYD, Ph.D.

See also: Labor: Overview; Social Science Research on American Childbirth Practices

See **Guide to Related Topics:** Childbirth Practices and Locations

Resources

Abrahams, Roger D. (1973). "Ritual for Fun and Profit (or The Ends and Outs of Celebration)." Paper delivered at the Burg Wartenstein Symposium No. 59, on "Ritual: Reconciliation in Change," Wenner-Gren Foundation for Anthropological Research, New York.

Babcock, Barbara. (Ed.) (1978). *The Reversible World: Symbolic Inversion in Art and Society.* Ithaca, NY: Cornell University Press.

Davis-Floyd, Robbie E. (1987a). "Obstetric Training as a Rite of Passage." *Medical Anthropology Quarterly 1* (3): 288-318.

———. (1987b). "The Technological Model of Birth." *Journal of American Folklore 100* (398): 93-109.

———. (1988). "Birth as an American Rite of Passage." In Karen Michaelson (Ed.) *Childbirth in America: Anthropological Perspectives.* Beacon Hill, MA: Bergin and Garvey, pp. 153-72.

———. (1990). "Ritual in the Hospital: Giving Birth the American Way." In Phillip Whitten & David Hunter (Eds.) *Anthropology: Contemporary Perspectives.* 6th edition. Glenview, IL: Scott Foresman, pp. 275-85.

———. (1990). "The Role of American Obstetrics in the Resolution of Cultural Anomaly." *Social Science and Medicine 31*(2): 175-89.

———. (1992). *Birth as an American Rite of Passage.* Berkeley, CA: University of California Press.

McManus, John. (1979). "Ritual and Human Social Cognition." In Eugene G. d'Aquili, Charles D. Lauglin, & John McManus (Eds.) *The Spectrum of Ritual.* New York: Columbia University Press, pp. 216-48.

Merchant, Carolyn. (1983). *The Death of Nature: Women, Ecology, and the Scientific Revolution.* San Francisco: Harper and Row.

Moore, Sally Falk & Myerhoff, Barbara. (Eds.) (1977). *Secular Ritual.* Assen and Amsterdam: Van Gorcum and Co.

Rothman, Barbara Katz. (1982). *In Labor: Women and Power in the Birthplace.* New York: W.W. Norton and Co. (Reprinted in paperback under the title *Giving Birth: Alternatives in Childbirth.* (1985). New York: Penguin Books.

Turner, Victor. (1974). *Dramas, Fields, and Metaphors: Symbolic Action in Human Society.* Ithaca, NY: Cornell University Press.

———. (1979). "Betwixt and Between: The Limited Period in Rites de Passage." In William A. Lessa & Evon Z. Vogt (Eds.) *Reader in Comparative Religion.* 4th edition. New York: Harper and Row, pp. 234-43.

HUSBAND-COACHED CHILDBIRTH. *See instead* BRADLEY METHOD: HUSBAND-COACHED CHILDBIRTH

See instead BRADLEY METHOD: HUSBAND-COACHED CHILDBIRTH

HYPERTENSION

Hypertension in pregnancy refers to blood pressure readings greater than 140/90 or elevation of 30 points systolic (upper number) and/or 15 points diastolic (lower number) above the mother's baseline. Hypertension may be pre-existing, known as essential hypertension, or may develop in the latter half of pregnancy, known as gestational or pregnancy-induced hypertension (PIH).

Essential hypertension causes known risks to the baby, such as growth retardation (because the fetus does not get enough oxygen and nutrients due to vasoconstriction), and to the mother, such as increased propensity to develop pre-eclampsia/eclampsia. A woman with pregnancy-induced hypertension also runs these risks, but the causes may include factors in diet and lifestyle, rather than underlying physical pathology. Therefore, at the first sign of elevated blood pressure during pregnancy, care providers often take a thorough social and personal history to identify any areas of imbalance or disruption.

In general, when pressure is mildly elevated, the following measures may help: (1) moderate exercise, which stimulates circulation so that blood vessels may stretch and pressure decline; (2) diet high in protein, complex carbohydrates, and vitamins and minerals, which maintain a healthy metabolism more resistant to the physical demands of pregnancy and stress in general; (3) periodic relaxation, using either meditation, visualization, or other techniques; (4) increased rest, including five-minute relaxation breaks as well as a regular nap daily and adequate sleep every night; (5) emotional clearing through counseling or discussion with one's care provider or other support person of any ongoing problems or upsetting circumstances; (6) strict avoidance of stimulants, including caffeinated beverages like coffee, black tea or soft drinks; chocolate; nicotine; and cocaine. Some cough and cold medicines also contain caffeine—over-the-counter medications should generally be avoided or cleared as harmless by one's care provider; and (7) use of herbal teas and preparations, particularly hops tincture or capsules (which are sleep inducing) or skullcap, chamomile, and valerian blends, which serve to relax. These are harmless in pregnancy when taken in moderation and with the advice and guidance of someone qualified.

When blood pressure becomes so high as to exceed normal limits, as stated above, bed rest on the left side several times daily is recommended to enhance kidney function and minimize chances that the condition will progress to pre-eclampsia. There is, in fact, some debate and confusion as to whether hypertension can exist independently of pre-eclampsia; although the two are often closely linked, they appear to be distinctly separate conditions. ✱ ELIZABETH DAVIS

See **Guide to Related Topics:** Pregnancy Complications

Resources

Davis, Elizabeth. (1987). *Heart and Hands: A Midwife's Guide to Pregnancy and Birth*. San Francisco: Celestial Arts.

Gaskin, Ina May. (1989). *Spiritual Midwifery*. Summertown, TN: Farm Publishing.

HYPNOSIS FOR CHILDBIRTH*

Hypnosis has been shown to be an effective means of decreasing medical complications in labor and facilitating normal delivery by addressing the emotional and psychological issues surrounding pregnancy and birth. Instead of trying to make childbirth painless through hypnosis, the Peterson method of hypnosis for childbirth emphasizes psychological preparation for *coping* with pain, and addresses anxieties about childbirth and the changes it will cause in a woman's life (Peterson, 1984; Peterson and Mehl, 1984, 1985). In addition, such body-centered hypnosis has been shown to bring about an increase in maternal self-esteem, maternal-infant bonding, increased confidence in mothering, and normal delivery outcome (Mehl, Donovan, and Peterson, 1988).

In the Peterson method of childbirth preparation, hypnosis is only used after several other activities have taken place. First, an interview is conducted in which a comprehensive history is gathered regarding the couple's relationship, previous childbirth experiences, plans for birth, family adjustment, etc. Next, the couple listens to a pre-recorded tape of a woman in labor in which pain is expressed clearly and audibly during contractions. This stimulates discussion of fears, allowing women and their partners to prepare psychologically and emotionally for childbirth. Pain coping is also promoted through an intense

* Copyright © 1992 by Gayle Peterson.

pinching exercise in which a woman learns to identify her individual style of coping with pain (visual, auditory, or somasthetic). Finally, an individually designed hypnosis tape is used in which the physically occurring processes of the body are used as anchors for suggestion in order to decrease the fear associated with the childbirth process and to resolve individual anxieties about motherhood. The physical process of labor later triggers the associated hypnotic messages; at this time the memory of the hypnotic birth journey is activated, leading many women to report that they feel as if they have already given birth as they relive phrases and images from the hypnosis experience while actually giving birth. (See *Body-Centered Hypnosis for Childbirth: A Training Videotape*, by Gayle Peterson, which includes a case example and full birth visualization.)

Women are more likely to give birth normally when prepared to cope with the pain of labor. The desire to reduce pain is a primary factor motivating most people seeking childbirth preparation, but it is only a small part of the body-centered hypnosis technique, which focuses on helping women cope with pain and reduce anxiety, as well as normalizing the childbirth process.

Body-centered hypnosis as developed by Peterson stimulates an experience of mastery in the pregnant woman for the childbirth experience. The sensations of the birth journey are encoded in the memory areas of the brain, along with suggestions for coping with pain. Body-centered hypnosis encourages subjects to actively experience bodily sensations rather than just relaxing and absorbing hypnotic suggestions passively. Subjects become active participants in the hypnosis process. The Peterson method is similar to the method of Milton Erickson in that it attempts to tap the individual's motivation to create positive suggestions (Zeig, 1982). The Peterson method, however, has greater emotional impact upon the childbirth process and relates specifically to the physiological sensations of childbirth.

✱ GAYLE PETERSON, Ph.D., L.C.S.W.

See also: Breath Control in Labor; Labor: Overview; Pain Relief in Labor: Nondrug Methods

***See* Guide to Related Topics:** Childbirth Practices and Locations

Resources

Hilgard, E. & Hilgard, J. (Eds.) (1975). *Hypnosis in the Relief of Pain*. Los Altos Hills, CA: William Kaufman, Inc.

LaMaze, F. (1958). *Painless Childbirth*. New York: Pocket Books.

Mehl, L.E., Donovan, S. & Peterson, G.H. (1988). "The Role of Hypnotherapy in Facilitating Normal Birth." In P. Freyburgh & M.L. Vanessa-Vogel (Eds.) *Prenatal and Perinatal Psychology and Medicine*. Park Ridge, NJ: Parthenon.

Peterson, G.H. (1984). *Birthing Normally*. Berkeley, CA: Shadow & Light.

———. (1987). "Prenatal Bonding, Prenatal Communication, and the Prevention of Prematurity." *Pre- and Peri-Natal Psychology* 2 (2): 87-92.

———. (1989). *Body-Centered Hypnosis for Childbirth: A Training Videotape*. Berkeley, CA: Shadow & Light.

Peterson, G.H. & Mehl, L.E. (1978, Oct). "Some Determinants of Maternal Attachment." *American Journal of Psychiatry 135* (10): 1168-73.

———. (1984). *Pregnancy as Healing*. Berkeley, CA: Mindbody Press.

———. (1985). *Cesarean Birth: Risk and Culture*. Berkeley, CA: Mindbody Press.

Zeig, J. (1982). *Ericksonian Approaches to Hypnosis in Psychotherapy*. New York: Bruner-Mazel.

Zeig, J. & Lankton, S. (Eds.) (1988). *Developing Ericksonian Hypnosis*. New York: Bruner-Mazel.

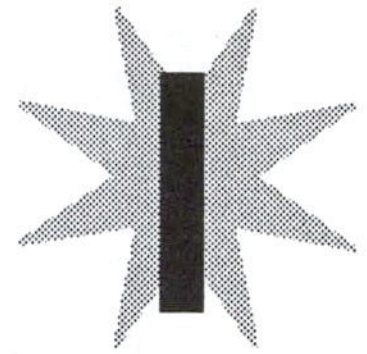

IMAGING TECHNIQUES

The technology that is used most often to create images of the fetus in pregnancy is ultrasound imaging. Ultrasound is sound of very high frequency, too high for humans or animals to hear. The most commonly used type of ultrasound imaging device uses small pulses or "beeps" of ultrasound to create a moving image of the fetus and the woman's internal organs. Such an image that shows movement as it is taking place is called a "real-time" image. The ultrasound is directed into the abdomen of the pregnant woman using a small device, called a "transducer," that is moved across the woman's abdomen. The sound waves are reflected at rates that depend on the density of the body part, and the information from these reflected waves is used to create the moving image.

Ultrasound is commonly used in "external fetal monitors" and in certain hand-held devices for making fetal heart tones audible. In the case of fetal monitors, what is produced is not a visual image of the fetus image, but audio signals that make fetal heart sounds audible. These heart sounds are then represented graphically. Major studies have shown that monitoring with the electronic fetal heart monitor does not improve the outcome of labor and delivery for either low-risk or high-risk pregnancies. One of the reasons that many hospitals continue to use the monitor is that they are experiencing a nursing shortage and one nurse can watch several monitors simultaneously but can only examine one laboring woman at a time.

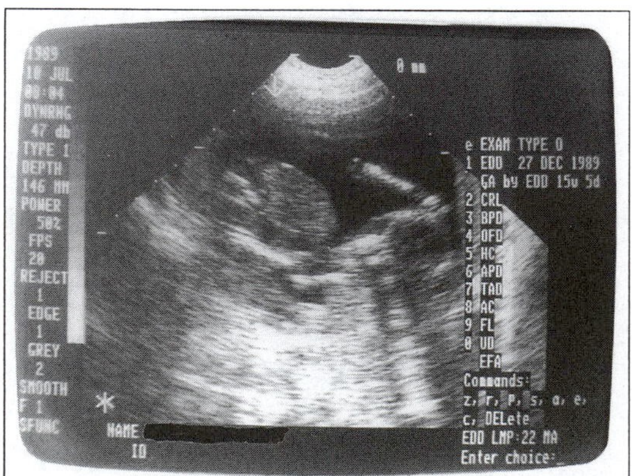

An ultrasound image of a fetus.

Imaging devices that use ionizing radiation, such as x-ray and CT scan (computed tomography) devices, are not used in pregnancy because the use of x-ray in pregnancy was shown to be dangerous to the fetus; x-ray exposure made it more likely that the fetus would develop cancer as a child. There is also a new technology that has occasionally been used with pregnant women: magnetic resonance imaging (MRI). (This technology used to be called "NMR," for nuclear magnetic resonance, but the name was changed because the word "nuclear" made people fear that radioactive substances were used in it.) This technology uses magnetic fields that are 1,000 times the strength of the earth's magnetic field to create images.

What are the risks of using these devices? It is known that ultrasound can produce changes in human tissue. For example, ultrasound waves can be used as part of a program of physical therapy to warm muscles. Ultrasound imaging has been used in pregnancy for several decades with no *known* "acute" harm—that is, harm that can be recognized soon after imaging. This may be because there has been no harm, or it may be because the harm is subtle or will not show up until years later. There have been no *systematic* studies of even the acute effects of low-dose pulsed ultrasound, and there has been very little study of possible effects that might occur years after imaging (Statmeyer and Christman, 1982). Because there is no registry of who has received ultrasound while in the womb, it would be difficult to do such a study.

In the case of MRI it is not known if any changes to human tissue result from exposure to an unvarying magnetic field; then again, researchers have very little experience with the effects of such enormous magnetic fields on mature adults, much less developing fetuses. There is a difference between saying that there are *no* risks and saying that there are no *known* risks. This difference is even more significant if, as in the case of MRI or in the case of the long-term effects of low-dose pulsed ultrasound, research has not been done on the subject. Largely because some risks of ultrasound are uncertain, the American College of Obstetrics and Gynecology has recommended *against* using ultrasound imaging in every pregnancy, even without any special reasons for doing it. A panel of experts at the National Institutes of Health (NIH) made a similar recommendation in 1984, saying that the use of ultrasound for fetal diagnosis should be limited to 28 medical indications. The following sorts of conditions are among those that many experts regard as indications that imaging should be done: excessive bleeding or other evidence of difficulties with the placenta, including the possibility that the placenta may be blocking the birth canal; suspected multiple birth; suspected abnormality in the fetus; woman's abdominal size does not match the projected due date; and a need to check the baby's position at time of birth if complications (such as breech presentation) are suspected. Ultrasound imaging is also regularly used as an aid in amniocentesis to help to properly position the needle that draws out the amniotic fluid.

There are risks associated with almost every medication or medical intervention, including aspirin and bed rest. The question is whether the risks are worth running in view of the advantages that may be gained by using the technology. The question is whether the information to be gained from ultrasound imaging is worth the relatively unknown risk of long-term effects that it presents.

It may be more necessary now than it was even a decade ago for individual patients to raise questions about the use of imaging technology, especially in pregnancy and childbirth. First, although there is an emphasis on obtaining a patient's informed consent for surgery and procedures that are known to carry a significant risk, this requirement does not extend to most diagnostic procedures. It is unlikely that a physician has ever asked a patient for informed consent before ordering a blood test or an x-ray. Usually, a physician will simply order the test or tell a patient to have it performed. A good physician will often take time to explain the nature of each test and what it is for, but this is not always done *unless the patient asks questions*. There have been some cases in which lawsuits have been brought against physicians for not doing ultrasound imaging even though there were no indications that there was a problem with the pregnancy. Although physicians were not found negligent in these cases, some physicians may recommend imaging only to protect themselves against being sued. In that case, it will be even more important for patients to discuss the reasons for imaging with their physicians when such testing is suggested to make sure that it is done only when needed and not simply to give the physician added legal protection, or to satisfy some person's curiosity to "see the baby."

✷ CAROLINE WHITBECK, Ph.D.

See also: Electronic Fetal Monitoring; Prenatal Diagnosis: Overview; Ultrasound in Obstetrics: A Question of Safety

See **Guide to Related Topics:** New Procreative Technologies; Prenatal Diagnosis and Screening

Resources

Baruch, Elaine, d'Amado, Amadeo, & Seager, Joni. (Eds.) (1988). *Women, Embryos, and Ethics Exploring the New Reproductive Technologies.* New York: Haworth Press.

Haverkamp, A. & Orleans, M. (1982). "An Assessment of Electronic Fetal Monitoring." *Women and Health 7* (3, 4): 115-34.

Holmes, H.B., Hoskins, B., & Gross, M. (1981). *Birth Control and Controlling Birth: Women-Centered Perspectives.* Clifton, NJ: Humana.

———. (1981). *The Custom-Made Child? Women-Centered Perspectives.* Clifton, NJ: Humana.

Luthy, David A. et al. (1987, May). "A Randomized Trial of Electronic Fetal Monitoring in Preterm Labor." *Obstetrics and Gynecology 69* (5): 687-95.

Patychuck, Dianne. (1985, Fall). "Ultrasound: The First Wave." *Healthsharing*: 25-28.

Rothman, Barbara Katz. (1986). *The Tentative Pregnancy.* New York: Viking.

Statmeyer, M.E. & Christman, C.L. (1982). "Biological Effects of Ultrasound." *Women and Health 7* (3, 4): 65-81.

Whitbeck, Caroline. (1988). "Fetal Imaging and Fetal Monitoring: Finding the Ethical Issues." *Women and Health 13* (1-2): 47-57.

———. (1991). "Ethical Issues Raised by New Medical Technologies." In Judith Rodin & Aila Collins (Eds.) *The New Reproductive Technologies.* Hillsdale, NJ: Lawrence Erlbaum Publishers, pp. 49-64.

IMMUNIZATIONS. *See instead* VACCINATIONS

IN VITRO FERTILIZATION FOR MALE INFERTILITY

In vitro fertilization (IVF), the procreative technology that was originally developed to bypass the blocked or missing Fallopian tubes of infertile women, is now also the treatment of choice in cases of male infertility due to low sperm count, poor sperm motility, or badly shaped sperm. Extra-corporeal fertilization works in male infertility because a *very* small amount of good sperm is needed to fertilize the egg in a Petri dish. The semen are washed to remove impurities, examined under a microscope to select the best sperm, and then microinjected into ova in a Petri dish. In male infertility cases, the woman may be physiologically fertile, but nonetheless, she is the one who has to undergo the hormonal stimulation, sonograms, and intravaginal or intra-abdominal procedures, often under general anesthesia, that the use of IVF entails. All the man has to do is produce sperm on demand.

The extent of male infertility in the population of couples undergoing treatment for infertility has surprised experienced clinicians. The famed Jones Institute of Reproductive Medicine reported that of a group of 52 couples in whom no fertilization had occurred, there was no obvious cause of failed fertilization in 40.4 percent. After reassessing sperm morphology with new criteria, they were able to diagnose sperm abnormalities in 61.5 percent of the men, with combined sperm and egg anomalies in 13.4 percent (Oehninger et al., 1988).

Surgical treatment and aspiration of semen has been used to correct or bypass male anatomical problems in a small number of infertile men (Spark, 1988). Despite its low success rate (only about 15 to 25 percent of infertile women have babies with IVF, and the rate is lower in cases of male infertility), the use of IVF in male infertility cases is now considered one of the most effective treatments: one that, according to the conclusion of a review paper, "opens up an area which will allow the treatment of a substantial population of infertile couples for whom before there was no effective treatment" (Yates and de Kretser, 1987). From a medical perspective, however, the situation is complicated by the fact that IVF treatment is undergone not by the person with the physiological problem, but by his female partner.

What are the risks, for a physiologically healthy woman, of undergoing IVF? In addition to the risks of surgery and infection (Holmes, 1988), a report from Israel (Ashkenazi et al., 1987) of two cases of iatrogenic tubal adhesions in female infertility led the authors to caution against its use in male infertility cases, arguing that the side effects of the treatment could prevent the patient from conceiving spontaneously in a subsequent attempt at becoming pregnant with the same or possibly another man. The authors' advice is: "It might be advisable to counsel the couple to attempt AID [donor insemination] prior to IVF and, possibly, avoid mechanical infertility" (244). AID, however, like adoption, is not likely to be the first choice of a couple if there is any possibility of producing a biological child of their own (Lasker and Borg, 1987).

In all IVF and related protocols, women are subject to most of the procedures and usually considered the primary patient. Women tend to take the initiative in seeking treatment for failure to conceive—they are the ones who know with each menstrual period that they have not gotten pregnant, and they usually have been to gynecologists at some time during their adult lives. In general, women usually see physicians more frequently than men do, while men tend to ignore physical difficulties that have not incapacitated them.

Patterns of disclosure suggest that couples are more reluctant to admit problems with infertility when the man is physiologically unable to inseminate than when the woman is unable to conceive. Sexual dysfunction seems to be a common reason why couples present themselves for infertility treatment and may be why there are so many "waiting list" pregnancies, pregnancies occurring spontaneously while awaiting treatment (Roh et al., 1987). It may also be the reason why the husband's inability to masturbate to ejaculation on demand is a perennial problem in IVF clinics the world over. A wife who wants a baby with her partner would be most reluctant to jeopardize her chances by insisting that the infertility workup start with an examination of his sperm, although physiologically that would seem to be the easiest place to begin. Once in treatment, however, she must involve her male partner.

For infertile women and those couples who have been unable to determine the cause of their procreative problems, these new technologies have often represented a valuable physiological, psychological, and social resource. However, in those cases where the couple's inability to conceive is clearly a male problem, the woman may feel coerced into the treatment, since she must undergo the greater part of these procedures.

✱ JUDITH LORBER, Ph.D.

See also: Donor Insemination; Egg Retrieval; Infertility: Overview

See **Guide to Related Topics:** Infertility; New Procreative Technologies

Resources

Ashkenazi, J. et al. (1987). "Ovum Pickup for *In Vitro* Fertilization: A Cause of Mechanical Infertility?" *Journal of In Vitro Fertilization and Embryo Transfer* 4: 242-45.

Callan, V.J. et al. (1988). "Toward Understanding Women's Decisions to Continue or to Stop *In Vitro* Fertilization: The Role of Social, Psychological, and Background Factors." *Journal of In Vitro Fertilization and Embryo Transfer* 5: 363-69.

Holmes, H.B. (1988). "*In Vitro* Fertilization: Reflections on the State of the Art." *Birth* 15: 134-45.

Lasker, J.N. & Borg, S. (1987). *In Search of Parenthood.* Boston: Beacon Press.

Lorber, J. (1987). "*In Vitro* Fertilization and Gender Politics." *Women and Health* 13: 117-33.

———. (1989, Fall). "Choice, Gift, or Patriarchal Bargain? Women's Consent to *In Vitro* Fertilization in Male Infertility." *Hypatia*: 23-36.

Oehninger, S. et al. (1988). "Failure of Fertilization in IVF: The 'Occult' Male Factor." *Journal of In Vitro Fertilization and Embryo Transfer* 5: 181-87.

Roh, S.I. et al. (1987). "*In Vitro* Fertilization and Embryo Transfer: Treatment-dependent versus Treatment-independent Pregnancies." *Fertility and Sterility* 48: 982-86.

Spark, R.F. (1988). *The Infertile Male: The Clinician's Guide to Diagnosis and Treatment.* New York: Plenum.

Williams, L.S. (1988). "'It's Going to Work for Me.' Responses to Failures of IVF." *Birth* 15: 153-56.

Yates, C.A. & de Kretser, D.M. (1987). "Male-factor Infertility and *In Vitro* Fertilization." *Journal of In Vitro Fertilization and Embryo Transfer* 4: 141-47.

INFANT CARRIERS

Once, while in a desert town in Morocco, I watched a toddler climb onto his mother's back, assisting her by holding on as she bent over and tied a large decorative shawl tightly around the two of them. When the shawl was tied the toddler was securely in place. The shawl aided the toddler in straddling his mother's back while allowing both his and his mother's arms and hands to be free.

Women have devised all sorts of convenient and comfortable methods to carry their young children. Methods of carrying infants and children vary among cultures and depend on weather conditions, materials available, and locale. The role of women and the beliefs regarding child care all influence the way we carry our young. In the West it seems that some variation of the carriage has been used for a long time. During medieval times in Europe, when the poor took their children to work with them in the fields, they used small carts or "waynes" to transport their infants too young to walk but too heavy to carry. Most women, however, like the Moroccan woman I observed, carry their young children.

Wrapping a large piece of material is a common and universal way to carry an infant. It is used by women to aid in carrying infants and children in front, on their backs, or alongside on their hips. This method has cultural variations, but the idea is the same. The mother's hands are free while the infant is securely in place and close to its mother.

There are variations on the shawl around the world. In rural Japan children are strapped onto the backs of their mothers with a long sash called an "ombu." The ombu is crossed in front of the mother and then crisscrossed above the baby's buttocks and brought around the mother's waist, where the sash is securely tied in front. In Himalayan villages babies are carried in their mothers' arms for the first six weeks, then are transferred to her back and held by a shawl. Among the Aymara of Peru and Bolivia, the baby is tightly bound with a belt until the eighth or ninth month and carried in a wide shawl or large square cloth called an "awayu." The fabric design of the awayu is simple for everyday use and more decorative for fiestas. The women of the highland tribes of south Colombia carry small children suspended on their backs in blue woolen blankets held with broad woven bands called "chumbes." The Sherente child of South America is supported by shoulder bands and straddles its mother's hips, or the child sits behind its mother in a sling that is wrapped around its mother's head. Net bags or slings are common carriers among South Pacific Islanders. The Apinayé of South America use carriers in which the infant sits on a girdle wide enough to accommodate it beside its mother's body, while its legs dangle out in front of it. Some carrying methods seem to be the most practical given the circumstances. The Copper Eskimo mother carries her baby inside the hood of her fur parka on the back of her head.

Except in the warmer southern regions, cradles were used as carriers by many native North American tribes. The native North Americans created a device that bound their infants and served as a cradle but primarily as a carrier. These cradles differed in form, technique, and decoration among tribes and regions. The materials used were tree bark, animal skin, flat sticks that were woven into baskets, or dugout wood. Along the north coast of Peru, the baby is also carried on the back of its mother in a small cradle that is made of wood or wild cane. The baby is not bound but is held in by a net that allows it to move its legs freely.

An American adaptation of the shawl carrier in which the infant is held close to the body is the "Snugli™." The Snugli was invented by Ann and Mike Moore of Evergreen, Colorado. In 1964, after arriving home from a Peace Corps assignment in Togo, a country in western Africa, Ann decided to imitate the infant carrier used by the women there for her own children. She noticed that babies carried close to their mothers in a shawl kept quiet, and their mothers were calm. She found the shawl too difficult to manage and asked her mother, Lucy Aukerman, to sew a cloth pouch with waist and shoulder straps. When people saw her using this comfortable carrier they started asking her about it and began requesting carriers for themselves. Almost 30 years later the Snugli, and imitations of it, are as common on the streets of the U.S. as the stroller or carriage.

The baby carriage is a comfortable bed on wheels. It is the most popular mode of transporting young in the West. The baby carriage became popular in England in the mid-19th century. These early carriages were used to pull small children too heavy to carry but too young to walk any distance. Infants were always carried in the arms. The carriages, which were popular with the well-to-do, were pulled by footmen or older children. Those with less money used small chairs on wheels, which were also pulled. Stick wagons were used by poorer families. The stick wagons were heavy and unwieldy and often tipped over. They were pulled by the father. In fact, women did not pull carriages; when they did not have men to help, they carried their babies in their arms.

It was not until the 1840s that the design of the carriage changed from one that was pulled to one that was pushed. These carriages became popular, and it became acceptable for women to be seen pushing them. The first push carriages were intended only for older children to sit up in. Very small infants were still carried in the arms. Then in the 1880s carriages were made that allowed babies to lie down. The style and wheel size of these carriages changed over time, but otherwise these large carriages with rigid bodies remained basically the same for almost 100 years.

These large baby carriages persisted until the 1960s when they were replaced by lightweight, folding carriages that offered a comfortable ride for the baby and could be easily stored in the trunk of the family car. The present-day strollers are all basically the same and come in two varieties: a lightweight umbrella model with few frills and a heavier combination carrier/stroller that converts from a carriage for infants to a stroller in which toddlers can sit up.

A unique variation of the stroller is the "Racing Stroller™." This is a tripod-shaped stroller for jogging parents invented by Phil and Mary Baechler. The Racing Stroller comes in several different models to accommodate different needs. One model is extremely durable and can be used for long jogs; another model is good for jogging in a city. A third model carries twins, and two other models can transport disabled children.

The "Gerry™," a device made of canvas and supported by a metal frame, allows one to carry larger babies on one's back. This doesn't seem to be as popular as the carriers used for smaller infants. Although not based on any hard empirical research, but on my own observations, this type of carrier is typically used by men. Women still seem to be more comfortable with the stroller, especially after the baby is no longer an infant.

Recently, I watched a mother walking down the street holding her baby in what is referred to as a carrier, which is the removable body part of the carriage/stroller. The carrier appeared to be heavy since she had to switch it back and forth from arm to arm. It dangled from her arm, which caused it to occasionally hit against her legs. The baby jumped reflexively with each bump of the carrier. If the baby wasn't being jarred from the bang of the carrier against the mother's leg, it was swinging from the movement of the mother's walk or swinging wildly with each transfer from arm to arm. What an absurd and seemingly uncomfortable way in which to carry a baby. Although there are merits for an attachment that removes easily from a carriage/stroller, walking down a city street is not one of them. With all the varieties of carriers to choose from, this certainly seemed to be the least desirable for both mother and baby.

✱ DIANE D'ALESSANDRO, R.N.

See also: Swaddling

See **Guide to Related Topics:** Baby Care

Resources

Bodnar, Janet & Kalnen, Bertha. (1990, Feb). "Upscale Wheels for the Diaper Set." *Changing Times*: 55-58.

Dick, Diana. (1987). *Yesterday's Babies: A History of Baby Care*. London: The Bodly Head Ltd.

Englblum, Cathie. (1983, Jan 31). "What Has a Pouch, Two Legs and Two Free Hands? A Snugli Parent!" *People*: 60.

Orr, Rachel. (1987, Nov). "Merrily They Roll Along." *Nation's Business*: 65.

Steward, Jilian H. (Ed.) (1963). *Handbook of South American Indians.* New York: Cooper Square Publishers, Inc.

INFANT FEEDING AND CARE: NINETEENTH AND TWENTIETH CENTURIES, UNITED STATES

Infant care practices reflect cultural and societal values, as well as contemporary scientific and technological knowledge. Even seemingly biologically based feeding practices are sensitive to these factors. For centuries, the typical infant diet consisted of milk of the mother or a wet nurse. But with the spread of 18th-century Enlightenment philosophy, infant diet was just one aspect of infant care that changed. Rather than seeing children as miniature adults with an inborn capacity for evil that needed to be disciplined, Enlightenment philosophers depicted children as unformed, highly malleable individuals requiring close care and nurturing, ideally from their mothers. Mothers came to be considered the primary caregivers, directly involved in infant care, rather than supervising baby nurses; most especially, mothers were to nurse their infants. Thus, a new perspective on children led to declining acceptance of wet nursing.

In the 19th century, other factors affected infant care. Employment opportunities in the areas of manufacturing, clerical work, and sales attracted potential wet nurses to other, often more desirable work situations. Moreover, wet nurses and baby nurses were frequently drawn from the lower- or working-class and, after the mid-19th century, immigrant groups. Upper and upper-middle class families and their physician-advisers were less willing to invite such women into their homes.

In the last third of the 19th century, researchers in the emerging specialty of pediatrics focused their attention on infant diet, particularly on the analysis of human milk, in order to determine the best food for babies. Human milk, they found, varied dramatically from woman to woman, with each mother's milk showing significant variation over time. This led some pediatricians to create cow's-milk formulas that they believed would ensure a stable, healthful diet for baby. Manufacturers followed with their own prepared bottle formulas. In this same period, science and medicine were gaining in prestige. Concerned mothers sought the best, most scientific and up-to-date advice for raising their children. Not surprisingly, increasing numbers of women turned to bottle feeding. Some used formulas designed by a physician and prepared in a milk laboratory; others bought prepared infant foods or filled their infants' bottles with condensed, evaporated, or cow's-milk formulas prescribed by a physician or published in an infant care manual or women's magazine.

These alternative information sources suggest a transformation in infant care practices dating from the late 19th century. Infant care was becoming both commercialized and "medicalized." Mothers, perhaps following doctors' orders, could purchase bottles of many designs, rubber nipples (unavailable before the development of vulcanized rubber), and sterilizers.

Feeding equipment was only one small part of the expanding market. With the growth of the commercial sector in American society, manufacturers produced a vast array of items from rattles and diapers to baby carriages. Mass-produced items often replaced domestically produced items; mass production created new products and made more products available to the average consumer. Advertisements in Sears, Roebuck catalogs from the 1890s to the present document the amazing increase in the number and type of products sold for infants and infant care. Commercialization did not sweep away class and ethnic differences, but it did accelerate a homogenization such that today, for example, the overwhelming majority of infants are dressed with disposable diapers.

Furthermore, while previously mothers' information came primarily from family and neighbors, women at the turn of the century could and did turn to many other sources. By the 1890s, the recognition of excessive infant mortality rates spurred governmental and private philanthropic agencies to produce publications and offer classes in proper, scientific infant care for mothers and young girls. As part of their promotions, manufacturers provided infant care advice. Proctor and Gamble, for example, printed and distributed a booklet entitled "How to Bring up a Baby: A Hand Book for Mothers," written by a trained nurse, Elizabeth Robinson Scovil (c.1906, 1920). While describing treatment for a sore throat, the publication also extolled the virtues of Ivory soap. In addition, now mothers found information in the popular press and women's magazines. Furthermore, doctors who had previously seen very few if any pediatric cases redefined their roles to encompass not only treatment of the ill child, but also care of the well one. Pediatricians and general practitioners gave advice on infant feeding, toilet training, bedroom architecture, as well as the care of the sick child. They advised private patients and wrote child care manuals and magazine columns. Additional books and magazines were written by laypersons who often stressed that their advice was based on the latest scientific and medical breakthroughs.

This shift from domestic information networks to medical practitioners and scientific pronouncements reflected the growing stature of science and medicine in American culture. It also arose from demographic and technological changes and medical advances. America is a highly mobile society; family was not always nearby to provide support and advice. Increased urbanization and the developments of extensive railroad systems, the automobile, and the telephone made it easier and less expensive to reach a doctor. Concern for urban milk and food supplies fostered technological solutions to adulteration and improved preservation. Increasingly sophisticated understanding of the germ theory and deficiency diseases added to the physician's success in some areas of treatment and encouraged mothers to depend more on medical advice. By the second decade of this century, regularly scheduled checkups at well-baby clinics and with private physicians were becoming the norm.

Infant care practices in the mid-20th century differed greatly from those of earlier centuries. Infants were fed under supervision of doctors who frequently prescribed bottle feeding as well as orange juice and cod-liver oil for the important vitamins discovered a few decades earlier. Mothers took their children for periodic checkups for immunizations and advice that ranged beyond physical care to the psychological.

Many factors that fostered changes in infant care are with us today. While many worry over the negative effects of commercialization and medicalization, society must be careful to balance this justifiable concern with the obvious benefits, such as immunizations and safe commercial milk, that advances in science and medicine can provide.

✱ RIMA D. APPLE, Ph.D.

See also: Breastfeeding: Historical Aspects; Diapers: Environmental Concerns; Formula Marketing; Nipples, Artificial; Pediatrics, History of

See **Guide to Related Topics:** Baby Care; Infant Feeding

Resources

Apple, Rima D. (1987). *Mothers and Medicine: A Social History of Infant Feeding.* Madison, WI: University of Wisconsin Press.

Cable, Mary. (1975). *The Little Darlings: A History of Child Rearing in America.* New York: Charles Scribner's Sons.

Hoffert, Sylvia D. (1989). *Private Matters: American Attitudes Toward Childbearing and Infant Nurture in the Urban North, 1800-1860.* Urbana, IL: University of Illinois Press.

Ladd-Taylor, Molly. (1986). *Raising a Baby the Government Way: Mothers' Letters to the Children's Bureau, 1915-1932.* New Brunswick, NJ: Rutgers University Press.

McMillen, Sally G. (1990). *Motherhood in the Old South: Pregnancy, Childbirth, and Infant Rearing.* Baton Rouge, LA: Louisiana State University Press.

Meckel, Richard A. (1990). *Save the Babies: American Public Health Reform and the Prevention of Infant Mortality, 1850-1929.* Baltimore: Johns Hopkins University Press.

INFANT FUNERALS: CONTEMPORARY PRACTICES

The Mormon Cemetery in Omaha, Nebraska, contains an impressive statue. A pioneer couple stand together, long cloaks billowing in the wind, the father's hand holding a shovel. As you approach the statue, you realize you are looking directly down into the tiny grave of a baby. Your immediate reaction is to look instantly upward—directly into the faces of the grieving parents. Once seen, it is never forgotten.

In the days of Mormon winter quarters, many babies died. Parents worked together. The mother bathed and dressed her dead baby. The father built a small casket, dug the grave, and held the little box while the mother placed their baby inside. Together they buried their child and mourned.

As society became more industrialized, it became more technical. People got the strange idea that mothers were better off not seeing a dead baby. Everyone else—father, doctor, nurses, funeral directors—could see the baby, but the mother was skirted away, ignored, and forgotten. Later, when she asked questions, did strange things, and worried, society thought *she* was the odd one.

Today the value of grieving for infants is acknowledged, and parent participation in some type of ceremony to say goodbye is encouraged. There are several guidelines that have been found valuable:

- Allow parents to see, hold, touch, and name their baby. Allow them all the time they need. These parents will never sign permission slips for school or put pictures drawn by their child on their refrigerator. The papers they sign concerning the death and funeral of their baby will be the only official acts they perform as parents. They should not be rushed.
- Take pictures—in the nursery, in the hospital room, with the parents, at the funeral home.

- Ask if the parents want their baby baptized. A drop of water in each wedding ring is a meaningful symbol.
- Let parents dress and prepare their baby for the service. Have baby powder and lotion handy.
- Suggest that the parents play baby music during the visitation and before or during the service.
- Encourage the parents to write a letter to their baby, and if they want it read or want to read it at the funeral, make the necessary arrangements.
- Parents need to plan the service, not other relatives. If the mother is hospitalized, a service can be held in her room and the funeral director can go to the hospital instead of insisting that the parents come to the funeral home. Most parents have found it helpful to include their other children in the planning of the service, asking them to draw a picture to put into the casket and letting them see and even hold their little sibling.
- Symbolize saying goodbye. Despite environmentalist concerns, balloon releases are popular. At the cemetery, family members and friends each release a helium balloon into the air. Most importantly, the service belongs to the parents. They deserve all the time and support they need.

✱ JOY JOHNSON

See also: Pregnancy Loss: Family Response; Stillbirth

***See* Guide to Related Topics:** Pregnancy Loss and Infant Mortality

Resources

Eddy, Mary Lou & Raydo, Linda. (1990). *Making Loving Memories.* Omaha, NE: Centering Corporation.

Ferguson, Dorothy. (1990). *Little Footprints: A Memory Book for Babies Who Die.* Omaha, NE: Centering Corporation

Johnson, Joy. (1986). *Newborn Death.* Omaha, NE: Centering Corporation.

S.H.A.R.E. (1989). *Bittersweet, Hello-Goodbye.* Springfield, IL: Prairie Lark Press.

INFANT MORTALITY STATISTICS: UNITED STATES

Infant mortality is an important indicator of the health of a nation, as it is associated with a variety of factors such as maternal health, quality of and access to medical care, socioeconomic conditions, and public health practices (Institute of Medicine, 1985, 1988; Hughes et al., 1989).

Infant mortality is defined as the death of an infant within one year of its birth. Statistics on infant mortality in the United States are derived principally from information reported on death certificates and birth certificates filed in the state vital statistics offices and compiled into a national database by the National Center for Health Statistics (NCHS), a component of the Centers for Disease Control, U.S. Department of Health and Human Services (National Center for Health Statistics, 1989a). In 1988, there were 3,909,510 live births registered in the United States and 38,910 deaths to infants before their first birthday. The infant mortality rate was 10.0 infant deaths per 1,000 live births, the lowest final rate ever recorded in the United States (National Center for Health Statistics, 1990a).

Infant mortality in the United States has declined approximately tenfold since 1900, when approximately one out of 10 infants died within the first year of life (Shapiro, Schlesinger, and Nesbitt, 1968). Infant mortality declined rapidly during the first half of this century. In 1950, the infant mortality rate was 29.2, one-third the 1900 rate. The rate of decline slowed from 1950 to 1964; the 1964 infant mortality rate of 24.8 was only slightly lower than the rate of 1950. Beginning in 1965, the rate of decline in infant mortality increased again, although there is new evidence of a slowdown in the rate of decline since 1980. (See Figure 1.)

Figure 1. Infant Mortality Rates by Race: United States, 1950-88

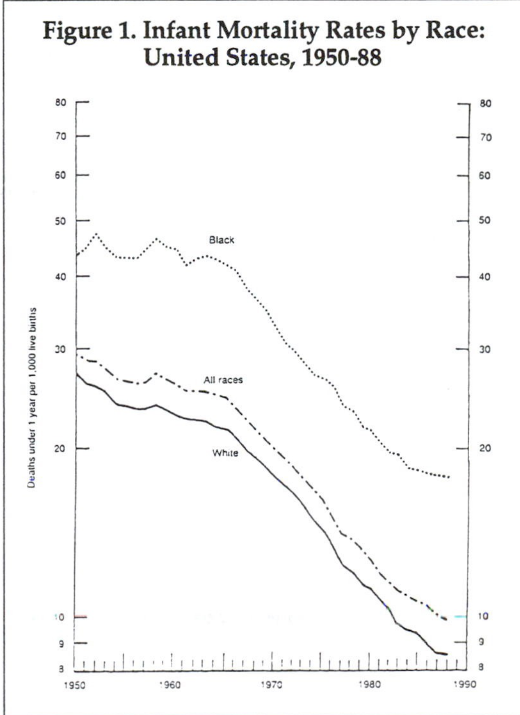

Despite this progress, the international ranking of the United States in infant mortality has fallen from 6th in 1950, to 12th in 1960, to 22nd in 1986 (International Statistics Staff, 1990). In fact, the 1986 infant mortality rate of 10.4 was exactly twice the rate of 5.2 for number one ranked Japan (National Center for Health Statistics, 1990b). This is because, since 1950, infant mortality has declined more rapidly in a number of other countries than in the United States.

Infant deaths are usually divided into two categories according to age: neonatal and postneonatal. Neonatal deaths are those that occur during the first 27 days of life, and postneonatal deaths are those that occur between 28 days and 1 year of age. In 1988, 63.5 percent of all infant deaths occurred during the neonatal period. The neonatal mortality rate was 6.3 deaths for infants under 28 days of age per 1,000 live births, while the postneonatal mortality rate was 3.6 deaths for infants between 28 days and 11 months per 1,000 live births (National Center for Health Statistics, 1990a).

It has generally been believed that different factors influence the child's survival during these two periods. Factors associated with prenatal development, heredity, and the birth process were considered dominant in the neonatal period; environmental factors, such as nutrition, hygiene, and accidents, were considered more important in the postneonatal period. Recently, however, the distinction between these two periods has blurred due in part to advances in neonatology, which have enabled more very small, premature infants to survive the neonatal period (National Center for Health Statistics, 1989b).

Although infant death is now a relatively rare event in the United States, large differentials in the risk of infant death exist between different subgroups of the population. In 1988, the mortality rate for black infants was 17.6 infant deaths per 1,000 live births, more than twice the rate of 8.5 for white infants. The infant mortality rate for male infants was 11.0, almost 25 percent higher than the rate of 8.9 for female infants (National Center for Health Statistics, 1990a).

One of the most important risk factors for infant mortality is low birth weight (a weight of less than 2,500 grams or 5.5 pounds at birth). The risk of infant death is more than 20 times greater for a low birth-weight infant than for a normal birth-weight infant. In fact, about 60 percent of all infant deaths in the United States occur in the less than 7 percent of infants who are born at low birth weight (National Center for Health Statistics, 1990c). Other factors associated with an elevated risk of infant death are teenage childbearing, out-of-wedlock births, late or no prenatal care, and low educational attainment of the mother (Institute of Medicine, 1985, 1988; Hughes et al., 1989).

Since 1979, cause-of-death data in the United States have been classified according to the *International Statistical Classification of Diseases, Ninth Revision*, published by the World Health Organization (World Health Organization, 1977). The 10 leading causes of death to infants are shown in Table 1. In 1988 more than half of all infant deaths in the United States were due to one of the four leading causes of infant death: congenital anomalies, Sudden Infant Death Syndrome, disorders

Table 1. Deaths under 1 Year and Infant Mortality Rates for the 10 Leading Causes of Infant Death: United States, 1988

[Rates per 100,000 live births]

Rank order	*Cause of death* (Ninth Revision International Classification of Diseases, 1975)	*Number*	*Rate*
...	All causes	38,910	995.3
1	Congenital anomalies .740–759	8,141	208.2
2	Sudden infant death syndrome .798.0	5,476	140.1
3	Disorders relating to short gestation and unspecified low birthweight .765	3,268	83.6
4	Respiratory distress syndrome .769	3,181	81.4
5	Newborn affected by maternal complications of pregnancy .761	1,411	36.1
6	Accidents and adverse effects .E800–E949	936	23.9
7	Newborn affected by complications of placenta, cord, and membranes .762	907	23.2
8	Infections specific to the perinatal period .771	878	22.5
9	Intrauterine hypoxia and birth asphyxia .768	777	19.9
10	Pneumonia and influenza .480–487	641	16.4
...	All other causes .Residual	13,294	340.0

relating to short gestation and unspecified low birth weight, and respiratory distress syndrome.

✱ MARIAN MACDORMAN, Ph.D. and
KATE PRAGER, Sc.D.

See also: Low Birth Weight: United States

See **Guide to Related Topics:** Pregnancy Loss and Infant Mortality

Resources

Hughes, Dana et al. (1989). *The Health of America's Children: Maternal and Child Health Data Book.* Washington, DC: Children's Defense Fund.

Institute of Medicine, National Academy of Sciences. (1985). *Preventing Low Birthweight.* Washington, DC: National Academy Press.

———. (1988). *Prenatal Care: Reaching Mothers, Reaching Infants.* Washington, DC: National Academy Press.

International Statistics Staff, National Center for Health Statistics. (1990). "Feto-Infant Mortality Data Base." Unpublished data.

National Center for Health Statistics. (1989a). *Vital Statistics of the United States, 1987, Vol. II, Mortality, Part A.* Hyattsville, MD: Public Health Service.

———. (1989b). Technical Appendix to *Vital Statistics of the United States, 1987, Vol. II, Mortality, Part A.* Hyattsville, MD: Public Health Service.

———. (1990a). "Advance Report of Final Mortality Statistics, 1988." *Monthly Vital Statistics Report 39* (7), supplement. Hyattsville, MD: Public Health Service.

———. (1990b). *Health, United States, 1989.* Hyattsville, MD: Public Health Service.

———. (1990c). *Public Use Data Tape Documentation—Linked Birth/Infant Death Data Set: 1985 Birth Cohort.* Hyattsville, MD: Public Health Service.

Shapiro, Sam, Schlesinger, Edward R., & Nesbitt, Robert, Jr. (1968). *Infant, Perinatal, Maternal, and Childhood Mortality in the United States.* Cambridge, MA: Harvard University Press.

World Health Organization. (1977). *Manual of the International Statistical Classification of Diseases, Injuries, and Causes of Death, Based on the Recommendations of the Ninth Revision Conference, 1975.* Geneva, Switzerland: World Health Organization.

INFANT MOVEMENT

Several groups of researchers, therapists, and educators are looking at infant developmental movement using two different points of view: (1) infant movement as nonverbal communication and (2) infant movement as perceptual, neuromuscular skeletal skill.

The movement an infant makes is a statement of what he or she is experiencing at that moment. This movement statement is projected into the environment and often elicits a response from the environment/caretaker that further influences the infant's experience. Experience leads to movement response that acts as nonverbal communication and elicits a response from the environment that becomes part of the infant's experience. The infant's own movements and the manner in which those movements are perceived partially determine the infant's experience of his or her environment, caretaker, and perception of himself or herself and the world. Either altering those movements or the perception of those movements may influence the child's/caretaker's experience and perceptions of self and other. For example, a child arches backwards when held. The caretaker may perceive that movement as an attempt by the infant to push away from him or her. The caretaker may respond by not holding the baby or by tightening his or her muscles when holding the baby. He or she may feel rejected and may feel rejecting toward the baby. The baby may in turn perceive the caretaker's handling as uncomfortable or may be deprived of stimulation by not being held. The cause of the original movement could simply be that the infant has more tone in the back of the body than in the front of the body and arches backward simply because of the increased tone. This interaction could be changed (1) if the caretaker could view the infant's movement statement differently; (2) if the infant could balance his or her extensor/flexor tone; or (3) if the caretaker could learn how to use body rhythm, tone, or positioning to hold the child more comfortably for them both.

Infant movement can also be viewed as the development of motor ability in terms of perceptual, neuromuscular skeletal coordination, and the way in which motor development patterns the body/mind/emotional system. As the infant moves, myelin, an insulating substance, is laid down along the nerve pathways involved in that particular movement. The more myelin that is laid down along a particular pathway, the easier and faster nerve impulses travel along that pathway and the easier and faster that particular movement pattern becomes. An analogy is the wiring of a house. Once the house is wired, electricity can be used along those pathways. If electricity is needed in other areas, those areas need to be rewired before electricity can be used. In the body, if a new movement pattern is used, a new nerve pathway needs to be found. If that movement pattern is used often enough, those nerves also become myelinated and that movement pattern becomes easier.

In his work with fetal ultrasound, Prechel (de Vries, Vosser, and Prechel, 1986) has discovered fetal movement patterns that are specific and reliably recognizable. He has begun to consider the possibility of developing a prediction scale that could be used to predict babies that are compromised by looking at movement *in utero*; if a fetus does not develop specific complex movements at age-appropriate times that fetus may be compromised.

Advocates of some philosophies of infant motor development look at their role as guiding infants and caretakers through difficult, inefficient, or stuck movement patterns that may pose a problem in later life: For example, if a child is always carried on the hip of the caretaker with one of the infant's hips elevated and rotated, that child may develop a pattern of elevating and rotating that hip; crawling on one foot and one knee; and always leading with one foot and elevating one hip when walking, a pattern that will lead to inefficient movement, decreased performance ability, and most likely injury imbalance or pain.

Advocates of another philosophy of infant motor development look at their role as facilitating the development of self-esteem and independence in infants by helping them to actualize the next step in motor development. The infants can be successful at manipulating their own bodies for their own purposes; they can get the toy they are reaching for, turn from front to back, move across the floor.

Some philosophies advocate developing a super baby, one who has optimal motor patterning, optimal intelligence, and optimal performance ability.

Infant development educators may work with the infants, the caretakers and infants, or the whole family. They may use discussion, role playing, movement, touch, sound, video playback, photography, play, manipulation of the environment, and/or movement patterning in which movement of the infant or the movement interaction between caretaker and infant is physically or verbally guided by the practitioner. Each approach has a unique way of looking at fetal/infant developmental movement patterns.

✱ SANDRA JAMROG, C.C.E., R.M.T., M.A.

See also: Chiropractic Care; Newborn Intelligence; Newborn Senses; Swaddling

See **Guide to Related Topics:** Baby Care

Resources

Cohen, Bonnie Bainbridge. (1989). "The Alphabet of Movement, Part 1 and 2." *The Contact Quarterly* 14 (2): 20-38. The Contact Quarterly, P.O. Box 603, Northampton, MA 01061.

———. (1989). "The Alphabet of Movement, Part 2." *The Contact Quarterly* 14 (3): 23-38. The Contact Quarterly, P.O. Box 603, Northampton, MA 01061.

de Vries, K.I.P., Vosser, G.J.A., and Prechel, H.F.R. (1986). "Fetal Behavior in Early Pregnancy." *European Journal of Obstetrics and Gynecology and Reproductive Biology* 21: 271-76.

Doman, Glenn. (1990). *How to Teach Your Baby to Read.* New York: Random House.

Kestenberg, Judith S. (1975). *Children and Parents.* New York: Jason Aronson.

Lipsitt, L.P. & Rovee-Collier, C.K. (1981). *Advances in Infancy Research, Vol. 1.* Norwood, NJ: Ablex.

———. (1983). *Advances in Infancy Research, Vol. 2.* Norwood, NJ: Ablex

Murphy, James. (1975). "The Use of Non-Verbal and Body Movement Techniques in Working with Families with Infants." *Journal of Material and Family Therapy* 5 (4): 61-111.

Pikler, Emmi. (1988). *Labt Mir Zeit. [Give Me Time.]* Munich: Pflaum Verlag & Co.

Prechel, Heinz F.R. & Hopkins, Brian. (1986). "Developmental Transformations of Spontaneous Movements in Early Infancy." *Early Human Development* 14: 233-38.

Stern, Daniel. (1974). *The First Relationship: Infant and Mother.* Cambridge, MA: Harvard University Press.

INFANTICIDE

Infanticide is any behavior calculated to lead to the death of a baby or child and most commonly refers to killing children under two years of age. Infanticide has been found to exist universally—in every society, on every continent, at every level of cultural complexity. It serves many different functions, but most commonly has been used to control the population, space children, regulate the sex ratio, and eliminate motherless or illegitimate infants, or children with birth defects (Williamson, 1978).

Infanticide generally is practiced for economic reasons, rather than as an expression of hostility or violence. The methods most often used are suffocation, abandonment, and exposure (Williamson, 1978). While other methods have been used (such as poisoning, beating, or stabbing), almost all societies favor more passive methods (Langer, 1974).

Infanticide is most often used to control the population in order to adjust to the economic resources of the society. There are three methods of population control in societies without contraception: sexual abstinence, abortion, or infanticide (Williamson, 1978). While there are some cultures in which sexual abstinence is the norm for certain periods of time (such as while a child is nursing), abstinence is not widely practiced. Many cultures have used abortion techniques for thousands of years, but infanticide is usually more effective and less dangerous to the mother's life. As abortion techniques improve and contraception becomes available in a society, infanticide becomes less prevalent and less socially acceptable.

Population control is a necessary element in almost all societies, as a way of keeping the population within the limits of food production capacity. Infanticide, as a form of population control, has been practiced largely in pre-agricultural societies, in which there exists a delicate balance between food and water resources and the population. These societies often have a strong cultural belief that a child is not fully human until accepted as a member of the social group (from a few days to a few years after birth). Infanticide before social initiation into the group has been considered acceptable (Williamson, 1978). Infanticide has also been used in post-agricultural societies (such as Imperial Japan, pre-Communist China, and medieval Europe) as a method of population control when food production capacities are reached (Langer, 1974).

Infanticide is also used in many societies to space children in a family effectively. Decisions about keeping a child are often made by the parents and are based on considerations such as the number, sex, and age of older siblings; the age of the mother; and the productive capacity of the family as a whole (Williamson, 1978). In many societies, it has been considered acceptable to kill a child if his or her older sibling is still nursing. When the number of children in a family is limited, each child has a better chance of surviving.

By studying sex ratios in a variety of societies, it is clear that infanticide often functions to select children based on their gender. At birth, the ratio of males to females is almost equal. However, in many societies, males are seriously overrepresented in the adult population. While many societies do not engage in systematic sex selection, those that do select against female babies (Miller, 1981). This can be explained by several reasons. Male babies are favored as a productive asset to the family. Also, by selecting against female babies, the number of potential mothers in a society is limited, contributing to population control. Furthermore, female babies can be seen as a drain on family resources. In certain sections of India, for example, female babies of higher castes were killed, in order to avoid payment of the high dowries expected when the child married (Miller, 1981). In the Eskimo culture, hunters are virtually the sole providers of food. Families usually only choose to keep females after they have already had several boys. Also, because Eskimo hunters face many dangers, the sex ratio would quickly become uneven if all female children were allowed to live, and the hunters could not provide for all of the extra women and children (Williamson, 1978). The Eskimo sex selection of children through infanticide results in population control, child spacing, and regulation of the sex ratios.

Babies that are deformed, motherless, or illegitimate have also been killed throughout history. Babies born with birth defects are often killed so that the parents can focus their attention on children with a better chance of growing up. Multiple births, children of mixed race, and children with birth defects have often been considered "bad luck," or a sign of some evil. In many societies, babies whose mothers die are buried with them if no one else can care for the baby.

Illegitimate children are also often killed. Most societies generally disapprove of illegitimate children and do not allow them to take a proper place in the society. Mothers of illegitimate children also often do not have the resources to provide for their children. In Europe and the United States, illegitimate children have composed a large proportion of infanticides. For example, in England in the 13th century, the infant mortality rates of illegitimate children were twice as high as those of legitimate children (Kellum, 1974). As recently as 1887, over 60 percent of all homicides in England and Wales were committed against babies under one year of age, although babies only composed 3 percent of the population overall (Rose, 1986).

Although many studies of infanticide either focus on infanticide in so-called "primitive" cultures (Apthekar, 1931) or on infanticide in Western society (Hoffer and Hull, 1981; Rose, 1986), it is clear that the reasons behind infanticide tend to be similar from society to society. Often economic resources are the determining factor in the decision to keep or not keep a child. However, as abortion becomes medically safer and contraception becomes more widely available and effective in a society, infanticide occurs less often.

✷ JOYA MISRA

See **Guide to Related Topics:** Pregnancy Loss and Infant Mortality

Resources

Apthekar, Herbert. (1931). *Anjea: Infanticide, Abortion, and Contraception in Savage Society.* New York: William Godwin.

Hausfater, Glenn & Hardy, Sarah Blaffer. (Eds.) (1984). *Infanticide: Comparative and Evolutionary Perspectives.* New York: Aldine Publishing.

Hoffer, Peter C. & Hull, N.E.H. (1981). *Murdering Mothers: Infanticide in England and New England 1558-1803.* New York: New York University Press.

Kellum, Barbara. (1974). "Infanticide in England in the Later Middle Ages." *History of Childhood Quarterly: The Journal of Psychohistory 1* (3): 367-88.

Kohl, Marvin. (Ed.) (1987). *Infanticide and the Value of Life.* Buffalo, NY: Prometheus Books.

Langer, William. (1974). "Infanticide: A Historical Survey." *History of Childhood Quarterly: The Journal of Psychohistory 1* (3): 343-65.

Miller, Barbara D. (1981). *The Endangered Sex: Neglect of Female Children in Rural North India*. Ithaca, NY: Cornell University Press.

Rose, Lionel. (1986). *The Massacre of the Innocents: Infanticide in Britain 1800-1839*. London: Routledge and Kegan Paul.

Williamson, Laila. (1978). "Infanticide: An Anthropological Analysis." In Marvin Kohl (Ed.) *Infanticide and the Value of Life*. Buffalo, NY: Prometheus Books.

INFERTILITY: CROSS-CULTURAL AND HISTORICAL ASPECTS

There are wide variations in the incidence of infertility throughout the world. Infertility rates range from as low as 1.5 percent in Thailand to as high as 42.5 percent in some parts of Africa (Belsey and Ware, 1986). It is not clear what accounts for such vast differences, but one reason is almost certainly variations in the prevalence of sexually transmitted diseases.

Virtually all childlessness in traditional societies is due to infertility (Poston and Trent, 1984). Not all cultures share the same definition of what it means to be childless. In traditional Korea and Taiwan, where a son was required to ensure family continuity, having no sons had virtually the same social consequences as being childless (Pasternak, 1972).

Infertility has been attributed to many causes (Greil, 1991). The Aowin people of Ghana diagnose infertility as being due to witchcraft, to nonobservance of prescribed behavior, to disrupted social relationships, or to quarrels between matrilineal kin (Ebin, 1982). Most cultures have viewed infertility as primarily a woman's problem.

Cultures vary widely with regard to their beliefs about appropriate solutions for infertility (Greil, 1991). In many societies, men whose wives have borne no children may legitimately divorce them. In a number of cultures, a man whose wife has had no children may take a second wife. Cures for infertility open to the traditional Taiwanese peasant woman included making appeals to the gods, consulting a diviner to read her "flower fortune," trying herbal remedies, and adopting a female child in order to encourage the birth of a son (Wolf and Huang, 1980). In some cultures adoption has been so common that up to half of all households have included adopted children.

People throughout the world stigmatize the infertile. Among the Ashanti of Africa, an infertile man is called "wax penis" (Rattray, 1923). The South American Cagaba refer to an infertile woman as a "mule" (Tschopik, 1951). Sandelowski (1990) suggests that, in America, the infertile have long been and still are held responsible for their own problems.

The recent history of infertility in America and Europe is primarily a history of the gradual replacement of traditional modes of understanding and dealing with infertility by a medical model (Greil, 1991). Throughout the 19th century, the infertile looked to accoucheurs (birth attendants) and gynecologists for relief from infertility, but these professionals did not have a lot to offer. The repertoire of cures offered to infertile women in the first half of the 19th century included "change of air," sea bathing, sexual abstinence, and rest (Lewis, 1986). From the mid-19th century through the early 20th century, most cases of female infertility were attributed to displacements of the uterus or to cervical stenosis, an abnormal narrowing of the cervical canal. These conditions were treated sometimes with surgery and sometimes with more conservative means (McLane and McLane, 1969).

What did the infertile do in the absence of effective medical treatment? Some women continued to use some of the herbal remedies employed in the 18th century. Some may have used patent medicines like Lydia Pinkham's "Vegetable Compound," which advertised, "There's a baby in every bottle" (Stage, 1979). Reliance on nonmedical cures for infertility continued well into the 20th century; in the 1930s, hundreds of sterile women took away "magic pebbles" from the courtyard of the home of the Dionne quintuplets in the hope of bearing a child (Gebhard, 1976). Because parents often died before the end of their childrearing years, because apprenticeship of young children was quite common, and because working mothers often placed young children in the homes of both relatives and strangers, people interested in raising children not biologically their own were likely to find it relatively easy to do so in the 19th century.

The development of modern conceptions of reproductive technology in the 1920s and 1930s did not have much practical impact on the treatment of infertility until the mid-1960s. In the 1950s, the most effective treatment for infertility in the minds of many ob/gyns was still to "let nature take her course." This attitude was reinforced by the widespread acceptance of Therese Benedek's theory that infertility, like other feminine complaints, was emotional rather than medical in its origins (Ehrenreich and English, 1979).

The early 1960s saw the first clinical trials of drugs that proved very effective in dealing with ovulatory problems. By the end of the decade, ovulation problems had gone from being intractable to being highly solvable, so much so that it was in this area of fertility treatment that the highest pregnancy rates were being achieved. Since that time, medical technology for treating infertility has expanded dramatically, as has the demand for services (Aral and Cates, 1983; Scritchfield, 1989; Greil, 1991).

Recent social trends have acted to sharpen the demand for infertility services. The tendency on the part of middle-class American couples to delay childbearing has meant that a larger proportion of middle-class couples are childless than has been the case in the past. The trend toward delayed childbearing has meant that many women are now discovering their infertility at an older age when less time remains on the "biological clock." The advent of birth control technology may have given the infertile a stronger sense that conception is something that can be conquered via technology. Increased media attention to the issue of infertility helps to popularize the view that infertility is something that can now be brought under control. Increased demand for medical services may also be related to the decreasing availability of nonmedical solutions to the problem of involuntary childlessness, such as adoption.

Several factors have affected the availability of providers of medical services for infertility. A decline in the fertility rate has resulted in a drop in demand for obstetrical services. When the supply of obstetricians exceeds the demand, ob/gyns may be inclined to specialize in other kinds of services. Other reasons why some ob/gyns are drifting away from obstetrics include concern over the rising cost of malpractice insurance, greater reluctance to be on call at night, and increasing specialization in medicine generally. Physicians may also have been encouraged to devote increased attention to infertility by the increased prestige that has come to infertility as a specialty as a result of publicity surrounding *in vitro* fertilization and other "high-tech" treatments.

✱ ARTHUR L. GREIL, Ph.D.

See also: Infertility: Overview; Infertility: Social and Demographic Aspects

See **Guide to Related Topics:** Infertility

Resources

Aral, Sevgi O. & Cates, Willard, Jr. (1983). "The Increasing Concern with Infertility: Why Now?" *Journal of the American Medical Association 250*: 2327-31.

Belsey, M.A. & Ware, Helen. (1986). "Epidemiological, Social and Psychosocial Aspects of Infertility." In Vaclav Insler and Bruno Lunenfeld (Eds.) *Infertility: Male and Female.* Edinburgh, Scotland: Churchill Livingstone, pp. 631-47.

Ebin, V. (1982). "Interpretations of Infertility: The Aowin People of Southwest Ghana." In Carol P. MacCormack (Ed.) *Ethnography of Fertility and Birth.* London: Academic Press, pp. 141-59.

Ehrenreich, Barbara & English, Deirdre. (1979). *For Her Own Good: 150 Years of the Experts' Advice to Women.* Garden City, NY: Anchor.

Gebhard, Bruno. (1976). "The Interrelationship of Scientific and Folk Medicine in the United States of America since 1850." In Wayland D. Hand (Ed.) *American Folk Medicine: A Symposium.* Berkeley, CA: University of California Press, pp. 87-97.

Greil, Arthur L. (1991). *Not Yet Pregnant: Infertile Couples in Contemporary America.* New Brunswick, NJ: Rutgers University Press.

Lewis, Judith Schneid. (1986). *In the Family Way: Childbearing in the British Aristocracy, 1760-1860.* New Brunswick, NJ: Rutgers University Press.

McLane, Charles M. & McLane, Midy. (1969). "A Half Century of Sterility 1840-1890." *Fertility and Sterility 20*: 853-70.

Pasternak, Burton. (1972). *Kinship and Community in Two Chinese Villages.* Stanford, CA: Stanford University Press.

Poston, Dudley L., Jr. & Trent, Katherine. (1984). "Modernization and Childlessness in the Developing World." *Comparative Social Research 7*: 133-53.

Rattray, R.S. (1923). *Ashanti.* Oxford, England: Clarendon Press.

Sandelowski, Margaret. (1990). "Fault Lines: Infertility and Imperiled Sisterhood." *Feminist Studies 16*: 33-51.

Scritchfield, Shirley A. (1989). "The Social Construction of Infertility: From Private Matter to Social Concern." In J. Best (Ed.) *Images of Issues: Typifying Contemporary Social Problems.* New York: Aldine de Gruyter, pp. 99-114.

Stage, Sarah. (1979). *Female Complaints: Lydia Pinkham and the Business of Women's Medicine.* New York: Norton.

Tschopik, Harry, Jr. (1951). "The Aymara of Chucuito, Peru: Magic." *Anthropological Papers of the American Museum of Natural History 44*: 133-308.

Wolf, Arthur P. & Huang, Chieh-shan. (1980). *Marriage and Adoption in China, 1845-1945.* Stanford, CA: Stanford University Press.

INFERTILITY: DIAGNOSIS AND TREATMENT

A couple is considered infertile if they fail to conceive after trying for 12 months. The Office of Technology Assessment (U.S. Congress, 1988, 4, 51) found that 8.5 percent of all U.S. couples aged 15 to 44 were infertile. Primary infertility means the couple never had a child; secondary infertility means that they cannot conceive now, despite having had one or more biological children. Some 35 percent of infertility cases can be traced to the female partner, 35 percent to the male, and 20 percent to both; 10 percent of the cases are untraceable (idiopathic) (Bellina and Wilson, 1985, xvi).

Self Diagnosis and Treatment.

Intercourse. Be sure to do intercourse correctly. When trying to conceive, it is important for couples to remember that there is a correct way to have sexual intercourse. It may be helpful to consult and follow instructions in a sex education manual.

Ovulation regularity. It is helpful for a woman trying to conceive to find out if she ovulates regularly by taking basal body temperature and checking cervical mucus for several months (Berger, Goldstein and Fuerst, 1989, p. 114). (*See* "Natural Family Planning.") If she is not ovulating, she can first try to improve her lifestyle through moderate exercise, good diet, and abstention from smoking and drug use.

Ovulation timing. The woman trying to conceive should pinpoint ovulation in advance, using an over-the-counter test, and then time sexual intercourse to coincide. It can be beneficial to vary intercourse frequency within the fertile period: more frequent (twice in one night) or less frequent (every three days), with partial (not total) abstention otherwise.

Lubrication. Couples trying to conceive should not use lubricants, jellies, or cremes during intercourse. If lubrication is really necessary, saliva or egg white can be used.

Douching. A woman trying to conceive should never use a douche before or after intercourse but should instead rest and relax for at least 20 minutes following intercourse.

Minimally Invasive Professional Diagnosis and Treatment.

Screening for infections. Both partners should be tested for sexually transmitted diseases and yeast infections (using blood tests and swabbings from the vagina and cervix) (*see* "Sexually Transmitted Diseases") and should use the antibiotics or cremes prescribed. If all findings are negative and the woman ovulates regularly, she should ask for a two-week prescription of a broad-spectrum antibiotic like doxycycline or tetracycline, and then be tested for disease organisms again three months later.

Semen analysis. The male partner should get a semen analysis. If results are abnormal, and the woman ovulates regularly, then the woman should not seek any additional medical treatment while her partner is being treated (however, treatments for "male factor" are not very effective).

Post-coital (Sims-Huhner) test (PCT). If possible, couples wishing to conceive should have sexual intercourse close to the ovulation date and then go to the doctor within six hours. Swabs taken from the cervix will reveal whether sperm are actively moving in the thin and elastic mucus (Bellina and Wilson, 1985, pp. 161-65; Frisch and Rapoport, 1987, pp. 110-12; Berger, Goldstein, and Fuerst, 1989, pp. 107-09).

Artificial insemination. Even with poor semen, artificial insemination with the partner's sperm sometimes works, and if the male has an extremely low count or no sperm at all, donor sperm may succeed. If the PCT shows poor sperm activity in the cervical mucus, then intrauterine insemination (insertion of semen via the cervix directly into the uterus) may work (Berger, Goldstein and Fuerst, 1989, pp. 226-28). (*See* "Donor Insemination.")

Steroid hormone blood tests. Both partners should have these (unfortunately expensive) tests. The woman's testing should occur three times during her menstrual cycle, and should include LH, FSH, estrogen, progesterone, and prolactin (Bellina and Wilson, 1985, pp. 159-61; Berger, Goldstein, and Fuerst, 1989, pp. 115-17). These tests help locate a problem in ovaries or in the pituitary gland (which controls ovary functioning).

Fertility drug treatment. If the sperm are viable but the woman is not ovulating, a doctor may prescribe a fertility drug to induce ovulation. The most common such drugs have been clomiphene citrate (Clomid,® an estrogen mimic), pure follicle-stimulating hormone (FSH), and menotropin (Pergonal®, a mix of luteinizing hormone and FSH, extracted from the urine of menopausal women). Pure FSH and Pergonal® are expensive and need closer monitoring than Clomid®. Now various mimics of a hormone produced by the hypothalamus, the gonadotropin-releasing hormone, are often used to induce ovulation. Also, bromocriptine (an ergot derivative) may be prescribed when the pituitary gland produces too much prolactin. All of these drugs have side effects (Holmes, 1988, pp. 37-52; Klein and Rowland, 1988; Scialli, 1988). To avoid multiple pregnancies, it is advisable for the woman to ask the doctor to use very low doses. She should never exceed the prescribed dose and should watch out for side effects including moodiness. Intercourse should be timed to the induced ovulation time.

Drug treatment for endometriosis. If endometriosis is the problem, drug treatment is less invasive than surgery, but usually less effective. Drugs used, especially Danazol, have side effects. (*See* "Endometriosis.")

Ultrasonography. Clinicians may use an ultrasound probe that sends sound waves through the abdominal wall, but more commonly they will use a vaginal probe. The ultrasound picture on a video screen may reveal how eggs are developing in the ovary. Adverse effects of diagnostic ultrasound have not been reported; studies performed thus far were not designed to detect such effects (Dunn, 1985; Scialli, 1988).

Invasive Professional Diagnosis and Treatment. Whatever the invasive treatment, it is wise for the woman to have her partner or a friend with her, at the very least after treatment, but also before and during treatment if possible. It is also useful to ask the doctor to provide the name of a previous patient willing to talk about what to expect: pain, drugs used, attitude of nurses, etc. Although tranquilizers should be avoided whenever possible, their use during these procedures may be advisable. The woman and her doctor should clear up all genital infections before any invasive procedure.

Endometrial biopsy (EB). This test detects luteal phase defect, i.e., whether the uterus lining (the endometrium) is ready for an embryo to implant (Bellina and Wilson, 1985, pp. 165-66). It also monitors fertility drug effectiveness. EB is a painful office procedure timed during the luteal phase of the menstrual cycle, one to four days before expected menstruation (American Fertility Society, 1986, p. 8; Wild, Sanfilippo, and Toledo, 1986; Berger, Goldstein, and Fuerst, 1989, 141-42). The doctor grasps the cervix with a tenaculum, inserts a tube into the uterus, and scrapes some cells from the endometrium. Because of the pain, EB may be done along with another test that requires anesthesia. Later side effects are uterine cramping and sometimes bleeding (Brown and Kammeyer, 1986). Risks of EB include false positive results (leading to unnecessary drug treatment), uterine perforation, passage of vaginal infections into the uterus, and abortion of an embryo starting to implant (Brown and Kammeyer, 1986; Wild, Sanfilippo, and Toledo, 1986; Holmes, 1988; Scialli, 1988).

Hysteroscopy. This procedure is performed to reveal and possibly correct defects inside the uterus. A hysteroscope (a thin optical tube with another channel for instruments) is passed through the cervix, after the doctor distends the uterus with a gas or a sugar solution. The patient usually has general anesthesia—often a laparoscopy is also performed. Hysteroscopy can reveal fibroids, intrauterine scarring (Asherman's syndrome) (Frisch and Rapoport, 1987, pp. 139-401; Pellicer, 1988), and partitions in the uterus; these structures may be excised through the scope (Siegler and Lindemann, 1984; Scialli, 1988). Risks of hysteroscopy (and most surgery) include: blood vessel puncture, hemorrhage (during the procedure or later), anesthesia accidents, allergic reactions, pelvic infections, and uterine perforation. Rare complications specific to hysteroscopy result from the distending medium: embolism, heart rhythm changes, water in the lungs, and rupture of a Fallopian tube (Bellina and Wilson, 1985, pp. 173-74; Holmes, 1988, p. 27; Scialli, 1988).

Hysterosalpingography (HSG). After injection of an x-ray opaque dye through the cervical canal, HSG is the x-ray or fluoroscope monitoring of the Fallopian tubes to check for blockage (American Fertility Society, 1986, pp. 14-15; Wolf and Spatano, 1988; Berger, Goldstein, and Fuerst, 1989, pp. 134-35). To minimize the excruciating pain during injection, throughout the procedure, and afterwards, patients often receive analgesics or tranquilizers (Acton, Devitt, and Ryan, 1988). Risks include oil droplets traveling to the lungs, granular tumors in the tubes, false positives, false negatives, radiation damage to the ovaries, adhesions (Bellina and Wilson, 1985, p. 137), and internal spread of vaginal infections (Holmes, 1988, pp. 22-23). Usually HSG correctly detects blocked tubes (Snowden, Jarret, and Dawood, 1984); patients occasionally become pregnant right afterwards (Acton, Devitt, and Ryan, 1988).

Uterotubal insufflation. To check for Fallopian tube blockage, the doctor pumps carbon dioxide gas into the uterus via the cervix and then listens with a stethoscope to hear whether the gas escapes from the tubes. Shoulder pain also indicates that gas is passing through (American Fertility Society, 1986, p. 13; Scialli, 1988).

Laparoscopy. In this procedure, a laparoscope, a fiber optic telescope, is inserted through the abdomen near the navel to detect adhesions or endometriosis on pelvic organs, to retrieve eggs, and to perform chromotubation and certain surgeries (Bellina and Wilson, 1985, pp. 174-78; American Fertility Society, 1986, p. 16; Berger, Goldstein, and Fuerst, 1989, p. 137-42). Shoulder pain afterwards comes from pneumoperitoneum—the filling up of the abdomen with gas under pressure to push up the abdominal wall—which is necessary for egg retrieval and laser surgery. Chromotubation (or hydrotubation), like HSG, involves injecting dye through the cervix (dye escaping from the Fallopian tubes is observed through the laparoscope). Risks of laparoscopy include those from anesthesia, such as vomiting, allergic reactions, and respiratory arrest, and those from surgery, such as hemorrhage, organ perforation, adhesions, and infection (sometimes resurgence of pelvic inflammatory disease) (Dugan, 1985; Holmes, 1988, pp. 29-33; Scialli, 1988).

Laser and microsurgery. Surgery under a microscope often succeeds in reversing tubal ligation, rebuilding damaged tubes, and removing tissue of endometriosis. A laser is faster and does less damage to surrounding tissues than scalpel surgery. Sometimes lasers can be used via a laparoscope or through the cervix (to remove fibroids or partitions in the uterus); however, most laser and microsurgery requires an abdominal incision (Bellina and Wilson, 1985, ch. 24; Berger, Goldstein, and Fuerst, 1989, pp. 192-204).

* HELEN BEQUAERT HOLMES, Ph.D.

See also: Infertility: Overview
See **Guide to Related Topics:** Infertility

Resources

Acton, Christine M., Devitt, Jacinta M., & Ryan, Elizabeth A. (1988). "Hysterosalpingography in Infertility—An Experience of 3,631 Examinations." *Australia and New Zealand Journal of Obstetrics and Gynaecology 28*: 127-33.

American Fertility Society (AFS). (1986). *Investigation of the Infertile Couple.* Birmingham, AL: American Fertility Society.

Bellina, Joseph H. & Wilson, Josleen. (1985). *You Can Have a Baby: Everything You Need to Know about Fertility.* New York: Crown Publishers, Inc.

Berger, Gary S., Goldstein, Marc, & Fuerst, Mark. (1989). *The Couple's Guide to Fertility: How New Medical Advances Can Help You Have a Baby.* New York: Doubleday.

Brown, F.H. & Kammeyer, S.E. (1986). "Office Gynecologic Procedures." *Primary Care 13* (3): 493-511.

Dugan, Kathleen. (1985). "Diagnostic Laparoscopy Under Local Anesthesia for Evaluation of Infertility." *Journal of Gynecologic and Neonatal Nursing 14* (5): 363-66.

Dunn, F. (1985). "A Brief Provacative Statement on Ultrasound Bioeffects." *Ultrasound in Medicine and Biology 11*: L95-96.

Frisch, Melvin J. & Rapoport, Gayle. (1987). *Getting Pregnant: Over 1,000 of the Most Important Questions and Answers about Fertility Problems and How to Have a Baby.* Tucson, AZ: The Body Press.

Holmes, Helen Bequaert. (1988). "Risks of Infertility Diagnosis and Treatment." In Vol. IV: Social and Medical Concerns, Contractor Documents, for Congress of the United States, Office of Technology Assessment. *Infertility: Medical and Social Choices.* Washington, DC: U.S. Government Printing Office.

Klein, Renate & Rowland, Robyn. (1988). "Women as Test-sites for Fertility Drugs: Clomiphene Citrate and Hormonal Cocktails." *Reproductive and Genetic Engineering 1* (3): 251-73.

Pellicer, Antonio. (1988). "Hysteroscopy in the Infertile Woman." *Obstetrics and Gynecology Clinics of North America 15* (1): 99-105.

Scialli, Anthony R. (1988). "Risks of Infertility Diagnosis and Treatment." In Vol. IV: Social and Medical Concerns, Contractor Documents, for Congress of the United States, Office of Technology Assessment. *Infertility: Medical and Social Choices.* Washington, DC: U.S. Government Printing Office.

Siegler, A.M. & Lindemann, H.J. (Eds.) (1984). *Hysteroscopy: Principles and Practice.* Philadelphia: J.B. Lippincott.

Snowden, E.U., Jarret, J.C., & Dawood, M.Y. (1984). "Comparison of Diagnostic Accuracy of Laparoscopy, Hysteroscopy, and Hysterosalpingography in Evaluation of Female Infertility." *Fertility and Sterility 41*: 709.

U.S. Congress, Office of Technology Assessment. (1988). *Infertility: Medical and Social Choices.* Washington, DC: U.S. Government Printing Office.

Wild, R.A., Sanfilippo, J.S., & Toledo, A.A. (1986). "Endometrial Biopsy in the Infertility Investigation: The Experience at Two Institutions." *The Journal of Reproductive Medicine 31* (10): 954-57.

Wolf, David M. & Spatano, Robert F. (1988). "The Current State of Hysterosalpingography." *RadioGraphics 8* (6): 1041-58.

INFERTILITY: OVERVIEW

Approximately 2.3 million American couples are infertile—unable to conceive or carry a pregnancy to term after one year of unprotected intercourse. Hormonal, structural, genetic, environmental, and immunological factors can cause infertility, as can infections and lifestyle. In approximately 30 percent of the cases, male infertility is a major factor, and in another 20 percent, a contributing factor.

The most common causes of infertility in women are ovulatory problems, blocked or damaged Fallopian tubes, and endometriosis. In men, the most common causes of infertility are problems with sperm quality or production; these problems may result from hormonal imbalances or such structural problems as varicoceles (varicose veins of the testes) or obstructions in the vas deferens or epididymis that prevent sperm from reaching the testis and/or the penis.

Other important but less common causes of infertility in both sexes include genetic or chromosomal abnormalities and environmental factors, such as exposure to diethylstilbestrol (DES) *in utero* or to radiation. Infertility can also result from excessive exercise, weight loss, weight gain, drug or alcohol use, as well as sexually transmitted diseases and other infections.

Physical causes can be found in approximately 95 percent of the cases of infertility. Psychological factors may play a role in a man's ability to have or maintain an erection, or in a couple's frequency or timing of intercourse. However, there is no scientific evidence to prove that psychological or emotional factors cause infertility. Although stress can sometimes interfere with ovulation, fertility drugs easily correct for stress-induced ovulatory problems. Stress is primarily the *result*, not the *cause*, of infertility.

Male infertility should be diagnosed and treated by a urologist who has had special training in male-factor infertility or by an andrologist (a physician who specializes in male reproduction). Women ideally should be diagnosed and treated by a fertility specialist who is a reproductive endocrinologist (usually an ob/gyn with specialized postgraduate training in reproduction). Although most ob/gyns have some training in female infertility, they do not have the necessary expertise to diagnose and treat many of the more difficult cases. Unfortunately, there are fewer than 400 certified reproductive endocrinologists in the United States, and they are usually located in large urban areas and medical centers. If a reproductive endocrinologist is unavailable, the next best choice would be an ob/gyn who has a special interest in, and devotes at least 50 percent of his or her practice to, infertility.

Regardless of who has the fertility problem, the woman is usually treated alone or in conjunction with her partner. Fertility or ovulation-inducing drugs are usually the first course of treatment when structural problems are ruled out. A woman with or without ovulatory problems may be able to conceive even when her partner has a low sperm count if her fertility is enhanced with these drugs. They are relatively safe as long as the patient is carefully monitored by her physician. Fertility drugs are also occasionally prescribed by urologists for men.

Infertility caused by a blocked tube or endometriosis in a woman, or a varicocele or vasectomy in a man, is often successfully treated surgically. However, any surgical procedure not only carries the risks of postsurgical infection, but complications from the general anesthesia and the surgery itself. Another option for blocked tubes is *in vitro* fertilization (IVF); previously a surgical procedure, it is now done under local anesthesia. In IVF, eggs are retrieved vaginally under ultrasound guidance and mixed with sperm in a test tube or Petri dish, where fertilization takes place. The resulting embryos (no more than four) are then transferred to the woman's uterus through her vagina. Additional embryos can be frozen (cryopreserved) for future use. IVF is also now recommended for endometriosis, unexplained infertility, and male-factor infertility when traditional treatments fail.

GIFT (gamete intrafallopian tube transfer), a surgical procedure, is sometimes done in place of IVF if the woman has healthy Fallopian tubes. For these women, GIFT seems to have a higher success rate than IVF. In GIFT, the sperm and egg, before they fertilize, are surgically placed in a Fallopian tube—the place where fertilization occurs under normal circumstances.

Donor eggs can be used when a woman no longer ovulates or has a genetic condition she does not want to risk passing on to her offspring. The donor takes fertility drugs, then has the egg removed vaginally as in IVF. The egg is mixed with the recipient's husband's sperm (donor sperm can also be used), and the embryo is transferred vaginally into the recipient's uterus. She, if successful, will then carry and give birth to a baby not genetically related to her. The donor can be anonymous, or a friend or relative, depending on a woman's or couple's preference and a program's philosophy.

Artificial insemination with donor sperm can be done when a man has too few or no sperm, or his sperm are incapable of fertilizing his partner's egg. Most physicians will only deal with anonymous, frozen sperm (freezing helps protect against AIDS), and many refuse to inseminate unmarried or lesbian women. These women, and those wishing to use known donors, often successfully inseminate themselves with sterilized syringes. However, because fresh sperm are used, there is the risk of contracting AIDS unless the donor is carefully screened.

The newest treatment for male infertility is micromanipulation (or microfertilization) of the sperm. In this procedure, still in its experimental stage, a few sperm are microsurgically placed directly into the zona (outside layer) of an egg. When perfected, this procedure will theoretically make it possible for a man with very few sperm to fertilize his partner's egg.

Couples who insist on some genetic connection to their child might also opt for surrogate motherhood (which allows the couple to have a child genetically related to the husband) or a surrogate carrier (which allows a couple to have a child genetically related to both of them). These options, however, present legal, ethical, and social issues that differ from donor eggs and sperm in that they require one woman to go through the experience and risks of pregnancy and childbirth for the benefit of another. Many couples who fail to conceive are able to successfully resolve their infertility by adopting or remaining childless.

✱ JOAN LIEBMANN-SMITH

See also: DES: Diethylstilbestrol; Donor Insemination; Egg Retrieval; Endometriosis; *In Vitro* Fertilization for Male Infertility; Infertility: Cross-Cultural and Historical Aspects; Infertility: Diagnosis and Treatment; Infertility: Social and

Demographic Aspects; Pelvic Inflammatory Disease

See **Guide to Related Topics:** Infertility; New Procreative Technologies

Resources

Andrews, Lori B. (1984). *New Conceptions.* New York: St. Martin's Press.

Liebmann-Smith, Joan. (1989). *In Pursuit of Pregnancy.* New York: Newmarket.

Stangel, John J., (1988). *The New Fertility and Conception: The Essential Guide for Childless Couples.* New York: New American Library.

INFERTILITY: SOCIAL AND DEMOGRAPHIC ASPECTS

Infertility is the inability to conceive a child or to successfully carry a child to term. Most medical specialists consider a couple to be infertile if they have failed to conceive after 12 months of unprotected intercourse. Using this definition, the National Survey of Family Growth found that 2.3 million married couples were infertile in 1988 (Mosher and Pratt, 1990). This figure represents 7.9 percent of all married couples at that time. Several studies conducted in England have shown that anywhere from 24 to 28 percent of women there have had difficulty conceiving at some point in their lives.

In approximately 80 to 90 percent of couples who present themselves for medical treatment, it is possible to discover a clear medical reason (or reasons) for a couple's infertility. Although the general public tends to see infertility as the woman's problem, the man or the woman or both may have the reproductive impairment. Most studies of people attending infertility clinics have reported that a male factor is involved in from 20 to 40 percent of those cases where a cause for the failure to conceive can be identified.

Medical practitioners generally differentiate between "primary infertility" (involuntary childlessness) and "secondary infertility" (infertility experienced by couples who already have at least one biological child). Primary infertility accounts for only 30 percent of infertility among American couples (Hirsch and Mosher, 1987).

Increased media coverage in recent years has given the impression that the incidence of infertility has been rising dramatically. In fact, this is not the case. The incidence of infertility actually declined from 3.0 million in 1965 to 2.4 million in 1982, where it has remained. On the other hand, the number of childless infertile couples doubled from .5 million to 1.0 million in the same time period (Mosher, 1987; Mosher and Pratt, 1990). Since female fertility declines with increasing age, the current trend in American society toward delayed childbearing means that a larger percentage of infertile couples than before are childless when they discover their infertility. Because the tendency to delay childbearing is most pronounced among those with greater educational and occupational attainment (Rindfuss, Bumpass, and St. John, 1980) the trend toward an increasing proportion of cases of primary infertility is occurring primarily among the white middle class.

Of the women identified as infertile in 1988, 58.7 percent reported that they had been to a physician or a clinic to seek treatment (Mosher and Pratt, 1990). Women with primary infertility are approximately twice as likely as those with secondary infertility to seek treatment. While reproductive impairments are actually more common among blacks and those with lower incomes, it is whites and those with higher incomes who are most likely to seek treatment (Mosher, 1982; Hirsch and Mosher, 1987; Kalmuss, 1987).

The proportion of infertile women who have decided to seek medical treatment has increased dramatically in recent years. Office visits for infertility almost tripled between 1968 and 1984, rising from about 600,000 to about 1.6 million over 16 years. Office visits for men have remained at virtually the same level as before (U.S. Congress, 1988).

Social and Emotional Consequences. Infertility is a health problem that can have far-reaching effects on life satisfaction, well-being, and psychological adjustment (Mazor and Simons, 1984; Salzer, 1986; Lasker and Borg, 1987; Menning, 1988; Shapiro, 1988; Greil, 1991). In American society, parenthood is seen as an integral part of the transition to adult status. Studies of American women show that approximately 90 to 95 percent see childlessness as an undesirable state for themselves and for others. Because of the great importance attached to the childbearing and parenting roles, infertility can become the symbol of a catastrophic role failure. Some authors have likened the response of the infertile couple to grief.

Infertility can come to permeate every aspect of the lives of the infertile, especially infertile women. Television commercials, chance encounters with passers-by, conversations at work, and insensitive comments by friends and relatives all serve to dramatize for the infertile their involuntary exile from normalcy. In response, many attempt to withdraw from the world by avoiding situations where they are likely to be reminded of their infertility. Feeling that only those who share their experience are really equipped to understand, many infertile women and men turn to infertile friends and to self-help groups like Resolve, Inc., for support.

The infertile also find that treatment regimens take over their lives. Treatment of infertility is often expensive, time-consuming and invasive. The infertile often experience infertility as a chronic condition that never seems to leave. On the other hand, few infertile people are ever told they have no chance to conceive. The fact that many of the infertile have a realistic hope for a child can make infertility hard to accept and can lead the infertile, especially infertile women, to become very treatment-oriented. Medical practitioners often attend to the medical aspects of infertility without paying sufficient attention to the social and emotional aspects. Concerns about feelings of loneliness and of failure are sometimes acknowledged but are rarely addressed.

There is now considerable evidence to suggest that infertility is experienced differently by women and men. Women are more likely than men to experience infertility as a devastating threat to identity, about which they think often and from which they cannot easily escape. Husbands, especially those without reproductive impairments, are more likely to regard infertility as an unfortunate circumstance, but as one that can be put into perspective and dealt with. For many couples, these gender-based differences in the experience of infertility are one source of frustration and tension within the couple relationship. Women sometimes see their partners as callous and unaffected by infertility, while men sometimes see their partners as "overreacting" and unable to put things in perspective.

Tension within the couple often has a major impact on sexuality. The need to schedule intercourse often removes the spontaneity and romance from it. Infertile couples sometimes feel that the treatment regimen invades their privacy. The act of intercourse itself can become a potent reminder of the couple's inability to conceive.

✱ ARTHUR L. GREIL, Ph.D.

See also: Infertility: Cross-Cultural and Historical Aspects; Infertility: Diagnosis and Treatment; Infertility: Overview

See **Guide to Related Topics:** Infertility

Resources

Greil, Arthur L. (1991). *Not Yet Pregnant: Infertile Couples in Contemporary America.* New Brunswick, NJ: Rutgers University Press.

Hirsch, Marilyn B. & Mosher, William D. (1987). "Characteristics of Infertile Women in the United States and Their Use of Fertility Services." *Fertility and Sterility 47*: 618-25.

Kalmuss, Deborah S. (1987). "The Use of Infertility Services among Fertility-impaired Couples." *Demography 24*: 575-85.

Lasker, Judith N. & Borg, Susan. (1987) *In Search of Parenthood: Coping with Infertility and High-Tech Conception.* Boston: Beacon.

Mazor, Miriam D. & Simons, Harriet F. (Eds.) (1984). *Infertility: Medical, Emotional and Social Considerations.* New York: Human Sciences Press.

Menning, Barbara Eck. (1988). *Infertility: A Guide for Childless Couples.* 2nd edition. Englewood Cliffs, NJ: Prentice-Hall.

Mosher, William D. (1982). "Infertility among U.S. Couples, 1965-1976." *Family Planning Perspectives 14*: 22-27.

———. (1987). "Infertility: Why Business Is Booming." *American Demographics 9*: 42-43.

Mosher, William D. & Pratt, William F. (1990). "Fecundity and Infertility in the United States, 1965-88." Advance Data from Vital and Health Statistics, no. 192. Hyattsville, MD: National Center for Health Statistics.

Rindfuss, Ronald R., Bumpass, Larry, & St. John, Craig. (1980). "Education and Fertility: Implications for Roles Women Occupy." *American Sociological Review 45*: 431-47.

Salzer, Linda P. (1986). *Infertility: How Couples Can Cope.* Boston: G.K. Hall.

Shapiro, C.H. (1988). *Infertility and Pregnancy Loss: A Guide for Helping Professional.* San Francisco: Jossey-Bass.

U.S. Congress, Office of Technology Assessment. (1988). *Infertility: Medical and Social Choices.* Washington, DC: U.S. Government Printing Office.

INFERTILITY PREVENTION

Every woman should think carefully about her method of birth control (Frisch and Rapoport, 1987, ch. 12). The pill and injectables (like Depo-Provera and Norplant) may disrupt menstrual cycles for months after discontinuation, and young women should never use them until regular cycles are well established. From an IUD, germs or abrasion may cause or exacerbate pelvic inflammatory disease (PID), an infection of the internal organs. Tubal ligation is only about 60 percent reversible. Barrier methods (cervical sponge, cervical cap, the diaphragm, spermicidal jellies, condoms) are safer for preserving fertility, even though one or another may occasionally trigger allergic reactions or irritate the cervix or vagina.

A woman should be tested for endometriosis if severe cramping accompanies her menstrual period, especially if it is combined with lower back pain, leg cramps, bleeding between periods, or pain during intercourse. The only certain diagnosis for endometriosis, unfortunately, is an invasive procedure: laparoscopy (Bellina and Wilson, 1985). Both for comfort and to preserve fertility, endometriosis should be treated by drugs or surgery.

Vitally important to promoting fertility is avoiding sexually transmitted diseases (STDs) or infections that enter via the cervix—these often lead to adhesions and PID (Bellina and Wilson, 1985, pp. 236-37). Often-symptomless STD infections prevent pregnancy. When symptoms occur, they may be odorous vaginal discharges or sores on the genitals. Chlamydia, gonorrhea, mycoplasma, ureaplasma, and hemophilus can directly cause PID; herpes, trichomonas, and yeast infections may make intercourse painful; syphilis may affect the fetus. Herpes, chlamydia, and venereal warts infect babies during delivery (except in cesarean delivery). All of these infections, except herpes, can be and should be cured before PID or vaginal pain damages reproductive potential. Every sexually active woman should have tests for STDs annually unless both she and her partner are strictly monogamous.

To preserve fertility, women must remain alert to medical and occupational hazards. When possible, they should avoid x-rays, abdominal surgery, anesthetic gases, pesticides, manufacturing chemicals, radioactivity in hospitals and laboratories, and long hours in front of video terminals. Several months after any abdominal procedure, including abortion, women should have a doctor check for infections and adhesions.

✱ HELEN BEQUAERT HOLMES, Ph.D.

See also: Endometriosis; Male Factors in Pregnancy Outcome; Pelvic Inflammatory Disease; Sexually Transmitted Diseases

See **Guide to Related Topics:** Infertility

Resources

Bellina, Joseph H. & Wilson, Josleen. (1985). *You Can Have a Baby: Everything You Need to Know about Fertility*. New York: Crown Publishers, Inc.

Berger, Gary S., Goldstein, Marc, & Fuerst, Mark. (1989). *The Couple's Guide to Fertility: How New Medical Advances Can Help You Have a Baby*. New York: Doubleday.

Frisch, Merlvin J. & Rapoport, Gayle. (1987). *Getting Pregnant: Over 1,000 of the Most Important Questions and Answers about Fertility Problems and How to Have a Baby*. Tucson, AZ: The Body Press.

INFORMED CONSENT IN LABOR

Women in labor may be faced with having to make a number of decisions that could not have been anticipated or anticipated in specific detail, from the use and timing of analgesic to the need for cesarean delivery. Especially for those under the care of physicians in hospitals, the moral and legal requirements for informed consent apply. Yet, there is a presumption on the part of many physicians that women in labor, because of emotional stress or physical pain, are not competent to give informed consent. Informed consent is therefore by-passed in many cases, either by requiring the pregnant woman to give blanket consent prior to hospital admission or by proceeding as if there were no decisions to be made. There is an issue, then, of the role of the woman and the role of her physician in making decisions during labor (Ladd, forthcoming).

Informed Consent. Self-determination or autonomy is generally recognized as a fundamental moral value (Applebaum, Lidz, and Meisel, 1987, p. 21) and has been explicitly recognized in American law as applying to the medical context since Justice Benjamin Cardozo's opinion in the 1914 Schloendorff case: "Every human being of adult years and sound mind has a right to determine what shall be done with his own body" (Faden, Beauchamp, and King, 1986, p. 123). The requirements for informed consent include: (1) that the physician disclose all information that a reasonable person would need in order to make a decision, including risks and benefits; (2) that the consenter be competent; (3) that the consenter understand the information provided; and (4) that the consent be given voluntarily and without coercion (Meisel and Roth, 1983, pp. 271-72).

Exceptions to the requirement of informed consent can be made under the following conditions: (1) if the patient explicitly waives the right to be informed or to make decisions; (2) if the physician invokes therapeutic privilege, i.e., believes that disclosing information would be injurious to the patient's well-being; (3) if there is a life-threatening emergency, where time or the condition of the patient does not permit the usual process of informing and consenting; or (4) if treatment is court-ordered (Applebaum, Lidz, and Meisel, 1987, pp. 66-81).

Competency and Voluntariness of Women in Labor. Typically, obstetricians have doubted women's capacity to make rational, informed decisions while in labor. For example,

> I think you have to decide about analgesics *before* labor. I say that because it's almost too hard a decision to make while you're *in* labor...It's almost not fair to expect someone whose feelings are so intense to think rationally. (Bursztajn et al., 1981, pp. 373-74)

However, this claim seems to be supported only by anecdotal evidence, and the one recent published empirical study concludes that "the majority of laboring women are at least as mentally and physically competent to give consent as pre-operative patients" (Grice et al., 1988).

There may be more serious question about the actual degree of consent a pregnant woman has during labor, however. Typically, a hospital patient who does not want to give consent for a procedure can, if necessary, dismiss one's physician, discharge oneself from a hospital even against medical advice, or simply refuse or delay a proposed treatment. None of these options is feasible for women in active labor. Further, if blanket permission, that is, a signed permission form stating that "I consent to those procedures which my physician deems necessary" is required for hospital admission, that amounts to a coerced waiver of rights for all those women who, for geographic or economic reasons, do not have a choice of birthing facilities. Courts have accepted as evidence of implied consent the fact that a woman has not actively objected or has cooperated with various medical procedures (Knapp, 1990), ignoring the physical and psychological factors that may actually be quite coercive and can lead a woman to passively accept what she truly objects to.

Conclusion. The demedicalizing of childbirth by limiting the use of high technology, employing midwives, etc., should go a long way to resolving some of the issues surrounding informed consent. There are also some efforts being made to change the attitudes of physicians by encouraging the model of shared decisionmaking and promoting "preventive ethics" in the doctor-pregnant woman relationship (Chervenak and McCullough, 1990).

✱ ROSALIND EKMAN LADD, Ph.D.

See also: Research Issues in Childbirth; Rights of the Pregnant Patient

See **Guide to Related Topics:** Legal Issues

Resources

Applebaum, Paul S., Lidz, Charles W. & Meisel, Alan. (1987). *Informed Consent: Legal Theory and Clinical Practice.* New York: Oxford University Press.

Bursztajn, Harold et al. (1981). *Medical Choices, Medical Chances: How Patients, Families, and Physicians Can Cope with Uncertainty.* New York: Delta/Seymour Lawrence.

Chervenak, Frank A. & McCullough, Laurence B. (1990). "Clinical Guides to Preventing Ethical Conflicts between Pregnant Women and Their Physicians." *American Journal of Obstetrics and Gynecology 162* (2): 303-07.

Faden, Ruth R. & Beauchamp, Tom L. with King, Nancy M.P. (1986). *A History and Theory of Informed Consent.* New York: Oxford University Press.

Grice, S.C. et al. (1988). "Evaluation of Informed Consent for Anesthesia for Labor and Delivery." (abstract). *Anesthesiology 69* (3A): A664.

Knapp, Robert M. (1990). "Legal View of Informed Consent for Anesthesia during Labor." (letter). *Anesthesiology 72* (1): 211.

Ladd, Rosalind Ekman. (1989). "Women in Labor: Some Issues about Informed Consent." In Laura Purdy & Helen Bequaert Holmes, *Feminist Medical Ethics: New Perspectives.* Bloomington, IN: Indiana University Press (forthcoming); *Hypatia 4* (3): 37-45. Reprinted.

Meisel, Alan & Roth, L.H. (1983). "Toward an Informed Discussion of Informed Consent: A Review and Critique of the Empirical Studies." *Arizona Law Review 25*: 265-346.

ISRAEL

In all of the religious and cultural groups that make up contemporary Israeli society (Jewish immigrants from all over the world, Moslems, and Christians), bearing children has utmost importance. Indeed, setting up public maternity services for prenatal, intranatal, and postnatal care has been one of the earliest actions of the country's health care system.

Maternity care in Israel is public and mostly free of charge. By and large, adequate medical care is available to all women residing in the country, regardless of place of residence and economic status.

Care for pregnant women is provided for a nominal fee, through a system of community-based Family Health Stations. Women are seen by public health nurses and by obstetrician-gynecologists throughout their pregnancies. They are advised and referred to central laboratories for various screening tests, such as Tay Sachs, EFT, and amniocentesis (available free to women over 35, or with another proven risk factor; other women can obtain amniocentesis for a fee, in several licensed private laboratories). Other screening tests, such as CVS, are available only through special referrals to the few medical centers providing them. Great concern for healthy newborns results in the rather liberal use of ultrasound screening during pregnancy whenever there is the slightest suspicion of irregularity in fetal development. Private physicians can be used for prenatal care, for a full fee, but tests are to be obtained through the public health care system.

Childbirth education classes are taken by an increasing number of women and couples, yet by fewer women from lower socioeconomic backgrounds than their more educated and affluent counterparts. Classes are offered at Family Health Stations and by private instructors, affiliated with the Israeli Childbirth Education Association (an affiliate of the British National Childbirth Trust, NCT) or with ASPO (American Society for Psychoprophylaxis in Obstetrics). These organizations also provide afterbirth and breastfeeding classes and counseling. In recent years, literature of pregnancy and childbirth, from abroad and from local organizations and hospitals, has become available to women, gradually transforming them from passive patients to health care consumers.

The public health system provides services for childbirth in maternity wings of regional general hospitals and in maternity hospitals. Women are to register during pregnancy at the hospital of their choice for the birth. In large urban areas there is a choice between several hospitals, yet most scarcely populated regions offer only one hospital with a maternity wing. Still, a small number of women in these regions manage to exercise choice: the relatively small size of the country and the fragmented structure of its health care system make it possible for women to show up at hospitals of their choice located in different geographical regions. The few private hospitals also attract women from distant areas. In the latter, fees for childbirth are only partly covered by the State.

Childbirth in one of the regional public hospitals is referred to as "public delivery" and is the choice of most Israeli women. Labor, delivery, and postpartum care are provided by hospital physicians and nurse-midwives not previously seen by the woman. The law forbids physicians to care for their private patients in public hospitals, thus the fragmentation of care between pregnancy and childbirth, even for women opting for private prenatal care. Private deliveries, with the physician (or midwife) of the woman's choice, are available in only private hospitals.

Very few midwives practice privately, attending childbirth only; they cannot provide prenatal care in the mainstream maternity care system, though they meet their patients several times during pregnancy. Even fewer attend home births. There is no support for home birth among midwives and obstetricians from the public maternity care system, nor do Israeli women seek this option in high numbers. There is a lack of back-up services from physicians and hospitals, and strong opposition from professional organizations. Practicing medicine without a proper license is outlawed, so lay midwifery is practically nonexistent.

Hospitals differ only slightly in labor and delivery management practices. There is a general tendency to intervene to speed up labor and birth by various manual and technological means. Women spend most of their labor in bed, attached to an IV. Instrumental deliveries are common and episiotomies are routine, with frequent subsequent infections. In spite of such frequent interventions, the rate of cesarean sections is claimed to be lower than in industrialized countries, and the rate of vaginal births after cesarean (VBACs) higher. Both phenomena may be explained by the fact that the health care system is public and yields no personal financial rewards to physicians for performing unnecessary operations.

Conditions in hospitals vary from appalling (old buildings, crowding, lack of private showers) to modern, pleasant, and humane. Hospitals with physical conditions allowing for privacy encourage partners to stay with women in labor and delivery, provided there are no complications. Few hospitals offer rooming-in arrangements, and most newborns spend their first few days largely away from their mothers. Most nurses and physicians are convinced of the superiority of breastfeeding over bottle-feeding, yet they let the mothers choose the preferred feeding method. Several hospitals recently established education and support programs for breastfeeding, which allow nursing on demand and counseling for mothers.

The few small private maternity hospitals offer an alternative for childbirth. Women who want (and who can afford) to choose the attendant (physician or midwife) and have more choice in the management of childbirth (e.g., regarding birth position, having the newborn at their side) opt for these services.

Mother and newborn services, such as well-baby checkups, immunizations, feeding counseling, and developmental tests, are provided at local Family Health Stations. Early introduction to solid foods has been the customary advice to new mothers, yet a small number of pediatricians (mostly in large urban areas) now advise mothers to breastfeed for the first six months of life. The British NCT and La Leche offer breastfeeding counseling and support groups for new mothers in most of the country. New mothers create networks as they meet at the local Family Health Station or in support groups.

Largely in response to outside influences, the existing infrastructure of maternity services has been greatly improved over the past 20 years, as have behaviors and attitudes of health care recipients. American medicine has strongly influenced medical advances and consumer behavior. European influences are less evident, yet some demand for nontechnological alternatives to maternity care, including home birth, has recently emerged. As the potential for adequate maternity care already exists, the continuity of processes already begun can ensure its success.

✷ AHUVA WINDSOR, Ph.D.

See **Guide to Related Topics:** Cross-Cultural Perspectives

IUD: INTRAUTERINE DEVICE

An intrauterine device (IUD) is an object placed within the uterus to prevent pregnancy. Physicians in several countries experimented with IUDs in the early 20th century. In the United States experimentation was initially limited by law, and later by the association of infections and perforations with IUD use.

By the middle of the 1960s, historical developments encouraged new interest in the IUD. Control of international populations had become a goal and a real possibility with the development of oral contraceptives. The desire of women to control their procreative power helped create a mass market for modern contraceptives. So when doubts were raised about the safety of oral contraceptives, the IUD attracted attention as a possible alternative. The promise of a profitable international market contributed to a rush of innovations and new products by the end of the decade.

One IUD—the Dalkon Shield—became infamous. Hundreds of thousands of women reported injuries associated with its use, and many died. Although the problems with the Dalkon Shield are often thought to have been exclusive to that device, all of the problems have been associated with other IUDs, and all IUDs have been associated with serious injuries, infections, and their sequelae. These include septicemia; septic abortion; massive pelvic adhesions; ectopic pregnancy; appendicitis; infertility; pelvic, uterine, tubal, or ovarian abscess; fetal infections; embedding of the device in uterine tissue; perforation of the uterus, bladder, intestine, peritoneum, or appendix; and strangulation of the intestine. Injuries may lead to hysterectomies, ovariectomies, bowel or bladder surgery, and the attendant risks and complications. All IUDs have a failure rate, and pregnancy with an IUD is dangerous to the woman and to the fetus. Infection, injury, or pregnancy with an IUD can lead to fatal complications.

Studies indicate that an inflammatory reaction occurs when any foreign object is present in the uterus. Some researchers believe that it is the inflammatory reaction that prevents pregnancy with an IUD. That reaction involves the presence of macrophages, cells that emit a substance that suppresses the immune system and makes the uterus particularly susceptible to infectious organisms. The surface of the IUD may become an ecological niche that harbors and grows bacteria. Infectious organisms may be transmitted through the cervix or through the blood stream. They include gonorrhea, but are more commonly the type found in strep infections, pneumonia, gum disease, and dental cavities. A sexually monogamous woman with a monogamous partner may be protected from sexually transmitted infection, but no woman can protect herself from infection transmitted through her blood stream from other parts of her body to her uterus. The availability of antibiotics does not protect women who use IUDs because extensive and severe injuries can occur from low-grade infections that may not be detected in time to administer antibiotics. Risk to an individual woman from IUD-related injury, infection, or pregnancy cannot be projected from statistics drawn from the entire population of IUD users; the degree of risk to an individual is unknown.

For a brief period in the 1980s, most IUDs were removed from the market in the U.S. (though they continued to be sold abroad) because women who were injured by the Dalkon Shield and other IUDs were filing successful lawsuits against manufacturers and insurance companies. Now IUDs are available in the United States again, but women who use them must sign forms releasing the manufacturers, their insurers, and health care providers from liability if injuries occur.

✷ NICOLE GRANT, Ph.D.

See **Guide to Related Topics:** Contraception

Resources

Advisory Committee on Obstetrics and Gynecology, U.S. Food and Drug Administration. (1979). Document #017-012-00276-5.

Elias, Julian. (1985, May). "Intrauterine Contraceptive Devices." *The Practitioner 229*: 431-36.

Fisher, Sue. (1988). *In the Patient's Best Interest: Women and the Politics of Medical Decisions.* New Brunswick, NJ: Rutgers University Press.

Grant, Nicole. (forthcoming). Dalkon Shield study. Columbus, OH: Ohio State University Press.

Haire, Doris. (1984). *How the FDA Determines the "Safety" of Drugs: Just How Safe is "Safety?" A Report Released to the Congress of the United States.* Washington, DC: National Women's Health Network.

Hallatt, Jack G. (1976, Jul 15). "Ectopic Pregnancy Associated with the Intrauterine Device: A Study of Seventy Cases." *American Journal of Obstetrics and Gynecology 125* (6): 755-58.

Hartmann, Betsy. (1987). *Reproductive Rights and Wrongs: The Global Politics of Contraceptive Choice.* New York: Harper & Row.

Scott, William C. (1978, May 15). "Pelvic Abscesses in Association with Intrauterine Contraceptive Device. *American Journal of Obstetrics and Gynecology 131* (2): 149-56.

Stadel, Bruce V. & Schlesselman, Sarah. (1984, Feb). "Extent of Surgery for Pelvic Inflammatory Disease in Relation to Duration of Intrauterine Device Use." *Obstetrics and Gynecology 63* (2): 171-77.

Vessey, M.P. et al. (1981, Mar 14). "Pelvic Inflammatory Disease and the Intrauterine Device: Findings in a Large Cohort Study." *British Medical Journal 282*: 855-56.

I.V.F. FOR FEMALE INFERTILITY. *See instead* INFERTILITY: OVERVIEW

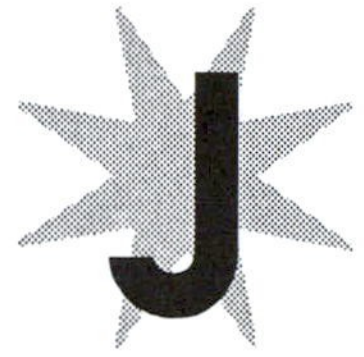

JAPAN

Japan is arguably the world's safest place in which to be born, with an infant mortality rate of 6 per 1,000 births; the national cesarean rate is 7 percent (Ministry of Health and Welfare, 1984; UNICEF, 1986). Universal access to prenatal, postpartal, and well-baby care is available through local governments. Pregnant women are entitled to one free liter of milk per day. While national health insurance does not cover the cost of a normal birth, the local government pays a stipend to residents to defray the expense. Public health nurses visit any new mother who mails a request card at the time of delivery. Pregnancies are registered at the local municipal government office (Engel, 1989).

This report reflects the sociocultural shift since World War II from an agrarian society to a highly centralized, industrial, technologically based economy. Gender role fulfillment is the basis for marital relations in Japan (Imamura, 1987). Ninety-eight percent of Japanese women marry; over 40 percent of marriages are arranged, particularly when a woman has not married by the age of 25. Half of Japanese women quit working when they marry, and a "honeymoon baby," conceived within the first year of marriage, is an ideal. The mother's investment in the child's well-being is total from before conception throughout the rest of the woman's life. From the time she becomes engaged she may change her style of dress and give up smoking, beer, and soft drinks to maintain an environment optimal for pregnancy (Lebra, 1984). Virtually 100 percent of expectant mothers seek early and regular prenatal care.

Excellent outcomes are believed to reflect universal literacy, universal compliance with care, a virtual absence of deliveries to teen mothers, a virtual absence of drug and alcohol abuse by pregnant women, and a middle class comprising 95 percent of the population; a low incidence of cephalopelvic disproportion is due to the value placed on a weight gain of just 18 pounds so that the baby will be small (*see* "Low Birth Weight: United States") and to the racial homogeneity that minimizes variation in female pelvises. Because of women's tremendous investment in successful pregnancy outcomes, abortion is readily sought when a fetal complication is suspected, though prenatal diagnostic testing is not widely practiced. The decision to abort is not unemotional: Most Buddhist temples have many marked and adorned fetal graves.

Pregnant women tend to withdraw from daily activities over the course of their pregnancies, culminating in a return to their mother's home during the eighth month. Women abstain from caffeine, avoid exposure to loud noise, and are urged to refrain from stressful mental activity. From the fifth month, a maternity sash is worn under the clothing to keep the fetus warm. Pregnant women wear knee socks because, in traditional Chinese medical practice, keeping the feet warm promotes uterine health. Thrombophlebitis is very rare among Japanese women. Prenatal exercise is just now beginning to be promoted.

Birth is the domain of women. Japanese fathers remain on the job when the mothers return to their natal home, and they may not see their newborns until the second postpartal month when they arrive to bring their wives home. Labor is endured in silence, to uphold the husband's family honor, with no use of anesthesia or analgesia for a vaginal delivery or episiotomy repair. The experience of pain is believed to enhance the value the mother places on her child. Japanese women are encouraged to eat complete meals during labor for energy to push.

Ninety-nine percent of births occur in hospitals or private birth clinics, attended by physicians. The remaining 1 percent occur in nurse-midwife clinics. Women tend to be admitted on their due dates, with labor often induced within just a couple days beyond the due date. Nearly universal procedures include the enema, episiotomy, and intermittent urinary catheterization just before the head is delivered. In addition, Japanese nurse midwives, by whom labor and delivery settings are staffed, practice perineal massage to stretch the tissues.

Long recuperations are valued. Rooming-in is not practiced extensively, reflecting the value placed on maternal rest. After a week or 10 days in the hospital, the new mother spends up to two months at her mother's home resting. Breastfeeding is nearly universal, but it is not exclusive. If the mother is sleeping when the infant is hungry it is expected that the grandmother will feed it infant formula from a bottle. The priority given recuperation is believed to account for the low incidence of uterine disease among older Japanese women.

Japanese babies are positioned on their backs so that they will not suffocate in the blankets. They are immersed in bath water from the first day of life with no ill effects on umbilical stump healing. Circumcision is not practiced. Japanese women do not bathe until lochia seros ceases, and they do not wash their hair during the first postpartal week. This may reflect the lack of a purified water supply and the use of unheated bathhouses until recent decades, as well as the current practice of families sharing the same bath water.

Japanese mothers tend to stay inside with their babies for the first 100 days of life. It is uncommon for mothers of preschoolers to work. Mothers sleep with their youngsters, commonly until the child reaches 10 years of age or until the next child is born. Sons are more highly valued than daughters, and it is often said that it is better to have a daughter first so that mothering skills are perfected by the time a son is born. The mother-son relationship continues to be the dominant family relationship throughout the son's life.

✱ NANCY C. SHARTS-ENGEL, R.N., Ph.D.

See **Guide to Related Topics:** Cross-Cultural Perspectives

Resources

Engel, N.S. (1989). "An American Experience of Pregnancy and Childbirth in Japan." *Birth 16* (2): 81-86.

Imamura, A.E. (1987). *Japanese Housewives: At Home and in the Community*. Honolulu: University of Hawaii Press.

Lebra, T.S. (1984). *Japanese Women: Constraint and Fulfillment*. Honolulu: University of Hawaii Press.

Ministry of Health and Welfare. (1984). *Statistics Related to Maternal and Child Health in Japan*. Tokyo: Maternal and Child Health Division, Children and Families Bureau, Ministry of Health and Welfare.

UNICEF. (1986). *The State of the World's Children, 1987*. Oxford, England: Oxford University Press.

JAUNDICE, NEWBORN

There are three basic types of jaundice that can affect newborns: physiological, pathological, and breastmilk. Jaundice, a yellowing of the skin and sometimes the whites of the eyes, can be benign or life-threatening depending on the type and severity.

Approximately half of all newborns develop a condition known as physiological jaundice. This usually harmless type of jaundice is a normal reaction to a baby's adjustment to life outside the uterus. While in the womb, the fetus needs additional red blood cells to receive adequate oxygen from the mother. After birth, the baby's liver begins to break down and excrete these cells. Bilirubin, an orange pigment, is a by-product of this process and starts to build up in the bloodstream if the infant's immature system is unable to metabolize it effectively. This causes the baby to turn yellow about the second or third day of life. Most cases of physiological jaundice are mild and disappear within a week or two.

Jaundice becomes dangerous when the level of bilirubin rises too high, causing brain damage called kernicterus. Premature, sick, and low birthweight babies are most at risk for developing kernicterus. The level of bilirubin can be measured with a blood test or by using an icterometer, a device that is simply pressed against the skin (Brewer and Greene, 1981). Twenty mg of bilirubin per 100 ml of blood is generally accepted as the threshold for development of kernicterus, though many practitioners begin treatment when bilirubin is as low as 9 mg. Bright light decomposes bilirubin, so naked, blindfolded babies are placed under "bililights" for phototherapy treatment. Phototherapy may last for hours or days until an acceptable bilirubin level is achieved. Along with increased hospital costs, side effects may include separation of mother and child, interference with breastfeeding, lack of visual stimulation, diarrhea, dehydration, vitamin deficiency, skin rashes, and fever. Severe jaundice may require a complete blood transfusion.

Many experts believe that phototherapy for otherwise healthy, full-term infants is overused and that the same results can be achieved at home without the trauma of separation and other side effects. Home treatment includes exposing the unclothed baby to indirect sunlight several times a day and frequent breastfeeding. Vitamin E (Korte and Scaer, 1984) and herbal remedies (Weed, 1986) may also prove beneficial. If phototherapy is deemed necessary, bililights can be rented from a medical supply company for home use.

Pathological jaundice differs significantly from physiological jaundice because it results from liver disease, infections, or maternal/fetal blood incompatibilities. This rare type of jaundice appears within the first day of life and requires immediate medical attention to prevent brain damage and possible death.

Breastmilk jaundice is very rare, occurs around the fifth day, and may persist for several weeks. Though caused by breastmilk, neither weaning nor any other treatment is required if the baby is active and nursing well. There has never been a case of brain damage reported from breastmilk jaundice.

Jaundice has also been linked to routine vitamin K shots for newborns, drug use during pregnancy and birth, bruising during birth, and poor pregnancy diets. Avoiding the above may prevent jaundice in newborns. ✱ CASSIE LUHRS, C.C.E.

See **Guide to Related Topics:** Baby Care

Resources

Brewer, Gail Sforza & Greene, Janice Presser. (1981). *Right from the Start*. Emmaus, PA: Rodale Press.

Gaskin, Ina May. (1987). *Babies, Breastfeeding and Bonding*. South Hadley, MA: Bergin and Garvey Publishers.

Korte, Diana & Scaer, Roberta. (1984). *A Good Birth, A Safe Birth*. New York: Bantam Books.

Simkin, Penney, & Edwards, Margot. (1979). "When Your Baby Has Jaundice." Seattle: Pennypress.

Stewart, David. (1981). *The Five Standards for Safe Childbearing*. Marble Hill, MO: Napsac Reproductions.

Weed, Susan, S. (1986). *Wise Woman Herbal for the Childbearing Year*. Woodstock, NY: Ash Tree Publishing.

KELSEY, FRANCES. *See instead* THALIDOMIDE

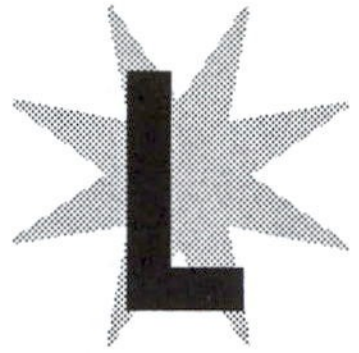

LABOR: OVERVIEW

Human labor is the process by which the muscles of a woman's uterus (womb) contract, or tighten, so that the cervix, or opening of the uterus, thins out (effacement) and opens up (cervical dilation) to about 4½ inches. The laboring woman can then push the baby from the uterus down the vagina to be born.

Each woman's labor is unique so it is not possible to predict what it will be like. Many factors determine labor's characteristics, for example, the position of the baby in the mother's pelvis, the size of the baby, the length and strength of the uterine contractions, whether labor is induced artificially (which often results in a more abrupt onset and tumultuous course of labor), and whether a woman is having her first baby (in such cases, labor is usually longer). Some women have quick and relatively painless labors, whereas others have labors that are difficult and painful. Most women's labor experiences fall somewhere in the middle. Also, where a woman gives birth (home, hospital, or birth center), who her birth attendant is (physician or midwife), and whether the birth attendant practices medical management of labor or uses a physiological approach will all affect labor. Even if a woman has taken excellent care of herself during pregnancy and educated herself for what to expect during labor, she still cannot plan for what she will experience (for example, the amount of pain she will have) during labor; she can, however, make careful choices about where she will give birth and who her birth attendant will be, realizing that both of these factors will influence her labor.

Women who have prepared themselves by attending childbirth education classes and have read and learned about how to cope with labor are likely to find labor more satisfying and manageable than women who begin labor scared, frightened, and uninformed. Having a companion present during labor has been shown to be important in improving labor outcome and in providing the woman with emotional and physical support. Usually this person is the baby's father, but a friend, family members, or a "monitrice" (a person who specializes in giving support during labor) may also be present. All women, whether or not they have had childbirth preparation, need careful explanations in nonmedical terms throughout labor about what is happening. This is true whether labor is normal or there are complications. Women, too, should not wait for caregivers to provide information but should ask questions and express worries. Otherwise, fear and tension can impede labor's progress.

A hormone called oxytocin is pivotal in causing labor to begin; the most obvious sign that labor has begun is an increase in the frequency and intensity of uterine contractions. Although the uterus is contracting during pregnancy (Braxton Hicks contractions), pregnancy contractions don't open the cervix, whereas labor contractions do. When a woman starts labor, there are signs that help her know it is time. Her contractions may start to have more of a pattern (for example, coming every 10 to 15 minutes), and they gradually get closer together and harder; the bag of waters that surrounds the baby inside the uterus may break so that there is a trickle or gush of water; she may have bloody "show," which is a little blood mixed with mucus that comes out of the cervix as it starts to open; and/or she may be aware of low back pain or more abdominal discomfort. Her mood may change, too, so that she is excited but also feels some apprehension about what lies ahead.

Some women have a burst of energy just prior to or early in labor. Mild diarrhea is common, which is nature's way of emptying the rectum and making more room for the baby to pass down the vagina.

Labor is divided into four stages. Stage one is from the first true contraction of labor until the cervix is completely open (dilated) to 10 cm (4.5 in). As the first stage of labor progresses, contractions become closer together, more intense, and longer so that by the end of the first stage they are quite frequent and hard. The second stage is from complete dilation to the time of birth. During second-stage labor the contractions usually ease up somewhat in intensity and strength, and the sensations of the baby moving down the vagina (stretching, pressure, burning, fullness) are predominant. The third stage is when the placenta and amniotic membranes (afterbirth) are delivered. During third-stage labor, when the baby has been born, the woman usually feels marked relief from discomfort. Stage four is the hour after birth.

First-stage labor is the longest of the three stages. It is divided into three parts or phases: early or latent, active, and transition.

During much of the early phase, when effacement and dilation of the cervix to 3 to 4 cm is occurring, the woman may be quite comfortable and able to go about her normal life, pausing at the contractions to relax with them and do slow deep breathing. If, however, she has induced labor, the early phase is often more intense, with contractions close together even though the woman's cervix is not yet very dilated. During spontaneous early-phase labor, the woman may feel uncertainty that she is really in labor because often the contractions initially are about the same as Braxton-Hicks contractions. The contractions may be 20 to 30 minutes apart (but sometimes as close as every 5 to 8 minutes), mild enough in intensity that the woman can walk and talk during a contraction, and typically last for 20 to 40 seconds. It is not unusual for the early phase of labor to last 8 to 12 hours or longer. Many women feel excited, but at the same time, they may be mildly apprehensive, sociable, and experience an energy surge. This is a time of adaptation, of getting used to labor contractions and their pattern. Women are usually most comfortable at home, keeping in contact by phone with their birth attendant. Checking into the hospital or birth center early in labor is usually unnecessary, unless there are complications or the bag of waters has spontaneously broken (ruptured); checking in early often results in unnecessary intervention to "speed things up." Further, women who labor in hospital settings are usually confined to bed, have intravenous fluids started, and have an electronic fetal monitor attached (usually two belts that are placed around the woman's abdomen) to record the baby's heartbeat and the strength of uterine contractions. These procedures restrict freedom of movement despite the fact it is known that moving around and changing positions during labor assist in labor's normal progress. Therefore, unless there are complications that require medical attention, staying home in early labor, moving and carrying on normal activities, taking a warm bath, eating lightly, drinking fluids, and relaxing and sleeping are all helpful. The woman's partner, family, and/or friends can best assist her by keeping her company and providing reassurance and love.

The active phase of labor is the period from 3 to 4 cm dilation until 7 cm. Women, however, can experience the characteristics of active phase early in labor, especially if they have induced labor. The predominant characteristics are contractions that are more intense, longer, and closer together. Typically they occur less than five minutes apart and last as long as a minute. The woman becomes deeply involved in her body's sensations and in coping with the contractions. Her expression is more sober, and she may be flushed. She typically shows restlessness and increased body tension, so that her breathing rate during contractions may quicken. She talks much less and is verbally preoccupied with her discomfort and her wish for labor progress. She is more detached from others than early in labor, she perspires, and her mouth is dry. She has no doubts now that she is in labor!

Transition, or the period from about 7 to 10 cm dilation of the cervix, usually lasts less than an hour. Transition is considered by many women to be the most intense and challenging time in labor. Contractions usually come very frequently (every two to three minutes) and last from 45 to 90 seconds, often feeling quite hard from the beginning, whereas earlier in labor there may have been a more gradual build-up of intensity. The woman may be very restless or, alternately, almost motionless. She often wants to hold on to someone, but at the same time may be irritable and resist being touched. Her face and neck are flushed (similar to an athlete who is expending a lot of energy), she will probably exhibit a sleepy, faraway quality between contractions, and she may experience a variety of physical changes: trembling, shaking, leg cramps, nausea, back and hip pain, burping, or perspiring. By this time she is very preoccupied with feelings of pain, pressure, and hoped-for relief. She may be loud and demanding in her requests for assistance. With the amount of work required of her now, it is normal that she may find relief by making sounds such as grunts, groans, and deep throaty noises. However, making sounds that are shrill and high-pitched can increase the woman's tension level rather than providing a release. As in active phase, a woman needs the continuous presence of helpers to assist with pain relief, movement, and position changes; to remind her to empty her bladder; to encourage her as she copes with each contraction; and to provide emotional reassurance of progress and that labor is normal. Many women find relief by immersing themselves in a Jacuzzi or tub of water. Toward the end of transition, some women start to feel rectal pressure and fullness and may have an urge to begin pushing. Usually this occurs when the cervix is almost open, and gentle pushing now can result in the cervix opening completely. However, if the woman feels like pushing much earlier in labor, she should try changing positions (for example, moving to her hands and knees) and resist the urge because pushing too early can result in swelling of the cervix and impede labor's progress. If her membranes (bag of waters) have not yet ruptured, they may spontaneously break during transition or early in second-stage labor or may be ruptured artificially by her birth attendant.

When the cervix is dilated to 10 cm, second-stage labor begins. Although the baby has only a distance of about four inches to descend down the vagina to be born, the process can be slow. This is because the baby's head must turn inside the pelvis to a position where the back of the head is directly against the pubic bone of the mother, and also because the vaginal tissues must stretch and make room for the baby's descent. Contractions may be somewhat shorter (45 to 60 seconds) and less intense than during transition. For women having their first baby, second-stage labor commonly lasts one to two hours, but it may be shorter or longer. For women who have previously given birth, second-stage labor usually is less than a half-hour. For any one woman, the length of second-stage labor depends on many factors, such as how resistant her vaginal tissues are to the stretching that is required, her pelvic bone structure, the size of the baby and its position within the woman's pelvis, whether she has a strong urge to push, and whether she has had medication that abolishes the urge to push.

Although second-stage labor begins when cervical dilation is complete, this does not necessarily mean that it is time to push. Some women are ready to push immediately because they have a strong bearing down urge (which occurs when the baby's head presses against stretch receptors during the descent down the vagina). Others, quite normally, develop an urge to push over a period of time so that early in second-stage labor they may not feel like pushing; by the end of second stage they usually experience a strong urge and are bearing-down with full effort. The time of "waiting" or "peace" before the urge to push becomes irresistible can be used by the woman to refresh herself, to rest, and to prepare for the hard work of pushing. It is also a time when she can try different positions for pushing and review some of the sensations she is likely to feel as the baby moves down the birth canal.

Some women get a "second wind" during second stage, regaining sociability and energy, and they may find there is less discomfort and actual relief when they push. Others experience the sensations of second stage as very painful and the hardest time in labor. Many women are surprised at the stretching fullness, pressure, and burning that occur with the baby's descent. Some find it easier to gradually ease into pushing rather than immediately pushing with full effort, so that they can become used to the feelings. It is not unusual and is quite normal for women to need time for emotional readiness during second stage, to think once more about their decision to have a baby, and to not feel ready to push until they have done so.

When labor is normal and the mother and baby are healthy, letting second-stage labor get underway gradually, according to the woman's physical and emotional responses, makes sense. Instead, with medically managed childbirth, second-stage labor is often viewed as an urgent situation where the woman must push as hard as she can and finish as quickly as possible, usually within two hours. There is not, however, evidence that this approach results in a better outcome and, in fact, it may cause physiologic stress for both mother and baby.

When a woman first begins to push, she may be uncoordinated and need to shift her energy from being passive (trying to cope with contractions) to being active and pushing her baby down the birth canal. Pushing is done during contractions, not between. Because some contractions are harder than others (this is true throughout labor), sometimes she will push hard and other times her pushing will be less vigorous.

She may need assistance in finding a position that is tolerable (seldom are any very comfortable), whether that be lying on her side, squatting, standing, on all fours, or semi-sitting. In no circumstance should she lie flat on her back. As she feels an urge to push, she will usually hold her breath spontaneously for five to six seconds as she bears down, or exhale with bearing down, making low guttural noises that reflect her effort. Other noises she may make during or in between contractions are low moans and groans. If her noises become high-pitched and shrill, she is probably feeling frightened and scared. When this occurs, her caregivers should provide reassurance; pain-relieving strategies, such as warm, wet compresses applied to her perineum; and direction about how she can position herself and push more effectively.

If a woman does not have an urge to push, she will need direction in pushing. This is especially common if she has had an epidural block or another local anesthetic that interferes with the bearing-down reflex. Sometimes a change of position, such as squatting, will increase the urge to push so that she is better able to work with her body. But occasionally the urge never occurs, making her job harder because she has to push despite the absence of an instinctive urge to do so.

If the woman is having her baby in a birthing room or at home, she will not be moved as the time of birth approaches. In many hospitals, however, women are moved to a delivery room for the birth. As the baby's head is born (with a breech, the delivery is usually by cesarean), the woman may feel a great release of pressure and let out a spontaneous cry. She may feel relief, exhilaration, and/or be aware of how tired she is.

The birth of the placenta, or afterbirth, occurs during third-stage labor—usually within a period of 5 to 20 minutes. Contractions are still occurring but usually are much less noticeable. The woman may have to push several times to deliver the placenta. Often medication (oxytocin) is given to encourage the placenta to detach from the side of the uterus. Putting the baby to breast helps the placenta separate from the uterus because with nipple stimulation the hormone oxytocin is released in the mother's body, causing the uterus to contract and release its contents. During third-stage labor the woman is often quite alert to her surroundings and events, whereas in second-stage labor she focuses very much on herself and what is happening in her body.

The fourth stage of labor refers to the hour after birth when the woman and her new baby are watched carefully to make sure all is normal. The woman's uterus is massaged frequently so that it remains firm and well contracted, because this reduces the amount of bleeding from the placental site. Her blood pressure, temperature, and pulse are checked to make sure they are normal. Early urination is encouraged. Women often feel wide awake and excited although they may be quite exhausted, hungry, and thirsty, and have chills that shake their entire body.

Fourth stage is a time—often referred to as "bonding" time—for family members to be together with the new baby. Although in the past babies were often taken from the parents to be observed in a nursery, when childbirth has been normal and the baby is healthy, the hour after birth should be one of privacy for the family, an opportunity to become acquainted with their baby. ✱ SUSAN MCKAY, R.N., Ph.D.

See also: Hospital Birth: An Anthropological Analysis of Ritual and Practice; Posture for Labor and Birth; Social Science Research on American Childbirth Practices

See **Guide to Related Topics:** Childbirth Practices and Locations

Resources

Kitzinger, Sheila. (1987). *Your Baby, Your Way: Making Pregnancy Decisions and Birth Plans.* New York: Pantheon.

———. (1989). *The Complete Book of Pregnancy and Childbirth.* Westminister, MD: Knopf.

———. (1989). *How It Really Feels.* Kirkwood, NY: Putnam.

Korte, Diana & Scaer, Roberta. (1990). *A Good Birth, A Safe Birth.* New York: Bantam.

McCartney, Marion & van der Meer, Antonia. (1990). *The Midwife's Pregnancy and Childbirth Book—Having Your Baby Your Way.* New York: Holt.

McKay, Susan. (1986). *The Assertive Approach to Childbirth.* Minneapolis: International Childbirth Education Association.

Simkin, Penny. (1989). *The Birth Partner: Everything You Need to Know to Help a Woman through Childbirth.* Boston: Harvard Common Press.

Todd, Linda. (1987). *Labor and Birth: A Guide for You.* 2nd edition. Minneapolis: International Childbirth Education Association.

LABOR ASSISTANTS

In choosing the hospital over the home as the place to give birth, American women relinquished control over this life-changing event. Historically, women had been cared for by other women, including midwives, during pregnancy and birth in their own homes. In the early part of the 20th century, women began to enter hospitals to give birth in hopes of controlling the dangers of childbirth. In doing so, they gave up their control over not only their environment but their choice of who to have around them while they gave birth. Indeed, by the 1950s, over 90 percent of women gave birth in hospitals. Birth was now controlled by obstetricians, who were mostly male.

Although there has been a resurgence of midwifery in North America, over 95 percent of women are still cared for by obstetricians. There is often no one of the woman's choosing in the birth room to mother the mother. In this vulnerable state and without support it is no wonder that only 10 percent of the 3.5 million American women who give birth each year do so naturally (Perez and Snedeker, 1990). Individualized, continuous care during birth is often lacking in this birth environment, which is dominated by machines. In hopes of replacing this vital missing link, a group of women—professional labor assistants—have entered the birthplace.

The labor assistant, monitrice, or doula is a guardian of normal birth. Her job is to educate families, support women during birth, and serve as an advocate for women's choices about their births. Doulas, from the Greek meaning "in service of," provide emotional and physical support to the laboring woman. Monitrices, from the French meaning "to watch over attentively," combine nurturing with clinical skills. They have the ability to assess both fetal and maternal well-being.

The labor assistant is often called upon to assist the mother at home prior to birth. She will assess the signs of active labor and, if she has clinical skills, will do vaginal exams and listen to fetal heart tones. Her presence and the knowledge she brings with her often help the mother to avoid a "too early" trip to the hospital.

In a birth environment dominated by machines, drugs, and tests, one of the most important functions of the labor assistant is to serve as an advocate for the laboring woman. When the laboring woman and her partner are in a vulnerable and often stressed state, the labor assistant provides them with information and advice and often interprets what others have said so that the family may make informed choices. Through her skillful communication she helps the hospital staff see and respect the laboring woman's birth plan.

With a labor assistant in attendance, the laboring woman's chances of delivering her child without the use of unnecessary drugs and interventions are much greater than if she and her mate went alone into the hospital environment. The presence of the doula or monitrice inspires confidence in their own abilities: she adds to their strengths instead of accentuating their weaknesses. She helps the laboring woman to believe in herself and her ability to birth her baby. The monitrice or doula helps turn a routine hospital event into a life event filled with feelings of joy, pride, and fulfillment.

✱ PAULINA G. PEREZ, R.N., B.S.N., ACCE-R

See also: Doula; Evolution of Human Birth; Labor Partner; Social Science Research on American Childbirth Practices

See **Guide to Related Topics:** Caregivers and Practitioners

Resources

Herzfeld, Judith. (1985). *Sense & Sensibility in Childbirth.* New York: Norton & Company.

Hodnett, Ellen & Osborn, Richard. (1989). "A Randomized Trial of the Effects of Monitrice Support during Labor: Mothers' Views Two to Four Weeks Postpartum." *Birth 16* (4): 177-84.

Kennell, J. et al. (1988). "Medical Intervention: The Effect of Social Support during Labor." *Pediatric Research 23*: 211.

Klaus, M. et al. (1986). "Effects of Social Support during Parturition on Maternal-Infant Morbidity." *British Medical Journal 293*: 585-87.

Perez, Paulina & Snedeker, Cheryl. (1990). *Special Women: The Role of the Professional Labor Assistant.* Seattle: Pennypress.

Shearer, Beth. (1989, Spring). "Birth Assistant: New Ally for Parents-to-Be." *Childbirth Educator*: 26-31.

Sosa, R. et al. (1980). "The Effects of a Supportive Labor Companion on Perinatal Problems, Length of Labor, and Mother-Infant Interaction." *New England Journal of Medicine 303*: 597-600.

LABOR PARTNER

A labor coach is a knowledgeable benefactor who guides and lovingly directs the woman through childbirth. (Eileen Frederick in "Coaching." *Childbirth Education, Practice, Research and Theory.* 1988)

Throughout history, women have been supported during childbirth by a companion, usually another woman (Jones, 1985). Over the past 30 years, the labor companion, through formal preparation in childbirth education classes, has taken a more active role in partnering the woman through labor and delivery. Birth partner, labor coach (Bing, 1967), significant other, labor assistant, monitrice, doula (Raphael, 1976), or ombudsman are various terms describing the husband, lover, baby's father, friend, relative, or professional who undertakes the role of supporter, guide, teammate, and caretaker of the laboring woman.

The birth partner's physical and emotional roles begin during the pregnancy (Simkin, 1990) as the couple make preparations for the baby, attend childbirth education classes, learn the facts pertaining to childbirth and the birth environment (hospital or home), visit and meet the physician or midwife, and discuss their birth preferences. In classes, they learn the various skills to help them share and participate in the emotional and physical events surrounding the birth. During pregnancy, the woman is encouraged to maintain her physical health through proper nutrition, exercise, and rest (Cain, 1990). As a couple, they practice the relaxation, breathing, and comfort techniques learned in the classes (Bing, 1967). This practice enables them to work more confidently as a team, to understand and change the mother-to-be's noneffective response to tension or pain, and to recognize the words or touch to which she best responds and to thereby utilize during labor.

The physical presence of the labor coach during labor ensures that the mother-to-be has the companionship of someone she knows and trusts, and upon whom she can depend as intermediary or friend. Studies of birth experience components concluded that the husband's (partner's) presence and participation reduce pain perception (Block, Block, and Shrock, 1975) and the ability of the mother to experience ecstasy and peak emotional experiences (Tanzer, 1972).

Being empathetic, timing contractions for duration and interval, offering verbal cues, listening to the mother-to-be's needs, and acknowledging her discomfort, together with providing information on her progress, feedback on her use of relaxation skills (Shrock, 1984), helpful advice, positive reinforcement, and reassurance and encouragement to maintain breathing and muscle release during (and complete rest between) uterine contractions, are some aspects of the many-faceted emotional support the partner can give.

In his or her unique position of prior knowledge of the mother-to-be, the birth partner can better cope with her varying moods through labor and adjust the environment for her physical comfort (Simkin, Whalley, and Keppler, 1984). He or she can encourage an upright position or ambulation if feasible, organize pillows to maintain flexed and released limbs, and remind her to maintain circulation by changing position and emptying her bladder often. The birth partner adjusts in relation to her changing moods and body temperature, providing ice chips, liquids, brow mopping when warm, or extra blankets when cool. Maintaining privacy or changing light intensity contribute toward more effective laboring.

Love and support are communicated through voice tone and concise directions, with focus on present behavior rather than future anxieties, and through physical caring and touch: holding, caressing, and massaging, and providing counterpressure and body support during pushing. The labor partner most importantly is a buffer between the laboring woman and the medical staff to both relay her needs and their instructions. With the partner's presence at the birth, a deeper emotional bond (Klaus and Kennell, 1983) is often forged between mother and partner and partner and child.

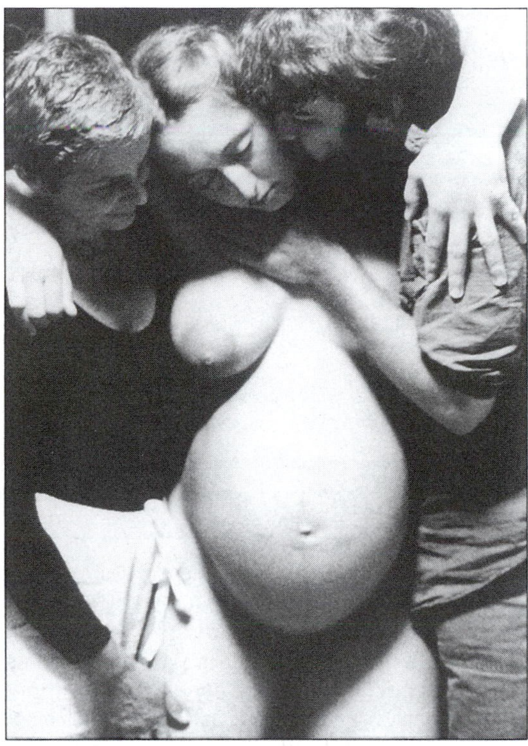

Laboring woman with partner and midwife. Photo courtesy of Kip Kozlowski.

✷ PAMELA SHROCK, Ph.D.

See also: Bradley Method: Husband-Coached Childbirth; Doula; Evolution of Human Birth; Labor Assistants; Social Science Research on American Childbirth Practices

See **Guide to Related Topics:** Caregivers and Practitioners

Resources

Bing, E. (1967). *Six Practical Lessons for Easier Childbirth.* New York: Bantam Books.

Block, R., Block, C., & Shrock, P. (1975). "The Effect of Support of the Husband and Obstetrician on Pain Perception and Control in Childbirth." *Birth and Family Journal* 2 (2).

Bradley, R. (1974). *Husband-Coached Childbirth.* New York: Harper and Row.

Butler, M., Luther, D., & Frederick, E. (1988). "Coaching: The Labor Companion." In F. Nichols & S. Humenick. (Eds.) *Childbirth Education, Practice Research and Theory."* Philadelphia: Saunders, pp. 275-90.

Cain, K. (1990) *Partners in Birth: Your Complete Guide for Helping a Mother Give Birth.* New York: Warner Books.

Jones, C. (1985). *Sharing Birth: Father's Guide to Giving Support during Labor.* New York: Quill/William Morrow.

Klaus, M. & Kennell, J.H. (1983). *Bonding: The Beginnings of Parent-Infant Attachment*. New York: C.V. Mosby.
Perez, Pauline. (1990). *Special Women: The Role of Professional Labor Assistants*. Seattle: Pennypress, Inc.
Raphael, D. (1976). *The Tender Gift: Breastfeeding*. New York: Schocken Books.
Shapiro, Jerrold Lee. (1987). *When Men Are Pregnant: Needs and Concerns of Expectant Fathers*. New York: Impact.
Shrock, P. (1984). "Relaxation Skills: Update on Problems and Solutions." *Genesis 6* (5).
Simkin, P. (1990). *Partners in Birth*. Seattle: Pennypress, Inc.
Simkin, P., Whalley, J., & Keppler, A. (1984). *Pregnancy, Childbirth and the Newborn*. Deephaven, MN: Meadowbrook Pub.
Tanzer, D. (1972). *Why Natural Childbirth?* New York: Doubleday.

LACTATION, INDUCED

Induced lactation is the establishment of a milk supply in a nulliparous woman, that is, one who has never given birth (Riordan, 1983). In practice this term is also used when a woman who has previously lactated re-establishes a milk supply many months or years after lactation has ceased (Anderson, 1986). Induced lactation is almost invariably undertaken for a foster or an adopted child.

In the course of a normal pregnancy, estrogen, progesterone, prolactin, and the adrenal corticol steroids cause the alveoli and ducts in the breasts to increase in both size and number (Riordan, 1983). Following the birth and expulsion of the placenta, the hormonal balance shifts. While estrogen and progesterone go down, prolactin goes up and signals the alveoli to produce milk (Hormann, 1989). As long as the baby sucks, the breasts will continue to make milk. When sucking slows down or stops, so does milk production. Renewed sucking or frequent, regular breast stimulation can start the process again or for the first time. If it has been some time since the woman lactated, if she is inducing lactation following weaning of an older baby or toddler, or if she has never had a pregnancy, alveoli and milk ducts will have involuted (or never experienced the changes associated with pregnancy) and it may take considerable time to establish even a modest milk supply.

Induced lactation depends on stimulation, on the mother's motivation and perseverance, and on the baby's cooperation. Some women use natural or artificial galactogogues, milk-inducers—fenugreek, chaste root, basil, and ginseng have long histories as natural galactogogues (Fleiss, 1988; Hormann, 1989). Estrogen/progesterone combinations to simulate pregnancy prior to the arrival of the baby (Waletzky and Herman, 1976) have been tried by some physicians. Chlorpromazine (Jelliffe and Jelliffe, 1978) and oxytocin (Lawrence, 1989) are commonly used in conjunction with the baby's sucking to enhance milk production. There has been little evidence that galactogogues per se are very helpful, but they frequently have a positive psychological effect—"sympathetic magic" Jelliffe calls it—on the mother or on her medical provider. This effect must be weighed against the known side effects of each of these drugs (for both mother and baby) when deciding whether to employ a galactogogue.

Psychology plays a critical role in induced lactation. There will be very discouraging periods when there appears to be little or no milk produced. The baby may be reluctant to take the breast or may be at times frustrated at the modest production. It is helpful for mothers inducing lactation to have as the first priority establishing a close nursing relationship with their babies. This is an achievable goal for most women with very young babies, and it is not uncommon for babies

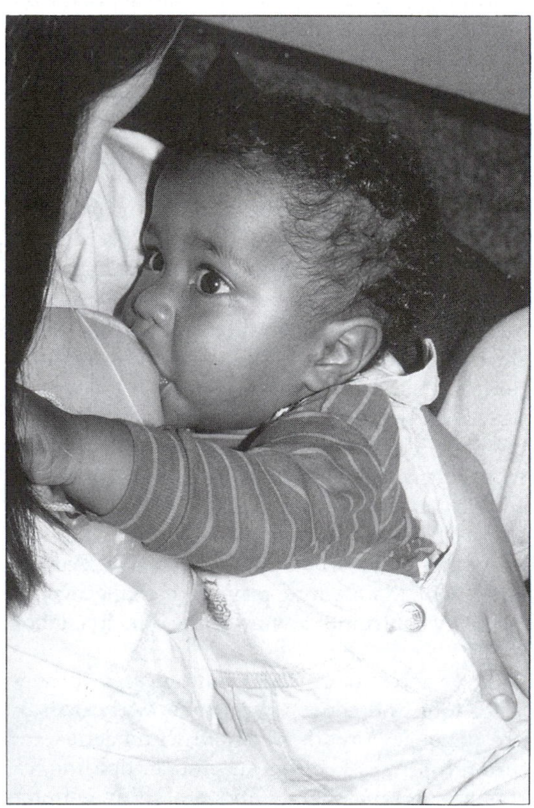

A mother nursing her 11-month-old adopted son, using the Medela Supplemental Nursing System.Photo taken by Marta Starnfeld; © Marta Guoth-Gumberger.

over six months to take to the breast if the mother has sufficient patience. Women inducing lactation should be prepared for their babies to be reluctant to suck at the breast at first and should be reassured that this reluctance is not a personal rejection—any more than a breastfed baby's refusal to take a bottle is a rejection of his or her mother. Babies need time to learn new skills, and resistance during the learning period is to be expected.

Milk supply plays a very secondary role in induced lactation. Nearly every woman, given sufficient stimulation and time, will produce some milk (Hormann, 1977). Lawrence suggests an average of four weeks from beginning stimulation until the appearance of the first drops of milk (Lawrence, 1989). In a study of 240 adoptive mothers (Auerbach and Avery, 1981), all of the mothers had some milk, but only somewhat over a third were able to breastfeed exclusively at any time in the nursing experience. Milk supply in induced lactation is reported to be very much higher in some developing countries (Phillips, 1971; Jelliffe and Jelliffe, 1978; Hormann, 1989). It is generally held that there are psychological factors built into these societies that make lactation of any sort easier than in industrialized countries, but there has been little research.

A woman inducing lactation can expect a considerable investment of her time and energy. She may begin with breast massage and stimulation several weeks or even months before her baby arrives. If she is going to try a course of hormones to encourage her body to "believe" that it is pregnant, it should be during the time prior to the baby's arrival. Once the baby comes, he or she needs to be offered every possible chance to nurse—at least every two hours in the daytime and through the night. The breast should be offered to comfort as well as to feed. As much as possible, pacifiers and the bottle should be avoided to minimize nipple confusion and provide an incentive for the baby to suck at the breast. Formula feeding will almost always be necessary to ensure that the baby has an adequate intake of fluid and calories. Ideally, formula should be given by spoon, cup, eyedropper, or via a specially designed nursing supplemental system that delivers the milk at the mother's breast. Women inducing lactation need a great deal of practical and emotional support. Usually this is best accomplished with a referral to a mother support group, such as La Leche League, or a breastfeeding counselor with experience in helping women induce lactation.

Success in induced lactation is seldom defined by milk supply, though, as seen above, some milk is almost always present. Duration of nursing is a more reliable indicator of success in these cases. In an early study (Hormann, 1977) 23 of 65 adoptive mothers nursed at least 6 to 12 months. Thus in the mid-1970s this group had already achieved the six-month 35 percent breastfeeding goal set by the Surgeon General's office for 1990 (U.S. Department of Health and Human Services, 1984). In a study just a few years later (Auerbach and Avery, 1981) 90 percent of the adopted infants were sill nursing at six months, and 80 percent at one year. By this standard, adoptive mothers are among the most successful nursing mothers. Their view of themselves confirms this. Seventy-five percent of the adoptive mothers in the 1981 study and 82 percent of the mothers in the 1977 study viewed the experience as a successful one that they would do again and recommend to others.

✷ ELIZABETH HORMANN

See also: Relactation

See **Guide to Related Topics:** Adoption; Infant Feeding

Resources

Anderson, Kathryn. (1986). "Breastfeeding Your Adopted Baby." Franklin Park, IL: La Leche League Information Sheet #55.

Auerbach, K.G. & Avery, J.L. (1980). "Relactation: A Study of 366 Cases." *Pediatrics 65*: 236.

———. (1981). "Induced Lactation: A Study of Adoptive Nursing by 240 Women." *American Journal of Disabled Children 135*: 340.

Fleiss, Paul. (1988). "Herbal Remedies for the Breastfeeding Mother." *Mothering 48*.

Hormann, Elizabeth. (1977). "Breastfeeding the Adopted Baby." *Birth and Family Journal 4* (4).

———. (1987). *After the Adoption*. Old Tappan, NJ: Revell.

———. (1989). *When You Nurse Your Adopted Baby*. Cologne, Germany.

Jelliffe, D. & Jelliffe, E.F.P. (1978). *Human Milk in the Modern World*. New York: Oxford University Press.

Lawrence, Ruth. (1989). *Breastfeeding: A Guide for the Medical Profession*. St. Louis: C.V. Mosby.

Phillips, Virginia. (1971). "Non-Puererpal Lactation Among Austrailian Aboriginal Women." *New Zealand Parents' Centres Bulletin*.

Riordan, Jan. (1983). *A Practical Guide to Breastfeeding*. St. Louis: C.V. Mosby.

U.S. Department of Health and Human Services. (1984). "Report of the Surgeon General's Workshop on Breastfeeding and Human Lactation." Washington, DC.

Waletzky, L.R. & Herman, E.C. (1976). "Relactation." *American Family Practice 14*: 69.

LAMAZE. *See instead* PSYCHOPROPHYLACTIC METHOD (LAMAZE)

LANGUAGE OF BIRTH

Even the most seemingly neutral terms for procreative processes are defined by stressing the "active male, passive female" dichotomy. "Ovum" is defined as a "female germ cell which, generally only after fertilization, develops into a new member of the same species." "Spermatozoon," on the other hand, is "the male germ cell, found in semen, which penetrates the ovum, or egg, of the female to fertilize it; it . . . moves with a swimming action."

Only the father can "beget." The mother simply "gets," and what she gets is "impregnated," "knocked up," "with child." Each of these has its own trajectory of linguistic development, none of which takes into account the biological reality of the vagina as an active, grasping organ that aids in procreation. The female is a field, to be plowed and planted:

GREEK: *aro* to plow, to sow, to beget, to enjoy
arotron, plow; *arotra*, genitals
arotros, cornfield, procreation
aroura, woman who receives seed and bears.

SANSKRIT: *langala*, plow; *langula*, penis.

Sperm is the carrier and producer of life, so woman is field and child is seed to be planted. This planted seed becomes fruit of the womb, and may even be discovered in the garden. Slavic folktales have babies found among the cabbages, explicit in the French *planter des choux*—to plant a cabbage, generate a child. Eastern European folktales stress the maternal element: The stork, ostensible deliverer of babies, actually migrates each fall to its swamp home in the Nile *delta*, Greek for "door" and symbol of the female since the Paleolithic Era. The sense of delta/door is in the Bible's "go in unto her," a euphemism for sexual union.

In ancient days the role of the father in procreation was not understood, as is reflected in conception stories of Greek mythology: Natural processes of wind, rain, lightning, or the ocean are impregnators. These were incorporated as attributes of Zeus; thus Danae became pregnant by the rain shower (of gold), and Hera by the wind. And into the 20th century, Trobriand Islanders believed that women should avoid bathing in the sea at high tide, lest they become pregnant.

The word "conceive" is another example of the aggressive underpinnings of language. The Middle English *conceiven* and Old French *conceivre*, *conciver* derive from the Latin *concipere*, meaning to receive, take in. But *concipere* is formed out of another kind of taking altogether: *con* = *com* (together) + *capiō*, *capere*—to take, lay hold, seize.

Similarly, the Old Norse *knoka* and Anglo-Saxon *cnocian* became knock: "to strike with a sounding blow, to rap upon a door to gain admittance, to copulate with, to make pregnant; to knock a child (or an apple) out of." In American English, "knocked up" is then "to drive upwards by knocking, to impregnate," and shares meaning with "knock-down drag-out" (fight), "knocked" (exhausted), and "knocked out" (unconscious).

The Swollen Vessel. The word "pregnant" derives from the Latin *pregnans*, *pregnantis*—heavy with young. The word is formed from the prefix *prae-* (before) + *gnasci* (to be born), and thus refers to prebirth mode. However, another meaning was added: "mentally fertile, prolific of ideas; inventive," thus subsuming reproduction under production control. (It is interesting to note that the Thesaurus entry for "pregnant" ends its two lines with a cross-reference to "production," whose entry occupies almost a full page (*Roget's College Thesaurus*, 1962). Language, like a woman, is pregnable, subject to capture, as a fortress; able to be attacked; assailable, or vulnerable.)

LATIN: *gerō, gerere/gestāre/gestatus* → gestate: to carry
ferrō, ferre → *fertilis* → fertile: to bear
gravis, heavy (gravity) → gravid: pregnant

ANGLO-SAXON: *beran*, to bear, carry

GERMAN: *Geburt*, to carry a fetus

A pregnant woman can also be said to be propagating, multiplying, procreating, reproducing, and breeding. Most interesting in this connection is the concept of "increasing," which means to swell or grow in size or number. The womb swells in response to the previous swelling of a different, masculine organ; the idea is that semen = yeast. Unleavened bread is thus virgin bread, suitable for Old Testament sacrifices.

HEBREW: *shā'ar*, to swell → sēor, yeast-cake

INDO-EUROPEAN base: *bhrue*, to swell, ferment → bread

ANGLO-SAXON: *hlāf*, loaf →
hlāford, loaf-ward (protector) → lord

Kneading in the yeast should thus be performed with "fervor," from the Latin *ferveo, fervere* (to boil, be hot, ferment, glow). The twin notions of yeast fermentation and heat are joined in the baking of the bread. The Greeks and Romans shaped baked goods into replications of genitalia; "split-rolls" were female. And the Old Norse word *kaka,* meaning "cake," includes the honey cake, shaped like a baby. The honey cake in Greece was called *plakous,* from which derives the Latin word *placenta,* making the mother's body the true land of milk and honey. This constellation of meanings has been degraded into the slang expression "She has a bun (or a cake) in the oven," which reduces the woman yet again to a repository or production unit.

Upon examination, some phrases that are usually devalued as polite euphemisms turn out to have positive connotations. The word "expecting," for example, derives from the Latin *expectare,* a compound of *ex-,* meaning "out," and *spectare,* meaning "to see." The prospective mother spends a lot of her time doing exactly that: looking forward, planning, anticipating. "In the family way" shares this meaning, as "way" implies travel along a particular path, a course of action. The "way of the family" represents a major change, a journey taken, as all such adventures are, one step at a time. The base definition of "family" as mother and child refers to an emotional reality: We need a separate expression, "family man," to connote a male who is devoted to his wife and children. There is no parallel expression, "family woman": a mother's dedication is both required and assumed.

Deliverance. We have seen that the language of procreation is not neutral. Even more weighted are terms for the actual birthing process, and most blatant is the word "deliver," from the Latin *deliberare,* to set free. *Webster's New World Dictionary* (1966) lists nine definitions:

1. To set free or save from evil, danger, etc.
2. To assist at the birth: the doctor *delivered* the child
3. To give forth or express in words: *deliver* a speech
4. To give up or hand over; transfer
5. To give out, distribute: *deliver* the mail
6. To give forth: the well *delivers* much water
7. To strike (a blow)
8. To throw or toss: the pitcher *delivered* a curve
9. [Colloq.] To cause votes to be directed towards. . . .

It isn't always clear just who is being "rescued" or "set free." Such language reflects the current view of pregnancy: Woman is incidental; delivering babies is what doctors do.

But they didn't always. In fact, the word "obstetrics" derives from *obstetrix,* meaning "midwife," a compound of *ob-* (in front of) and *stare* (to stand) that literally means "she who stands before." The word "midwife" itself is the Anglo-Saxon *mid + wif,* meaning "with wife," "woman with," "woman assisting."

Cultural variances in the birthing process have been recorded throughout history, starting with Exodus 2:16-19, in which Pharaoh ordered Hebrew midwives to attend those "upon the stools" (to kill male children at birth). The midwives responded that Hebrew women were lively and didn't wait for the midwife; there is also the implication that they didn't use the birthing stool. Written Egyptian shows an older, different delivery style: The hieroglyph for "birth" is a kneeling woman.

By the 16th century, there were "lying-in hospitals" for birthing, as in the French *accoucher,* meaning "to put to bed," and the German *eines Kindes liegen,* meaning "to lie down for a child." Women were said to be "in confinement" or "brought to child-bed."

Words referring to birth show two distinct orientations, as though what is in fact a joint effort to mother and child must be linguistically differentiated. Thus we have from the Latin *partiō, partīre* (to share, divide, distribute), "to bear," "to bring forth," and from the Latin *pario, parere* (to come forth, appear), "to emerge," "to arrive." The unity of mother and child is thus physically and verbally separated: *separō, separāre* (to be born asunder, to be severed by birth); as reflected in the Old English *sundrian,* to force apart or divide by rending, cutting.

Once the birth process begins, the female, who moments before was in a "delicate condition" (tender or feeble in constitution, weakly, pregnant), finds herself "in labor and travail." The latter word has a tremendous linguistic load: from the Late Latin *tripalium,* a compound of *tria* (three) and *palus* (a stake), it refers to a specific torture instrument. The Late Latin verb *tripaliāre* (to torment) continues the association of inflicted pain.

The word "labor," on the other hand, connotes a natural process, referring both to hard work and the pain of muscular contractions in the specific task of childbirth. "Labor" can also be used to speak generally of something being "labored" or "laborious," made or done with great effort, but sometimes a "labor of love." The woman who "bears" (carries, endures, pushes, sustains the burden of) must alternately "bear up," "bear down," and "bear with" the whole process.

Baby Talk. Social relations are clearly indicated in the way people talk about babies. Verbal labeling indicates the appropriate content of each relationship, as different words connote different stages of development, as well as varying conceptions of when "it" becomes a human being. Precisely when this occurs is debatable, clearly shown in continuing disagreements about procreative choice. "Personhood" is ascribed differentially, depending upon the term one uses.

In more recent history, the critical event is "quickening."

HEBREW: *rōsh*, to shake, move, stir

GREEK: *skirtaō*, to leap, spring, bound

GERMAN: *Ursprung*, origin, primordial jump
Absprung, to leap away from

ANGLO-SAXON: *ofspring* offspring: child or children;
cwicu, alive.

The word "embryo" is used to refer to the human organism in the first three months after conception; for the rest of the gestation period, "fetus" is the appropriate term. The word "child" is now applied indiscriminately, but in Greek, Latin, and Old English, it originally meant "fetus, the uterine being." Its developmental chain shows a progression from "round swelling" to "womb" to "fetus" to "offspring."

The word "infant," from the Latin *infans* (speechless) is duplicated in the Polish *niemowle*. Greek has two terms: *teknon* (that which has been generated) and *nēpios* (without mind or reason, silly). The Anglo-Saxon verb *beran* (to carry or bear) produced Old English *bearn*, Old High German and Gothic *barn*, and the more recent Scottish *bairn*. What is significant is that all of these words, from the Greek and Latin onward, are neuter. Personhood was not achieved even at birth but occurred later.

In many societies, the infant was inspected at birth by the elders; only the whole and healthy were returned to the mother to be suckled. This is echoed in the Old English *halic*, *hal* (sound and well) from which derive "holy," "wholeness," "health."

In some cultures, being born is merely the first step to personhood, especially for boys. Tales of Zeus incubating Dionysus in his thigh or giving birth to Athena, fully grown, from his forehead, are acted out in formal rituals of "initiation" (from the Latin *īnire*, to go in). The delta/door of the mother, by which the father had "gone in unto her" and through which the son had "appeared," must be negated and the child born again, this time of the father.

The word "son" is another linguistic anomaly, out of the Indo-European base *sonu-s* (to give birth, to produce). Note the absence of gender designation. The implication is, then as now, that "son," like "man," is the unmarked category, the norm, and that one has not "produced" until a son is born. "Daughter," on the other hand, is a different sort of anomaly, unique among descriptors of females: an independent word, not derived from masculine forms. ✷ DONNA JORDAN

See **Guide to Related Topics:** Literature and the Arts

Resources

Lewis, Charlton T. (1918). *Elementary Latin Dictionary*. New York: American Book Co.

Oxford English Dictionary. (1989). Prepared by J.A. Simpson and E.S.C. Weiner. Oxford, England: Clarendon Press.

Partridge, Eric. (1970). *A Dictionary of Slang and Unconventional English*. 7th edition. New York: McMillan.

Poynton, Cate. (1989). *Language and Gender: Making the Difference*. Oxford, England: Oxford University Press.

Roget's College Thesaurus. (1962). New York: The World Publishing Company.

Thass-Thienemann, Theodore. (1973). *The Interpretation of Language: Volume I: Understanding the Symbolic Meaning of Language; Volume II: Understanding the Unconscious Meaning of Language*. New York: Jason Aronson, Inc., Publishers.

Thorn, Barrie & Henley, Nancy. (Eds.) (1975). *Language and Sex: Difference and Dominance*. Rowley, MA: Newbury House Publishers, Inc.

Webster's New World Dictionary. College Edition. (1966). New York: The World Publishing Co.

LEBOYER METHOD

Dr. Frederick Leboyer (1918-), a French obstetrician, described a method of delivery in his book *Birth without Violence* (1976) that is relevant mainly to the infant, not to providing coping mechanisms for women in labor. Leboyer claimed that he had relived his own birth (with this claim he lost much credibility with the U.S. medical establishment). As a result of his experience, he devised a "gentler" method of bringing babies into the world. With the Leboyer method of delivery, instead of bright lights and a lot of noise in the delivery room, the lights are dim, voices hushed. Instead of turning the baby upside down and spanking it, the baby is gently placed on the mother's abdomen. Instead of clamping the umbilical cord immediately, the cord is allowed to stop pulsating, which takes a couple of minutes, before it is clamped, allowing a small additional volume of blood into the baby.

The best-known element of a Leboyer-style delivery is the bath. Soon after birth the newborn is immersed in a body-temperature bath. Many newborns whose bodies have been tense relax in this more familiar medium, unscrew their faces, open their eyes, and begin to look around. Depending on whose book you read (Leboyer, 1976; Berezin, 1980; Odent, 1984a, 1984b), either the obstetrician, the father, or the mother holds the baby while it is in the bath. In this country, the father is the most likely candidate for the job, and many observers see the bath as a beautiful way to involve the father right at the beginning in behavior that is likely to increase attachment to the newborn. One observer, however, has remarked that "the symbolic reemergence from the amniotic fluid and the rebirthing by the father's hands is the male improvement over the female's birthing" (Rothman, 1982, p. 100).

Two controlled studies by the same team at McMaster University Medical Centre (Nelson et al., 1980; Saigal et al., 1981) in which women were randomly assigned to have Leboyer or "conventional" deliveries found no differences in the state of the newborn during its first hour of life; in both groups, newborns spent most of this time in the "quiet alert" state, in which the newborn is receptive to contact with other human beings. It must be noted, however, that the "conventional" delivery described in these studies is a "gentle" conventional birth, meaning that the philosophy, if not the particular techniques, of the Leboyer method are being adopted. Leboyer and others who follow his gentle birth principles have said that it is not the particular techniques they use that are important, but the philosophy of attending to the enormous sensitivity and needs of the newborn; in fact, Odent (1984a) goes so far as to say that others may start to adopt the techniques without the philosophical view and not achieve the same ends. Or, as Leboyer (1976) puts it, without love, there is only skill. Klaus and Kennell (1976) found the same problem in the implementation of their findings on maternal-infant bonding. They recommended that parents be allowed to engage in the attachment process with their babies directly after birth, since babies' unusually receptive quiet-alert state seems to have been designed for this purpose. What has happened is that in many American hospitals, "bonding time" has been implemented—certainly an improvement over the routine separation of parents and newborns—but with someone timing it with a stopwatch and rushing in to whisk the baby off to the newborn nursery after the requisite bonding has occurred. The philosophy is just not there. And women who have been unable to see their babies within one hour of birth—if, for example, they have had a cesarean section with general anesthesia—have been made to feel that they have "failed at bonding." Klaus and Kennell have expressed dismay at some of the negative consequences of these distortions of their work.

Although Leboyer focuses on the needs of the newborn, it seems likely that there are psychological benefits to the birthing woman as well, particularly if contrasted with standard birthing practices that separate mother and infant routinely. One study found that laboring women expecting a Leboyer-style delivery had significantly shorter first-stage labors (averaging 7.5 hours) than women who expected a standard delivery (14 hours) (Nelson et al., 1980, p. 657).

✱ MARTHA LIVINGSTON, Ph.D.

See also: Newborn Intelligence; Newborn Pain; Newborn Senses; Rebirth

See **Guide to Related Topics:** Baby Care; Childbirth Practices and Locations

Resources

Berezin, N. (1980). *The Gentle Birth Book.* New York: Simon & Shuster.

Klaus, M.H. & Kennell, J.H. (1976). *Maternal-Infant Bonding.* St. Louis: C.V. Mosby.

Leboyer, F. (1976). *Birth without Violence.* New York: Alfred A. Knopf.

Nelson, N.M. et al. (1980). "A Randomized Clinical Trial of the Leboyer Approach to Childbirth. *New England Journal of Medicine* 302: 655-60.

Odent, M. (1984a). *Birth Reborn.* New York: Pantheon.

———. (1984b). *Entering the World: The De-Medicalization of Childbirth.* New York: Marion Boyars, Inc.

Rothman, B.K. (1982). *In Labor: Women and Power in the Birthplace.* New York: W.W. Norton & Co.

Saigal, S. et al. (1981). "Observations on the Behavioral State of Newborn Infants during the First Hour of Life: A Comparison of the Leboyer and Conventional Methods." *American Journal of Obstetrics and Gynecology 139*: 715-19.

LEGISLATION AFFECTING MATERNITY CARE*

The Maternity Information Act, which was enacted in New York State in 1989, is proof that women's groups can win against tremendous opposition if individual members of the groups understand the importance of their active participation in the effort. The New York District II of the American College of Obstetricians and

* Copyright © 1992 by Doris B. Haire.

Gynecologists bitterly opposed this bill, as did the New York State Medical Society, the State Nursing Association, and the State Hospital Association. Organized medicine was stunned at their defeat. What was the secret of the women's groups' success? Working well with other consumer groups concerned with health care and being accurate and concise in all communications with legislators.

Having an effect on state legislation is not as complicated as most people assume. Many are put off by the term "lobbying," thinking it is something people do in the interest of big business. In fact, lobbying in its purest form is the process of educating legislators as to the need for a proposed bill. While lobbying a bill may require one or two visits to the state capitol, much can be done from home. A simple handwritten letter or note from a constituent to his or her respective state representatives or state senators carries far more weight than one might assume. Legislators are interested in issues that are popular among their voting constituencies. While trips to the state legislature will become necessary as the bill goes through the process of becoming a law, it does not take bus loads of people to do the lobbying. Above all else it takes teamwork and a willingness to fight again if the bill doesn't make it through the legislature the first year it is introduced. (Most bills take more than one year to become enacted into law.)

The Maternity Information Act directs the New York State Commissioner of Health to require that every hospital distribute an informational pamphlet to each prospective maternity patient at the time of preadmission and, upon request, to the general public. This pamphlet is prepared by the commissioner and contains information describing maternity-related procedures performed at each respective hospital and such other information as is deemed appropriate by the commissioner.

The law requires hospitals to make public their annual rates of:

- cesarean sections, primary and repeat
- women with previous cesarean sections who have had a subsequent successful vaginal birth
- deliveries in birthing rooms
- deliveries by certified nurse-midwives
- fetal monitoring listed on the basis of auscultation, external and internal
- births using forceps, listed on the basis of low forceps and mid-forceps delivery
- births using breech vaginal delivery
- vaginal births using analgesia
- vaginal births using anesthesia, including general, spinals, epidurals, and paracervicals
- births using induction of labor
- births using augmentation of labor
- births using episiotomies
- mothers breastfeeding upon discharge

Bringing about changes in laws regulating maternity care requires organization, but the job is made easier because most women know more about the subject than most legislators. True, physicians as a whole tend to fight against bills that provide added protection for the patient, but in this case women have the advantage in lobbying for legislation affecting maternity care, because in general they are the only ones who have had direct experience with childbirth.

If a legislator will plead your cause by sponsoring or signing on as a secondary sponsor for the bill you are proposing, the following steps are recommended:

1. Obtain a printed guide to the legislature of the state. One with photographs of the legislators is helpful. A local newspaper editor can provide information on how to get one, as can the local chapter of the League of Women Voters.
2. Organize your thoughts by preparing a concise "memorandum of support" listing the reasons the bill is needed. It should be kept short (not more than two pages) and easy to scan.
3. Write the bill in everyday language. Lobbyists should not sound like lawyers. If a legislator agrees to sponsor the bill, his or her aide will make any necessary changes in language.
4. Make a list of groups that might support the bill. Send each group a copy of the proposed bill and memorandum of support. (In the successful effort to pass the Maternity Information Act, the support of the following groups was absolutely essential: the New York Public Interest Research Group, the National Women's Health Network, the International Childbirth Education Association, the Cesarean Prevention Movement, and the Black Women's Health Project.)
5. Take time to consider the wording of the proposed bill carefully before sending it to the legislators. Make sure that the bill is well constructed and says exactly what you want to say.

6. Be realistic. Is the implementation of the bill practical? Is it likely to get through the ways and means committees? What are the likely financial costs to the state if the bill is passed? Is passage of the bill likely to save the state money?
7. Determine where opposition to the bill will come from. Try to look at the implications of the bill from the opposition's point of view and do your best to find information that will help to overcome opponents' objections.
8. Convince those who share your concerns of the importance of letting their respective legislators know how they feel about the bill by contacting them at their home office or in the state capitol.
9. Try to choose primary sponsors of the bill from the leadership of both houses of the legislature. For example, if the majority of the members of the state house of representatives or assembly are Democrats, they should ask a Democrat to be the primary sponsor of the house or assembly bill. (The primary sponsor of the bill must be willing to work for the bill's passage.) If the majority of the senate members are Republicans they should ask a Republican to be the primary sponsor of the bill in the state senate.
10. Ask the sponsors of the bill to send copies of any letters or memoranda of support and of opposition they receive regarding the bill. Then update your own memorandum of support, addressing the opposition's complaints, and send copies to the legislators sponsoring the bill and to those from whom you are seeking support.
11. Keep colleagues current and informed. Send each group a copy of the updated memo of support and any memo of opposition received, and ask them to send copies to their colleagues. It is important that they are made to feel that they are an integral part of the effort. There is nothing like a memo of opposition from a contentious group to keep the "troops" moving forward.
12. When the time comes for your colleagues to contact their respective legislators, they should be reminded that if they are not sure of the name of their state senators and representatives (or assemblymen or women) they can obtain that information from their local newspaper office or League of Women Voters.
13. Remind colleagues that it is always best if they speak directly with their legislators. A legislative aide may agree wholeheartedly with the logic of a bill, but the cold fact is that the legislator may be under pressure from opposing factions that are politically important to him or her. Insisting on talking to the legislator directly will help to impress upon him or her the urgency of your concern.
14. Think about appearance. When the time comes to show up at the capitol it is of utmost importance that everyone attending look professional—no slacks, no knapsacks, etc. While some mothers may want to take along their babies, it is important that almost everyone be free to go back and forth between the senate and the house (or assembly) to speak to the legislators as they travel between their offices and legislative floors.
15. Have everyone prepare in advance little notes with their respective signatures which read, "May I speak with you for a moment?" The legislator's name can then be written in with the same pen above the note and handed to one of the remarkably obliging sergeants at arms, who will pass it to the appropriate legislator. It is amazing how agreeable legislators are to being called from the floor to speak to members of the public in the lobby. If meeting the legislator for the first time, it is helpful to have previously seen his or her picture in a legislative guide.

As mentioned earlier, much can be done by lobbyists at home, but there are certain critical times when it may help to be near the scene of action. For example, a bill may be held up by opposing legislators in the rules committee of either house. The rules committee determines whether a proposed bill is in conflict with other laws on the books. If there is no such conflict or opposition, the bill is then referred to the legislative floor to be voted on. Sometimes a bill will be held up in the appropriations committee on the grounds that the costs of implementing the bill would be prohibitive. It's up to the lobbying group to show that it would not be.

The bill comes to the floor for a final vote within a few days after the rules committee puts it on the legislative calendar. If the lobbyists' bill is passed, those groups who participated in the mutual effort should let those legislators who actively supported the bill know how much their efforts were appreciated.

Finally, a bill has just been passed by the New York Legislature that, establishes the first State

Board of Midwifery in the United States. The bill establishes midwifery as a separate profession in the state; provides an appropriate regulating body for midwifery practice; and authorizes a study of those policies that affect the recruitment, education and practice of professional midwifery.

✱ DORIS B. HAIRE

See **Guide to Related Topics:** Legal Issues

LESBIAN MOTHERS

Although the 1970s and 1980s have made up what has been called the lesbian baby boom (Riley, 1988a), some theorists argue that lesbian mothers may be traced back to the origin of the family itself (Cavin, 1985). Lesbian mothers cross all class, racial, ethnic, nationality, and physically able lines. Lesbian mothers live in heterosexual marriages or alternative family structures. Prior to the Lesbian Feminist Movement, most lesbian mothers became parents via heterosexual intercourse. The women's, civil rights, and lesbian/gay movements of the 1960s and 1970s gave confidence to lesbian feminists to parent children. Sperm banks and adoption agencies became accessible to single parents, giving lesbians more options for having children.

Lesbian mothers are creating new family forms and are potentially a force for change in sexist, racist, and heterosexist societies. They can be lesbians in the lesbian community and mothers in the heterosexual world, but they find little support for lesbian motherhood in either world. In patriarchal cultures, where motherhood is extolled as the primary role for women and lesbianism is tabooed, lesbian mothers are in a double bind. Lesbian mothers of color and multiracial families also face racism.

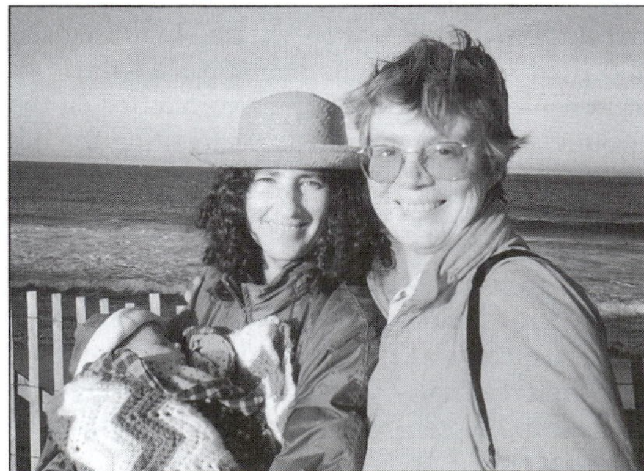

A proud and happy lesbian couple and their new baby. Photo courtesy of Laura Zeidenstein, C.N.M.

Options for Parenting. Alternative fertilization (donor insemination), as a form of woman-controlled conception (O'Donnell et al., 1979), is the process of introducing a donor specimen of sperm, either fresh or frozen, into the woman's vagina at or near the time of ovulation with the intention of fertilizing the ovum (ova). The issue of whether to use a known or unknown donor has important repercussions. Issues to explore with a known donor include: Will the donor be involved in parenting? How will the lesbian mother(s) protect herself (themselves) if the donor desires custody of the child(ren)? With an unknown donor, the central issue is: How much information about the donor will be available to the child(ren)? The AIDS pandemic has changed donor options. It is imperative to take thorough sexual histories and to screen for human immunodeficiency virus (HIV) antibodies and all sexually transmitted diseases (STDs) in donor semen. Frozen semen should be quarantined until it is tested two times, six months apart, with negative results.

Other options besides alternative fertilization include heterosexual intercourse, foster parenting, legal guardianship, combined families, and nonbiological parenting.

Family Configurations. Lesbian mothers challenge traditional heterosexual family structure and are pioneer developers of new family forms. Lesbian parent configurations may include: (1) a single woman with one or more child(ren); (2) two women lovers with one or more child(ren); (3) two or more friends with one or more child(ren); (4) a combined family consisting of two or more families coparenting each other's children; (5) an extended lesbian family consisting of a single lesbian or lesbian couple with one or more child(ren) and other friends and/or ex-lovers actively involved in childrearing; and (6) extended biological family (Pies, 1988). Lesbian family forms are developing so quickly that descriptive language lags far behind.

Birth Mother. The birth mother has many considerations, beginning with how she will become pregnant. Heterosexist attitudes of coworkers, family of origin, and health care providers may make this process stressful. Once pregnant, she is vulnerable and may find herself "coming out" all over again, but this time as a pregnant lesbian, then again later as a lesbian mother. Heterosexual assumptions, visibility of pregnancy, and invisibility of her lesbianism may challenge her own identity. A knowledgeable and supportive network of caregivers is vital. Hospital policies and staff often refuse lesbian parents labor support and postpartum visitation privileges. Recent research suggests that health care providers are often insensitive to lesbian health care needs (Hume, 1983; Johnson and Palermo, 1984; Olesker and Walsh, 1984; Stevens and Hall, 1988; Harvey, Carr, and Bernheine, 1989; Garceau, 1990; Loischild, 1990; Zeidenstein, 1990). These studies sampled predominantly white subjects; few studies of lesbian mothers of color have been done, except for Dr. Marjorie Hill's research on childrearing attitudes of black lesbian mothers (Hill, 1987).

Coparenting. Patriarchal definitions of the family are challenged by the lesbian coparent. "Nonbiological mother" is the most common term used to describe the coparent, although this gives a sense of negation or "of being made out of teflon" (Clausen, 1987). Other terms include "comother," "social mother," "other mother," and "second female parent" (Riley, 1988). Some families invent their own terms. New terminology is needed to describe this rapidly evolving kinship role. According to anthropologist Claire Riley, lesbian families are creating a new female parent: "Lesbians are changing the American kinship system. The alienation, stress and isolation that the new female parent experiences is due to lack of social and legal recognition" (Riley, 1988). This stress is sociological, rather than psychological. Generally, the second female parent's lesbianism is visible, while her motherhood is invisible. She may experience tremendous pain when her parenting role is not recognized by colleagues, family of origin, neighbors, and friends who are not lesbian/gay parents. In a society where she has no legal or social recognition, strong social support networks with other lesbian families are crucial.

Legal Issues. Legal recognition of parenthood for both mothers is sought by lesbians. Such recognition would give both parents equal rights under the law and recognize the "potential equalization of power fundamental to lesbian/gay relationships" (Polikoff, 1987). Legal concerns of lesbian parents include the custody rights a donor has to the child and the custody rights of the social mother in lesbian "divorce" cases. Individual state laws concerning parent-child relationships should be understood before using donor fertilization. The best protection against future legal problems is a "donor-recipient agreement" (Pies, 1988). Lesbian parent couples may want legal parent status for both parents, but no state allows an unrelated adult to adopt a child unless the birth parent waives all parental rights. Several documents may protect lesbian parental relationships: a will nominating the social mother as guardian in the event of the biological mother's death; a nomination of guardianship; a parental agreement between the birth mother and the social mother that recognizes the social mother's parental role and responsibility in the event of separation; and a medical consent form giving the co-mother medical authority (Pies, 1988).

✱ LAURA ZEIDENSTEIN, C.N.M., M.S.N.

See also: Donor Insemination

Resources

Alpert, Harriet. (Ed.) (1988). *We Are Everywhere: Writings by and about Lesbian Parents.* Freedom, CA: The Crossing Press Feminist Series.

Boston Lesbian Psychologies Collective. (Eds.) (1987). *Lesbian Psychologies, Explorations, and Challenges.* Chicago: University of Illinois Press.

Bozett, F.W. (Ed.) (1987). *Gay and Lesbian Parents.* New York: Praeger.

Bradford, J. & Ryan C. (1988). *The National Lesbian Health Care Survey.* Washington, DC: National Lesbian and Gay Health Foundation.

Cavin, Susan. (1985). *Lesbian Origins.* San Francisco: Ism Press.

Clausen, Jan. (1987). "To Live Outside the Law You Must be Honest: A Flommy Looks at Lesbian Parenting." In Sandra Pollack & Jeanne Vaughn. (Eds.) *Politics of the Heart: A Lesbian Parenting Anthology.* Ithaca, NY: Firebrand Books, 333-42.

Curry, H. & Clifford, D. (1985). *A Legal Guide for Lesbian and Gay Couples.* 3rd edition. New York: Nolo Press Self-Help Law Books.

Garceau, L. (1990). *Lesbian Health Care: Knowledge Levels of and Heterosexist Bias in Initial Assessment of Female Clients by Nurse-Midwives and Nurse Practitioners. Master's thesis, Yale School of Nursing, New Haven, CT.*

Harvey, S.M., Carr, C., & Bernheine, S. (1989). "Lesbian Mothers: Health Care Experiences." *Journal of Nurse Midwifery 34* (3): 115-19.

Hill, Marjorie. (1987). "Child-rearing Attitudes of Black Lesbian Mothers." In Boston Lesbian Psychologies Collective. (Eds.) Lesbian Psychologies, Explorations, and Challenges. Chicago: University of Illinois Press, pp. 215-26.

Hitchens, Donna J. (1982). *Lesbian Mother Litigation Manual.* (Lesbian Rights Project, 1370 Mission St., 4th Floor, San Francisco, CA 94103).

Hume, B.J. (1983). *Perspectives on Women's Health: Disclosure Decisions, Needs and Experiences of Lesbians.* Master's thesis, Yale School of Nursing, New Haven, CT.

Johnson, S.R. & Palermo, J.L. (1984). "Gynecological Care for the Lesbian." *Clinical Obstetrics and Gynecology 27* (3): 724-31.

Jullion, Jeanne. (1985). Long Way Home: The Odyssey of a Lesbian Mother and Her Children. New York: Cleis Press.

Loischild, Judith R.M. (1990). *The Experiences and Health Care Needs of Childbearing Lesbians.* Master's thesis, Yale School of Nursing, New Haven, CT.

O'Donnell, M. et al. (1979). *Lesbian Health Matters.* (Santa Cruz Women's Health Collective Publication, 250 Locust St., Santa Cruz, CA 95060).

Olesker, E. & Walsh, L.V. (1984). "Childbearing among Lesbians: Are We Meeting Their Needs?" *Journal of Nurse-Midwifery 29* (5): 322-29.

Pies, Cheri. (1988). *Considering Parenthood, Second Edition*. San Francisco: Spinsters/Aunt Lute.

Polikoff, Nancy D. (1987). "Lesbian Mothers, Lesbian Families: Legal Obstacles, Legal Challenges." In Sandra Pollack & Jeanne Vaughn (Eds.) *Politics of the Heart: A Lesbian Parenting Anthology*. Ithaca, NY: Firebrand Books, pp. 325-32.

Pollack, Sandra & Vaughn, Jeanne. (Eds.) (1987). *Politics of the Heart: A Lesbian Parenting Anthology*. Ithaca, NY: Firebrand Books.

Riley, Claire. (1988a, Fall). "American Kinship: A Lesbian Account." *Feminist Issues*: 75-94.

———. (1988b). "The Significance of Second Female Parent Role in Lesbian Families." Paper presented at the 89th Annual Meeting of the American Anthropological Association, Phoenix, AZ.

Stevens, P.E. & Hall, J.M. (1988). "Stigma, Health Beliefs, and Experience with Health Care in Lesbian Women." *Image: Nursing Scholarship 20* (2): 69-73.

Zeidenstein, Laura. (1990). "Gynecological and Childbearing Needs of Lesbians." *Journal of Nurse-Midwifery 35* (1): 10-18.

LOW BIRTH WEIGHT: UNITED STATES

The incidence of low birth weight (LBW) (less than 2,500 grams or 5½ pounds) has been carefully monitored in the United States because it is a major predictor of infant morbidity and mortality. The birth certificates of the 50 states and the District of Columbia provide data on birth weight, as well as related demographic and health information for the mother and infant, which are reported to the National Center for Health Statistics, Centers for Disease Control.

Between 1975 and 1985, the incidence of LBW declined by 9 percent, from 73.9 to 67.5 low birth-weight babies per 1,000 live births, but 86 percent of this decline occurred between 1975 and 1980 (Taffel, 1989). (See Table 1.) Although LBW declined for both white and black births between 1975 and 1980, the decline was nearly twice as much for white (9 percent) as for black (5 percent) births. The decline in LBW rates in the 1980 to 1985 period was 1 percent or less for both white and black births.

The overall rate of LBW increased from 67.5 in 1985 to 69.3 in 1988, but this was wholly a reflection of the 4 percent rise in the rate for black births (from 124.2 to 129.7); white LBW rates were no higher in 1988 than in 1985 (56.4) (National Center for Health Statistics, 1990).

In recent years, growing attention has been paid to the incidence of very low birth weight (VLBW) (less than 1,500 grams or 3 pounds 4 ounces) because infants weighing this little are at greatest risk of dying or of having a serious illness. Infants weighing less than 1,500 grams make up only about 1 percent of all live births, but they account for almost 40 percent of all infant deaths (Hogue et al., 1987).

VLBW remained almost unchanged between 1975 and 1980 (11.6 very low birth-weight babies per 1,000 live births in 1975, compared with 11.5 in 1980), but increased by 5 percent (from 11.5 to 12.1) from 1980 to 1985. (See Table 1.) The increase in VLBW between 1980 and 1985 was about twice as much for black as for white babies (9 percent compared with 4 percent). VLBW rates for white births remained fairly stable in the 1985 to 1988 period (9.4 in 1985 compared with 9.3 in 1988), but rose by 5 percent for black births (from 26.5 to 27.8).

Concomitant with the decline in low birth weight in the 1975 to 1985 decade was a reduction in the proportion of babies born weighing 2,500 to 3,499 grams and a distinct shift to birth weights of 3,500 grams (7 pounds 12 ounces) or more. (See Table 2.) By 1985, 41 percent of newborns weighed at least 3,500 grams, up from 37 percent in 1975. Because the increase in higher birth weights was of about the same magnitude for white as for black births, there was no narrowing of the racial difference. In 1985, as in 1975, the proportion of white newborns weighing at least 3,500 grams was 1.7 times the comparable proportion of black newborns (44 percent compared with 26 percent in 1985). These proportions remained almost unchanged between 1985 and 1988.

A common theme in the study of low birth weight is the substantial and persistent difference in low birth-weight risk between black and white babies. In 1975, black babies were 2.1 times as likely as white babies to have a birth weight of less than 2,500 grams. Low birth weight declined more

Table 1. Rates of Low and Very Low Weight, by Race of Child: United States, Selected Years, 1975-88

(Rates per 1,000 live births)

Year	Low birth weight 1/			Very low birth weight 2/		
	All races 3/	White	Black	All races 3/	White	Black
1975	73.9	62.6	130.9	11.6	9.2	23.7
1980	68.4	57.0	124.9	11.5	9.0	24.4
1985	67.5	56.4	124.2	12.1	9.4	26.5
1986	68.1	56.4	125.3	12.1	9.3	26.6
1987	69.0	56.8	127.1	12.4	9.4	27.3
1988	69.3	56.4	129.7	12.4	9.3	27.8

1/ Less than 2,500 grams (5 pounds 8 ounces)
2/ Less than 1,500 grams (3 pounds 4 ounces)
3/ Includes races other than white and black

Table 2. Number of Live Births and Percent Distribution by Birth Weight, According to Race of Child: United States, Selected Years, 1975-88

Race of child and year	All live births	All birth weights	Less than 1,000 grams	1,000-1,499 grams	1,500-1,999 grams	2,000-2,499 grams	2,500-2,999 grams	3000-3,499 grams	3,500 3,999 grams	4,000-4,499 grams	4,500 grams or more
		Birth Weight									
All races 1/	Number 2/	Percent distribution									
1975	3,144,198	100.0	0.5	0.6	1.4	4.8	17.9	37.9	27.4	7.8	1.6
1980	3,612,258	100.0	0.5	0.6	1.3	4.4	16.3	37.0	29.1	8.9	1.8
1985	3,760,561	100.0	0.6	0.6	1.3	4.2	15.9	36.7	29.6	9.2	1.9
1986	3,756,547	100.0	0.6	0.6	1.3	4.3	15.9	36.7	29.5	9.2	1.9
1987	3,809,394	100.0	0.6	0.6	1.3	4.3	16.0	36.7	29.5	9.1	1.9
1988	3,909,510	100.0	0.6	0.6	1.3	4.4	16.0	36.6	29.4	9.2	1.9
White											
1975	2,551,996	100.0	0.4	0.5	1.2	4.1	16.2	37.8	29.3	8.6	1.8
1980	2,898,732	100.0	0.4	0.5	1.1	3.7	14.6	36.6	31.1	9.9	2.1
1985	2,991,373	100.0	0.4	0.5	1.1	3.6	14.1	36.1	31.7	10.3	2.2
1986	2,970,439	100.0	0.4	0.5	1.1	3.6	14.2	36.1	31.6	10.3	2.1
1987	2,992,488	100.0	0.4	0.5	1.1	3.7	14.2	36.1	31.6	10.3	2.1
1988	3,046,162	100.0	0.4	0.5	1.1	3.7	14.2	36.1	31.7	10.3	2.1
Black											
1975	511,581	100.0	1.1	1.2	2.6	8.1	25.7	38.4	18.4	3.8	0.7
1980	589,616	100.0	1.2	1.2	2.5	7.6	24.3	38.4	19.8	4.3	0.8
1985	608,193	100.0	1.4	1.2	2.4	7.4	23.6	38.4	20.3	4.5	0.8
1986	621,221	100.0	1.4	1.3	2.5	7.4	23.6	38.2	20.3	4.5	0.8
1987	641,567	100.0	1.5	1.3	2.4	7.5	23.5	38.0	20.4	4.5	0.9
1988	671,976	100.0	1.5	1.3	2.5	7.7	23.4	37.8	20.3	4.6	0.9

1/Includes races other than white and black
2/Includes births with unknown birth weight, which are excluded from the computation of the percent distribution

for white than for black births in the 1975 to 1985 period, increasing the racial differential to 2.2. It remained at this level in 1986 and 1987 but increased to 2.3 in 1988.

Although relatively more black than white mothers are represented in subgroups at high risk of LBW (unmarried, less than 20 years of age, with less than 12 years of education, or with late or no care during pregnancy), this only partly explains the greater risk of LBW for black babies. Regardless of age of mother, month that pregnancy prenatal care began, years of schooling completed, or marital status, black mothers are generally twice as likely to have a LBW baby and two to three times as likely to have a VLBW baby (Taffel, 1989). Although increased years of schooling lowers the risk of low birth weight for both black and white babies in high-risk categories, the racial gap in LBW incidence actually increases with added years of schooling.

One of the major reasons for the more than double incidence of low birth weight among black babies is their high risk of being born prematurely (before 37 completed weeks of gestation). Although the percentage difference for incidence of low birth weight for black premature births was only 12 percent higher than for white premature births in 1988 (42.2 percent compared with 37.7 percent), black babies were more than twice as likely to be born prematurely in that year (18.3 percent of black births, compared with 8.5 percent of white births). The racial disparity in low birth weight is even more evident for term and postterm infants. For infants born at term (37 to 41 weeks of gestation), 6.1 percent of black babies compared with 2.6 percent of white babies weighed less than 5½ pounds. For infants born postterm (gestations of 42 weeks or longer), 4.5 percent of black infants and 1.8 percent of white infants were of low birth weight (National Center for Health Statistics, 1990).

The differential between black and white women in the risk of bearing a low or very low birth-weight baby after controlling for age, education, marital status, and prenatal care may to some extent reflect differences in personal finances, health status, and lifestyle. Black women are generally more likely than white women of similar pre-pregnancy weight to gain less than 16 pounds during pregnancy—well below current guidelines (Taffel, 1986). Black married women who have had at least one child are more likely to work during pregnancy than are white married women who have had the same number of children, and they are more likely to be blue-collar workers (Makuc, 1983). Also, black mothers have a lower average family income than do white mothers at comparable levels of education (Kleinman and Kessel, 1987).

There are undoubtedly many other racial differences in nutritional status, lifestyle, and environmental conditions, not yet quantified, that have an important impact on birth weight. Beginning with the 1989 data year, a wealth of new information relevant to the etiology of low birth weight became available from the revised U.S. Standard Certificate of Live Birth, implemented by almost all states in 1989. Included on the new certificate are questions relating to medical risk factors of pregnancy, such as anemia and cardiac disease, and lifestyle factors—tobacco and alcohol use and weight gain during pregnancy—that are closely related to birth weight. This new information, combined with other socioeconomic and health data from birth certificates, should help clarify the reasons for the persistent and large racial differential in the incidence of low birth weight.

✱ SELMA TAFFEL

See also: Infant Mortality Statistics: United States; Premature Birth: Prevention; Teenage Childbearing: Trends in the United States

See **Guide to Related Topics:** Pregnancy Loss and Infant Mortality

Resources

Hogue, C.J.R. et al. (1987). "Overview of the National Infant Mortality Surveillance (NIMS): Project Design, Methods, Results." *Public Health Rep 102* (2): 126-38.

Kleinman, J.C. & Kessel, S.S. (1987). "Racial Differences in Low Birth Weight." *New England Journal of Medicine 317* (12): 749-53.

Makuc, D. (1983). "Employment Characteristics of Mothers during Pregnancy." *Health, United States, 1983.* National Center for Health Statistics. Washington, DC: Public Health Service.

National Center for Health Statistics. (1990). "Advance Report of Final Natality Statistics, 1988." *Monthly Vital Statistics Report 39* (4). Supplemental. Hyattsville, MD: Public Health Service.

Taffel, S.M. (1986). "Maternal Weight Gain and the Outcome of Pregnancy, United States, 1980." *Vital Health Statistics 21* (44).

———. (1989). "Trends in Low Birth Weight: United States, 1975-85." *Vital Health Statistics 21* (48).

LULLABIES AND CRADLE SONGS

Lullabies exist in virtually every society. Some define lullabies strictly as songs about sleep (Hawes, 1974). While their primary function is to induce sleep in infants and small children, lullabies also serve as an introduction to music and as a means of intimacy between parent and child. On a deeper level, they contain some aspects of interest to many scholars. Musicologists note that lullabies have influenced the works of such composers as Bach, Byrd, and others. Psychologists and educators are also interested in how lullabies are related to the early development of infants and small children. On a broader scale, sociologists, folklorists, and anthropologists have all speculated on what these tunes can tell them about their respective cultures.

Musicological Aspects. Most musicologists consider lullabies folk music—that is, music that is handed down orally from generation to generation. Often in this type of transmission, certain aspects, such as melody and lyrics, are embellished, changed, or omitted by individual performers over a long period of time. Thus, it is likely that many versions of the same lullaby can coexist. There have been attempts over the last century to preserve certain lullabies in large anthologies. However, these are usually versions that were either arranged by a specific author or indicative of how the song was typically done at one time, and should therefore not be regarded as the definitive version of a particular lullaby.

Like other folk genres, lullabies have been utilized as a basis for the composition of "classical" music, especially during the 19th century, when the concept of the Folk (or Volk) gained ideological and artistic prominence. Character pieces such as the French berceuse and German wiegenlied featured the soft timbre, the gentle rhythm, and the sing-song melodic features characteristic of most European lullabies. Among some of the more well-known composers of these genres were Chopin ("Berceuse," op. 57), Grieg ("Badriat," op. 65, no. 5), and Balakiev ("Berceuses for Piano").

Lullabies have also served as a basis for popular compositions. Songs such as "The Coal Black

Rose" sold widely in the form of sheet music during the 1830s, while in recent times, tunes such as "Mockingbird" (recorded in 1974 by James Taylor and Carly Simon) have also done well. Some composers have forsaken traditional songs and have instead used the characteristically gentle rhythmic and tonal motion of this folk genre to create new songs (e.g., B.J. Thomas's "Rock 'n' Roll Lullaby").

Psychological Aspects. Singing a lullaby to a small child usually entails many different activities. Besides vocalizing, the performer also looks at the child, cuddles him or her, and perhaps makes gentle rocking motions. All of these actions provide the baby with tactile, visual, and aural stimulation. For this reason, lullabies aid in some aspects of development and well-being. The intimacy of lullaby singing can be a factor in the child's sense of security, as well as a means of emotional bonding between it and the performer.

Children are capable of developing aural sensibility at a very early age, and this sensibility is connected to both the development of speech and musical perception. For example, a baby is able to determine the volume of and localize a sound within the first 10 minutes after birth, and within 24 hours can distinguish various sounds. "Musical babble" (imitation of musical sounds) as opposed to speech babble (imitation of the spoken word) can happen between 4 and 18 months. Because of the link between speech and musical vocalizations, some experts advocate singing lullabies as well as reading to infants and young children, ascribing to the Piagetian belief that "the more a child has seen and heard, the more he will want to see and hear," which implies that during infancy, both of these activities stimulate unconscious learning (Brand, 1985).

Other Aspects. While the lullaby itself might be universal, each culture tends to lend its own flavor to the content of each song. For example, the Hopi of North America do not perceive rhythm in strict metrical patterns. Thus, their lullabies do not contain strong pulses and might not even coincide with the rocking motion of the cradle. On the other hand, the lullabies of western Africa contain strong polyrhythmic organizations that parallel the rest of their musical output, while lullabies originating in western Europe emphasize pitch organization and metered rhythm.

Lyrics can also provide valuable insight into class interactions, especially in cases where the performer is not a parent, but a servant. Erick Masuyama writes about one particular Japanese village (Itaskui) in which lullabies are traditionally sung by lower-class nannies to children of aristocratic families. A typical example:

> I hate to baby-sit a baby.
> I am hated by my master because the baby cries.

Masuyama goes on to talk about the desperation felt by the young women torn from their families, too poor to care for them, and then placed in a strange environment (Masuyama, 1989).

Here, lullabies allow the performer to express safely resentment she may have toward a frustrating occupation and an unsympathetic employer. But even when sung by parents, lullabies often give the performer a chance to say the unsayable. In this regard, even such time-honored songs as "Rock-a-Bye Baby" contain elements of the macabre with its vivid image of a child crashing "cradle and all" from the treetops. A more recent example (sung to the tune of "Freres Jacques"):

> Beating babies with a blackjack
> Is such fun. Is such fun.
> How I love to beat them. How I love to beat them.
> Yum, yum, yum.
> Yum, yum, yum. (Goldberg, 1983)

Groups of lullabies and other children's songs can often reveal extended insights into the workings of a larger social system. For example, the *Mother Goose* rhymes explain much about pre-industrial British culture. Basic agrarian economy is illustrated in songs such as "Little Bo Peep," "Baa Baa Black Sheep," and "Three Blind Mice," while elements of social stratification (kings, gentlemen, knights, etc.) appear in many more.

✱ EHRICK LONG, M.M.

See also: Newborn Intelligence; Newborn Senses

See **Guide to Related Topics:** Baby Care

Resources

Baker, William J. (1975). "Historical Meaning in Mother Goose: Nursery Rhymes of English Society before the Industrial Revolution. *Journal of Popular Culture 9* (3): 645-52.

Brand, Manny. (1985, Mar). "Lullabies that Awaken Musicality in Infants." *Music Educators Journal 71*: 28-31.

Brown, Maurice. (1980). "Lullaby." In Stanley Sadic. (Ed.) *The New Grove Encyclopedia of Music and Musicians 11*: 314. London; New York: Macmillan Publishers.

Goldberg, Millie. (1983). "Frères Jacques (variation)." *New York City Lullabies* (audiocassette). Julia Lebentritt and Karen Pearlman, producers. New York: Song Bank.

Hawes, Bess L. (1974). "Folksongs and Function—Some Thoughts on the American Lullaby." *Journal of American Folklore 87* (344): 140-48.

Masuyama, Erick. (1989). "Desire and Discontent in Japanese Lullabies." *Western Folklore 48* (2): 144-48.

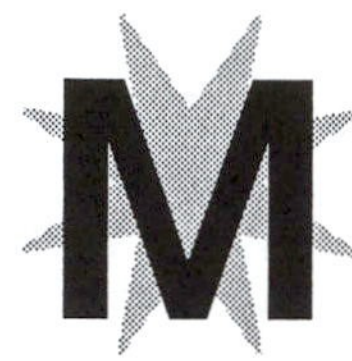

MALE FACTORS IN PREGNANCY OUTCOME

Women are held more accountable for a healthy birth outcome than their partners. This societal attitude can result in undue anxiety, depression, and feelings of inadequacy in new mothers. On a larger scale, a scientific and medical research bias that sways public attitudes and influences employment and health policy can be observed.

Media coverage relating to women, alcohol, and Fetal Alcohol Syndrome is an excellent example of targeting women for punitive action. Studies indicating that alcohol "damages" women more readily than men have captured front page coverage. One very small-scale research project concluding that the female digestive system is unable to metabolize alcohol as efficiently as the male's earned an editorial in the *New England Journal of Medicine* (Kolata, 1990). Inaccurate statements about women's biology and their sole responsibility in creating "perfect" children have resulted in threats to civil liberties in such areas as equal employment, privacy, and equal protection under the law.

Although rarely discussed in the media, research has demonstrated that there are definite male factors that can lead to a less than optimal birth outcome. Studies have shown a relationship between chronic drinking in men and abnormal sperm production and testicular atrophy (Rosett and Weiner, 1984). Dr. Devra Lee Davis, a scholar in residence at the National Academy of Sciences, stated, "You don't have to be Sigmund Freud to figure out there are cultural factors to say why we have paid so much attention to the female and so little to the male" (Blakeslee, 1991).

A recent article in the *New York Times* announced a new research emphasis on possible paternal contribution to birth defects, especially as related to the fathers' occupation (Blakeslee, 1991). Previously, the theory was that a "defective sperm" would not be strong enough to go the distance to fertilize an egg. But it is now known that there are tiny hairs in the female reproductive tract that help move *all* sperm along the Fallopian tubes. Also, since sperm production is an ongoing process during a male's lifetime, sperm cells may be particularly vulnerable to genetic damage from external sources during their division. Some toxins, such as anesthetic gases, radiation, lead, solvents, vinyl chloride, airborne pollutants, and pesticides, could cause genetic mutations or other changes in sperm. These damaged sperm may succeed at fertilizing an egg that will become a fetus with a birth defect or perhaps have a predisposition to some form of cancer.

There are three ways that drugs, chemicals, and physical agents can act through the father. Male fertility can be affected, either through decreased sperm cell count or depressed performance. A substance can be carried in the semen in very small amounts and thus expose the egg. The substance can also damage the sperm cell itself at any point in its development.

The U.S. Supreme Court recently heard a case that challenged a policy in which employers could bar fertile women from jobs that might endanger a fetus. This case was brought before the Court over a "fetal protection policy" at a Milwaukee manufacturer of automobile batteries. The policy barred women who could not provide medical evidence of infertility from jobs involving exposure to lead. The Court's conclusion was that this type of policy is unconstitutional and discriminatory, in that it offers men personal choice in their work options but not women (Greenhouse, 1991). Judith Lichtman, president of the Women's Legal Defense Fund, stated, "Employers have used women as the scapegoat of their failure to properly evaluate the harm caused by workplace hazards to both men and women" (Greenhouse, 1991).

✷ PAT RICHTER, M.P.A.

See also: Pregnancy and Social Control

Resources

Blakeslee, Sandra. (1991, Jan 1). "Connection Hinted Between Birth Defects and Sperm Damage." *New York Times*: A1.

Greenhouse, Linda. (1991, Mar 21). "Court to Review Fetal Safety Plan." *New York Times*: A1.

Kolata, Gina. (1990, Jan 11). "Study Tells Why Alcohol Is Greater Risk." *New York Times*: A1.

Rosett, Henry L. & Weiner, Lyn. (1984). *Alcohol and the Fetus*. New York and Oxford: Oxford University Press.

MATERNAL MORTALITY

In 1940, one out of every 266 pregnant women in the United States died from pregnancy or childbirth; for every 100,000 live births in the country that year, approximately 376 women died from maternal causes (National Center for Health Statistics, 1990). (See Figure 1.) Since that time, deaths related to pregnancy and childbirth have become rare in this country, so that now the chance of dying from pregnancy or childbirth is one in 12,500 (330 women died in 1988, which is approximately eight deaths per 100,000 live births) (National Center for Health Statistics, 1990). Most maternal deaths can be prevented; in fact, health experts estimate that up to 75 percent of these deaths can be prevented. This dramatic decrease in maternal mortality has occurred for several reasons. First, women today are better nourished and generally are in better health than women were 50 years ago. Second, the common causes of maternal death have been reduced through medical advances such as new surgical and anesthesia techniques for cesarean section, powerful antibiotics to prevent and fight infections, and intravenous fluids and blood transfusions to treat bleeding. Third, new methods for diagnosing pregnancy earlier and for monitoring and detecting problems such as placental abnormalities, ectopic pregnancy, etc., earlier reduce maternal complications. Last, the development of strategies to reduce maternal death has taken place through concerted efforts by maternal mortality committees, state medical societies, and state health departments, and has led to a better understanding of the causes of maternal death (Thoms, 1960; Marmol, Scriggins, and Vollman, 1969; Antler and Fox, 1976; Rochat, 1980).

Figure 1. Maternal Mortality Rates by Year, United States, Selected Years, 1940-1988

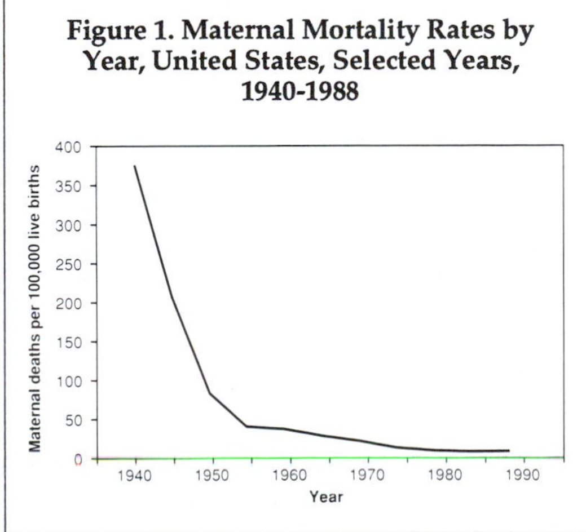

Source: National Center for Health Statistics

The recommended international definition of a maternal death is the death of a woman occurring during pregnancy or within 42 days after pregnancy has ended, regardless of the duration and site of pregnancy, from any cause related to, or aggravated by the pregnancy, or its management, but not from accidental or incidental causes (World Health Organization, 1977). Other definitions of maternal mortality include a death during pregnancy or after the end of pregnancy up to one year (Kaunitz et al., 1985; Ellerbrock et al., 1988). Studies have shown that by limiting the definition of maternal death to 42 days, 11 percent of maternal deaths are missed, therefore a one-year definition is recommended (Rochat et al., 1988; Fortney, 1990). Maternal mortality rates (also referred to as maternal mortality ratios) are calculated as the number of maternal deaths in a given year divided by the number of live births in that year, multiplied by a constant (usually 100,000). Maternal mortality rates in the United States are expressed as per 100,000 live births.

The number and characteristics of maternal deaths are derived from information reported on death certificates filed in state vital statistics offices. National statistics, compiled from death certificates, are published by the National Center for Health Statistics of the Centers for Disease Control. The Division of Reproductive Health, Center for Chronic Disease Prevention and Health Promotion, Centers for Disease Control, conducts national epidemiologic studies using information from maternal death certificates and from medical and other sources.

Even though maternal deaths rarely occur, some subgroups of women are at higher risk than others for this type of death. For example, women of minority races, women over 30 years of age, women who do not receive prenatal care, unmarried women, and women with less than a high school education are all at higher risk. In the United States, the risk of maternal mortality is a significant problem for minority women. Since 1940, the mortality rate for women of black and other races has remained three to four times the rate for white women (Atrash et al., 1990). (See Figure 2.)

Women who are 30 years and older also have a higher risk of maternal death than women who are less than 30 years old (Buehler et al., 1986; Atrash et al., 1990). (See Figure 3.) Currently there is a trend towards an increase in childbearing among women who are in their 30s and 40s. Many women have delayed childbearing to pursue an education or career. Fortunately, childbearing is much safer now for older women than it was years ago, yet women over 30 years still have higher rates of maternal death than younger women. Women aged 30 to 34 years have about twice the risk of maternal death as women aged 20 to 24 years; women who are 34 to 39 have almost a fourfold increased risk; and women aged 40 years and older have almost a ninefold greater risk than do women aged 20 to 24 years. Older women can reduce their chances of problems in pregnancy and childbirth by seeking prenatal care. Prenatal care is a key factor in ensuring a healthy pregnancy (Institute of Medicine, 1985). Women who receive no prenatal care have a risk of maternal death that is almost six times the risk for women who have received any amount of prenatal care. Women who receive early and consistent prenatal care have the lowest risk of maternal death (Koonin et al, 1991).

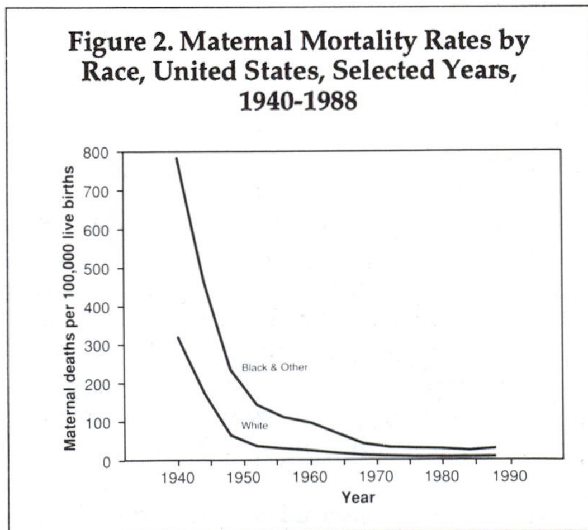

Source: National Center for Health Statistics

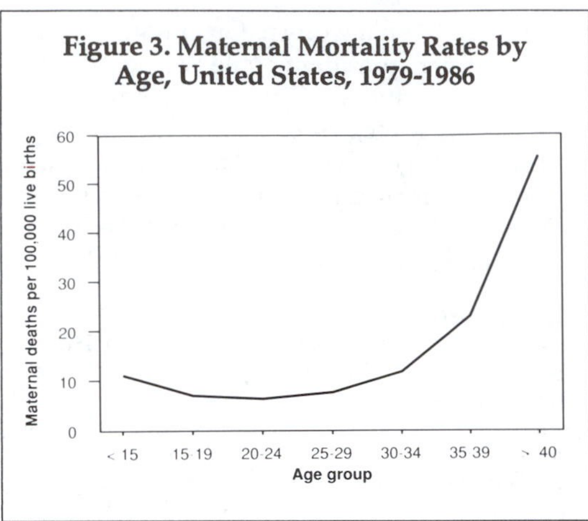

Source: H.K. Atrash et al., 1990.

Unmarried women have almost a three times higher risk of maternal death than married women. The risk of maternal death for unmarried women is much more pronounced for white women than for black women (Atrash et al., 1990).

As the level of education increases, the risk of maternal death decreases. Overall, women 20 years and older who did not complete high school have the highest maternal death ratios. Women who have attained more than 12 years of education have the lowest risk of dying among all age groups (Koonin et al., 1991). Women with higher educational levels may be more likely to recognize a pregnancy early and to seek prenatal care. They may also eat healthier foods and practice better health habits than less-educated women.

The major causes of maternal death differ for the various outcomes that result from pregnancy. (See Table 1.) For women who had a live birth, the leading causes of death were pulmonary embolism (blood clot that migrates to the lung), pregnancy-induced hypertension complications (high blood pressure that arises during pregnancy and causes such conditions as pre-eclampsia and eclampsia), and hemorrhage (primarily excessive uterine bleeding that occurs after the baby is born). For women whose pregnancy ended in a stillbirth, the leading causes of death were hemorrhage (primarily from abruptio placentae, which is the premature separation of the placenta from the uterine lining before the birth of a baby), pregnancy-induced hypertension complications, and pulmonary embolism.

Among women whose pregnancy ended in an ectopic (tubal) pregnancy, almost 90 percent of maternal deaths were caused by hemorrhage that resulted from a rupture of the ectopic site. In 1986, 73,700 ectopic pregnancies occurred among

Table 1. Cause of Maternal Death by Outcome of Pregnancy, United States, 1979-1986

	Outcome of Pregnancy															
Cause of Death	Live birth		Stillbirth		Ectopic		Abortion *		Molar		Undelivered		Unknown		Total	
	No.	%	No.	%	No.	%	No.	%	No.	%	No.	%	No.	%	No.	%
Hemorrhage	249	18.3%	89	33.9%	305	88.9%	43	34.7%	2	14.3%	30	20.5%	81	20.7%	799	30.2%
Embolism	370	27.1%	47	17.9%	10	2.9%	24	19.4%	2	14.3%	60	41.1%	106	27.1%	619	23.4%
Pregnancy-induced hypertension	307	22.5%	59	22.4%	1	0.3%	1	0.8%	2	14.3%	17	11.6%	92	23.5%	479	18.1%
Infection	101	7.4%	22	8.4%	6	1.7%	35	28.2%	2	14.3%	8	5.5%	28	7.2%	202	7.6%
Cardiomyopathy	53	3.9%	4	1.5%	0	0.0%	1	0.8%	0	0.0%	2	1.4%	30	7.7%	90	3.4%
Anesthesia complications	65	4.8%	3	1.1%	4	1.2%	11	8.9%	0	0.0%	0	0.0%	3	0.8%	86	3.3%
Other	218	16.0%	39	14.8%	17	5.0%	9	7.3%	6	42.9%	29	19.9%	51	13.0%	369	14.0%
Total Maternal Deaths	1363	100.0%	263	100.0%	343	100.0%	124	100.0%	14	100.0%	146	100.0%	391	100.0%	2644	100.0%

* Includes spontaneous and induced abortion

women aged 15 to 44 years in the United States (Lawson et al., 1989b). In that same year, 36 maternal deaths were reported that were related to ectopic pregnancy. On the basis of those numbers, 49 deaths occur for every 100,000 ectopic pregnancies each year. Women of black and other minority races have a risk of dying from ectopic pregnancy that is more than twice the risk for white women.

For women who died after an abortion (spontaneous or induced), the major causes of death were hemorrhage from uterine bleeding or infection. Since the 1970s, very few women have died from the complications of a spontaneous or induced abortion in the United States. In 1972, there were 90 abortion-related deaths in this country. Of those, 25 were related to spontaneous abortions, 24 to legally induced abortion, 39 to illegally induced abortion, and 2 could not be classified. In 1985, only 14 abortion-related deaths were reported. Of these, 6 were related to spontaneous abortion, 6 were related to legally induced abortion, 1 was related to an illegally induced abortion, and 1 could not be classified. The risk of death related to legally induced abortion has dropped dramatically, from about four deaths for every 100,000 legal abortions performed in 1972 to less than one death per 100,000 in 1985 (Lawson et al., 1989a).

Overall, maternal mortality occurs infrequently in the United States, however, many deaths are preventable. In addition, a racial gap persists. New causes of maternal deaths, such as those related to HIV (human immunodeficiency virus) infection (Koonin et al., 1989) and illicit drug use (Syverson et al., 1991), are now emerging. Greater efforts are being made to understand the factors that lead to maternal death and to educate physicians and the public about ways to prevent maternal mortality for all women.

✱ LISA M. KOONIN, M.N., M.P.H., and HANI K. ATRASH, M.D., M.P.H.

See also: Infant Mortality Statistics: United States

Resources

Antler, J. & Fox, D.M. (1976). "The Movement toward a Safe Maternity: Physician Accountability in New York City, 1915-1940." *Bulletin of the History of Medicine 50* (4): 569-95.

Atrash, H.K. et al. (1990). "Maternal Mortality in the United States, 1979-1986." *Obstetrics and Gynecology 76* (6): 1055-60.

Buehler, J.W. et al. (1986). "Maternal Mortality in Women Aged 35 Years or Older: United States." *JAMA 255* (1): 53-57.

Bureau of the Census. (1943). *Vital Statistics of the United States, 1940, Part I.* Washington, DC: United States Department of Commerce, United States Government Printing Office.

Ellerbrock, T.V. et al. (1988). "Pregnancy Mortality Surveillance: A New Initiative." *Contemporary Obstetrics and Gynecology 31* (6): 23-34.

Fortney, J.A. (1990). "Implications of the ICD-10 Definitions Related to Death in Pregnancy, Childbirth, or the Puerperium." *World Health Statistics Quarterly 43* (4): 246-48.

Institute of Medicine. (1985). *Preventing Low Birthweight.* Washington, DC: National Academy Press.

Kaunitz, A.M. et al. (1985). "Causes of Maternal Mortality in the United States." *Obstetrics and Gynecology 65* (5): 605-12.

Koonin, L.M. et al. (1989). "Pregnancy-associated Deaths due to AIDS in the United States." *JAMA 261* (9): 1306-09.

Koonin, L.M. et al. (1991). "Maternal Mortality Surveillance, 1979-1986." Centers for Disease Control. CDC Surveillance Summaries, *Morbidity and Mortality Weekly Report* 40 (SS-2).

Lawson, H.W. et al. (1989a). "Abortion Surveillance, United States, 1984-1985." Centers for Disease Control. CDC Surveillance Summaries, *Morbidity and Mortality Weekly Report* 38 (SS-2): 11-45.

Lawson, H.W. et al. (1989b). "Ectopic Pregnancy in the United States, 1979-1986." Centers for Disease Control. CDC Surveillance Summaries, *Morbidity and Mortality Weekly Report* 38 (SS-2): 1-10.

Marmol, J.G. Scriggins, A.L., & Vollman, R.F. (1969). "History of the Maternal Mortality Study Committees in the United States." *Obstetrics and Gynecology 34* (1): 123-38.

National Center for Health Statistics. (1990). Advance Report of Final Mortality Statistics, 1988. *Monthly*

Vital Statistics Report. 39 (7 supp.) Hyattsville, MD: Public Health Service.

Rochat, R.W. (1980). "Maternal and Perinatal Statistics." In S. Aladjem (Ed.) *Obstetrical Practice*. St. Louis: C.V. Mosby).

———. (1981). "Maternal Mortality in the United States of America." *World Health Statistics Quarterly 34* (1): 2-13.

Rochat, R.W. et al. (1988). "Maternal Mortality in the United States: Report from the Maternal Mortality Collaborative." *Obstetrics and Gynecology 72* (1): 91-97.

Syverson, C.J. et al. (1991). "Pregnancy-related Mortality in New York City, 1980 to 1984: Causes of Death and Associated Risk Factors." *American Journal of Obstetrics and Gynecology 164* (2): 603-08.

Thoms, H. (1960). *Our Obstetric Heritage: The Story of Safe Childbirth*. Hamden, CT: Shoe String Press.

World Health Organization. (1977). *Manual of International Statistical Classification of Diseases, Injuries and Causes of Death*. 9th revision. Geneva, Switzerland: World Health Organization.

MATERNAL SERUM ALPHA-FETOPROTEIN SCREENING

Over the past decade, the maternal serum alpha-fetoprotein (MSAFP) screening test has been introduced into the prenatal care market by both non-profit and commercial genetic laboratories and is now routinely offered to all women during pregnancy. This screening test is used to signal maternal risk for several fetal disabilities, including neural tube disorders (spina bifida and anencephaly), open ventral wall conditions (omphalocele and gastoschisis) and Trisomy 21 (Down's syndrome).

The MSAFP screening test is performed between 15 and 18 weeks of pregnancy, counting from the first day of the last menstrual period. AFP, produced by the fetal liver, is passed into the amniotic fluid through the placenta into the maternal blood circulation (serum), where it can be measured. Since the AFP level increases each week during pregnancy, the timing of the test is extremely important. Results are usually obtained within one week.

Maternal serum AFP screening is not itself a diagnostic test. Because it is a *screening* test it cannot determine with certainty whether a condition exists. It can only be used to identify those women for whom further diagnostic tests, such as ultrasound and amniocentesis, may be helpful. Approximately 5 percent of initial maternal serum samples will be abnormal even in the presence of a healthy fetus. Common causes of an abnormal result include the miscalculation of gestational age or the presence of twins. Accuracy is dependent upon the experience of the laboratory technicians performing the test as well as the accuracy of the clinical information accompanying the blood sample. It is necessary for the laboratory to have trained staff who are aware of the special responsibilities associated with the screening process.

The MSAFP test kit was originally regulated by the U.S. Food and Drug Administration (FDA) and restricted to use in research settings. The FDA received numerous comments from physicians and laboratories opposing the restrictions, and deregulation occurred in 1984. In 1985, the Department of Professional Liability of the American College of Obstetricians and Gynecologists (ACOG) issued a liability alert stating that obstetricians ought to advise all prenatal patients of the availability of this screening test. A major upsurge in screening followed the issuance of this alert.

The introduction of this screening test into the prenatal care market has generated "AFP anxiety" and has changed the pregnancy experience (Burton, Dillard, and Clark, 1982; Blatt, 1988). It has also led to the increased use of other technologies, such as ultrasound and amniocentesis. Participation in MSAFP screening and prenatal genetic testing is voluntary. Necessary components for a comprehensive MSAFP screening program include the provision of culturally and linguistically appropriate written educational materials in early pregnancy, adequate prenatal genetic counseling (nondirective), and financial and geographic access to follow-up medical and support services.

An *enhanced* MSAFP screening test for Down's syndrome was introduced in the late 1980s. Using a variety of proprietary names (Fetoscreen, Triple Screen, AFP3, Trisomy Screening Profile, and AFP Plus), this test measures alpha-fetoprotein (AFP) in addition to two other biochemical markers: unconjugated estriol (uE3) and human chorionic gonadotrophin (hCG). Enhanced screening can identify 60 to 65 percent of fetal Down's syndrome versus 40 percent when screening for Down's syndrome with AFP alone. To date, biochemical screening with AFP and hCG, in combination with maternal age, is the most informative method of estimating maternal risk for fetal Down's syndrome. The usefulness of uE3 is still under investigation. ✱ ROBIN J.R. BLATT, M.S.

See also: Central Closure Defects; Prenatal Diagnosis: Overview

See **Guide to Related Topics:** New Procreative Technologies; Prenatal Diagnosis and Screening

Resources

Blatt, Robin J.R. (1988). *Prenatal Tests: What They Are, Their Benefit and Risks and How to Decide Whether to Have Them or Not.* New York: Vintage Books.

Blatt, Robin J.R. & Miller, W.A. (Eds.) (1981, Aut/Win). *The Genetic Resource* Special Issue on the Application of the MSAFP Screening Test. Massachusetts Department of Public Health: 8-27.

Burton, B.K., Dillard, R.G., & Clark, E.N. (1982). "Anxiety Associated with Maternal Serum Alpha-fetoprotein (AFP) Screening." *American Journal of Human Genetics*, 34:83A.

———. (1985). "Maternal Serum Alpha-fetoprotein Screening: The Effect of Participation on Anxiety and Attitude Toward Pregnancy in Women with Normal Results." *American Journal of Obstetrics and Gynecology 152:* 540-43.

Burton, B.K., Sowers, S.G., & Nelson, L.H. (1983). "Maternal Serum Alpha-fetroprotein Screening in North Carolina: Experience with More Than Twelve Thousand Pregnancies." *American Journal of Obstetrics and Gynecology 146*: 439-44.

Canick, J.A. et al. (1988). "Low Second Trimester Maternal Serum Unconjugated Oestriol in Pregnancies with Down's Syndrome. *British Journal of Obstetrics and Gynecology* (95): 330-33.

DiMaio, M.S. et al. (1987). "Screening for Fetal Down's Syndrome in Pregnancy by Measuring Maternal Serum Alpha-fetoprotein Levels. *The New England Journal of Medicine 317*: 342-46.

Haddow, J. (1985). "Identifying Fetal Disorders by MSAFP Screening." *The Practitioner 229.*

Haddow, J.E. (Ed.) (1990). "Prenatal Screening for Major Fetal Disorders." *The Foundation for Blood Research Handbook.*

Knight, G.J., Palomaki, G.E., & Haddow, J. (1986, Feb). "Maternal Serum Alpha-fetoprotein: A Problem with a Test Kit." *The New England Journal of Medicine 20*: 20.

———. (1987, Oct). "Assessing Reliability of AFP Test Kits." *Contemporary Ob-Gyn 30.*

Macri, J.N. et al. "Maternal Serum Down Syndrome Screening: Unconjugated Estriol Is Not Useful." *American Journal of Obstetrics and Gynecology* (162): 672-73.

Martin, A.O. & Liu, K. (1984). "Implications of 'Low' Maternal Serum Alpha-Fetoprotein Levels." *Journal of the American Medical Association (JAMA) 2252*: 1438-42.

Merkatz, J.R. et al. (1984). "An Association Between Low Maternal Serum Alpha-fetoprotein and Fetal Chromosomal Abnormalities." *American Journal of Obstetrics and Gynecology 148:* 886-94.

The New England Regional Genetics Group, Collaborative Study of Down Syndrome Screening. (1989). "Combining Maternal Serum Alpha-fetoprotein Measurements and Age to Screen for Down Syndrome in Pregnant Women under Age 35." *American Journal of Obstetrics and Gynecology 160*: 575-81.

Rothman, Barbara Katz. (1986). *Tentative Pregnancy: Prenatal Diagnosis and the Future of Motherhood.* New York: Viking Press.

Wald, N.J. et al. (1988). "Maternal Serum Screening for Down's Syndrome in Early Pregnancy." *British Medical Journal 297:* 883-87.

———. (1988). "Maternal Serum Unconjugated Oestriol as an Antenatal Screening Test for Down's Syndrome." *British Journal of Obstetrics and Gynecology 95:* 334-41.

MATERNAL THINKING

According to a "practicalist" conception of reason, thinking arises out of and is tested by "practices." "Maternal thinking" refers to the complex and variable mix of metaphysical attitudes, cognitive styles, epistemological tenets, and values that tends to arise from practices of mothering.

Practices are collective activities identified by their aims and by the consequent demands made upon practitioners who share those aims. Mothering varies radically across cultures; even within a narrow subculture there are usually sharp differences among mothers. However, there is a sufficient commonality among human children to define a maternal practice. All children are physically vulnerable and dependent upon adults for their safety and health. All children demand that their lives be preserved. Children grow in complex ways, changing radically, from infancy through adulthood. All children demand that their growth be fostered. Most social groups seem to believe that children do not "naturally" develop in acceptable ways. They demand of mothers, and mothers demand of themselves, that mothers train children to behave acceptably. The three demands to preserve life, foster growth, and raise acceptable children define maternal practice. To be a mother is to try to respond to these demands with protection, nurturance, and training rather than with neglect, assault, or indifference.

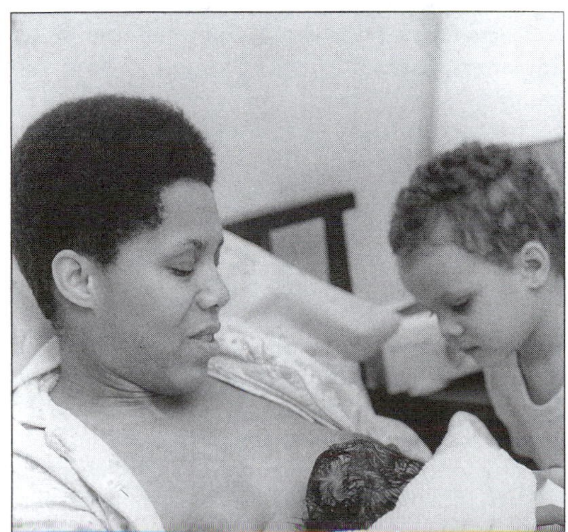

With each new child, maternal obligations become more complex. Photo courtesy of Harriette Hartigan/Artemis.

Although, for many people, mothering is a life- and mind-shaping commitment, people actually engage in mothering to different degrees at different times in their lives, depending upon the number and ages of the children mothered, the demands of nonmaternal projects, and the requirements of nonmaternal labor. Many people engage in mothering in appalling circumstances against almost insurmountable odds, battling poverty, bigotry, and tyranny in order to raise their children. Even fortunate mothers frequently fail to protect, nurture, and train. To be a mother is to commit oneself to a project of protection, nurturance, and training, despite the inevitable temptations and sense of failure that commitment brings in its wake.

On a daily basis, mothers think out strategies of protection, nurturance, and training. In quieter moments, many mothers reflect upon their practice as a whole. Although some mothers are more thoughtful than others, maternal thinking is no rarity. Like a scientist writing up an experiment, a historian assessing texts, or a critic working over a text, a mother engages in a discipline. She asks certain questions relevant to her aims and accepts certain criteria for the truth and adequacy of proposed answers. In the course of her work, she develops certain cognitive capacities and tends to acquire distinctive metaphysical attitudes toward, for example, nature, the body, birth, control, change, and emotion. Maternal thinking, like other disciplines, establishes criteria for determining failure and success, sets priorities, and identifies the virtues that the discipline requires. To *identify* a virtue does not presume that mothers are virtuous; like anyone else, mothers often fail in the projects they undertake. Rather, maternal thinking offers distinctive conceptions of virtue and of failure.

Mothering could become a gender-free (or gender-full) activity. Although biological differences between female and male mothers might survive in an egalitarian society, there is no reason to believe that these differences would make women (or men) better mothers. Similarly, although all mothering begins in female birth, giving birth is neither necessary nor sufficient to ensure a commitment to mothering. Nonetheless, there are practical, emotional, and conceptual links between the maternal and the womanly. Throughout history, and even currently in much of the world, most mothers are women. The work of all mothers, women and men, depends upon some woman's birthing labor. Because of the history of women's child caring and the relation of mothering to female childbearing, women who are not yet mothers are more apt than men to anticipate taking up mothering, while women who never choose or expect to take up mothering are more apt to identify with the passions and thinking of mothers. Accordingly, researchers trying to identify distinctive moral or philosophical "voices" arising from women's lives and work investigate maternal thinking. Correlatively, maternal thinking expresses, to a degree, women's ways of knowing.

While there may be enough commonality among children to identify maternal practices in many cultures, there is no such commonality among mothers. Mothers care for few or many children. Some have access to technological and medical services; some cannot expect their children to survive infancy. Mothers lead varieties of heterosexual, gay, lesbian, or celibate lives; form different kinds of families; and engage in all kinds of financially necessary or chosen nonmaternal projects. Every ethnic group, every oppressing or oppressed class has its mothers. Even if mothers tend to share a certain preoccupation with, for example, control, emotion, birth, or vulnerability, the details of cognitive style and concept differ radically.

Because of commonalities among children, it is possible to compare and contrast maternal practices and thinking. In many cases, the social location and political agendas of those researchers investigating maternal practice shape their ability to see similarities or differences and influence their decisions on which ones to highlight. Some have argued that notions like "the maternal" are creations of middle-class mothers and are oppressive to those whose experience they assimilate, especially to mothers struggling in abject poverty. By contrast, people responsive to the idea of maternal thinking anticipate a rich and heterogenous mix of concepts that can enliven many kinds of thinking about the natural and social world.

✱ SARA RUDDICK, Ph.D.

See also: Matrescence and Patrescence; Motherhood as Transformation

See **Guide to Related Topics:** Pregnancy, Psychological Aspects

Resource

Ruddick, Sara. (1989). *Maternal Thinking: Towards a Politics of Peace.* Boston: Beacon Press.

MATERNITY CLOTHES

In the world of the blue-collar worker prior to the 1940s, there was neither money, leisure, nor stimulus to cultivate an interest in fashion. The loose-fitting housedress was roomy enough to allow for body changes during pregnancy. For upper- and upper-middle class women, however, fashionable attire could be adapted at certain times to accommodate the growing fetus, while at other times this was impossible.

Between 1790 and 1820, and again from 1875 to 1920, designs were such that fashionable attire could be adjusted to allow for the changing proportions. Such modification enabled women to conceal their pregnancy and made it possible for them to participate in public life (Moore, n.d.; Arnold, 1968; Steele, 1988). In the 14th and 15th centuries, after plagues decimated a large part of the population in Europe, the "pregnant look" was the desirable look. The dress draped at the center of the body, simulating pregnancy (Batterberry and Batterberry, 1977, p. 99). The United States experienced a declining birth rate during the 1920s, the Depression, and the Second World War. In 1939, only two basic styles of maternity clothes existed, and these were matronly in color and feel. The clothes used cluttered necklines to shift the viewer's eyes from the abdomen to some less embarrassing location (Bartlett, 1936). In the 1940s, however, glamour and youthfulness became associated with maternity clothes. During the war years, in stories and headlines, *Vogue* publicized the pregnancies of the newly wed, young daughters of America's upper class (Bailey, 1981, p. 283).

Photo essays of pregnant celebrities and actresses helped define pregnancy as legitimate and glamorous. Rose Kennedy, wife of Ambassador Joseph P. Kennedy, was joined by star mothers, such as Rita Hayworth, Dorothy Lamour, Hedy Lamarr, Shirley Temple, Lana Turner, and Loretta Young. They were all depicted as wonderfully pregnant (Bailey, 1981, p. 282).

Vogue editors decreed that the vibrant, loose-fitting Hawaiian muu muu and the lively hand-embroidered dresses worn by Mexican peasant women were appropriate, elegant choices for pregnancy. Color was thus introduced as an important element of maternity dressing. In November 1943, *Vogue* offered eight specially designed styles, described as "all young, all pretty," including a puffed-sleeved Heidi outfit.

Youthfulness was also the emphasis of the January 1944 fashion section of *Good Housekeeping Magazine*, which was devoted to maternity clothing. Garments and details traditionally worn by young girls were adapted for maternity clothes, for example, the A-line jumper and the pinafore, ruffles, white puffed sleeves, the small Peter Pan collar, and candy stripes. For the first time in a magazine, very trim but pregnant women modeled the garments.

The outsize design features that had been used in the past to obscure pregnancy were declared obsolete. Women could now be revealed as undeniably pregnant. The category "maternity clothes" as a distinct listing made its appearance in 1947 in *The Reader's Guide to Periodic Literature*.

A 1948 *Life* magazine story featured pregnant Lauren Bacall with her husband, Humphrey Bogart. The article noted that she "even ventured successfully into shorts" and featured a picture of the actress wearing them. According to the article, Bacall believed that the "figure irregularities" of expectant motherhood should be decorated instead of concealed ("Maternity Clothes," 1948). In 1950, for the first time, the ready-to-wear market made available to the pregnant woman all types of clothing: playclothes, slacks, cocktail dresses, and shorts (Warden, 1950). Maternity dress acquired greater acceptance when Paris couture houses offered fashions that made participation in public life while pregnant acceptable. One of the major new designs offered by French designer Yves St. Laurent was the Trapeze style, which made the abdomen the focus of attention. A similar style was offered again in 1958 by Dior (Lessing, Bruer, and Stimson, 1963). The sack, too, a loose and unbelted style, made pregnancy or the pregnant look a virtue. Both Balenciaga and Givenchy featured it in their 1957 collections in fabrics that were firm, reinforced, and interfaced in every possible way. Like turtles, pregnant women were encased and provided with a measure of protection. Between 1953 and about 1963, two sources of dress were thus available to pregnant women: maternity apparel specifically designed for pregnant women and "regular" fashionable attire, with styles that could be worn during pregnancy.

This celebration of reproduction peaked between 1954 and 1964, when each year close to four million babies were born in the United States. This baby boom put a great economic strain on individual families and on the nation. For a time elementary schools could not be constructed fast enough, and the quality of elementary education declined as schools operated on half sessions.

Early in the 1960s the new fashion celebrated the thin and juvenile ideal. It was no longer possible to wear fashionable attire during pregnancy. An article in the May 4, 1963, issue of *Business Week* expressed the hope that Jacqueline Kennedy, the chic and fashionable wife of the president, might inspire more elegant maternity styles. She chose, however, to follow the Victorian precedent and go into seclusion. A slump in the design of maternity clothing occurred after the mid-1960s, reaching a postwar low in 1974.

The body-hugging fashions of the 1980s did not "allow" pregnancy. There were other times in history when fashionable attire made no such concession either, for example, between 1820 and 1870, when the tight-fitting bodice dominated fashion during the flapper era, and the Depression of the 1930s, when the boyish and then the long, lean look was the mode. Women awaiting the birth of a child were expected to stay out of sight (Steele, 1988; Yellis, 1969).

The production of maternity clothes was revitalized in the late 1970s when businesses learned that half of all pregnant women between the ages of 26 and 34 were working. To the retailer, it meant that there was now a group of consumers who were older, employed, and in need of clothing. Fashionable colors and styles were interpreted into maternity clothes, and in 1989, the number of births topped the four-million mark.

The variety of clothing now available to a pregnant woman makes it possible for her to both work and play. More important, perhaps, the availability of maternity clothing may not be dependent on the need for a population increase.

✱ RUTH RUBINSTEIN, Ph.D.

Resources

Arnold, Janet. (1968). "The Art and Construction of Women's Dresses, 1890-1914." In proceedings of the 15th Annual Conference of the Costume Society, *La Belle Epoque*. London: Victoria and Albert Museum.

Bailey, Rebecca Lou. (1981). *Fashions in Pregnancy: An Analysis of Selected Cultural Influences, 1850-1980.* Ph.D. dissertation, Michigan State University.

Bartlett, Florence C. (1936, Aug). "Dressing for Two." *Delineator 29:* 42-43.

Batterberry, Michael & Batterberry, Ariane. (1977). *Fashion: The Mirror of History.* New York: Greenwich House.

"Jacqueline Kennedy." (1963, May 4). *Business Week:* 18.

Lessing, Alice, Bruer, Rheid, & Stimson, Erma. (1963). *Sixty Years of Fashion.* New York: Fairchild Publications.

"Maternity Clothes." (1948, Oct). *Life 25:* 99-100.

Moore, Doris L. (n.d.). *Gallery of Fashion 1790-1822.* London: B.T. Batsford Ltd.

Steele, Valerie. (1988). *Paris Fashion: A Cultural History.* Oxford: Oxford University Press.

Warden, Helen. (1950, Mar 25). "Maternity Can Be Chic My Dear." *Collier's 125:* 26-F.

Yellis, Kenneth A. (1969, Spring). "Propserity's Child: Some Thoughts on the Flapper." *American Quarterly 21:* 44.

MATERNITY HOMES

Maternity homes for unwed mothers have changed remarkably little since their 19th-century beginnings: They have continued to remind women that pregnancy and childbearing out of wedlock violate sexual and social norms.

Models for maternity homes were the shelters for prostitutes opened in the 1830s and 1840s by female moral reform societies, which hoped that in an appropriately religious and domestic setting these fallen women would repent their sins and convert to a virtuous and Christian life. Most maternity homes were founded in the last third of the century by churches, especially the Roman Catholic Church and the Salvation Army, and by evangelical organizations, such as the Woman's Christian Temperance Union, the Young Women's Christian Association, and the National Florence Crittenton Mission. Like most Victorians, these founding organizations firmly opposed abortion and birth control, believing that they would encourage the "sin" of extramarital sexual activity. They also believed, however, that if a woman pregnant out of wedlock had fallen from God's grace, she could be reclaimed by religious conversion. Maternity homes therefore required that inmates remain cloistered for several months to receive religious instruction, so that their souls would be saved, and training in domestic skills, so that they could support themselves. Mothers were also required to keep their children since child care was believed to have redemptive powers, an idea popularized by Dr. Kate Waller Barrett, president of the National Florence Crittenton Mission. Pious matrons staffed the homes, and volunteer boards of women often managed the daily operations. Homes provided not only long-term shelter but medical care, and as childbirth moved out of the middle-class home into the hospital, many homes for unwed mothers developed into strictly medical facilities—that is, maternity hospitals for married patients.

Although figures on illegitimate births are unreliable, most women almost certainly bore their illegitimate children in public hospitals or in private residences, not in maternity homes. In 1923, according to a federal census, maternity homes had only 2,389 inmates, including infants. Nevertheless, the chief providers of maternity home care continued to open new institutions: In the early 1930s the Salvation Army had more than two dozen homes; the Catholic dioceses, 44; the National Florence Crittenton Mission, 65 (*Children*

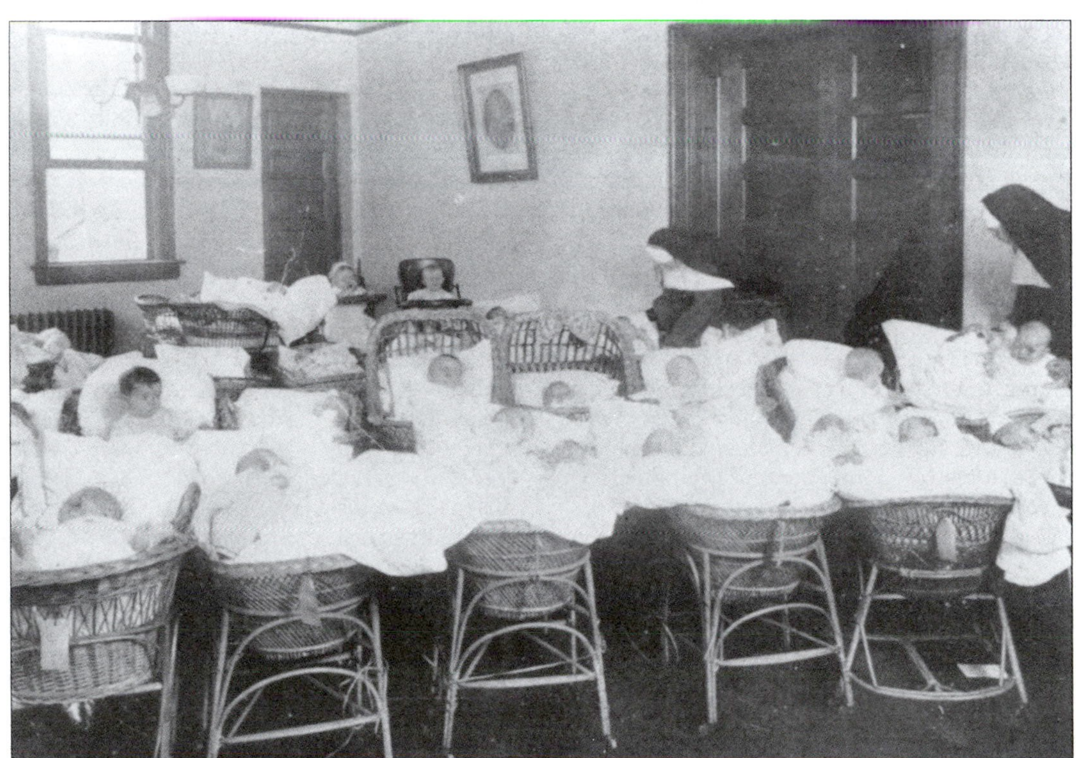

Like many homes for unwed mothers, St. Ann's Infant and Maternity Asylum (1873-1983) in Cleveland, Ohio, also developed a medical facility for married patients, St. Ann's Hospital. Photo reproduced with permission of the Archives of the Sisters of Charity of Saint Augustine.

under Institutional Care, 1927, p. 14; O'Grady, 1930, p. 141; Wilson, 1933, p. 4; McKinley, 1980, p. 139). Clients were predominantly working-class women, who paid no fees, and the homes were almost entirely privately funded since state and city governments would not spend tax monies on the institutional care of sexually delinquent women.

The Great Depression, however, dramatized the prohibitive expense of institutionalizing dependent persons, a historic practice already under fire from social workers. Accordingly, New Deal social insurance programs provided outdoor relief to some groups, including the elderly through old age insurance and children through Aid to Dependent Children (ADC). Strict guidelines for the allocation of ADC funds were designed to make it difficult if not impossible for an unmarried mother to receive this public support. Simultaneously, the medicalization of childbirth raised maternity home costs. The homes responded by shortening the customary six-month confinement and, more important, by raising their fees. As a result, the once-charitable institutions gradually became facilities used almost exclusively by middle-class women.

This new clientele, in turn, forced homes to change some long-standing practices. In the 1940s homes began to advise inmates to give up their children for adoption, a policy compatible with the respectable social background of the woman as well as the principles of the social workers who had begun to staff the homes. During the 1950s, as psychiatric casework gained prestige, middle-class pregnancy out of wedlock was interpreted not as a sin but as a psychological disorder; lengthy confinements were still required for therapy, however, as psychiatric counseling partially replaced religious devotions. By the late 1960s, middle-class women had gained access to birth control devices and by the early 1970s, to legal abortion, avoiding extramarital pregnancies and the necessity of maternity home care. Black women, who made up a growing proportion of unwed mothers, had never been served by maternity homes because administrators and social workers had assumed that illegitimate childbirth was accepted by the black community. Outpatient services, often publicly funded and much cheaper than residential care, therefore, became the preferred strategy for dealing with pregnancy out of wedlock.

The number of maternity homes declined from 201 (all but two privately funded) in the mid-1960s to 99 in 1980. During the 1980s, however, the Salvation Army and the Roman Catholic Church, long-time maternity home sponsors and opponents of abortion, were joined by other anti-abortion groups such as the National Right to Life Committee, which opened many new homes. As in the late 19th century, these facilities stressed religious conversion and job training but, because they were privately funded, could provide long-term shelter for only a tiny fraction of women who became pregnant out of wedlock (Pappenfort, 1970, Table 1; *New York Times*, July 23, 1989, p. 1, and May 13, 1990, p. 1). ✱ MARIAN J. MORTON, Ph.D.

See also: Adoption, Closed; Birthmothers

See **Guide to Related Topics:** Adoption

Resources

Abramowitz, Mimi. (1988). *Regulating the Lives of Women: Social Welfare Policy from Colonial Times to the Present.* Boston: South End Press.

Aiken, Katharine. (1980). "The National Florence Crittenton Mission, 1883-1925: A Case Study in Progressive Reform." Ph.D. dissertation, Washington State University.

Children under Institutional Care, 1923-1927. (1927). Washington, DC: U.S. Government Printing Office.

McKinley, Edward H. (1980). *Marching to Glory* New York: Harper and Row.

Morton, Marian J. (1988, Mar). "Fallen Women, Federated Charities, and Maternity Homes, 1913-1973. *Social Service Review 62*: 63-82.

New York Times. (1989, Jul 23): 1, 25.

New York Times. (1990, May 13): 1, 22.

O'Grady, John. (1930). *Catholic Charities in the United States.* Washington DC: National Conference of Catholic Charities.

Pappenfort, Donnell M. (1970). *A Census of Children's Residential Institutions in the United States, Puerto Rico, and the Virgin Islands.* Chicago: Aldine.

Pascoe, Peggy, (1990). *Relations of Rescue: The Search for Female Moral Authority in the American West.* New York: Oxford University Press.

Sedlack, Michael. (1982, Sept). "Youth Policy and Young Women, 1870-1972." *Social Service Review 56*: 448-64.

Wilson, Otto. (1933). *Fifty Years' Work with Girls, 1883-1933.* Alexandria, VA: National Florence Crittenton Mission.

MATRESCENCE AND PATRESCENCE

A most dramatic time in any adult's life occurs at the birth of the first child, a time of deep psychological and cultural change. Becoming a mother, *matrescence*, and becoming a father, *patrescence*, are terms coined (Raphael, 1966) to highlight and distinguish this reproductive stage previously viewed by social scientists largely from the newborn's vantage. Matrescence and patrescence are rites of passage similar to those life stages so brilliantly demarcated by the French sociologist Van Gennep (1960) as adolescence, marriage, and death. The terms define a period beginning sometime during pregnancy and continuing for many months after birth. Yet even Van Gennep recognized that "its duration varies among different peoples" (Van Gennep, 1960, p. 43); the rites, ceremonies, events, and timing when both mother and father are acknowledged as parent are remarkably diverse

For example, in the United States middle-class women assume the role of mother from the moment they leave the hospital. Not so in India where the mother is embraced by many helpers who allow her a longer space of time to ease into this role. Matrescence is heralded with joy, but the possibility in many cultures that the child may not survive limits the ceremonies and celebrations until the baby is older and has gotten past the critical months. In India, it is a pattern for the young mother, preferably attended by her own mother, to deliver at her natal home where she is permitted to continue in the role of daughter and does not need to assume the responsibility of motherhood until a few months later, when she returns to her husband's village. Even then, the mother-in-law may take over much of the mothering role, not allowing her son's wife to make decisions about the welfare of the grandchild.

A difference even exists between social and physiological puberty during these great changes in a person's life. Van Gennep noted that "in Rome social puberty precedes physiological puberty, and in Paris it follows physiological puberty" (1960, p. 66). Similarly, matrescence, which involves both a physiological and cultural phenomenon for women, may have physical responses in men similar to that which has been recorded for some males during their wife's pregnancy (Mirsky, Kaplan, and Broh-Kahn, 1950).

The Tikopia envision the experience of birth in a very broad context. They herald it as a time when "a mother is born," "a father is born." They recognize a baby's arrival as creating "a house of aunts" or "a house of grandparents" (Firth, 1960).

Ethnographic descriptions of the ritual and rites during this time have the newborn as the focal point—a grandmother bathes the neonate, others chant oaths to ward off illness, the baby is given a haircut or an icy bath, or women join together to sing in behalf of the newborn. Researchers record secret birth spells carried out by the mother's brother, or religiously based premises agreed to by a co-padre or co-madre, who files in bearing culturally proscribed edibles and a clear knowledge of who is to eat which food under what conditions.

Mention of the new mother in much of the traditional anthropological literature tends to be limited to descriptions of her movements—she sits up or lies down; or to her care—she is warmed by a fire or covered by ashes; or in regard to her pattern of breast-feeding—she begins after saying a prayer or before confessing a previous sexual indiscretion. Much is made of her confinement, which has her housebound for an exact number of days in cultures without calendars. In reality, the matrescent/patrescent periods represent a far more complex set of behaviors, full of stress as well as joy.

Since this interval has only recently been recognized, in order to clarify its meaning, it will be necessary to observe who the participants are, what their functions are, how the economic status of the family determines and shapes the behavior of others, what people do to substitute personnel and gifts under difficult circumstances, and what support systems coalesce around the new father and the mother during this extraordinary stage in their lives. ✷ DANA RAPHAEL, Ph.D.

See also: Bonding; Motherhood as Transformation

See **Guide to Related Topics:** Pregnancy, Psychological Aspects

Resources

Firth, Raymond. (1960). "Ceremonies for Children and Social Frequency in Tikopia." *Oceania 27* (1): 25.

Mirsky, I. Arthur, Kaplan, Stanley, & Broh-Kahn, Robert H. (1950). "Pepsinogen Excretion (Uropepsin) as Index of the Influence of Various Life Situations on Gastric Secretion. *Life Stress and Bodily Disease.* Vol. 29 of the 1949 Proceedings, Association for Research in Nervous and Mental Diseases.

Raphael, Dana. (1966). The Lactation-Suckling Process within a Matrix of Supportive Behavior. Unpublished Ph.D. dissertation, Columbia University, New York. (Microfilm number 69-15, 580.)

Van Gennep, Arnold. (1960). *The Rites of Passage.* (Translated by Monika B. Vizedom and Gabrielle L. Caffee). London: Routledge and Kegan Paul.

MECONIUM

Meconium is the first stool excreted by the infant. It is characterized by its sticky consistency and dark green to black color. The typical infant passes meconium within 12 hours after birth. On occasion, an infant exposed to stress during the intrauterine period may pass meconium prior to birth. Intrauterine excretion of meconium, as well as failure to excrete meconium within 48 hours after birth, are frequently signs of an abnormal condition.

Meconium begins to form in the fetal intestine between the 13th and 16th week of gestation as the fetus begins to swallow amniotic fluid. The swallowed amniotic fluid enters the fetal digestive system. There, the water is reabsorbed into the fetal-placental circulatory system. The nondigestible elements of the amniotic fluid, such as lanugo hair and epithelial cells, are mixed with secretions from the gastrointestinal mucosa, liver, and pancreas, including bile pigments, fatty acids, and mucus, to form meconium. While the formation of meconium begins early in the gestational period, it normally remains in the lower gastrointestinal tract or colon until the onset of peristalsis after birth.

The passage of meconium prior to birth is frequently associated with fetal distress. When the fetus experiences a time of stress *in utero*, especially a hypoxic episode, the fetal anal sphincter may become relaxed, allowing the escape of meconium into the intrauterine environment and resulting in meconium staining of the amniotic fluid. Meconium-stained fluid is seen in 5 to 15 percent of births and is usually associated with term or postterm infants who are small for gestational age (SGA). These infants are frequently depressed and require resuscitation at birth.

Meconium staining of the amniotic fluid may result in temporary discoloration of the infant's skin and nails. More alarming are the increased rates of morbidity and mortality associated with Meconium Aspiration Syndrome, which is seen in 10 to 30 percent of infants with meconium-stained fluid (Rossi et al., 1989). Meconium aspiration is thought to occur with the onset of respiratory activity; however, the incidence of intrauterine aspiration has not been ruled out. When meconium is aspirated into the lungs, it results in obstruction of the small airways, leading to signs of respiratory distress (e.g., grunting, tachypnea, and retractions) within the first hour of life. Infants exhibit chest overdistention and an increased anterior/posterior diameter or a barrel-chest appearance. Continued obstruction of the airways may result in a pneumothorax, and the presence of a foreign substance in the lung fields may produce a chemical pneumonitis. Consequently, meconium aspiration remains a significant cause of neonatal morbidity and mortality (Rossi et al., 1989).

Anticipation is the most important step in reducing the incidence and complications of meconium aspiration. The most important intervention in cases of meconium-stained amniotic fluid is to suction the nose and mouth prior to delivery of the infant's trunk and the onset of respiration. This removal of meconium from the mouth and nose before the initiation of breathing prevents the meconium from moving into the lungs and causing obstruction and respiratory distress. ✱ DEBORAH RAINES, M.S.N., R.N.C.

See **Guide to Related Topics:** Pregnancy, Physical Aspects

Resources

Behrman, R.E. & Vaughna, V.C. (1983). *Nelson Textbook of Pediatrics.* Philadelphia: W.B. Saunders Co.

Daga, A.S., Daga, S.R., & Patole, S.K. (1990). "Risk Assessment in Birth Asphyxia". *Journal of Tropical Pediatrics 36*: 34-39.

Desmond, M.M. et al. (1957). "Meconium Staining of the Amniotic Fluid." *Obstetrics and Gynecology 9* (1): 91-103.

Dickason, E.J., Shult, M.D., & Silverman, B. (1990). *Maternal Infant Nursing Care.* St. Louis: C.V. Mosby.

Fanaroff, A. & Martin, R. (1987). *Neonatal-Perinatal Medicine.* St. Louis: C.V. Mosby.

Perez, R.H. (1981). *Protocols for Perinatal Nursing Practice.* St. Louis: C.V. Mosby Co.

Rossi, E.M. et al. (1989). "Meconium Aspiration Syndrome: Intrapartum and Neonatal Attributes." *American Journal of Obstetrics and Gynecology 161* (5): 1106-10.

Schreiner, R. & Niceta, B. (1988). *Care of the Newborn.* New York: Raven Press.

MENSTRUAL EXTRACTION

Menstrual extraction is a method of removing the contents of the uterus by suction. A small cannula (4 mm flexible plastic tube) is inserted into the uterus and the contents suctioned into a jar with a hand pump, most commonly a syringe. The procedure takes 20 to 30 minutes. The usefulness of menstrual extraction is twofold: (1) as a way to lessen the menstrual flow, relieving women of the inconvenience and pain of menstruation, and/or (2) as an abortion technique.

Menstrual extraction was developed in the United States in 1971 as a way women could have active control of their periods and reproduction. The technique of menstrual extraction was developed in self-help groups that sought to empower women by demystifying simple body functions such as menstruation and early abortion. The primary method of extraction is the use of a simple and inexpensive device, the Del-Em, consisting of a cannula, Mason jar, 50 cc syringe, and connecting tubing. Menstrual extraction is intended to be carried out in a supportive atmosphere of women's self-help groups. Self-help groups believe menstrual extraction technology, including mild suction, a thin and flexible cannula, gentle movements, and a woman who is unanesthetized, makes the procedure safe for minimally trained laypersons to perform.

Menstrual extraction is carried out either at a woman's home or at the self-help group's meeting place. Three women are needed for the procedure: the woman who is to have the extraction and who often holds the syringe and controls the vacuum, the woman who observes the equipment, and the woman who inserts and moves the cannula. If its purpose is to remove menstrual fluid, the extraction takes place a few days before or on the first day of the period. As an abortion technique, menstrual extraction can take place up to the eighth week after a missed menstrual period.

The risks of menstrual extraction are hotly debated. Since the women involved in self-help groups do not keep records, a systematic study has not been undertaken. Overall the rates of infection and incomplete emptying of the uterus appear to be small. When it is performed carefully, the physical danger of menstrual extraction is reduced. The procedure takes on additional risk when attempted by untrained individuals outside of the self-help group setting.

Since the Supreme Court's decision in *Webster v. Reproductive Health Services*, women's interest in menstrual extraction has increased as many search for alternative abortion methods. Supporters of the extraction procedure are practically and politically motivated. They want women, especially low-income women, to be able to obtain abortions if the procedure becomes illegal. At the same time supporters are sending a message to the government conveying how important control of reproduction is for women. Women have the technology of abortion and will share this technology so that, if necessary, an underground network can be organized. In spring 1990, the Federation of Feminist Women's Health Centers released a 28-minute video "No Going Back: A Pro-choice Perspective" featuring a self-help groups learning to perform menstrual extraction. It is being distributed to women's groups nationwide.

✱ HEATHER D. BOONSTRA

See also: Webster v. Reproductive Health Services

See **Guide to Related Topics:** Abortion

Resources

Federation of Feminist Women's Health Centers. *A New View of a Woman's Body.* Available from the Federation of Feminist Women's Health Centers. (See "Appendix of Organizations and Resources.")

Federation of Feminist Women's Health Centers. (1990). "No Going Back: A Pro-choice Perspective." Video, 28 min. ($25.00).

National Women's Health Network. *Abortion Then and Now: Creative Responses to Restricted Access*. Available for $10.00 from National Women's Health Network. (See "Appendix of Organizations and Resources.")

MEXICO

Traditional beliefs in Mexico about pregnancy and childbirth have included the following:

- A baby born at seven months' gestation has a better chance of surviving than one born at eight months' gestation.
- A mother experiencing *susto* (shock or fright) can suddenly become diabetic, have her milk turn sour, or give birth to an ill baby.
- Vitamin pills make people fat (or cause them to gain weight). Therefore, weight-conscious pregnant women will avoid them.
- Dizzy spells or feelings of faintness are caused by abrupt *bajadas* (sudden dips) in blood pressure.
- Women pregnant during a lunar or solar eclipse will traditionally wear a key, coin, safety pin, or other metal object, preferably tied or on a sash of red ribbon over their belly button to protect their unborn from potential death, deformation, or retardation, which could ensue if exposed to the eclipse unprotected.
- Pregnant women are often referred to as (la) *gorda* ("fat," translated literally to English), or *enferma*, literally translated as "sick."
- A woman who carries her baby "wide," i.e., whose belly and hips become wider and fuller, is believed to be carrying a girl, while the woman whose uterus protrudes straight out, in a manner more compact and in front (*picudo*) is said to be carrying a boy.
- The most essential part of traditional prenatal care consists of the *sobadas*, or prenatal massages of the baby *in utero* and the mother's abdomen, performed by a midwife or healer to ensure that the baby is in good position; she will gently manipulate it if it is not.

At the time of birth, the traditional midwife in Mexico will encourage the woman to birth in a squatting or other position. However, a large number of midwives who received training or orientation from the government, as well as most doctors currently practicing, insist on the supine position during pushing, telling the woman it is "much easier" and that other positions provoke difficult tears.

Postpartum. The mother often wears a *faja*—a large bandage or cloth or type of girdle—about her middle to keep the "heat" in and help her organs to go back in place. She is to keep the "40 days" (*la cuarentena*); i.e., in the six weeks following birth she will stay in her home, dedicating herself to her baby and her own recuperation. To encourage abundant milk, postpartum women drink *atole*, a hot beverage made from ground corn or cornstarch, milk, and sugar. In general, new mothers are encouraged to eat hot and warmed foods, nothing cold after birth. Teas for milk flow include *anis estrella* (star anis), *hinojo* (fennel), and, in certain areas, *ixbud*. Babies are commonly given chamomile tea for colic.

Women often pass around a recipe for a liniment to be rubbed on their bellies in the first week postpartum, so as not to "lose heat" from the area or remain flabby. The liniment consists of rosemary (*romero*), camphor, and ether dissolved into a liter of grain alcohol and left to steep for several weeks prior to the birth. Other plants may be added, depending upon what region the woman is from.

Babies are traditionally kept well wrapped, and usually have their faces covered by a light blanket on their first outings, to protect from the *aires* (bad winds, drafts, dirt) and *mal ojo* (overly admiring gazes by others). The babies may also wear a flannel belly band or cotton gauze, mostly to prevent an "outie" belly button from forming. A bean may be placed on the cord stump before the *faja* is put in place to further ensure that the belly button won't later stick out.

✱ ALISON PARRA

See **Guide to Related Topics:** Cross-Cultural Perspectives

Resources

Cushing, Cindy. (1984). "Ser Partera." Austin TX: self-published pamphlet.

Mellado, V., Zolla, C., & Castanade, X. (1989). *La Atencion al Embarazo y el Parto en el Medio Rural Mexicano*. [Prenatal Care and Birth in Rural Mexico.] Mexico City: CIESS.

Parra, Alison. 1985. *Un Embarazo Sano* [A Healthy Pregnancy.] Unpublished manuscript.

Peredo, Miguel Guzman. (1985). *Medical Practices in Ancient America*. Mexico City: Ediciones EuroAmericanas.

MIDWIFE LICENSING

Whether legal or illegal, licensed or unlicensed, lay midwives have attended childbirths throughout American history. In colonial America, midwives worked under an incomplete system of municipal licensure. Most midwives were unregulated and allowed to practice without governmental intervention, for social norms held that healthy mothers and children were blessings from God, not the outcomes of medical management. Consequently, where licensure existed, the requirements focused on midwives' moral character and obligations, not their skills or training. Licensing regulations typically specified that midwives attend all who needed their services, reveal the truth about illegitimacy and infanticide, and foreswear abortions and magic. Civil and religious authorities rarely interfered in midwives' practices unless witchcraft or other heresy was suspected.

As these ideas about childbirth waned in the post-colonial era, so did moral licensure laws. Meanwhile, the number of physicians grew rapidly in free market 19th-century America. Increased competition pressured American physicians (who, like midwives, were unregulated and unlicensed) to seek clients in areas, like normal childbirth, that previously had not been considered within the medical sphere. Consequently, physicians argued that the pain and potential dangers of childbirth required their more knowledgeable assistance. By the mid-19th century, most upper- and middle-class women in northern cities were attended during childbirth by physicians.

Regular physicians escalated their attack on midwives around the turn of this century, as part of a larger campaign to improve the quality of health care and to eliminate competition. Physicians also hoped that eliminating midwives would force poor women to give birth in hospitals and thus provide medical students with necessary clinical experience. Playing on contemporary xenophobia, racism, and sexism, and on the public's growing respect for science, physicians argued that midwives (most of whom were immigrant or black women) were ignorant, uneducable, and a threat to American health. At the same time, physicians successfully pressed for restrictive medical licensing laws and more rigorous medical education, accentuating the difference between their backgrounds and those of midwives.

Yet medical opposition to midwifery was far from universal. Some physicians, especially in the South, argued that midwives should not be eliminated even if they provided only second-class care because too few doctors were willing to serve in rural communities, especially poor black ones. Similarly, many public health physicians concerned with the burgeoning numbers of poor immigrants in northern cities supported the New York Academy of Medicine's 1911 resolution promoting midwifery education and regulation. The following year, Dr. Abraham Jacobi advocated midwifery training and licensing in his presidential address at the national meeting of the American Medical Association. His endorsement failed to sway the opposition, and midwives in most areas continued to practice without formal training or supervision.

Public health supporters of midwifery achieved their greatest success in 1921 with passage of the Sheppard-Towner Maternity and Infancy Protection Act. Fourteen states chose to use some of the funds provided under the act for midwifery training and regulatory programs. However, funding for this legislation failed to gain renewal in 1929, and the midwifery programs soon disappeared.

Ironically, the doctors' battle to eradicate midwives succeeded only indirectly. By 1930, only Massachusetts, the center of the struggle, had outlawed lay midwifery. The rest of the states either ignored the dwindling practice of lay midwifery or adopted lenient registration statutes. These "granny midwife" laws usually limited midwives to uncomplicated births, prohibited them from using drugs or instruments such as forceps, and required that all births be registered. Few laws required formal training. Even fewer provided training beyond sporadic short courses, and many did not even require literacy. Because midwives' training was not upgraded, their status and popularity declined, and they essentially disappeared by the middle of the century. In contrast, the adoption of restrictive licensure for physicians, based on rigorous, scientific training enhanced their status and solidified their authority over childbirth and all other aspects of health care.

Yet in the last two decades, lay midwifery has re-emerged. Beginning in the 1950s, a small but vocal minority of women began talking about and acting on their dissatisfaction with how doctors were managing childbirth—the routine use of drugs for pain relief and augmenting labor, the refusal to allow husbands into delivery rooms, the separation of mother from newborn, and so on. These women's search for alternatives led to the rapid growth of the natural childbirth movement during the 1960s and 1970s and pressured hospitals to make at least some changes in how they handled childbirth.

The superficiality of these changes (as exemplified by the rising rate of cesarean sections) has led the most disenchanted consumers to seek home birth. Because few doctors or nurse-midwives would assist in home births, a new population of lay midwives has emerged to meet this demand. The legal status of these midwives varies greatly from state to state. Lay midwifery is clearly legal in several states and clearly illegal in others. In addition, it is effectively illegal in those states that still have lenient "granny midwife" laws on their books but no longer grant new licenses. In the remaining states, no statutes or court decisions unequivocally address lay midwifery. In these circumstances, lay midwives' freedom to practice depends on the politics and philosophies of prosecutors, judges, and regulatory boards. Consequently, midwives' legal status in these states will remain uncertain until either legislatures pass new laws or judges write new opinions on older laws that address midwifery.

States where lay midwifery is legal can be classified into three groups. Some, such as Arizona and South Carolina, have developed relatively rigorous licensure standards for those seeking to practice. Others, such as Texas, merely register, rather than license, midwives, setting only minimal requirements for practice. Finally, two states, Mississippi and Tennessee, officially permit any individual to practice midwifery and neither register nor license such practices.

✷ ROSE WEITZ, Ph.D., and
DEBORAH SULLIVAN, Ph.D.

See also: Midwifery: Overview; Midwifery and the Law; Midwives, Southern Black

See **Guide to Related Topics:** Caregivers and Practitioners; Legal Issues

Resources

Donegan, Jane B. (1978). *Women and Men Midwives: Medicine, Morality, and Misogyny in Early America.* Westport, CT: Greenwood Press.

Kobrin, Frances E. (1984). "The American Midwife Controversy: A Crisis of Professionalization." In Judith W. Leavitt (Ed.) *Women and Health in America.* Madison, WI: University of Wisconsin Press, pp. 318-26.

Litoff, Judy B. (Ed.) (1986). *The American Midwife Debate.* Westport, CT: Greenwood Press.

Sullivan, Deborah A. & Weitz, Rose. (1988). *Labor Pains: Modern Midwives and Home Birth.* New Haven, CT: Yale University Press.

Wertz, Richard W. & Wertz, Dorothy C. (1977). *Lying-In: A History of Childbirth in America.* New York: Free Press.

Wolfson, Charles. (1986). "Midwives and Home Birth: Social, Medical and Legal Perspectives." *Hastings Law Journal 37*: 909-67.

MIDWIFE-ATTENDED BIRTHS

Due to the escalating costs associated with childbirth and a movement away from the increasing application of new technologies in obstetrics, growing attention has been devoted to midwife-attended births (Allgaier, 1978; Bennetts and Lubic, 1982; Taffel, 1984; Scupholme, McLeod, and Robertson, 1986; Annandale, 1988; Rooks et al., 1989). Although midwives attended only 3.4 percent of births in the United States in 1988, the number of midwife-attended births has quadrupled since 1975, rising from 29,413 to 132,670. Most of this increase can be attributed to the increase in the number of midwife-attended births in hospitals. The number of births attended by midwives in hospitals rose nearly fivefold, from 19,686 in 1975 to 115,886 in 1988, while the number in nonhospital settings rose 73 percent from 9,727 to 16,784 over the same period. (See Table 1.) The proportion of midwife-attended deliveries varies greatly by state, ranging in 1988 from less than 0.1 percent in Kansas, Louisiana, Missouri, and Nebraska, to 8.6 percent in New Mexico.

Data from live-birth certificates of the 50 states and the District of Columbia provide a demographic profile of mothers attended by midwives. Women attended by midwives in hospital settings are more likely than those cared for by physicians to be black, under 20 years of age, unmarried, and less educated. Those mothers attended outside of hospitals by midwives, on the other hand, tend to be older white married women who are better educated than average and are having a third or higher-order birth. (See Table 2.) Regardless of where they deliver, women attended by midwives are more likely to be foreign-born and to begin prenatal care late. (See Table 2.)

Much concern has been voiced by health professionals about the safety of out-of-hospital births (Scupholme, McLeod, and Robertson, 1986; Rooks et al., 1989). Opponents have suggested that the unpredictability of obstetric emergencies necessitates the immediate availability and use of the latest life-saving medical technology and the expertise of physicians. Proponents have stated that low-risk mothers attended by certified nurse-midwives can deliver safely out of hospitals. Consequently, it is important to examine how babies of mothers attended by midwives fare as compared to babies of mothers who are attended by physicians in hospitals. One way to do this is to compare birth outcomes for the different groups.

Figure 1 indicates that for white births, a midwife-attended birth is less likely to result in a low birth-weight baby (i.e., one who weighs less than 2,500 grams) than a birth attended by a physician in a hospital. Similar results for black births are shown in Figure 2. These findings hold across all educational levels, indicating that these differences are not the result of differing educational

Table 1. Live Births by Place of Delivery, Attendant, and Race of Child: United States, 1975 and 1980-88

Year and race of child	Total	In hospital 1/				Out of hospital 2/			
		Physician	Midwife	Other	Unspecified	Physician	Midwife	Other	Unspecified
All races									
1988	3,909,510	3,740,213	115,886	13,668	2,661	8,975	16,784	10,640	683
1987	3,809,394	3,660,923	98,425	12,414	2,344	8,132	15,465	11,049	642
1986	3,756,547	3,617,281	89,810	9,311	3,266	9,400	15,398	11,408	673
1985	3,760,561	3,623,215	85,941	10,695	2,299	9,746	16,135	11,839	691
1984 3/	3,669,141	3,532,397	78,040	13,085	7,381	9,777	15,862	10,835	1,764
1983 3/	3,638,933	3,508,666	71,617	12,532	6,845	10,215	15,406	11,662	1,990
1982 3/	3,680,537	3,560,644	63,062	11,936	6,554	10,296	14,375	11,855	1,815
1981 3/	3,629,238	3,490,919	55,537	13,303	31,823	10,998	12,754	11,794	2,110
1980 3/	3,612,258	3,499,959	51,576	17,456	7,379	11,992	11,093	11,630	1,173
1975 3/	3,144,198	3,026,024	19,686	7,122	64,069	11,265	9,727	2,960	3,345
White									
1988	3,046,162	2,921,170	82,789	9,469	1,897	6,075	15,878	8,355	529
1987	2,992,488	2,880,824	70,521	9,218	1,823	6,201	14,678	8,741	482
1986	2,970,439	2,864,957	64,379	6,634	2,923	7,336	14,593	9,113	504
1985	2,991,373	2,887,795	61,051	7,286	1,967	7,795	15,268	9,664	547
1984 3/	2,923,502	2,819,888	55,682	9,042	5,865	7,785	14,946	8,933	1,361
1983 3/	2,904,250	2,806,960	49,651	8,477	5,400	8,132	14,391	9,748	1,491
1982 3/	2,942,054	2,853,427	42,684	8,197	5,116	7,982	13,262	9,982	1,404
1981 3/	2,908,669	2,804,868	37,019	9,405	25,505	8,560	11,577	10,047	1,688
1980 3/	2,898,732	2,815,382	33,730	13,691	5,548	9,495	9,919	10,021	946
1975 3/	2,551,996	2,465,957	10,076	5,342	52,392	7,818	5,082	2,585	2,744
Black									
1988	671,976	639,037	24,180	3,372	678	2,482	486	1,625	116
1987	641,567	615,029	19,907	2,369	431	1,605	452	1,642	132
1986	621,221	596,089	18,924	1,989	278	1,668	497	1,652	124
1985	608,193	582,768	19,097	2,306	241	1,566	573	1,535	107
1984 3/	592,745	568,092	17,304	2,547	927	1,638	616	1,391	230
1983 3/	586,027	561,304	17,400	2,377	922	1,602	742	1,384	296
1982 3/	592,641	568,943	16,162	2,147	1,024	1,868	877	1,364	256
1981 3/	587,797	561,821	15,104	2,113	4,267	1,976	991	1,262	263
1980 3/	589,616	567,568	14,229	2,090	1,321	2,062	1,001	1,170	175
1975 3/	511,581	484,416	7,707	1,311	9,595	3,161	4,602	281	508

1/ Includes races other than white and black.
2/ Includes births with place of delivery not stated.
3/ Based on 100 percent of births in selected States and on a 50-percent sample

attainment distributions. For each educational attainment group, in-hospital physician-attended births have a higher percent low birth weight than do midwife-attended groups. Midwife out-of-hospital births are the least likely to be of low birth weight.

Because midwives screen their patients carefully throughout the prenatal care process and refer high-risk patients to physicians, it is not possible to determine whether or not midwives achieve better or worse outcomes than physicians do. These data do indicate that midwives, both in and out of the hospital, can safely manage low-risk pregnancies and labor and thus provide a safe alternative to the traditional in-hospital physician-attended birthing experience. More recent research indicates that delivery in birthing centers attended by midwives can also lead to relatively fewer cesarean sections and to savings in cost (Scupholme, McLeod, and Robertson, 1986; Rooks et al., 1989).

Table 2. Attendant and Place of Birth by Selected Characteristics: United States, 1988

Selected characteristics	Physician in hospital	Midwife in hospital	Midwife out of hospital
		Percent	
All births	100.0	100.0	100.0
Race of child			
White	78.1	71.4	94.6
Black	17.1	20.9	2.9
Age of mother			
Under 20 years	12.4	17.9	6.3
30 years or more	28.5	24.2	40.0
Marital status of mother			
Married	74.6	64.6	90.3
Unmarried	25.4	35.4	9.7
Years of school completed by mother 1/			
Less than 12 years	20.0	30.9	21.4
16 years or more	17.8	14.3	25.6
Birth order of child			
First order	41.6	39.8	25.5
Fourth or higher order	9.8	12.5	24.7
Nativity of mother			
Native-born	87.2	77.7	76.4
Foreign-born	12.8	22.3	23.6

1/ Excludes data for California, Texas, and New York State (not including New York City) which did not require reporting of educational attainment of mother.

The 1989 revision of the U.S. Standard Certificate of Live Birth permits a more comprehensive comparison of birth outcomes by attendant type. Previously, the birth certificate did not permit the differentiation of lay midwives from certified nurse-midwives. Consequently, the birth outcomes of mothers choosing these alternative attendants could not be examined separately. Also,

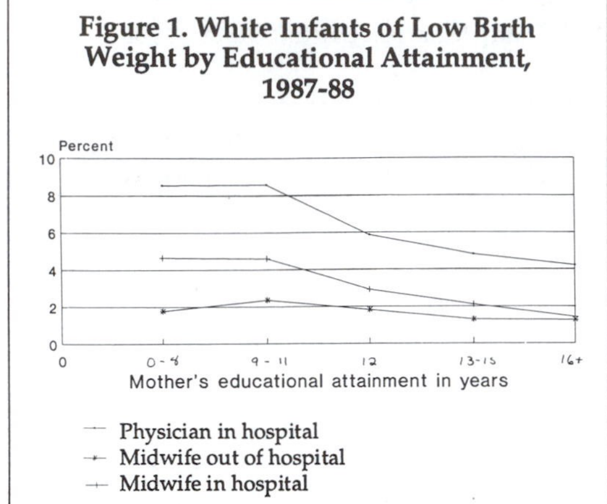

Figure 1. White Infants of Low Birth Weight by Educational Attainment, 1987-88

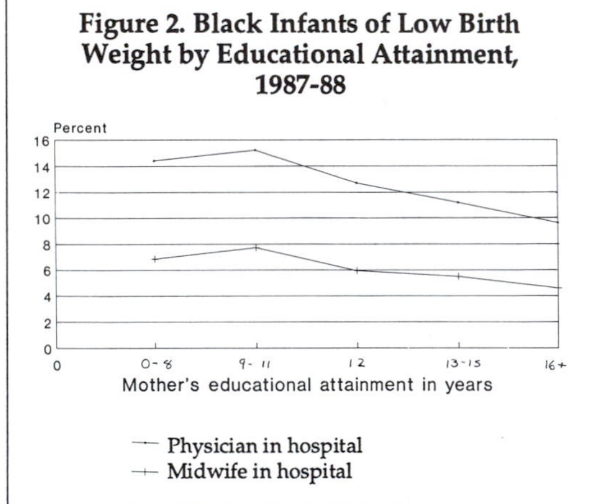

Figure 2. Black Infants of Low Birth Weight by Educational Attainment, 1987-88

the old certificate included only two designations for place of birth: in hospital and out of hospital. Birthing centers were included in either category depending on each state health department's determination. The revised certificate now separately identifies free-standing birthing centers, the mother's residence, and clinic or doctor's office as place of birth. The new certificate also includes questions relating to medical risk factors (e.g., anemia and cardiac disease) and lifestyle factors (e.g., alcohol and tobacco use), which permits comparison of outcomes for different risk groups by attendant. ✱ CAROLINE T. LEWIS, M.A.

See also: Midwife Licensing; Midwifery: Overview; Midwifery and the Law

See **Guide to Related Topics:** Caregivers and Practitioners

Resources

Allgaier A. (1978). "Alternative Birth Centers Offer Family-centered Care." *Hospitals 52:* 97-112.

Table 3. Percent of Live Births of Low Birth Weight by Attendant, Place of Birth, Educational Attainment, and Race of Child

Educational attainment and race	Physician in hospital	Midwife in hospital	Midwife out of hospital
White			
0-8	8.6	4.6	1.8
9-11	8.6	4.6	2.4
12	5.9	2.9	1.8
13-15	4.8	2.1	1.3
16+	4.2	1.4	1.3
Black			
0-8	14.4	6.8	*
9-11	15.2	7.7	*
12	12.7	6.0	*
13-15	11.2	5.5	*
16+	9.6	4.6	*

* Figure does not meet standard of reliability.

Annandale, E.C. (1988). "How Midwives Accomplish Natural Childbirth: Managing Risk and Balancing Expectations." *Social Problems 35* (2): 95-110.

Bennetts, A.B. & Lubic R.W. (1982). "The Free-standing Birth Centre." *Lancet 1:* 378-80.

Lewis, C.T. (1988). "A Current Perspective on Midwife-Attended Births." Paper presented at the annual meeting of the American Public Health Association, Boston.

Rooks, J.P. et al. (1989). "Outcomes of Care in Birth Centers." *New England Journal of Medicine 321*: 1804-11.

Scupholme, A., McLeod, A.G.W., & Robertson, E.G. (1986). "A Birth Center Affiliated with the Tertiary Care Center: Comparison of Outcome." *Obstetrics & Gynecology 67*: 598-603.

Taffel, S. (1984). "Midwife and Out-of-Hospital Deliveries, United States" National Center for Health Statistics. *Vital Health Statistics 21* (40).

MIDWIFERY: OVERVIEW

"Midwife," a word derived from Middle and Old English, means "with woman" (*Webster's*, 1938). It refers to the person, nearly always a woman, who is a primary caregiver to a woman during pregnancy, childbirth, and the month or so following birth. Women have been helping other women give birth from the beginning of time. The first reference to midwives in literature is found in the Bible in the book of Genesis. Historically, midwives have attended most births around the world. The French word for midwife—*sage femme*—is translated "wise woman," which reflects the larger role midwives have often played in the community. Frequently, they were the ones most knowledgeable about herbal medicine, anatomy, health and illness, childbirth, child care, and death. They were healers, advisors, and companions during life's most challenging passages. Their training filled the spectrum from grandmotherly neighbor who learned purely from experience to hospital-trained nurses with graduate degrees.

In 1972, the World Health Organization established an international definition of a midwife which states:

> A midwife is a person who, having been regularly admitted to a midwifery educational program duly recognized in the country in which it is located, has successfully completed the prescribed course of studies in midwifery and has acquired the requisite qualifications to be registered and/or legally licensed to practice midwifery.
>
> She must be able to give the necessary supervision, care and advice to women during pregnancy, labor and the postpartum period, to conduct deliveries on her own responsibility, and to care for the newborn and the infant. This care includes preventive measures, the detection of abnormal conditions in mother and child, the procurement of medical assistance, and the execution of emergency measures in the absence of medical help. She has an important task in counseling and education—not only for patients, but also within the family and community. The work should involve antenatal education and preparation for parenthood and extends to certain areas of gynecology, family planning and child care.
>
> She may practice in hospitals, clinics, health units, domiciliary conditions or any other service. (Davis, 1987)

In the United States midwives were the primary caregivers at births until the 1800s, when their numbers began to steadily decline. Political and social factors caused midwifery to all but disappear (Wertz and Wertz, 1977), although midwives continued to practice quietly, and sometimes secretly, especially in poor or rural areas. Childbirth became the realm of male physicians, who had invested much energy in discrediting the profession of midwifery. And in the 1900s, birth moved to the hospital.

For the most part, formal midwifery training was restricted to two schools. The first nurse-midwifery educational program was the Lobenstine Midwifery School, associated with the Maternity Center Association in New York City and established in 1931. The school was started in response

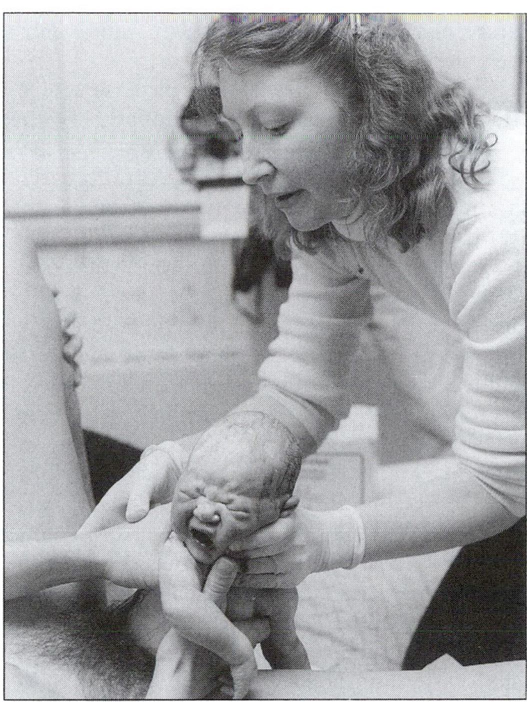

Birth with nurse-midwife at birth center. Photo courtesy of Harriette Hartigan/Artemis.

to a growing awareness that the U.S. had higher maternal and neonatal morbidity and mortality rates than did countries whose obstetrical care was centered around well-educated midwives. In 1925, Mary Breckenridge, a British-trained nurse-midwife, began to import midwives from England to serve the women and children of the rural Appalachians in Kentucky. The tremendous success of this program led to the establishment of a school, now called the Frontier School of Midwifery and Family Nursing, in 1939 (Varney, 1987).

At the same time, non-nurse midwifery continued to be practiced underground. These women were referred to as "lay midwives," suggesting that they were untrained and unskilled, despite the fact that they may actually have been highly experienced and skilled. No term has been universally accepted to describe non-nurse midwives. "Direct-entry midwifery," used in other countries to describe those who do not attend nursing school before receiving their midwifery training, became a popular title in the late 1980s.

In the early 1960s, nurse-midwives could practice legally in only four jurisdictions: New Mexico, Kentucky, New York City, and Maryland (Varney, 1987). But the late 1960s and early 1970s saw tremendous growth in the field of nurse-midwifery, as well as the re-emergence of direct-entry midwifery.

A number of factors led to this increase. Nurse-midwifery was recognized nationally by the medical profession for the first time (Varney, 1987). The nursing profession began to emphasize its autonomy and equality as a member of the health care team. Consumers were made more aware of the existence of CNMs through the popular media. CNMs were utilized in federally funded programs and became involved in gynecological and pediatric care, and state and federal health care agencies began their search for lower-cost methods of providing all health care services.

At the same time, there had been growing interest in natural childbirth, popularized by Drs. Lamaze and Bradley [*see* Bradley Method; Husband-Coached Childbirth; Psychoprophylactic Method (Lamaze)], who had in turn drawn from Grantly Dick-Read's *Childbirth without Fear* (1959) (*see* "Read Method: Natural Childbirth"). Not only were an increasing number of women interested in unmedicated childbirth, but the childbirth educators who provided support for them during labor were often radicalized by the hospital experiences they witnessed. They became consumer advocates for change in hospital birth; some became direct-entry or nurse-midwives, and many began to question the increasingly technological event that birth had become in the hands of the medical profession. Several movements also contributed to the increased interest in home birth and midwifery. Interest in "natural" and "organic" foods; a healthier lifestyle; do-it-yourself, "back-to-the-land" philosophies; and disenchantment with the medical profession and other established authorities led to the rise of the so-called "hippie midwife," immortalized in Ina May Gaskin's book *Spiritual Midwifery* (1975). The Farm Community of which she wrote also promulgated a spiritual approach to childbirth, which was shared by a growing number of other spiritual/religious groups. Their spiritual beliefs differed, but they all recognized a spiritual aspect to birth and emphasized the importance of including the family in this event. The 1970s also brought the re-emergence of feminism as a cultural and political force. Landmark books inspired and reflected this trend: *Our Bodies, Ourselves* by the Boston Women's Health Book Collective (1973), which championed respect for women by health care providers, empowerment of women through education about their bodies, and self-care, and *Immaculate Deception* by Suzanne Arms (1975), which questioned the medical profession's view of childbirth and the scientific validity of their practices. *Witches, Midwives and Nurses*, written by feminists Barbara Ehrenreich and Deirdre English (1973), reclaimed women's role as healers and exposed the political reasons for the demise of the midwife in the United States.

The beliefs of these various groups have permeated the philosophy and practice of midwives, leading to a new view of childbirth that rejects the concept that normal pregnancy is a medical condition requiring hospitalization and physician care. This Midwifery Model of birth, first coined by Barbara Katz Rothman, was fully defined in Steiger's *Becoming a Midwife* (1987). According to Steiger, the Midwifery Model:

> Sees pregnancy and birth as a fundamentally healthy process, which has many normal variations. It is a normal part of life, not a medical condition.
>
> Sees this process as doing best without interference and understands that attempts to control the process inevitably alter it and frequently harm it.
>
> Considers each woman and birth unique, calling for an individual, non-routine response.
>
> Calls for the use of the midwife's "heart and hands" (Davis, 1987), and her head (intellect and intuition), too.
>
> Sees the birth attendant's role as encourager, supporter, friend and, sometimes, guide, rather than as "manager." Women are best served when the same birth attendant provides care throughout pregnancy, birth and the postnatal period.
>
> Emphasizes nourishment, emotional support, "active birth" and other non-harmful techniques. They stress "dis-ease" prevention, self-care and exploration of feelings and their effect on physical processes.
>
> Believes the birth experience belongs to the family, not to the birth attendant. The focus is on the mother, baby and family rather than on mother, baby and birth attendant.
>
> Recognizes that choice of birthplace, birth attendant and other decisions about childbirth are basic rights of all women and their families.
>
> Regards knowledge as something to be shared freely with apprentices, other midwives, and pregnant women and their families. Elitism and competition are seen as undesirable traits, cooperation as the ideal.
>
> Holds the belief that midwives should be trained by other midwives, whether in schools or apprenticeships, and that midwives should be experienced, skilled and knowledgeable.
>
> Sees that, although the birth of a baby is the ultimate goal of pregnancy and labor, the process itself has intrinsic value and great importance in the life and psyche of each woman. Pregnancy and childbirth are not seen as distinct and separate from the rest of a woman's life, they are part

of the greater whole of her self-expression, sexuality, and emotional, psychological and spiritual development. Although the goal is still seen as important, this perspective makes midwifery less goal-oriented and more process-oriented than other models and becomes a major factor in the midwife's (and family's) decisions and choices.

Also sees the process of birth, and the environment into which the baby is born, as being vitally important to the physical and emotional health of the baby, potentially affecting his/her entire life.

Recognizes that pregnancy and birth are times of great and rapid change on many levels. Although she is not intrusive or controlling, each midwife must, as Elizabeth Davis says, take responsibility for maintaining a safe situation. This is done in many ways, including: detecting problems prenatally which indicate the need for a hospital birth; overseeing the labor process; using midwifery knowledge to prevent problems, to promote health, or to heal; knowing when and when not to take action; and observing carefully for early signs of conditions which suggest the need for consultation or referral.

Requires midwives to be accountable to one another (though some midwives practice in areas too isolated for regular peer review.)

Generally sees a spiritual aspect to childbirth and midwifery. (Steiger, 1987)

While this model offered a "new" view of childbirth, it was also, paradoxically, more traditional and brought a return of such ancient practices as home birth, herbal remedies, breastfeeding, unmedicated labor, and squatting for delivery.

Individual midwives may practice with a philosophy based purely on the Midwifery Model, or their attitudes may be influenced to varying degrees by the Medical Model of childbirth, depending on where they have been trained and where they have obtained clinical experience. Direct-entry midwives, especially, have rejected many common (yet scientifically unsupported) medical practices, such as routine use of episiotomies, IVs, perineal prep and shave, enemas, lithotomy position for delivery, confinement to bed for the duration of labor, medicated childbirth, and continuous electronic fetal monitoring. Individual certified nurse-midwives may identify more strongly with the philosophy behind their training as nurses, or they may identify more readily with the "midwife" component of their role and therefore perceive birth more in accordance with the Midwifery Model (Rothman, 1982).

Nurse-midwifery educational programs fall into two categories: certificate programs and those leading to master's degrees. Certificate programs, generally lasting 9 to 12 months, accept RNs who have not received a B.S. in Nursing. Master's degree programs require a B.S.N. and are generally completed in one and a half to two years. Certified nurse-midwife programs must be affiliated with institutions of higher learning and accredited by the American College of Nurse-Midwives. Training is generally obtained at hospital births. Graduates are eligible to sit for the ACNM's national examination, which certifies them to practice as certified nurse-midwives. The leading textbook for certified nurse-midwives is *Nurse-Midwifery* by Helen Varney (1980).

Certified nurse-midwives (CNMs) practice in a wide variety of settings, including hospitals, free-standing birth centers, and at home births. Some have concentrated on women's health care or primarily provide prenatal care in hospital and community clinics. CNMs deliver approximately 3 percent of babies in the U.S. (Korte and Scaer, 1990).

There are no national standards for the training and education of direct-entry midwives (DEMs) in the United States. Requirements vary from state to state. A wide variety of routes to education and practice have arisen to meet the needs of DEMs and the communities they serve. A number of schools, unaffiliated with other institutions, have arisen, some providing didactic and clinical training (such as the Seattle School of Midwifery), and others providing mostly clinical experience and on-the-job training (Maternidad La Luz in El Paso, Texas). Most DEMs are either self-trained or have trained through apprenticeship to individual practicing midwives, and some of the smaller schools are essentially expanded and formalized apprenticeships. Some apprenticeships have taken the form of correspondence courses, most notably the Midwifery Home Study Course. Since 1987, many apprenticeships have been based on Steiger's *Becoming a Midwife,* the first articulation of what a midwifery apprenticeship should entail. The leading direct-entry midwifery textbook is Elizabeth Davis's *Heart and Hands* (1987).

Direct-entry midwives practice primarily at home births and at privately run, free-standing birth centers. Hospital privileges are yet to become a reality and will most likely be limited to those states that license DEMs.

Midwives in 1990 assisted about 5 percent of all births in the United States. They face many political and legal obstacles as they struggle to retain or expand their scope of practice. Issues such as licensing, third-party reimbursement, the ability to practice without the supervision of a physician, malpractice insurance, establishing national core competencies for direct-entry midwives, and other concerns continue to challenge the political unification of midwives and their ability to practice autonomously. Many members of the medical profession have opposed the proliferation of midwifery, for economic, political, and philosophical reasons, despite the consistently good outcomes from midwife-attended births (Stewart, 1981). The five countries in the world with the lowest perinatal mortality rates have midwifery-based systems of providing pregnancy health care (Davis, 1987). The practice of midwifery has consistently been associated with higher birth-weight babies, lower cesarean rates, and drastically lower rates of medical intervention (Stewart, 1981; Korte and Scaer, 1990). While nurse-midwifery is now legally defined in all 50 states, direct-entry midwifery is legal in some states, illegal in some, and quasi-legal (not criminalized but not regulated by law) in a number of others. Direct-entry midwifery organizations in many states have established self-regulation, standards of practice, and certification exams in response to the lack of regulation and in an attempt to promote their identity as an independent profession.

Midwives from the ranks of both CNMs and DEMs combined forces in the 1980s to found the Midwives Alliance of North America. Along with other midwives throughout the world they struggle with the conflicts between preserving the Midwifery Model and gaining acceptance from the more politically powerful medical profession, between serving minorities of groups with specific needs unmet by other care providers and developing protocols and training that will perhaps make them more accessible to the mainstream of American women. ✷ CAROLYN STEIGER, C.M.

See also: Evolution of Human Birth; Midwife Licensing; Midwife-Attended Births; Midwifery and the Law; Midwives, Southern Black; Nurse-Midwifery: History in the United States; Obstetrics, History of; Social Science Research on American Childbirth Practices

See **Guide to Related Topics:** Caregivers and Practitioners

Resources

Arms, Suzanne. (1975). *Immaculate Deception.* Boston: Houghton Mifflin Company.

Baldwin, Rahima. (1986). *Special Delivery.* Berkeley, CA: Celestial Arts.

Boston Women's Health Book Collective. (1973). *Our Bodies, Ourselves.* New York: Simon and Schuster.

Bradley, Robert A. (1965). *Husband-Coached Childbirth.* New York: Harper & Row.

Davis, Elizabeth. (1987). *Heart and Hands: A Midwife's Guide to Pregnancy and Birth.* Berkeley, CA: Celestial Arts.

Dick-Read, Grantly. (1959). *Childbirth without Fear.* 2nd edition. New York: Harper & Row.

Ehrenreich, Barbara & English, Deirdre. (1973). *Witches, Midwives and Nurses: A History of Women Healers.* Oyster Bay, NY: The Feminist Press.

Gaskin, Ina May. (1975). *Spiritual Midwifery.* Summertown, TN: The Book Publishing Co.

Korte, Diana & Scaer, Roberta. (1990). *A Good Birth, A Safe Birth.* New York: Bantam Books.

Lamaze, Fernand. (1970). *Painless Childbirth.* Chicago: Henry Regnery.

Rothman, Barbara Katz. (1982). *In Labor: Women and Power in the Birthplace.* New York: W.W. Norton.

Steiger, Carolyn. (1987). *Becoming a Midwife.* Portland, OR: Hoogan House.

Stewart, David. (Ed.) (1981). *Five Standards for Safe Childbearing.* Marble Hill, MO: NAPSAC Reproductions.

Varney, Helen. (1987). Nurse-Midwifery. Boston: Blackwell Scientific Publications.

Webster's New International Dictionary of the English Language. (1938). Springfield, MA: G. & C. Merriam Co.

Wertz, Dorothy C. & Wertz, Richard. (1977). *Lying-In: A History of Childbirth in America.* Schocken: New York.

MIDWIFERY AND THE LAW

Direct-entry midwives are increasing in number in the United States. Direct-entry midwives are those who have entered their profession directly through self-study, apprenticeship, and/or midwifery school. Training is most often gained through a combination of these routes. Direct-entry midwifery is distinctly different from certified nurse-midwifery. Certified nurse-midwives (CNMs) are RNs with usually one additional year of hospital and academic training in obstetrics. Direct-entry midwives generally have independent home birth practices, whereas CNM practices are primarily centered in hospitals under physician supervision.

Almost every state in the U.S. has some historical and legislative basis for the practice of midwifery. As society shifted from home birth to hospital birth in the 1940s and then shifted again with a resurgence of interest in home birth in the 1960s, the legal and political climate for midwifery also changed. Twenty-one states have pending legislation that either clarifies old laws, amends recent ones, or creates an entirely new precedent for midwifery.

Political and legal climates for midwifery practice vary from state to state, but similarities exist in certain groupings of states. Five general categories have been used here to distinguish states with similar characteristics. Ten states have active licensure, certification, or registration processes. They are Alaska, Arizona, Arkansas, Louisiana, Montana, New Hampshire, New Mexico, South

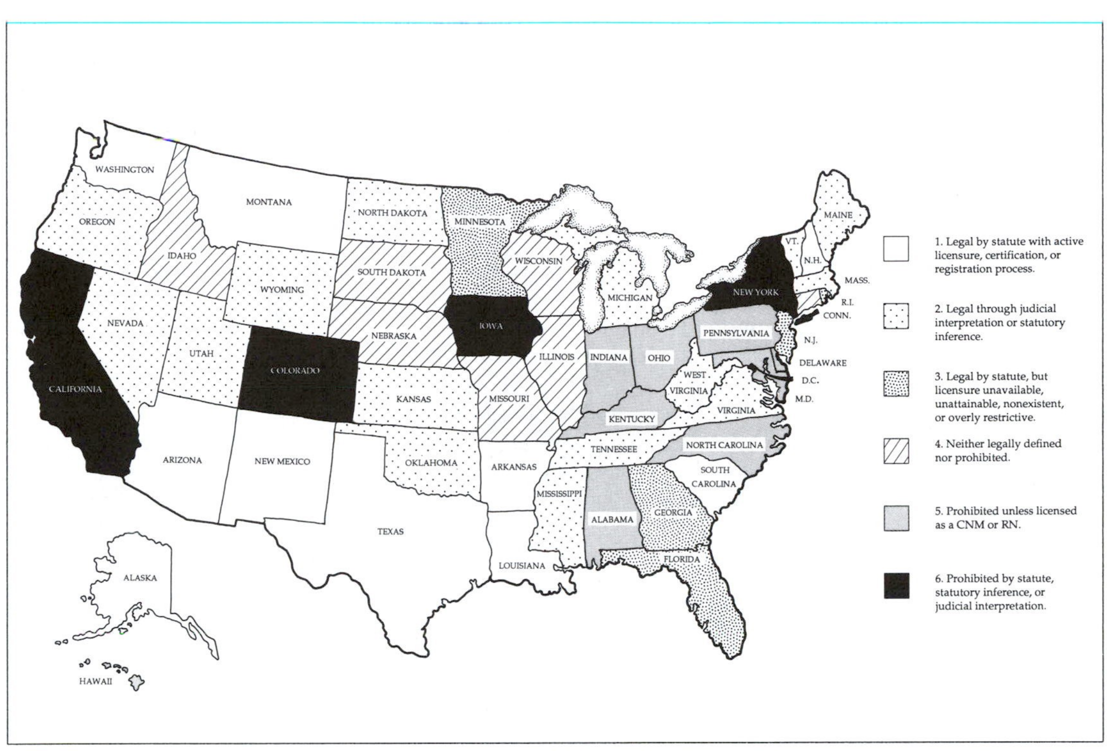

Ten states with licensure, certification, or registration processes

State	Basis of Legal Status	Pending Legislation
Alaska	1985 midwifery legalized, standards to be defined in upcoming legislature	Upcoming to clarify standards
Arizona	1982 law legalized midwifery and set specific standards	Current legislation clarifies unregulated practice
Arkansas	1987 law legalized midwifery practice and stipulated that midwives have emergency back-up plan	None pending
Louisiana	1988 licensing procedure finalized	None pending
Montana	1989 law legalizes midwifery and stipulates requirements	1991—to further clarify law
New Hampshire	1981 law defines midwifery and sets standards	1990 to legalize VBAC waiver
New Mexico	1980 old laws revised and regulations created	None pending
South Carolina	1981 statute updated 1931 law to include an advisory board	None pending
Texas	1983 law requires midwives to register annually; 1987 amendment includes a midwifery board	1991—for education standards
Washington	1917-1988 several statutes define midwifery practice; state licensing	None pending

Fifteen states that define midwifery's legality through judicial interpretation or statutory inference

State	Basis of Legal Status	Pending Legislation
Kansas	1984 court case permitted midwifery within certain parameters	1991
Maine	Attorney General opinion stating midwifery is not the practice of medicine	None pending
Massachusetts	1985 statute stating that no statutes prohibit midwifery except for nurses (CNMs not included in this restriction)	Ongoing
Michigan	1939 court decision distinguishes midwifery from the practice of medicine	None pending

State	Basis of Legal Status	Pending Legislation
Mississippi	Law states practice of midwifery is not prohibited and licenses are not required	None pending
Nevada	1982 Attorney General's opinion stated that midwifery did not need to be licensed	None pending
North Dakota	Two statutes: one defines the practice of medicine as treating illness, and one mentions midwives treating the eyes of newborns	None pending
Oklahoma	Law states that practicing medicine is treating disease and clarifies "lay"midwifery from CNM	None pending
Oregon	1977 Attorney General opinion recognizes midiwfery as distinct from RN and CNM certification; several other references in Oregon law	1991
Tennessee	Midwifery is exempted from the practice of medicine	None pending
Utah	1979 CNM act states that midwifery is not practicing medicine and that parents can choose attendant	None pending
Vermont	Statute requires midwives to sign birth certificates	None pending
Virginia	1977 statute allowed only midwives who currently held licenses to continue practice; however, a midwife was defined as someone who practiced for compensation	None pending
West Virginia	Midwifery practiced for compensation is a misdemeanor	None pending
Wyoming	1991 statute interpreted to mean that midwives can attend births but not give pre- or postpartum care	1991 to revise statute

Seven states with no legal definition or prohibition of midwifery

State	Basis of Legal Status	Pending Legislation
Connecticut	1983, obsolete law repealed	None pending
Idaho	No law	None pending
Illinois	Law judged unconstitutionally vague in 1990	Currently sought
Missouri	1959 law rescinded 1901 midwifery law	1990 and ongoing
Nebraska	No law	None pending
South Dakota	No law	None pending
Wisconsin	1953 statute rescinded 1909 midwifery law; no new law	Currently sought

Five states where midwifery is legal by statute, but licensure is unavailable, unattainable, nonexistent, or overly restrictive

State	Basis of Legal Status	Pending Legislation
Florida	1982 legalized midwifery and created licensure requirement; 1984 law restricted licensure to those holding current licenses	Currently sought
Georgia	1924 law governs midwifery practice; however, after 1976, health department no longer certified midwives	None pending
Minnesota	Law states attendance at childbirth is practicing midwifery; no current licensing procedure	1990 and ongoing
New Jersey	1982 legalizes midwifery but requires unobtainable licenses	None pending
Rhode Island	Midwifery licensure required for practice and currently only CNMs are granted licenses	None pending

Thirteen states and the District of Columbia with prohibition of midwifery through statutory restriction or judicial inference

State	Basis of Legal Status	Pending Legislation
Alabama	1976 act permitting only licensure of CNMs	1991
California	Statute defines midwifery as practice of medicine	Currently sought
District of Columbia	Law defines midwifery as the practice of medicine	None pending
Colorado	Statute defining midwifery as practice of medicine	1991 legislation; Supreme Court case pending
Delaware	1978; State Board of Health grants licenses only to CNMs	None pending

State	Basis of Legal Status	Pending Legislation
Hawaii	State licenses only CNMs	None pending
Indiana	1989 requires licensure of midwives; Medical Board licenses only CNMs	Currently sought Court case pending
Iowa	1978 Attorney General opinion; practicing midwifery is practicing medicine without a license	None pending
Kentucky	1975 law allows midwives with old permits to practice; new midwives must be CNMs	1992
Maryland	1981 statute restricts licensure to CNMs	None pending
New York	1972 Public Health law; midwifery considered practice of medicine	1990 and ongoing
North Carolina	1983 required midwives to be CNMs, with provision for those with old licenses (there is one such midwife)	None pending
Ohio	1967; midwives must be CNMs	None pending
Pennsylvania	1982 law requires midwives to be nurses	1990

Carolina, Texas, and Washington. In the majority of these states an extensive licensing process is required; however, in New Hampshire state licensure is voluntary, and in Texas only annual registration is required. Another 15 states define midwifery's legality through judicial interpretation or statutory inference. They are Kansas, Maine, Massachusetts, Michigan, Mississippi, Nevada, North Dakota, Oklahoma, Oregon, Tennessee, Utah, Vermont, Virginia, West Virginia, and Wyoming. With the exception of Mississippi, in which midwives practice in an oppressive medical climate despite midwifery's legality, the majority of these states have open, active midwifery communities. Also noteworthy in this category are Virginia and West Virginia, in which the law states that a midwife is someone who practices for compensation, simultaneously recognizing midwifery practice while restricting it by making receiving compensation a misdemeanor in West Virginia and by not offering current licenses in Virginia. Concurrently, the state health department in West Virginia is exploring the possibility of training midwives. Seven states do not legally define or prohibit midwifery. They are Connecticut, Idaho, Illinois, Missouri, Nebraska, South Dakota, and Wisconsin. Some of these states are actively seeking legislation, while others prefer the freedom of practice the absence of legislation can confer. In five states midwifery is legal by statute but licensure is either unavailable, unattainable, nonexistent, or overly restrictive. They are Florida, Georgia, Minnesota, New Jersey, and Rhode Island. Midwifery practice in these states may be compromised by uncooperative legislatures. Thirteen states and the District of Columbia prohibit direct-entry midwifery through statutory restriction or judicial inference. They are Alabama, California, Colorado, District of Columbia, Delaware, Hawaii, Indiana, Iowa, Kentucky, Maryland, New York, North Carolina, Ohio, and Pennsylvania. In nine of these states midwifery is allowed if practiced by an RN or a CNM, and in four of these states and the District of Columbia, midwifery is considered the practice of medicine. Most midwives' practices in these states are covert with two notable exceptions, California and Pennsylvania. Two hundred to 400 midwives practice openly in California, challenging the legal system through court cases (41 to date). Pennsylvania has a long history of midwifery in the Amish community. Thirty to 40 midwives practice openly and file birth certificates.

Forty-five states have midwifery organizations providing midwives with legal and political assistance, peer review, continuing education, standards of practice and protocols, newsletters, and training opportunities. Sixteen midwifery organizations have developed voluntary certification procedures. Another eight organizations are developing certification. Certification requires attaining certain competencies, writing an application, and taking an exam.

Approximately 1,780 direct-entry midwives practice in the United States. Of these, 1,306 have overt practices, while 474 practice covertly. In 10 states that collect birth attendant data, 10,004 births were attended by direct-entry midwives.

Consumers of midwifery care are tremendously important in any legal or political change. Thirty-eight states have powerful consumer communities that have lobbied for midwifery care. When the 1989 law legalizing midwifery care was passed in Montana, the judge who lifted a previous injunction against a midwife stated, "The people of Montana have spoken through their legislators."

Additional information can be found in *Midwifery and the Law*. To order send $19.95 to *Mothering*, P.O. Box 1690, Santa Fe, NM 87505. The 1990 edition of *Midwifery and the Law* contains extensive information on individual state midwifery communities, plus a reference section of national organizations, schools, and publications.

✱ MERIA LOEKS, L.M.

See also: Midwife Licensing; Midwife-Attended Births; Midwifery: Overview

See **Guide to Related Topics:** Caregivers and Practitioners; Legal Issues

MIDWIVES, SOUTHERN BLACK

The system of midwifery that survived in the South from slavery until recently empowered thousands of black women. Historically, in deep South states, the majority of midwives were black. These midwives provided care for countless black women as long as segregation and economic barriers prevented access to medical care. In an agrarian-based economic system that locked women into generations of sharecropping, tenant farming, segregated education, and discrimination in employment, black women had few opportunities to occupy positions of authority. Women who demonstrated skill and caring as midwives, however, could gain a degree of legitimacy, status, and prestige. In addition to being birth attendants, midwives were also spiritual authorities, personal confidantes, and healers.

While past contributions of individual midwives have been recognized on the community level, an understanding of the collective importance of midwifery practices is just beginning to emerge. The only known study to compare southern black midwife-attended births with physician-managed births found that empirically trained black midwives had excellent outcomes when caring for medically low-risk mothers in home deliveries in North Carolina (Burnett et al., 1980). Past medical descriptions of the so-called "granny midwife" as superstitious and backwards, which once monopolized the literature, now are being challenged. Organizations such as the National Women's Health Project and the Midwives Association of North America (MANA) are among the groups that have publicly recognized the contributions of the southern black midwife.

Significance. Southern black midwives acquired their skills through apprenticeships, the births of their own children, and the informal support they gave to family members and friends during their births. These midwives began their practices as part of the plantation system of medical care, which they provided for slaves and slaveholders (Savitt, 1978). The long-term survival of southern black midwifery practices reflects the myriad of social and cultural factors that have shaped the South. Poverty, malnutrition, and excess disease resulted in early death for many mothers and infants. Communities supported the indigenous system as a self-help mechanism until the civil rights movement and Medicaid reimbursement provided some access to medical services. By the end of the 1940s, when hospital-based physicians were attending the majority of white births, southern black midwives continued to care for the majority of black childbearing women in the South (Robinson, 1984). As recently as 1960, 46 percent of non-white births in Alabama still occurred outside of the hospital with midwives providing care in 80 percent of these births (Houde et al., 1982). Even when medical services were available, some women, black and white, preferred midwives because of personal sentiment, family tradition, cost, and negative experiences with medical care. Most recently, women with third-party insurance who desired to have their babies in nonmedical settings have turned to southern black midwives for care (Holmes, 1981). Severe disparities in access to quality health services also continue to exist in rural areas and elsewhere, forcing some women to face major barriers to maternity care.

The Medical Attack. In the 1920s and 1930s, health officials across the South recorded the largest number of practicing southern black midwives ever. In Mississippi, for example, the Mississippi State Supervisor of Midwives as part of the statewide maternity plan of 1921 to 1922 reported 4,209 midwives; 99 percent of them were "Negroes" (Ferguson, 1950). Racism and lack of economic incentives were major factors in medical tolerance of southern black midwives. Since doctors had political power and midwives didn't, physicians controlled the steps for regulation and outlawing of midwives (Ehrenreich and English, 1973). As part of tolerating midwifery practices, midwives were counted and forced to attend training sessions that focused mostly on cleanliness, morals, and Christian attitudes. County health departments set up supervisory structures that encouraged dependency and tried shifting authority from the community-empowered midwife to local health departments. Senior midwives were targeted for replacement by new recruits willing to accept the health departments' dictated standards for midwifery practice. The medically controlled model that was designed to take over the indigenous system has been called the "white folks' way" (Ferguson, 1950). Midwives sometimes called the indigenous system of midwifery care the "old time way" (Holmes, 1981)

The Indigenous System. Despite the aggressive attack on the traditional system of midwifery, several aspects of the indigenous system have survived. Midwives maintained their independent process for recruiting and training midwives. Community women determined who became midwives and provided them with training. Sometimes midwives encouraged their daughters to take up their practice once they retired. Senior midwives also encouraged women they observed helping in emergencies and attending births in the community as potential candidates for midwifery apprenticeships.

Another component of the indigenous system was the belief in spiritual influences in women's decisions to become midwives. These supernatural interventions were usually dreams or visions that initiated or confirmed a woman's decision to become a midwife. In addition to divine calls to practice, many midwives integrated spiritual practices into their midwifery work. Midwives prayed prior to attending births and during births (Holmes, 1984). The emphasis on carrying out God's will served to justify the tremendous sacrifices required for midwifery work and reinforced the confidence needed to negotiate with employers and families when needing to abandon other obligations for midwifery service. This spiritual focus also shifted attention from the practitioner or other social/cultural/environmental issues when midwives encountered difficulties. While faith was a source of strength for midwives when faced with challenges, it may also have effectively buffered harsh realities. Midwives also frequently accepted payment in kind or no payment at all because they viewed their work as God's work.

Through the community-based indigenous system, midwives could keep the "old time way" alive. Senior midwives provided information to their selected apprentices about the cultural traditions of midwifery practices. They learned to keep mothers actively "stirring" during labor, how to support mothers who wanted to use alternative birthing positions such as kneeling or stooping during birth, how to create a "hot" state for mothers in labor to stimulate birth, how to prepare hot pepper tea, how to bring down the afterbirth by having the mother sit on a pot of water containing drops of turpentine, how to bandage the abdomen in the postpartum period, and how to carry out other postpartum rituals. Midwives took special care of the afterbirth, for example. In "the old time way," a midwife would sprinkle salt on the afterbirth prior to burying it in the ground. Many midwives also provided pregnant women with the white or red clay that they craved during pregnancy. Geophagy was common in the South and midwives sometimes had clients in northern cities who craved southern quality earth, which the midwives dug up from favorite earth mounds and shipped to pregnant women.

When filling traditional midwifery roles, midwives might be expected to provide basic household assistance. Depending on the availability of family or other social supports, midwives might help with household chores such as the first wash. In the traditional system, the midwife might come back on the eighth day "to take the mother up." This involved taking the mother outdoors for the first time. Sometimes the mother would be required to drink a thimble of water or call the baby's name three times before returning to the house. One midwife in Alabama said she named babies when she carried them around the house after taking the mother up (Holmes, 1981). Younger midwives also learned important hand skills and techniques from senior midwives. Midwives were aware that without telephones, transportation, or access to medical facilities, they needed to be adept at turning babies *in utero*, attending multiple births, and in succeeding at manipulations to expel retained placentas. Special titles of respect for midwives such as "second doctor lady" reflected community recognition of midwifery skill (Holland, 1987).

Survival. Public health officials underestimated the strength of midwives' skills and their personal attributes in their initial attempts to disrupt the indigenous system. Despite the availability of public health department recruits to replace senior midwives, pregnant women continued to seek the care of midwives who were part of the traditional system (Mongeau, Smit, and Maney 1960). According to one anthropologist who studied midwifery practices in Florida, "Health Department personnel failed to take into account the established patterns at the community level, the elements of traditional practice attractive to clients and the self-confidence and influence of midwives in the community" (Dougherty, 1982).

To keep the indigenous system alive, midwives learned to satisfy health department regulators and covertly maintain midwife traditions. Sometimes midwives kept a midwifery bag for inspection by health officials and another bag that they actually used when attending births (Mongeau, 1973). While midwives listened to adamant nursing instructors inform them about the risks of women having babies on their knees, midwives continued to support those who wanted to kneel or stoop on a pallet (Holmes, 1981).

In the 1970s, state legislators moved to totally eradicate midwifery. The prerequisite for replacing midwives was now in place: Doctors could make some money for poverty care through Medicaid. Signs of the demise of the midwifery system had been apparent for some time. Past regulatory efforts greatly reduced the number of midwives who remained in practice; those remaining were targeted for ongoing harassment by health department officials who wanted them to quit or retire (Holmes, 1981). Many of the older midwives who were the strongest representatives of the indigenous system had died, and surviving midwives were geographically dispersed, competed among themselves, and had no political base. As the demise of the system became apparent, older midwives had difficulty attracting women with the skills and personal attributes of previous generations of midwives. Daughters of senior midwives and other young community women who exhibited midwifery potential and displayed the charisma of previous midwife leaders now could pursue a wide range of educational opportunities and careers. Community women who might have been strong advocates for midwives failed to rally to their support, partly because they associated midwives with the most oppressive decades of southern poverty and discrimination. Nevertheless, oral histories and other media reports are confirming the importance of midwifery roles (Stoney, 1959; Milton, 1985; Holmes, 1986; Greene, 1987; Gentry, 1988; Susie, 1988; Logan, 1989). As contemporary midwives and midwifery advocates seek avenues for supporting direct-entry and other independent midwives with varying experiences and backgrounds, southern black midwives could yet win back the political support needed for them to continue their practices.

✱ LINDA JANET HOLMES, M.P.A.

See also: Midwife Licensing; Midwifery: Overview; Midwifery and the Law

See **Guide to Related Topics:** Caregivers and Practitioners; Cross-Cultural Perspectives

Resources

Burnett, Claude A., III et al. (1980). "Home Delivery and Neonatal Mortality in North Carolina." *Journal of the American Medical Association 224* (24): 2741-45.

Dougherty, Molly C. (1982, Spring). "Southern Midwifery and Organized Health Care: Systems in Conflict." *Medical Anthropology*: 114-26.

Ehrenreich, Barbara & English, Deirdre. (1973). *Witches, Midwives, and Nurses: A History of Women Healers.* Brooklyn, NY: The Feminist Press.

Ferguson, James H. (1950). "Mississippi Midwives." *Journal of the History of Medicine* (5): 85-94.

Gentry, Dianne Koos. (1988). "Gladys Milton." In *Enduring Women.* College Station, TX: Texas A & M University Press, pp. 150-75.

Greene, Melissa. (1987, Nov). "All the Hours of the Night." *Country Journal*: 58-63.

Holland, Ida Mae Endesha. (1987, Jun). "Portrait of a Time: Granny Midwives." *Ms.*: 48.

Holmes, Linda J. (1981). Collected Oral Histories, Alabama. Unpublished transcripts.

———. (1984). "Alabama Granny Midwife." *The Journal of the Medical Society of New Jersey 81* (5): 389-91.

———. (1986). "African American Midwives in the South." In Pamela Eakins (Ed.) *The American Way of Birth.* Philadelphia: Temple University Press.

Houde, John et al. (1982) "Out of Hospital Deliveries in Alabama 1940-1980. *Journal of the Medical Association of the State of Alabama:* 20-25.

Logan, Onnie Lee as told to Katherine Clark. (1989). *Motherwit: An Alabama Midwife's Story.* New York: E.P. Dutton.

Milton, Gladys. (1985, Winter). "My Story." *The Practicing Midwife*: 5-10.

Mongeau, Beatrice. (1973). "The Granny Midwives: A Study of a Folk Institution in the Process of Social Disintegration." Ph.D. dissertation, University of North Carolina.

Mongeau, Beatrice, Smit, Harvey L., & Maney, Ann C. (1960). "The Granny Midwife: Changing Roles and Functions of a Folk Practitioner." *American Journal of Sociology 66*: 497-505.

Robinson, Sharon. (1984). "A Historical Development of Midwifery in the Black Community: 1600-1940." *Journal of Nurse-Midwifery 29* (4): 247-50.

Savitt, Todd, L. (1978). *Medicine and Slavery: The Diseases and Health Care of Blacks in Antebellum Virginia.* Urbana, IL: University of Illinois Press, pp. 182-84.

Stoney, George. (1959). "All My Babies Research." In Robert Huges (Ed.) *Film: Book I: The Audience and the Filmmaker.* New York: Grove Press, Inc., pp. 79-95.

Susie, Debra Anne. (1988). *In the Ways of Our Grandmothers: A Cultural View of Twentieth Century Midwifery in Florida.* Athens, GA: University of Georgia Press.

MISCARRIAGE

Miscarriage refers to a pregnancy that ceases to develop and is discharged from a woman's body before being viable, i.e., typically before 28 weeks' gestation. Miscarriages are differentiated from babies who are born alive but soon die (neonatal deaths) and full-term pregnancies in which a dead baby is born (stillbirths). The most commonly used medical term for "miscarriage" is "spontaneous abortion" (in contrast with "induced abortion"). Other medical and legal terms include "abortion," "fetal waste," and "fetal tissue." Pregnant women may use terms such as "dead baby," "ended pregnancy," or "a miss."

Miscarriages are extremely common, currently estimated at 20 percent of all U.S. women's pregnancies. Each year, between 600,000 and 800,000 U.S. women miscarry. Given that a woman is likely to have more than one pregnancy, the chances that she will have a miscarriage at some time in her life are very great. Miscarriages violate "the myth of procreative control," the idea that women can prevent and induce pregnancies at will, and thus have babies when they want to. Miscarriages also violate the individual woman's sense of her body's integrity.

Miscarriages are a possible outcome of first, as well as subsequent, pregnancies, even after a woman has given birth to numerous full-term normal children. Miscarriages occur in single women, married women, and lesbians; in young teenagers and middle-aged women; in women with poor or excellent prenatal care. Miscarriage is related to age—the likelihood of miscarrying is high for very young teenagers, reaches its lowest point (12 percent) for women around the age of 20, and increases to 41 percent for women pregnant at the age of 42. Thus, delayed childbearing, a common phenomenon of middle-class women whose involvement in education or work interferes with childbearing, increases the risk of miscarriage.

Miscarriage is also a highly likely outcome of pregnancies accomplished with the assistance of reproductive technology. As these technologies proliferate, so will the miscarriage experience. Miscarriages occur in women of all ages, races, and creeds and at every stage of pregnancy, although they are more common in early (between the 7th and 14th week of gestation) rather than late (between the 15th and 28th week) stages. Every pregnant woman should be prepared for miscarriage at any time.

Because people believe erroneously that miscarriages do not occur after the first trimester, some women do not divulge the fact that they are pregnant during that time. People are also superstitious about miscarriages and do not like to talk about them with pregnant women. As a result, pregnant women frequently know very little about them. Given the prevalence of miscarriages, it is unfortunate that women are so poorly informed and ill-prepared.

It is possible to be unaware that one is miscarrying because one is unaware that she is pregnant. A woman may experience an early miscarriage as a heavy menstrual period. Later miscarriages are equivalent to labor and delivery, topics that many women know little about in their first pregnancies. Women pregnant for the first time are thus relatively unprepared physically or emotionally for the miscarriage process. The possible speed and severe pain of a miscarriage make it imperative for women to be prepared.

The first signs of miscarriage typically are spotting and cramps. For a miscarriage to occur, the cervix must open and the forming fetus and placenta must be expelled. Typically, painful muscular contractions accompany the opening of the cervix, and a great deal of blood flow accompanies the discharge of products from the uterus.

Many women prefer to be in a hospital under medical care when these processes occur, but some women have poor access to hospital facilities. Medical personnel who examine a woman who is miscarrying will probably recommend that she be anesthetized during or after she completes the delivery process, that her cervix be dilated, and that the uterus be scraped of any placental remains. This process is called D&C—dilation and curettage—and is considered necessary in many cases to prevent infection. All invasive procedures, however, carry their own risk of infection. After this procedure and a short period of recovery, the woman is discharged from the hospital. It usually takes at least a week for the woman to regain her strength from this experience.

Between 1940 and 1970, physicians, primarily in the U.S., prescribed DES (the estrogen diethylstilbestrol) to prevent miscarriages. This synthetic hormone proved ineffective and tragically "raised the risk of genital abnormalities, especially vaginal cancer, in people exposed in utero" (Oakley, 1984, p. 194). (*See* "DES: Diethylstilbestrol"). Currently women receiving prenatal care who are at risk for miscarriage are prescribed bedrest (not always possible for women with multiple responsibilities and few supports), reduced activity, and cessation of sexual intercourse, although none of these prohibitions has been definitely linked with increasing the chances of averting miscarriage.

Medical practice differentiates between women who have miscarried only once or twice and those who have miscarried repeatedly. It is likely to leave uninvestigated the cause of a single or pair of miscarriages, much to the dismay of those women determined to understand the cause of death. The likelihood of a subsequent miscarriage increases after two such experiences. Repeat miscarriages can sometimes be traced to a cause (e.g., genetic abnormality or exposure to teratogens) that may be correctable. The cause of most miscarriages is not known, although most probably reflect a defect in the developing fetus rather than a problem in the woman or her partner (Pizer and Palinski, 1980). Male fetuses are more likely to be miscarried than are female fetuses. Miscarriages are sometimes inadvertently induced by the amniocentesis procedure. Since miscarriages may be induced by physical violence, and men who are violent to women are likely to beat their partners, particularly when their partners are pregnant, a pregnant woman in a relationship with a battering man has a high risk of miscarrying. (*See* "Violence against Pregnant Women"). There are numerous psychiatric and psychoanalytic theories that attribute miscarriages to unresolved psychological conflicts in the woman. Many women who miscarry blame themselves, particularly if they desired the child and received no medical explanation for the miscarriage.

Rituals designed to avoid miscarriages exist in almost all cultures (Reinharz, 1988a), but few rituals deal with what to do after a miscarriage has occurred. This lack deepens the grief and confusion of women and men who have experienced a miscarriage. In the contemporary U.S., some pro-life groups and women's mental health groups advocate disposing "fetal waste" with dignity, naming the "child," photographing the "miscarriage," or conducting a religious burial. It is important to separate these efforts from any plan that would deny women the right to induced abortions.

Hospitals typically provide little emotional support for miscarrying women and may place them insensitively in obstetrics wards. Unfortunately, some women must endure miscarriage alone, although miscarriage support groups for women and their partners are offered by some health centers and self-help organizations.

A miscarrying woman and/or her partner may be grief stricken and feel depressed and enraged. Other children in the family and grandparents may suffer from this loss as well and are frequently neglected. Unwelcome solicitous remarks such as "you were hardly pregnant," "you can always try to get pregnant again," or "you already have such nice children" invalidate the woman's experience. According to studies by Peppers and Knapp (1980a, 1980b), the grief experienced from miscarriage, stillbirths, and neonatal death are equivalent if the child was wanted. For other men and women, a miscarriage is a welcome relief from an unwanted pregnancy. The meaning of miscarriage can not be assumed.

✱ SHULAMIT REINHARZ, Ph.D.

See also: Pregnancy Loss: Family Response

See **Guide to Related Topics:** Pregnancy Loss and Infant Mortality

Resources

Berezin, N. (1982). *After a Loss in Pregnancy: Help for Families Affected by Miscarriage, A Stillbirth or the Loss of a Newborn*. New York: Fireside/Simon & Schuster.

Borg, Susan & Lasker, Judith. (1981). *When Pregnancy Fails: Families Coping with Miscarriage, Stillbirth and Infant Death*. Boston: Beacon Press.

Boston Women's Health Book Collective. (1985). *The New Our Bodies, Ourselves*. New York: Simon and Schuster.

Callahan, E.J., Brasted, W.S., & Granados, J.L. (1983). "Fetal Loss and Sudden Infant Death: Grieving and Adjustment for Families." In E.J. Callahan & K. McCluskey (Eds.) *Life-span Development Psychology: Non-normative Life Events*. New York: Academic.

Friedman, R. & Gradstein, B. (1982). *Surviving Pregnancy Loss*. Boston: Little, Brown.

Jimenez, Sherry Lynn Mims. (1982). *The Other Side of Pregnancy: Coping with Miscarriage and Stillbirth*. Englewood Cliffs, NJ: Prentice-Hall.

Lachelin, Gillian. (1985). *Miscarriage: The Facts*. New York: Oxford University Press.

Moriarty, D. (1952, Oct). "The Right to Mourn." *Ms. 15* (10): 79-84.

Oakley, Ann. (1984). *The Captured Womb: A History of the Medical Care of Pregnant Women*. Oxford: Basil Blackwell.

Panuthos, Claudia & Romeo, Catherine. (1984). *Ended Beginnings: Healing Childbearing Losses*. South Hadley, MA: Bergin & Garvey.

Peppers, L.G. & Knapp, R.J. (1980a, May). "Maternal Reactions to Involuntary Fetal/Infant Death." *Psychiatry 43*: 155-59.

———. (1980b). *Motherhood and Mourning: Perinatal Death*. New York: Praeger.

Pizer, Hank & Palinski, Christine O'Brien. (1980). *Coping with a Miscarriage*. New York: New American Library.

Reinharz, Shulamit. (1987). "The Social Psychology of a Miscarriage: An Application of Symbolic Interactionist Theory and Method." In Mary Jo Degan & Michael R. Hill (Eds.) *Women and Symbolic Interaction*. New York: Allen and Unwin.

———. (1988a). "Miscarriage: A Cross-Cultural Study of Women's Experience." In Dorothy Wertz (Ed.) *Research in the Sociology of Health Care*. Greenwich, CT: JAI Press.

———. (1988b). "What's Missing in Miscarriage?" *Journal of Community Psychology 16* (1): 84-103.

Welch, M.S. & Herrmann, D. (1980). "Why Miscarriage Is So Misunderstood: New Medical and Emotional Findings." *Ms. 13* (8): 14-22.

MISCARRIAGE: IMAGES IN THE ART OF FRIDA KAHLO

Images of childbearing, including conception, birth, the fetus, or miscarriage, are rare in the history of art, despite the universality of the subject. Some contemporary artists, particularly women, have explored the subject, but no artist has approached it with the riveting intensity and candor of the Mexican artist Frida Kahlo (1907-1954). An artist whose greatest strength was in self-portraiture, she literally reinvented the genre in her acutely painful images of her personal miscarriages.

Severe injuries that Kahlo sustained in a tragic bus accident in 1926 directly shaped her art. A streetcar slammed into the bus on which she was riding, fracturing her spine, breaking her right foot, and driving a handrail through her pelvis. She endured a life of intermittent pain and invalidism due to these injuries and underwent over 30 operations to correct them. She desperately wanted to have children, but as a result of the pelvic injury, she was unable to bear a fetus to term and suffered at least three known miscarriages.

Kahlo's tumultuous marriage to the famous Mexican muralist Diego Rivera and her love of Mexican folk art and popular tradition also greatly influenced her art. Rivera, whose affairs during their 25 years of marriage were legion (she paid him back in kind), had great respect for Kahlo's art. He once said: "In the whole history of art, Frida is the only example of a painter virtually tearing her breast and heart open in order to express the feelings in them and tell the biological truth . . . Frida is the first artist to portray the real act of birth since the black basalt sculptures of the Aztec masters" (Billeter, 1988).

By nature a theatrical and vivacious person with a sophisticated sense of humor, she lived life with an intensity and vigor that belied her semi-invalid state and chose to confront her pain head-

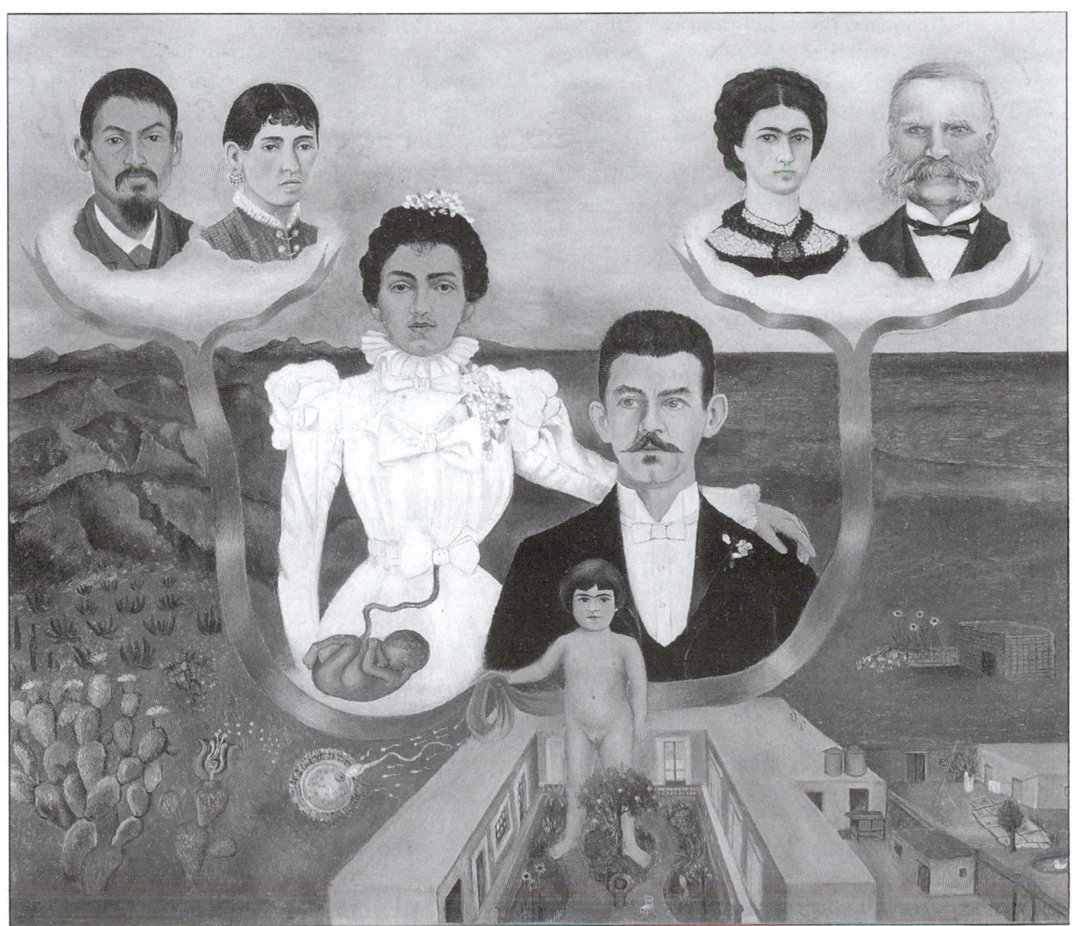

My Grandparents, My Parents, and I (Family Tree) (1936) by Frida Kahlo. [Oil and tempera on metal panel, 12⅛ x 13⅝.] Collection, The Museum of Modern Art, New York. Gift of Allan Roos, M.D., and B. Mathieu Roos.

on through her art. She painted to please only herself and to exorcise the demons of her existence. The small size and scale of her work suited that of an invalid, as she was often forced to paint while bedridden, using a specially built easel. She once explained: "I paint my own reality . . . The only thing I know is that I paint because I need to, and I paint always whatever passes through my head, without any other consideration" (Herrera, 1983).

A 1932 lithograph, "Frida and the Abortion," is based on Kahlo's first loss of a fetus, her pregnancy terminated by a therapeutic abortion. Frida stands naked and vulnerable, her tears of sorrow echoed in the tears of the moon and the blood dripping from her uterus, down her leg, to join with the earth below. The fetus is curled inside her, linked to a larger fetal image, resembling a baby Diego, by the umbilical cord wrapped around her leg. The hideous, monstrous side of nature responsible for her loss is represented by her deformed and discolored left hand and foot, and by the third arm sprouting from her left shoulder. The heart-shaped palette combines an image of her life's work with that of her sorrow, showing the two as inextricably linked.

In 1932, Kahlo suffered a miscarriage (in Detroit, where she had accompanied Rivera, who was working on a mural commission), which resulted in a 10-day hospital stay because of hemorrhaging. When she painted "Henry Ford Hospital" while recuperating, she directly addressed the miscarriage. Frida lies naked on blood-stained sheets, her abdomen still swollen, wholly given over to despair. A single tear rolls down her cheek. Floating in the air, but physically linked to her by a red string suggesting the umbilical cord, are several images, including a boy fetus (again resembling Rivera), a human pelvis, and a wilted flower. She endures the sorrow of this lost life alone, and her feeling of isolation is evident in the composition of the painting. The bed is stranded on a flat gray-green plain, far from the industrialized Detroit skyline and its inhabitants.

One of Kahlo's most anguished works is the portrayal of her own birth, titled "My Birth" or "Childbirth." This "real act of birth," which Rivera spoke of, is a graphic image of a shrouded mother in the throes of giving birth to an adult-size head. Both the mother and the "baby" appear to be dead. Kahlo's use of primitive elements make the grisly image more palatable to the viewer. "With fantasy, bright color, and charmingly naïve drawing, Frida distanced both the viewer and the artist from her painting's painful content" (Herrera, 1983).

In a 1936 painting, "My Grandparents, My Parents and I" (illustrated), Kahlo again portrayed herself. She is a young child standing in the courtyard of her home in Coyoácan (a suburb of Mexico City where she lived most of her life), holding a red ribbon, which connects her to the portraits of her parents and grandparents. The incongruous image of a fetus (possibly meant to be herself in the womb) rests outside her mother's body, on the white skirt of her dress. Below the fetus is a depiction of a sperm penetrating an egg. Kahlo portrays the cycle of life through the moment of conception, the fetus, the growing child, the parents, and the aging grandparents. With this painting she is looking back to happier times, before the quality of her life was shattered in 1926.

Kahlo became a cult figure in her native Mexico during her lifetime, due in part to her own efforts to create herself and in part to her artistic talent. Her early death in 1954 due to complications from pneumonia (after being weakened by a major spinal operation and the amputation of her right leg due to gangrene) served to increase her cult status. The cult of personality surrounding her life does not diminish the power of her intensely honest images of childbearing, which show how forcefully her life and her art were intertwined.

✷ MEREDITH DINGMAN SUTTON, M.A.

See **Guide to Related Topics:** Literature and the Arts; Pregnancy Loss and Infant Mortality

Resources

Billeter, Erika. (Ed.) (1988). *Images of Mexico: The Contribution of Mexico to 20th Century Art.* Dallas: Dallas Museum of Art.

Carter, Angela. (1989). *Images of Frida Kahlo.* London: Redstone Press.

Herrera, Hayden. (1978). *Frida Kahlo.* Chicago: The Museum of Contemporary Art.

———. (1983). *Frida: A Biography of Frida Kahlo.* New York: Harper and Row, Publishers.

Osborne, Margot. (Ed.) (1990). *The Art of Frida Kahlo.* Art Gallery of South Australia and Art Gallery of Western Australia, 1990 Adelaide Festival.

Zamora, Martha. (1990). *Frida Kahlo: The Brush of Anguish.* San Francisco: Chronicle Books.

MOLAR PREGNANCY

In about 0.7 percent of all pregnancies, a faulty embryo forms that is called a hydatidiform (cystlike) mole (lump of tissue). The chorion (outer layer) of this defective embryo aggressively invades the uterus wall to form an abnormal placenta. The resulting "trophoblast" secretes the pregnancy hormone human chorionic gonadotrophin (hCG). There are several variations.

Complete ("Classic") Hydatidiform Mole. The very rare complete mole is created when two sperm nuclei unite in a human egg (instead of the nuclei of one sperm and one egg). Sperm genes are programmed to make a trophoblast, not an embryo. Some trophoblast cells may pervade the body—the lungs especially—as emboli (clumps) in the blood. These cells secrete hCG and can invade blood vessels wherever they go. Such invasiveness is not cancer, although 2 to 5 percent of such moles do become cancerous.

Partial Hydatidiform Mole. The partial mole is created when two sperm nuclei plus an egg nucleus unite in a human egg, forming a defective embryo plus an abnormally invasive trophoblast. Partial moles are probably relatively common and underdiagnosed. Most abort spontaneously in the first or second trimester. They never progress to cancer and form no emboli, but an invasive trophoblast occasionally remains after the embryo aborts.

Gestational Trophoblastic Disease (GTD). This term includes complete moles; partial moles; the very rare choriocarcinoma (cancer of the chorion), which produces hCG; and placental site tumor, with little hCG production.

Symptoms and Diagnosis. Usually when a hydatidiform develops, vaginal bleeding, scanty to extensive, occurs in the second month of pregnancy. With a complete hydatidiform mole, the uterus is greatly enlarged. Other symptoms may be hyperthyroidism, ovarian cysts, toxemia of pregnancy, and severe vomiting. Blood hCG level is high, as in a twin pregnancy, but there is no fetal heartbeat. Ultrasound reliably distinguishes molar from normal pregnancies.

Treatment. After tests for migrated trophoblast, the pregnancy is terminated by suction curettage and the patient watched closely in the hospital for hemorrhage. For the next year, the patient must use contraceptives while her blood is periodically monitored to check for hCG from trophoblast.

Almost all partial moles are cured after abortion. But with about 20 percent of complete moles, trophoblast tissue remains; in about 4 percent of these cases, the tissue becomes malignant. Treatment (chemotherapy) is the same for malignant as for benign tumors. Methotrexate and actinomycin-D are considered very effective. Since these drugs' side effects are severe—sometimes dangerous, often not appearing during the first weeks—extensive hospitalization and astute, expert nursing observation are essential. Psychological impacts are formidable: loss of wanted pregnancy, enforced contraception, debilitating chemotherapy, and threat of death. Prognosis, however, is excellent because of accurate diagnostic methods, monitoring for hCG, and effective chemotherapy. ✱ HELEN BEQUAERT HOLMES, Ph.D.

See **Guide to Related Topics:** Pregnancy Complications

Resources

Berkowitz, R.S. (1988). "Diagnosis and Management of the Primary Hydatidiform Mole." *Obstetrics and Gynecology Clinics of North America 15* (3): 491-503.

Berkowitz, R.S., Goldstein, D.P., & Bernstein, M.R. (1985). "Natural History of Partial Molar Pregnancy." *Obstetrics and Gynecology 66*: 677-81.

Celeste, Sonya M. & Maureen D. Smith. (1986). "Gestational Trophoblastic Neoplasms." *Journal of Obstetric, Gynecologic and Neonatal Nursing 15* (1): 11-16.

Remy, J.C. (1989). "Trophoblastic Disease: 20 Years Experience." *International Journal of Gynecology and Obstetrics 28* (4): 355-60.

Szulman, A.E. (1988). "Trophoblastic Disease: Clinical Pathology of Hydatidiform Moles." *Obstetrics and Gynecology Clinics of North America 15* (3): 443-56.

MONITRICE. *See instead* LABOR ASSISTANTS

MORNING SICKNESS. *See instead* COMMON COMPLAINTS OF PREGNANCY

MOTHERHOOD AS TRANSFORMATION

Women move to motherhood in a linear way, through the nine-month pregnancy; the twelve-hour labor; the forty-five-second contraction; the slow, painful passage of the baby through the birth canal; the timeless wait for the first breath; the momentous reaching to take the baby; and the twenty-four-hour day, seven-day week of life with the child. Yet the linear view does not accommodate the depth of change that occurs in women as they become mothers. Transformation (Bergum, 1989), while taking linear time, involves change that is deep, complex, and dramatic, and may, as Neumann (1955, p. 32) stated, "reshape the woman's life down to its very depths." Transformation to mother is not seen as a succinct experience. Rather, transformation is a never-ending process, changing and developing each moment for women with children of varying ages: in the womb, as infants, school-age children, adolescents, or adults. Women, as mothers, live change.

The Decision. One way of conceptualizing the beginning of transformation is to examine the experiences and relations that are involved in the decision to have a child. The Latin origin of the word "decide" is *décídere,* meaning "to cut off." Does the decision to have a child cut off possibilities in life, by being "gobbled up," "bogged down," or "losing oneself," or "being dependent"? Or does the choice for the child cut off one way of being, by opening to something new, to being enriched, or to being blessed? Opening to the possibility of becoming a mother, in creating space in a woman's life for a child, is the beginning of change, the beginning of her transformation to mother.

The Presence of the Baby in One's Body. With the presence of the child in her body, a woman sees the world as changed and experiences that changed world in various ways. There is no possibility for a woman to become a mother without a child, nor is it possible for a fetus to become a child without a woman. Thus, the presence of the child transforms a woman to mother. Being "with child," a primordial relationship, is peculiar to women who carry within their own bodies the body of another. It is a relationship that develops over time as the baby and the mother grow together. Not only is the fetus bound to the woman through the nourishing pathways running through the umbilical cord, but baby and woman are truly one body. What affects the woman affects the child, and as the child evolves, so does the mother. They are one, an indissoluble whole, yet they are two: There is no closer union. Through the interrelatedness with the child in pregnancy, a woman begins to see herself as mother.

The Pain of Separation. Birth is a separation of mother and baby. Is it possible that the separation, and its accompanying pain, is a penetrating aspect of a woman's transformation? What is the role of pain in this transformation? To have experienced birthing pain offers the possibilities of self-knowledge, knowledge of one's limitations and capabilities. As women give birth to children, they, in a sense, birth themselves into a new life as a mother. Giving voice to women's pain, the pain of childbirth, assists women's use of the pain experience to express themselves and the reality of their world. It transforms women's experience of pain to something useful to them—they say, "I'm glad I had the experience. I can do anything now." Of course, pain should not be stoically endured by women for some psychological or physiological value, but by acknowledging and giving voice to pain, women may help themselves through it, to express themselves rather than let the pain defeat or belittle them. The pain of childbirth acknowledges the transformation that is occurring—the separation of baby and mother so that both may live their own lives.

The Sense of Responsibility. To decide to be responsive in a deep sense to life with children is to be open to its challenges and possibilities. The word "responsible" comes from the Latin *respondére,* meaning "to promise in return." To respond to the presence of the child, then, is to promise to look after that child, to be trusted by the child, to care for the child, and to always return. No longer acting only for herself, the woman is "one for the other." It is an awesome project. What has been a self-regulated, self-defined, and self-contained life is now suddenly broken by the experience of the Other, the child. And in taking responsibility for the child as Other, the woman is forced to be responsible also for herself. Here is the crunch, the dichotomy. How does a woman become responsible as a mother? For women, while they move toward a responsibility that transforms them (in their responsiveness to the positive "Other," the child), they are continually faced with the reality of their own "Other"-ness (a negative reality) in our patriarchal culture, which defines women as Other. Therefore, in exploring the theme of responsibility, the focus becomes divided: responsibility for the baby and responsibility for the woman.

Mindfulness to the Child. What is the experience of having a child on one's mind? How does the nourishing aspect of the mother-child bond transform the woman? Is it the transformation of woman to mother that connects a woman to her child in such a way that from thereafter the "child is always on her mind"? While the primary interest of mothers, early on, is the preservation and nourishment of this new life, it is not long before other interests, such as fostering the child's growth and shaping an acceptable child, also become important (Ruddick, 1983, pp. 219-23). These interests demand change on the part of the woman, which involves moving away from the child. It is through the Otherness of the baby, and seeing that Otherness, that the woman beings to understand herself in relation to that person. "Little ancestor, sweet baby, how you temper me, deepen. Like an ancient smithy working slowly" (Chesler, 1979, p. 281). To have one's mind full of thoughts of the child—while it may at times fragment thinking—pays respect to the child and enriches a mother's life. Living with children causes one to think of the nature of the world, a world as a community for children; having children on one's mind changes how one sees the world.

✻ VANGIE BERGUM, R.N., Ph.D.

See also: Bonding; Fetus, Maternal Experience of; Maternal Thinking; Matrescence and Patrescence

See **Guide to Related Topics:** Pregnancy, Psychological Aspects

Resources

Bergum, Vangie. (1989). *Woman to Mother: A Transformation*. Amherst, MA: Bergin & Garvey Publishers.

Chesler, Phyllis. (1979). *With Child: A Diary of Motherhood*. New York: Thomas Y. Cromwell.

Neumann, Erich. (1955). *The Great Mother: An Analysis of the Archetype*. Princeton, NJ: Princeton University Press.

Ruddick, Sara. (1983). "Maternal Thinking." In J. Trebilcot (Ed.) *Mothering: Essays in Feminist Theory*. Totowa, NJ: Rowman & Allanhead, pp. 211-30.

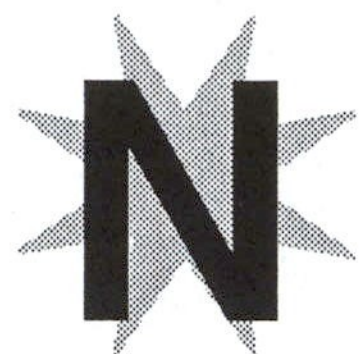

NAMING PRACTICES: GIVEN NAMES

Naming a child serves to make that child a part of the social world. A named child has a social identity. To know a child's name, in a sense, is to know who that child is. When the child is old enough to know his or her own name, that child, in a sense, knows who he or she is. The various processes by which adults select and apply names to children in different societies reveal something about how children are inducted into their societies, brought into their social worlds, and provided with a social identity. And the ways children are named differ radically from society to society.

Today, American children are provided with a "given name," one or more middle names, and a surname (usually the surname of the father). But this is not true in many other societies. In many underdeveloped societies children receive only a given, or personal name, and surnames are not used. Gradually, with the spreading influence of Western culture, more and more societies are using surnames, which in such cases often suggest high status. In several Asian societies (Thailand, Korea, China) children receive both surnames and given names, but the surnames come before the given names, thus suggesting the importance of family identity over personal identity. In several European and Moslem societies children receive given names along with what are called "patronyms," names referring to their fathers. In Russia, for example, the given name of the father (say, "Ivan") will be appended with a "ovich" or a "ovna," indicating that the child is the son or daughter of "Ivan." In Spain and a number of other Hispanic societies children receive given names followed by the surname of their father and the surname of their mother. In Moslem societies children do not receive surnames but, rather, receive given names followed by the given name of their father and by the given name of their father's father. In all of these cases, the familial identity of the child is emphasized.

American children are named immediately after birth or within one week of their birth. But this is not the case in other parts of the world. In many underdeveloped societies children are not named for months, or even years, after birth. Sometimes, when infant mortality rates are high, children are not named early to reduce the family's attachment to the child in case the child dies. On the Pacific island of Truk, for example, children are not named until they show signs of strength and health. But other societies delay naming children for other reasons. Korean children are not named for 100 days to avoid the notice of malevolent spirits. In many societies children are named when they reach some significant stage in socialization. In the American Southwest, Zuni children are named when they first begin to crawl. In Africa, Chagga children are named when their first tooth appears, and Wolof babies are named when their hair is first shaved. Finally, in some societies children are not named until their character or personality becomes evident, and the name is then descriptive of their character or personality.

Since giving a name to a child is an important part of giving that child an identity, just who names a child is often significant. In the United States it is the parents who tend to select given names for their children. About two-thirds of the time fathers and mothers jointly make these decisions, but about one-quarter of the time mothers make these decisions alone. In contrast, in underdeveloped societies it is often someone other than a parent who has the right to name a child, like a grandparent, an aunt or uncle, or a priest. In some societies a number of people each gives a child a name. A Hopi Indian child, for example, is given a name by his paternal grandmother, as well as from various paternal aunts. From these names the parents will eventually pick one.

In the United States parents typically have free choice in selecting their children's names. Exceptions to this tendency are Jews and Catholics. Jewish tradition requires the selection of a name of a deceased relative, while Catholic tradition requires the selection of a name from the Church's list of acceptable saints' names. Often today, however, Jewish and Catholic parents are ignoring these prescriptions. One pronounced tendency in naming American children is the use of names of relatives. About six of ten children receive a first or middle name from a relative; this is especially true of boys and first-born children, and especially common in the higher social classes. In other societies, naming children after relatives is also very common. A number of unusual choice techniques are also used in non-Western societies. Several societies select a name in a dream or by a process of divination. Often these techniques are believed to reveal what deceased person has been reincarnated in the child. Among the Lozi of central Africa, for example, names of ancestors are repeated and when the child cries as a name is spoken, this indicates that that ancestor has been reincarnated in the child. Other naming systems include naming children after the day of the week when they are born (Ashanti), naming children according to a religious calendar (Somali), and naming children according to a fixed sequence of names (Malaya).

Probably the most common bit of information contained in a personal name is the sex of the child. In approximately three of four societies in the world, names indicate a child's sex. In the United States, too, the vast majority of given names are sex-typed. Increasingly, however, female names in the United States are being derived from male names (e.g., Michelle, Christine, Nicole, Denise, Erica, etc.), while the opposite is rarely true. Also, in the United States there is a greater variety of women's names than men's names, and women's names tend to be more fashionable and to change more from decade to decade than men's names. American men's names, in contrast, tend to be much more traditional and exhibit less variety. This is especially true among the higher social classes. ✷ RICHARD ALFORD, Ph.D.

See also: Naming Practices: Surnames
See **Guide to Related Topics:** Baby Care

Resources

Alford, Richard. (1988). *Naming and Identity: A Cross-Cultural Study of Personal Naming Practices.* New Haven, CT: HRAF Press.

American Name Society, *Names.* (A journal devoted to the study of naming.)

Lebell, Sharon. (1988). *Naming Ourselves, Naming Our Children: Resolving the Last Name Dilemma.* Freedom, CA: The Crossing Press.

Stewart, George R. (1979). *American Given Names.* New York: Oxford University Press.

NAMING PRACTICES: SURNAMES

Most Americans follow the custom of patronymy when they assign family names, also known as last names or surnames. Patronymy ("father-naming") consists of two practices, maritonymy and patrilineal descent.

Maritonymy is the custom of a woman giving up her original family name at marriage and replacing it with her husband's. Patrilineal descent is the practice of giving a child born in wedlock its father's family name and thus tracing descent through the paternal line only. While these naming practices are more widespread than others, they are compelled only by tradition and perpetuated by the personal choices of married women and parents, not by law.

Family names as we know them today were not used in Europe until about the 11th century, and they didn't become common until the end of the 16th century. Women first started taking their husbands' names around the 13th century. But many isolated communities did not readily adopt patronymical surnames. They simply used first names or given names along with unfixed surnames, such as place names, patronymics (names derived from one's father's or other male ancestor's first name, such as Johnson, son of John, or Fitzgerald, son of Gerald), descriptive names, occupational names, or matronymics ("Sara, daughter of Rebecca").

All cultures exhibit a predominant systematic code governing the structure and derivation of names to which its members are expected to conform. Until recent times, idiosyncratic experimentation with naming structure or derivation was virtually unheard of.

While family naming codes tend to remain consistent across the generations within a given culture, these codes vary widely from culture to culture. The standard American patronymical codes of first name-middle name-father's surname for children and first name-middle name-husband's surname for married women are by no means universal.

Historical and contemporary cross-cultural examples of family naming systems other than patronymy abound. For example, while for centuries the communities around them were using patronymical last names, the Jews in the ghettos of central and Eastern Europe did not use fixed surnames. It wasn't until the late 18th and early 19th centuries that Jews had to choose or were given family names. Even when they did begin using last names, European Jews did not universally adopt the last name of their fathers. Very frequently children were given their mother's family name.

Norwegians also used patronymics at the time other European communities had converted to the last-name systems that resemble the one prevalent today. When Norwegians immigrated to the United States in the mid-19th century, they had to convert their patronymics and the names of their homeland family farms, which were also used as surnames, into patrilineal last names—hence, the large number of Hansens and Petersens. Relationship-to-father or -mother names are still in use in Iceland and the Shetland Islands.

Today, married Chinese women do not take husbands' family names and the present-day naming systems of Spain, Portugal, and other Latin countries provide males and females with both their fathers' and mothers' surnames for life.

Present-day American family naming practices are rooted in the English common law tradition that provided that people could call themselves whatever name they pleased and change their names at will as long as they didn't do so "for fraudulent purposes" or "interfere with the rights of others." Against this seemingly permissive legal backdrop, one reason patronymy has held sway over other potential, more sexually egalitarian naming systems is that only in recent history have women had independent legal control over property and the fate of their own children. Historically, patronymy, particularly its patrilineal component, which is based on the legitimacy of progeny, was a way of authenticating legal heirs.

Families continue to assign names patronymically by force of custom and because patronymy seems to be an efficient way of consolidating family ties, though a growing number of critics would say it does so at great expense. Patronymy collapses human bilineal origins into a unilineal naming system. While preserving the paternal line, it discards family names borne by females and thus suppresses the maternal line of descent.

Patronymy continues to be the dominant mode of family naming; however dissatisfaction with patronymy's limitations has given rise to widespread adoption of alternative ways of naming. Married women now keep their own family names in record numbers, which has in turn called into question the inevitability of passing only fathers' names on to children. Many parents are thus experimenting with giving children hyphenated surnames or a last name other than the child's father's.

✷ SHARON LEBELL

See also: Naming Practices: Given Names
See **Guide to Related Topics:** Baby Care

Resources

Hamilton, M.J. (1973). "Female Surnames and California Law." *Law Review: University of California, Davis 6*: 405-21.

Lebell, Sharon. (1988). *Naming Ourselves, Naming Our Children: Resolving the Last Name Dilemma*. Freedom, CA: The Crossing Press.

———. (1990, Jul 22). "Father Doesn't Always Know Best: Surname Systems Around the World." *San Francisco Chronicle*, p. 13.

Stannard, Una. (1973). *Married Women v. Husband's Names: The Case for Wives Who Keep Their Own Names*. San Francisco: Germainbooks.

———. (1977). *Mrs. Man*. San Francisco: Germainbooks.

NATURAL CHILDBIRTH. *See instead* READ METHOD: NATURAL CHILDBIRTH

NATURAL FAMILY PLANNING

Natural family planning is a form of birth control that relies on a woman's natural signs and symptoms of fertility. Used either to prevent or plan pregnancy, it involves observing and charting specific bodily signs in order to establish the time of ovulation. By estimating the times of fertility, one can avoid intercourse (or unprotected intercourse) to prevent pregnancy, or increase chances of pregnancy if the intention is to conceive.

The primary natural sign of fertility is a change in the body's basal temperature. Before ovulation, when the body is under the influence of the hormone estrogen, the waking temperature is low, usually around 97.5 to 98.5 degrees Fahrenheit. When ovulation takes place, a different hormone, progesterone, is released from the ovary, causing the basal temperature to rise to the range of 98 or 99 degrees Fahrenheit. When plotted on a graph-like chart, this temperature rise is quite apparent.

In addition, the change from estrogen to progesterone influence causes obvious changes in a woman's cervical mucus and in the cervix itself.

With rising estrogen, the cervical mucus, observed as a vaginal discharge, changes from scant, opaque, and sticky to profuse, clear, and slippery. At the height of estrogen production, this mucus often looks and feels like raw egg white and can be stretched in a shimmering thread. As soon as ovulation takes place and progesterone is released from the ovary, the mucus abruptly disappears or reverts to the scanty and opaque stage. Other signs of fertility include the internal position of the cervix, mid-cycle lower quadrant pain, breast tenderness, and changes in mood and libido.

The Natural Family Planning method of birth regulation incorporates very specific rules to determine when intercourse will be fertile or infertile. These rules must be studied carefully and followed meticulously in order for this method to be effective. As with any method of birth control, there is the risk of unintentional pregnancy, usually due to misuse of the method.

Some couples incorporate periodic abstinence into their relationship in order to prevent pregnancy during the naturally fertile days each month, and often report that it enhances their appreciation of intercourse. Others prefer to use barrier methods at this time. Certainly, women who are not in a stable, monogamous relationship need the health protection of condoms during all instances of intercourse.

Natural family planning takes more time and direct involvement than other methods of birth control, but it can be an interesting and educational personal study that many women find worth the effort. ✷ MARGARET NOFZIGER

See **Guide to Related Topics:** Contraception

Resources

Frances, J.T. (1981). "Biology of the Fertile Period." *International Journal of Fertility 26*: 143-52.

Nofziger, Margaret. (1988). *Signs of Fertility: The Personal Science of Natural Birth Control.* Nashville, TN: MND Publishing Co.

World Health Organization. (1967). "Biology of Fertility Control by Periodic Abstinence." Technical Report Series no. 360. Geneva: World Health Organization.

THE NETHERLANDS

While some may think of the Dutch as famous for their fine cheese or their magnificent tulip bulbs and gardens, among those concerned with childbearing issues, the greatest Dutch contribution is its midwifery. The Dutch people have, unique in the Western world, maintained a system of midwifery care with a high proportion of births at home; this home-based, midwifery-provided care has been associated with infant and maternal health that is among the very best in the world.

It is of course difficult to pinpoint any one factor that explains the unique Dutch situation. But one of the very important aspects has been the independent legal status of midwives. In marked contrast to the United States, in which midwives are, in most states, forced into a position of operating under the supervision of an obstetrician, Dutch midwives are independent professionals who call upon obstetrician specialists for referral and consultation as needed. With three years of professional training in a school of midwifery—distinct from nursing training—the midwives are fully qualified to provide independent care during normal pregnancy and childbirth. They may attend births in or out of hospitals.

Within the Netherlands, as elsewhere in the world, midwife-attended births show equal or better health results for the newborn, and achieve these results with far less intervention. For example, in a study of 1,034 infants born to low-risk women in the Nihmegen area, the neurological condition of the newborns was compared. Sixty-two percent of the women were attended by a midwife, 12 percent by a general practitioner, and 26 percent by an obstetrician. There were no differences in the neurological conditions of the infants in the different groups, but there were important differences in the interventions used in their births—and thus in the conditions of their mothers. Obstetric intervention has negative consequences, both physically and psychologically, for birthing women. In this study, not at all atypical, obstetricians used drugs (oxytocin) to stimulate and hasten the labor in 21.3 percent of the cases, compared with 4.5 percent of the cases attended by midwives. The general practitioners fell between the two, at 14.8 percent. Similarly, there were instrumental and operative deliveries for 16.0 percent of the obstetrician-attended births and 5.9 percent of the midwife-attended births, with the general practitioners again, at 8.6 percent, falling between the two (Treffers et al., 1990).

It should be noted that Dutch obstetricians have far lower rates of intervention than do American obstetricians. In the U.S. the cesarean section rate alone is now considerably higher than the combined rate of instrumental and operative deliveries reported by Dutch obstetricians. One possible explanation is that the very presence of the midwives and the high proportion of births at home have a balancing effect on obstetrical practice: women in Holland expect birth to be normal, and obstetricians in Holland are continually shown that birth is a normal, healthy process that can come to a healthy completion without intervention. Consider in contrast the American obstetrician, who may never in all of his or her years of training have even heard of anyone having a home birth.

Home birth, in Holland as elsewhere, is not simply a location, but includes a set of relationships as well. As the highly influential Dutch obstetrician G. Kloosterman has said:

> The advantages of home confinements are that in her own home the expectant mother is not considered a patient, but a woman, fulfilling a highly natural and personal task. She is the real centre around which everything (and everybody) revolves. The midwife or doctor and the maternity aide nurse are all her guests, there to assist her. This setting reinforces her self-respect and self-confidence. The modern hospital very often functions in an opposite way. The woman is the guest of the doctors and nurses in their home. She becomes a patient, dependent on people who like to mother her. The security of the hospital, so important in situations where interference is necessary, is of no use for the women who do not need any interference. The atmosphere in the hospital, on the other hand, weakens her self-confidence. This explains why in so many hospitals (and in so many countries with total hospitalization) the percentage of artificial deliveries is rising to such an extent that it is inconceivable that it occurs for good medical reasons. (1978)

With official Dutch policy acknowledging this relationship, obstetrical care is more readily tied to an ongoing understanding of birth as a nonmedical event, thus benefitting not only the approximately 40 percent of Dutch women who birth at home but the remaining 60 percent who birth in hospitals.

The Dutch approach to maternity care goes beyond the issue of home birth itself. Even when the actual birth takes place in the hospital, there is a vast difference between the Dutch and the American experience. The Dutch government actively values birth and the family: women are, as they are in most of the world, given long periods of paid maternity leave both before (6 weeks) and after (10 weeks) the birth. In the first, often hectic, days after a birth, the government supplies a maternity aide or "mothercraft nurse" to work in the home for eight days following birth. (Ed. note: See "Doula.") The maternity aide can provide practical services—answering the phone, getting young children off to school in the morning, preparing meals—that permit the mother and father to sleep, rest, and take care of the baby. The maternity aide also provides educational services in the optimal setting: the home in which the infant is being raised. It is one thing to learn to bathe a plastic doll in a special parent-education class and another thing to have a knowledgeable person with you as you bathe your own baby in your own home for the first few times. Similarly, breastfeeding assistance in the home and family setting is far more useful than a class or counseling session in a hospital.

Midwifery and home birth advocates in the United States and throughout the world look to the Netherlands as a source of knowledge, wisdom, and inspiration.

✱ BARBARA KATZ ROTHMAN, Ph.D.

See **Guide to Related Topics:** Cross-Cultural Perspectives

Resources

Kloosterman, G. (1978). "The Dutch System of Home Birth." In S. Kitzinger and M. Davis (Eds.) *The Place of Birth*. Oxford: Oxford University Press.

Lievaart, M. & De Jong, L. (1982). "Neonatal Morbidity in Deliveries Conducted by Midwives and Gynecologists: A Study of the System of Obstetric Care Prevailing in the Netherlands." *American Journal of Obstetrics and Gynecology 144*: 376-86.

Treffers, Pieter E. et al. (1990, Nov 7). "Home Births and Minimal Medical Interventions." *JAMA 264* (17): 2203-08.

van Arkel, W., Amen, A.J., & Bell, N. (1980, Summer). "The Politics of Home Delivery in the Netherlands." *Birth and the Family Journal 7* (2): 101-12.

World Health Organization. (1985). *Having a Baby in Europe*. Copenhagen, Denmark: World Health Organization.

NEURAL TUBE DEFECT. *See instead* CENTRAL CLOSURE DEFECTS

NEWBORN INTELLIGENCE

As soon as babies open their eyes they begin exploring the world around them, reaching out with the same hands and fingers that have been busy probing the uterine environment and the same senses of taste and hearing that they had been using for months before birth. They are "all eyes" and full of curiosity, sometimes arriving on the scene with robust signals of panic, pain, or anger, or, under more fortunate conditions, with feelings of surprise or joy written all over their faces.

Proving they are ready for social interaction, babies only minutes old can instantly imitate adult tongue and mouth gestures, and more important, can imitate adult expressions of happiness, sadness, and surprise—an instant dialogue suggesting they are already sensitive to how other people feel. Additional evidence for this quality of empathy can be seen in their discriminating reaction to crying sounds. Infants usually join the chorus of other crying infants their *own* age but are not moved by white noise, computer-simulated cries, a crying baby chimpanzee, or even a crying five-month-old baby. Significantly, when recordings of their *own* cries are heard, their heart rates go up and they stop to listen—an indication that they recognize themselves.

Newborns are extremely perceptive and communicative. They are able to both receive and send information. After a few days of breastfeeding experience they can identify their mother's distinctive underarm odor and distinguish between her used breast pad and a pad from another mother. They are expert face watchers and react quickly to signs of depression or grief, to the mother wearing a mask, or to the mother becoming strangely silent. In these ominous situations, babies struggle to set things right with distracting movements of face and body and by vocalizing.

Babies have a special gift for language, listening with amazing precision and sometimes moving their bodies in rhythm with speech. They can pick out their mother's voice reading a story, provided the reading is normal; if mothers read sentences in reverse, they no longer recognize which one is their mother, indicating that they have learned certain patterns of speech. Such lessons begin in the womb, a fact demonstrated by voice spectrographs. Sound prints of the first cry of a very premature baby can already be matched with voice characteristics of its mother. Thus, babies have a sharp ear for language. They recognize and seem to prefer stories that were read repeatedly to them *in utero.* Hearing tests show that babies hear the smallest sounds of speech better than adults do; this superiority lasts for the whole first year of life.

When only a few days old, French babies prefer to look at faces speaking French and Russian babies prefer to watch faces speaking Russian. One wonders how they can recognize and favor their mother tongue after only a few days outside the womb. They also seem to know how faces and voices should fit together—a skill requiring lip reading. For example, Scottish babies know which of two faces speaking Japanese is in synch with the sound they are hearing. At one month of age babies expect their mother's face and voice to match. They know something is wrong and look away if another voice comes from the mother's face or if the mother's voice is shown with another woman's face.

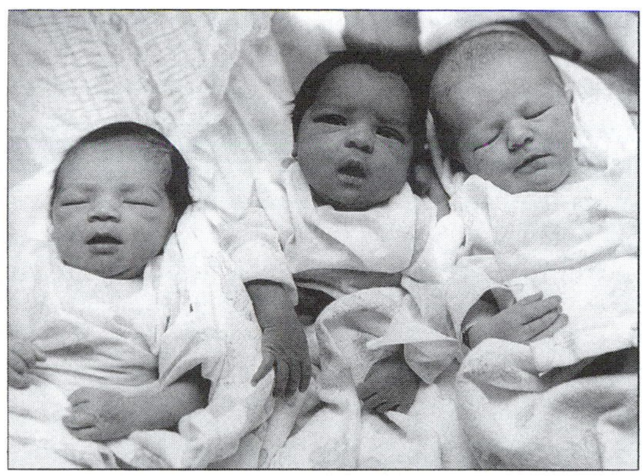

Newborns are perceptive and communicative. Photo courtesy of Harriette Hartigan/Artemis.

Newborns learn, perhaps as well as anyone can. In experiments before and after birth, babies have demonstrated classical conditioning, reward conditioning, imitation, and habituation—all of the formal ways that learning is tested. Even while in the womb babies have learned to recognize musical tunes like "Brahms's Lullabye," "Mary Had a Little Lamb," soap opera theme music, the cello line of a concerto, or phrases like "Breathe in, breathe out," apparently learned during childbirth preparation classes (Verny and Kelly, 1981).

Judging from the way infants plunge into psychology experiments, they enjoy learning and thrive on stimulation. If an experiment is too simple or dull, the babies will quit working; if new variables are introduced, they will show new interest and go on working long after the rewards have run out, apparently for the sheer pleasure of it. When a baby finally figures out how something works, he or she may break into a smile—a sure sign of cognitive satisfaction. Such actions have led some psychologists to assert that babies can think, formulate hypotheses, and use rational faculties to detect conjunctions between events and fit them into a predictive framework (Bower, 1989).

Babies dream. Brain wave studies of sleeping infants reveal the telltale rapid eye movements (REM) associated with dreaming. Tests show that newborns dream about half the time they are asleep, while premature babies of 30 weeks' gestation dream virtually *all* the time they are asleep. During dreams, muscles are activated, body and limbs quiver, and the face displays a range of adultlike emotions from pleasure to pain. Dreaming is a personal and creative process originating within the self and is a way of dealing with experience so far. Dreams can be pleasant or unpleasant. The very first smiles are usually seen in dreams, dreams we assume must be pleasant.

With the benefit of advanced sonography trained on eyes *in utero*, scientists have discovered that REMs begin about 21 weeks from conception. This means that dreaming is a common mental activity long before birth.

Perhaps the centerpiece of newborn cognition is memory, a faculty intrinsically involved in all learning, perception, communication, and dreaming. Thus, all evidence for these things is automatically evidence for memory. A dramatic example of excellent newborn memory is memory of birth itself. These memories, while controversial for almost a century, are now confirmed by children two or three years old who report their birth memories as soon as they can talk (Chamberlain, 1990). In addition, adults have recovered cogent memories of birth in a variety of psychotherapies using hypnosis or some other gateway to altered states of consciousness. These memories of birth reveal an intelligent, impressionable mind busily learning the mistakes of parents, nurses, and doctors. To avoid giving babies a bad start, adults will have to learn to be at least as intelligent as the babies themselves. ✱ DAVID B. CHAMBERLAIN, Ph.D.

See also: Lullabies and Cradle Songs; Newborn Senses

See **Guide to Related Topics:** Baby Care

Resources

Bower, Thomas G.R. (1989). *The Rational Infant: Learning in Infancy*. New York: W.H. Freeman.

Chamberlain, David B. (1990). *Babies Remember Birth*. New York: Ballantine Books.

Klaus, Marshall & Klaus, Phyllis. (1985). *The Amazing Newborn*. Reading, MA: Addison-Wesley.

Verny, Thomas & Kelly, John. (1981). *The Secret Life of the Unborn Child*. New York: Summit Books.

NEWBORN INTENSIVE CARE

Childbirth today is expected to result in a healthy, viable infant. The dramatic decline in infant mortality in recent generations gives rise to such optimism. Nevertheless, some infants are born critically ill, and it is these newborns who form the patient population for neonatal intensive care units (NICUs). Overwhelmingly, these patients are premature infants; in addition, a much smaller number suffer from either a specific defect, a birth trauma, or, more recently, from substance abuse or AIDS.

Premature birth is the greatest threat to infant life today and is the primary cause of death for infants in the first month of life. Risks associated with prematurity include immaturity of the lungs (respiratory distress syndrome or hyaline membrane disease), a fetal opening in the heart (patent ductus arteriosis), and bleeding in the brain (intraventricular hemorrhage). Newborns weighing less than 2,500 grams at birth are typically considered premature; those weighing 1,500 grams or less are considered to be of very low birth weight.

Numerous medical studies show improved survival rates for very premature newborns treated in NICUs, and practitioners today generally believe in aggressive care even for very low birth-weight infants. However, it is important to emphasize that the more premature the infant, the higher the risks of mortality (dying) and morbidity (illness). Furthermore, the lower the birth weight, the higher the chance of a surviving infant having permanent, serious disability. Thus, although a high percent of NICU patients are discharged in essentially normal condition, a certain percent—especially among those of lowest birth weight—are kept alive with serious permanent disability. It is these results that lead researchers to refer to the "mixed blessing" of such care.

Since the results of NICU treatment may be a "mixed blessing" for the infant, the family, and society in general, it is important to ask who makes the decisions about how aggressively to treat critically ill newborns. At present, these decisions are made primarily by physicians, with only peripheral input from families. The decisions

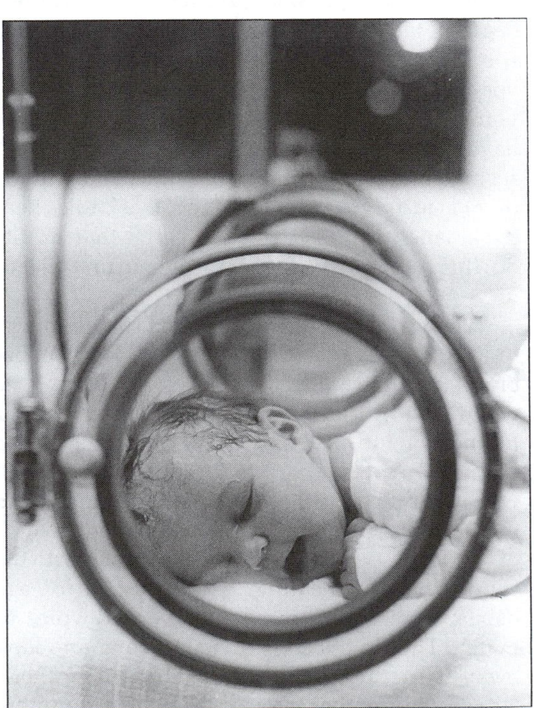

Newborn in incubator. Photo courtesy of Harriette Hartigan/Artemis.

about aggressiveness of care are made mostly within the NICU, and is shaped by the social organization of the work setting. Families are distanced from the NICU through a variety of mechanisms. Thus, largely professional and organizational concerns direct the decision making, despite the fact that ultimately the family will be responsible for the infant if it survives. In many hospitals, the professional and organizational concerns are such that the decision is almost always to intervene as aggressively as possible, no matter how dismal the prognosis; exceptions are exceedingly rare and occur in only exceptionally extreme circumstances (for example, multiple organ system failure combined with massive brain damage).

There is a voluminous literature on the ethical dilemmas of providing intensive care for infants on the edge of viability. While a number of important issues are raised in this literature, there are several crucial issues that do not receive adequate attention. One is the issue of the general condition of prematurity—the ethical literature tends to focus instead on cases of specific isolable defects. A second is the issue of overtreatment. Almost all of the ethical and public debate centers on the danger of undertreatment; very little attention is given to the equally problematic issue of overtreatment, indeed, even latent experimentation, performed on critically ill newborns. Third, little attention is given to the ethics of ignoring prevention.

Newborn intensive care has developed, like much of American medicine, as a curative approach to a largely preventable problem. There undoubtedly always will be some cases of prematurity. However, the rate of prematurity correlates, on a worldwide basis, with poverty. Impoverished pregnant women are far more likely than affluent women to have a premature, low birth-weight infant. It is utopian to suggest that poverty will be eliminated in the foreseeable future. However, specific detrimental conditions associated with poverty and poor birth outcomes—conditions such as hunger and malnutrition—have been effectively dealt with in the past and can be dealt with again; successful programs, curtailed or dismantled in recent years, could be reinstituted.

Newborn intensive care will continue to be a topic for debate, both because of the ethical dilemmas it raises and its high cost. The crucial issue, however, is not whether newborn intensive care should exist. Rather, the critical questions include these: Should newborn intensive care be allowed to deflect attention from prevention? Should its technology continue to be applied in an indiscriminate way? and, Who should be making the decisions since no one, including physicians, is a disinterested party? Additional issues in the 1990s are these: What is the proper approach to decision making if more stringent economic conditions prevail? Newborn intensive care may be a mixed blessing, but in the United States, it has been available to infants of all social classes through third-party payment; there is evidence that rationing of NICU services may occur as hospitals find uninsured and Medicaid patients a financial burden. What is the proper treatment approach to take with the increasing numbers of AIDS babies and substance-abuse babies that probably will be admitted to NICUs? Once again, it is important to note that although these conditions are preventable, the focus so far remains curative.

In conclusion, although many individual families with a premature infant feel that they have benefitted enormously from NICU services, some families among those with poor results are critical of the enterprise. One such mother, whose surviving, damaged child continues to suffer, announced bitterly on nationwide television that if she were faced again with the situation of premature labor that could not be controlled, she would go to the woods rather than the hospital to have the child, thus evading NICU intervention. Overall in the United States, NICUs have produced mixed results, have helped deflect attention from prevention, and have flourished within a broader social context that is insensitive to maternal-child health. It has proved easier to get resources to develop expensive NICUs than to get resources to provide basic preventive and support programs for women and their children.

✷ LYNDA LYTLE HOLMSTROM, Ph.D., and
JEANNE HARLEY GUILLEMIN, Ph.D.

See also: Ethics Committees; Premature Birth: Prevention; Prematurity and Low Birth Weight: An Alternative Management

See **Guide to Related Topics:** Special Needs Infants

Resources

Anspach, Renee R. (1987, Sept). "Prognostic Conflict in Life-and-Death Decisions: The Organization as an Ecology of Knowledge." *Journal of Health and Social Behavior 28*: 215-31.

Bogdan, Robert, Brown, Mary Alice, & Foster, Susan Bannerman. (1982). "Be Honest but Not Cruel: Staff/Parent Communication on a Neonatal Unit." *Human Organization 64*: 10-16.

Brown, J. Larry. (1989). "When Violence Has a Benevolent Face: The Paradox of Hunger in the World's Wealthiest Democracy." *International Journal of Health Services 19*: 257-77.

Guillemin, Jeanne Harley & Holmstrom, Lynda Lytle. (1986). *Mixed Blessings: Intensive Care for Newborns.* New York: Oxford.

Levin, Betty Wolder. (1985). "Consensus and Controversy in the Treatment of Catastrophically Ill Newborns." In Thomas H. Murray and Arthur L. Caplan (Eds.) *Which Baby Shall Live?* Clifton, NJ: Human Press, pp. 169-205.

Sosnowitz, Barbara G. (1984). "Managing Parents on Neonatal Intensive Care Units." *Social Problems 31*: 390-402.

Stinson, Robert & Stinson, Peggy. (1979). "On the Death of a Baby." *The Atlantic 244*: 64-72.

Wagner, Marsden G. (1986, Winter). "Infant Mortality in Europe: Implications for the United States." (Statement to the National Commission to Prevent Infant Mortality). *Journal of Public Health Policy 9*: 473-84.

NEWBORN PAIN

So many babies cry at birth that their signals of alarm are considered normal or even necessary. A strong cry is worth 2 points on the 10-point Apgar Scale hospitals use to evaluate a newborn's condition. [Ed. note: See Apgar] Nevertheless, perfectly healthy babies are sometimes born without any sign of pain, wearing unforgettable expressions of intense curiosity and interest on their faces. Some have been known to smile, which suggests that their smiles communicate genuine comfort and their cries genuine pain.

Health professionals commonly believe that pain is not serious for preemies or newborns because their brains and nervous systems are immature and incapable of attaching any meaning to pain or of registering it in memory. Largely because of this belief, pain is still a major feature of neonatal intensive care nurseries, neonatal surgery, standard hospital deliveries, and, for males, circumcision.

Current knowledge of the physiology of pain reaction indicates very early development going back to eight weeks after conception when the fetus will turn its face away from an irritating stimulus. Sensory receptors spread to the palms, soles, and parts of the arms and legs by 15 weeks and to all skin and mucous surfaces by the 20th week *in utero.* Corresponding development of brain connections provides every newborn baby with all the anatomical and functional components required for the perception of pain (Anand and Hickey, 1987). Cries of pain and protest have been heard as early as 21 weeks from conception.

After birth, pain can be measured by body movement, changes in heart rate, the presence of certain hormones in the blood stream, telltale facial expressions, and vocal sounds.

Newborn cries can convey a range of suffering, including physical pain, anger, hunger, and fear, which attentive mothers learn quickly. Unusual cries can announce illness, malnutrition, malformations, and hearing deficiencies. Very premature babies probably endure the most pain, due to the need for multiple punctures and catheter insertions, plus loud sounds and incessant lighting. Full-term babies run a shorter gauntlet of pain from trauma to the head, cold rooms, wiping of sensitive skin, injections to take blood and give vitamins, medication that stings the eyes, and being stretched out to measure.

Until recently, surgery on neonates was done without anesthesia in the belief that infants would not truly feel the pain or that the anesthetic itself might do more harm than the pain. Both assumptions are now considered false. Circumcision is still common, affecting over 40 percent of newborns in the U.S. Exhaustive measurements leave no doubt about the pain suffered. Although research has repeatedly shown that analgesics for circumcision are safe and effective, their use is still rare.

French obstetrician Frederick Leboyer was one of the first of his profession to accept the reality of newborn pain and to create a birthing process to avoid it. In his form of "gentle birth," the cutting of the cord is delayed, babies lie on their mothers undisturbed, light and sound are kept low, and, in time, the babies are offered a warm bath (Leboyer, 1976). ✱ DAVID B. CHAMBERLAIN, Ph.D.

See also: Circumcision Surgery; Leboyer Method; Newborn Senses

See **Guide to Related Topics:** Baby Care

Resources

Anand, K.J.S. & Hickey, P.R. (1987). "Pain and Its Effects in the Human Neonate and Fetus." *New England Journal of Medicine 317* (21): 1321-29.

Chamberlain, D.B. (1990). *Babies Remember Birth.* New York: Ballantine Books.

Gottfried, A.W. & Gaiter, J.L. (Eds.) (1985). *Infant Stress under Intensive Care.* Baltimore: University Park Press.

Leboyer, F. (1976). *Birth Without Violence.* New York: Alfred A. Knopf.

Lester, B.M. & Boukydis, C.R. (Eds.) (1985). *Infant Crying.* New York: Plenum.

Porter, F., Miller, R.H., & Marshall, R.E. (1986). "Neonatal Pain Cries: Effect of Circumcision." *Child Development 57*: 790-802.

NEWBORN SCREENING

Routine screening of newborns for treatable, inherited, metabolic disorders began in the 1960s. These disorders are caused by inherited biochemical defects, generally involving a deficiency of an intracellular enzyme that results in either an accumulation of certain metabolites or deficiency of the enzyme's product (Smith, 1988). Although several factors led to the development of newborn screening, the most significant was the introduction of the Guthrie bacterial inhibition assay for detecting phenylketonuria (PKU). This assay made newborn screening for PKU both feasible and highly cost-effective and led the way for mass newborn screening programs for a variety of metabolic disorders (Scriver et al., 1989). The first mandatory newborn screening program began in Massachusetts in 1963. Newborn screening tests now have been reported for more than 20 disorders (Therrell, 1988).

Legal guidelines governing newborn screening vary from state to state in terms of whether screening is mandatory or voluntary, as well as the types of disorders addressed (Andrews, 1985). Statutes governing newborn screening exist in 48 states and Washington, DC; only Delaware and Vermont have no statute. In the majority of states, newborn screening is mandatory, with provisions for refusal in all but five states (Arkansas, Iowa, Michigan, Montana, and West Virginia). Screening is voluntary in four states (Delaware, Maryland, North Carolina, and Oklahoma) and the District of Columbia (Andrews, 1985). Despite provisions in the majority of states to allow objection to screening on some grounds, few states require informed parental consent. Only three states (Maryland, Wisconsin, and Wyoming) and the District of Columbia require that parents and guardians be fully informed and be given the right to object.

Although all states that conduct newborn screening do screen for PKU, the number of additional conditions tested for varies by state (see Figure 1). The procedure for newborn screening is essentially the same regardless of the number of conditions included in the initial neonatal screen. Prior to the newborn's discharge from the hospital, a blood sample is obtained via a heel puncture and applied directly to filter paper. This sample does not require special handling or preservation and can be mailed in an envelope to the laboratory. If the original screen is positive, additional diagnostic studies are pursued (Smith, 1988). Typically, tests screen for seven diseases: Phenylketonuria (PKU); Congenital Hypothyroidism (CH); Galactosemia; Maple Syrup Urine Disease (MSUD); Homocystinuria; Biotinidase Deficiency; and Sickle Cell Disease.

Figure 1. National Screening Status Report

The National Screening Status Report lists the status of newborn screening in the United States. All infants in a state must be screened in order for a dot to be added.

	Phenylketonuria	Congenital Hypothyroidism	Galactosemia	Maple Syrup Urine Disease	Homocystinuria	Biotinidase	Sickle Cell Disease	Other
Alabama	•	•					•	
Alaska	•	•	•	•	•	•		2
Arizona	•	•	•	•	•		•	3
Arkansas	•	•						
California	•	•	•				a	
Colorado	•	•	•	•	•		•	3
Connecticut	•	•	•				a	
Delaware	•	•	•	•	•	•	•	
D.C.	•	•	•	•	•		•	
Florida	•	•	•					
Georgia	•	•	•	•	•		a	
Hawaii	•	•						
Idaho	•	•	•	•	•	•		
Illinois	•	•	•			•		2
Indiana	•	•	•	•	•		•	
Iowa	•	•	•	•			•	
Kansas	•	•						
Kentucky	•	•	•					
Louisiana	•	•					a	
Maine	•	•	•	•	•			
Maryland	•	•	•	•	•	•		
Massachusetts	•	•	•	•	•			1
Michigan	•	•	•	•		•	•	
Minnesota	•	•	•					
Mississippi	•	•						
Missouri	•	•	•				a	
Montana	•	•						
Nebraska	•	•						
Nevada	•	•	•	•	•	•		
New Hampshire	•	•	•	•	•			
New Jersey	•	•	•					
New Mexico	•	•	•	•	•		•	
New York	•	•	•	•	•		•	
North Carolina	•	•						
North Dakota	•	•						
Ohio	•	•	•		•			
Oklahoma	•	•						
Oregon	•	•	•	•	•	•		
Pennsylvania	•	•						
Rhode Island	•	•	•	•	•			
South Carolina	•	•					•	
South Dakota	•	•						
Tennessee	•	•					a	
Texas	•	•	•				•	
Utah	•	•	•					
Vermont	•	•	•					
Virginia	•	•	•	•	•	•	a	
Washington	•	•						2
West Virginia	•	•	•					
Wisconsin	•	•	•	•	•			3
Wyoming	•	•	•	•	•		•	3

a – Selected population.

1 – Toxoplasmosis
2 – Congenital adrenal hyperplasia
3 – Cystic fibrosis

Phenylketonuria (PKU). Phenylketonuria (PKU) is caused by an alteration or absence of the liver enzyme phenylalanine hydroxylase, which is involved in the conversion of the amino acid phenylalanine to tyrosine. Patients with classical PKU have elevated phenylalanine levels (>20 mg/daily) with decreased serum tyrosine levels. Untreated PKU results in profound mental retardation, seizures, psychotic behavior, and eczema. PKU occurs in approximately one in 12,000 live births. Infants diagnosed with PKU are treated by dietary restrictions of phenylalanine. The diet generally consists of an artificial substance, Lofenalac™ (Mead-Johnson), and natural food supplements that are low in protein. Initiating this diet in the first few weeks of life prevents the severe mental retardation previously seen in affected children. Careful supervision and ongoing management/follow-up are integral to effective therapy.

Congenital Hypothyroidism (CH). Congenital Hypothyroidism (CH) occurs in one in 5,000 births, and therefore is one of the most common preventable causes of mental retardation. Less than 5 percent of babies with CH show symptoms of the disease at the time of diagnosis. Symptoms include poor feeding, hypoactivity, constipation, dry skin, and a hoarse cry. Treatment consists of oral doses of thyroid hormone, which should be initiated by one month of age in order to prevent the onset of symptoms and mental retardation.

Galactosemia. Galactosemia is a metabolic abnormality of carbohydrate metabolism involving the enzymatic conversion of galactose to glucose esters. In the classic form, deficiency of galactose-1-phosphate uridyltransferase results in the accumulation of galactose-1-phosphate and galactose in blood. Galactose is one of the main building blocks of the disaccharide lactose, or milk sugar. Classic galactosemia causes failure to thrive, vomiting, jaundice, and an enlarged liver. If untreated, liver disease, cataracts, and mental retardation are the result. Early treatment by a diet free of galactose and lactose has been effective in preventing symptoms.

Maple Syrup Urine Disease (MSUD). Maple Syrup Urine Disease (MSUD) involves abnormal metabolism of leucine, isoleucine, and valine, three branched-chain amino acids that are found in increased levels in blood. Characteristics of the disorder are feeding difficulties, vomiting, lethargy, neurologic manifestations, and death by 10 to 14 days of age. A characteristic odor of maple syrup is often noticed in the urine of affected newborns. Dietary maintenance is difficult in MSUD, and even with treatment, children may develop neurological impairment.

Homocystinuria. Homocystinuria is a disorder of amino acid metabolism caused by a deficiency of the liver enzyme cystathionine synthetase. Its deficiency results in the accumulation of homocysteine and methionine in blood and urine. Estimates of incidence are from one in 88,000 to one in 310,000 live births. If untreated it is characterized by dislocation of ocular lenses, osteoporosis, tall-long limbed habitus, and thromboembolism. Mild to moderate retardation is found in approximately 50 percent of affected individuals. Treatment consists of dietary restrictions of protein intake.

Biotinidase Deficiency. Biotinidase Deficiency occurs in approximately one in 70,000 newborns. It is a disorder of biotin recycling that leads to multiple carboxylase deficiency. Signs and symptoms include convulsions, dermatitis, alopecia, hearing loss, mental retardation, and organic acidemia that can result in coma. Affected newborns are treated with oral doses of biotin (approximately 10 mg/daily).

Sickle Cell Disease (SS, SC and Sβ). Sickle Cell Disease is caused by synthesis of abnormal β-chains of hemoglobin. The gene for sickle cell anemia is present more often in individuals of black or Mediterranean ancestry, giving an incidence of sickle cell disease of one in 400 blacks and one in 600 total live births. Affected individuals may have overwhelming infections, chronic hemolytic anemia, pneumonia, enlarged liver and spleen, and bone marrow aplasia. The mortality rate is estimated at 13 to 14 percent under two years of age and 50 percent by age 20. Diagnosis during the newborn period is necessary to ensure appropriate medical management of patients (American Academy of Pediatrics, 1989).

Findings. Screening tests are usually repeated two weeks after birth to be certain no affected newborns are missed by the initial test (Gause, 1989). Findings are sent to the parents and the baby's health care provider. All seven diseases commonly screened for are inherited as autosomal recessive disorders, i.e., both parents have the same abnormal gene and pass it on to their baby. Once a child is diagnosed with one of these disorders, the parents have a 25 percent chance that subsequent children will also be affected. Should the parents wish, prenatal diagnosis by CVS or amniocentesis is possible for future pregnancies. Genetic counseling is recommended when a diagnosis is made. As DNA diagnosis techniques improve, they will be applied to screen for genetic diseases in newborns. ✱ ELIZABETH BALKITE, M.S.

See also: Genetics
See **Guide to Related Topics:** Prenatal Diagnosis and Screening

Resources

American Academy of Pediatrics, Committee on Genetics. (1989). "Newborn Screening Fact Sheets." *Pediatrics 83* (3): 449-64.

Andrews, L.B. (Ed.) (1985). *State Laws and Regulations Governing Newborn Screening.* Chicago: American Bar Foundation, National Center for Education in Maternal and Child Health.

Gause, Ralph W. (1989). "Newborn Screening Tests." March of Dimes Public Health Education Information Sheet.

Scriver, Charles R. et al. (1989). *The Metabolic Basis of Inherited Diseases.* New York: McGraw Hill.

Smith, Ann C.M. (1988). "Screening for Genetic Disease." *Genetic Applications: A Health Perspective.* Lawrence, KS: Learner Managed Designs.

Therrell, Brad. (1988). "National Screening Status Report." *Infant Screening 11* (1): 9.

NEWBORN SENSES

Can babies see, hear, taste, smell, and feel? The answers to these age-old questions have come only in the last two decades as a result of unprecedented scientific interest in babies. With the aid of new technology like the scanning electron microscope and intrauterine photography, ultrasound imaging and computer-assisted measurement of brain and body processes, we have learned much about life from conception to birth when the senses are developing. In addition, we have been able to watch the last three or four months of gestation in babies born extremely early and kept alive in high-tech nurseries. This growth period used to be completely hidden from view.

Skin sensitivity begins at about eight weeks after conception in the area of the face. From there sensitivity spreads first to the genitals and palms by 11 weeks, and finally to all skin and mucous areas by 20 weeks *in utero.* The sense of balance, needed to cope with the invisible forces of gravity and motion, also develops early. The necessary structures for this are in the fluid-filled semicircular canals of the ears, ready to use only 12 weeks after conception in a surprisingly active program of graceful exercises that can be seen under ultrasound. By the fifth month *in utero,* this system of equilibrium is adultlike.

The ability to taste things depends on a network of taste buds and nerve connections to the brain that is in place and working about 15 weeks after conception. What is available for tasting at that time is the fluid of the womb itself, containing a variety of sweet, salty, and bitter tastes. Radioactive tracers show the fetus swallowing 15 to 40 ml of this amniotic fluid per hour in the third trimester, from which some 40 calories of nourishment are derived each day.

If a few drops of bitter substance are injected into the womb, swallowing will come to a halt; swallowing may double if the drops are sweet. Taste buds are smart. The latest discoveries indicate that they function like microprocessors, integrating information from dozens of taste cells before sending off a coded message to the brain. By the time of birth, babies are as well equipped to taste as they will ever be. Tests show that they react to salt, sweet, sour, and bitter about the way adults do and have the same expressive facial reactions.

Hearing, which is vitally necessary for developing personal relationships and entering into the life stream of communication, is another early development dependent on structures in the ears and their connections to the brain. These are essentially in place halfway through pregnancy (20 weeks). In the womb, where sound is transmitted by both air and bone conduction, the most entertaining source of sound is the mother, who is broadcasting body and voice sounds around the clock. Elaborate sound spectrographs reveal that babies in the womb are taking language lessons, literally learning the speech characteristics of their mothers. Fathers can also be heard if they get close, speak slowly and deliberately, and raise their voices about an octave.

Experiments indicate that babies are startled and disturbed by loud sounds and prefer music that is quiet and harmonious. Normal newborns hear about as well as adults and in some ways better. In the whole first year of life, tests show, infants have hearing superior to adults for phonemes, the smallest units of speech. Brain wave measurements tell us that babies are listening even while asleep. Awake, they listen with amazing precision to adult speech, falling into rhythm with dancelike movements and showing a preference for sounds, tunes, and stories they heard in the womb. They discriminate between various crying sounds, reacting most to cries of babies their own age.

Newborns can use the sense of smell about as well as anyone. The place where odors register is a small area the size of a postage stamp at the roof of each nostril. Here, mucous-covered tissue contains a large number of receptor cells fringed with fine hairs pointing into the passageway through the nostrils. Another nerve monitors air more directly, functioning as a kind of instant smoke alarm. With this equipment babies will eventually learn hundreds of odors.

At birth, without any experience, babies already have a set of odor preferences quite similar to adults and show the same facial reactions to concentrated fish odors or rotten eggs (obviously unpleasant) and to banana, vanilla, chocolate, and strawberry (enjoyable). In a few days' time newborns can identify used from unused breast pads, and in a few more days, they can tell their own mother's breast pad from another mother's pad. Likewise, given a few days of breastfeeding, newborns can tell their own mother from other mothers by means of her distinctive underarm odor.

Of all the senses, vision is probably the most complex and important. Not long ago it was said that newborns were virtually blind; this was far from the truth. Being able to see involves the development and coordination of many parts: the eye itself, the muscles that move and adjust the eye, the specialized photoreceptors that are sensitive to light and color, the ocular nerve, and various relay stations to the brain. All are well advanced at birth, and babies are ready to use their eyes to acquire information with the first look. It will take two or three months before acuity and accommodation are perfect, but baby eyes are ready for all normal requirements. After all, they need to see their parents not read microfilm or freeway signs. The eye will continue to grow during the first two years, doubling the size of the retina and making all visual activity more efficient.

Newborns squint to protect their eyes from bright lights, but when the environment is friendly they are "all eyes," constantly scanning and searching for things to see, especially faces. They study their parents' faces with keen perception and can instantly mimic expressions of happiness, sadness, or surprise. When fully awake and alert, they will visually pursue a slowly moving target, showing depth perception and the awkward beginnings of eye-hand coordination. Given a choice of targets, newborns show their appetite for variety, complexity, color, and true-to-life angles and people. In their reaching out, they demonstrate intelligent coordination of all the senses, and perhaps even more important, reveal inner mental processes of interest and purpose.

✱ DAVID B. CHAMBERLAIN, Ph.D.

See also: Lullabies and Cradle Songs; Newborn Intelligence; Newborn Pain

See **Guide to Related Topics:** Baby Care

Resources

Bower, T.G.R. (1977). *A Primer of Infant Development.* San Francisco: W.H. Freeman.

Chamberlain, D.B. (1990). *Babies Remember Birth.* New York: Ballantine Books.

Klaus, M. & Klaus, P. (1985). *The Amazing Newborn.* Reading, MA: Addison-Wesley.

Osofsky, J. (Ed.) (1987). *Handbook of Infant Development.* New York: Wiley-Interscience.

NIPPLES, ARTIFICIAL

The artificial nipple, sometimes called a teat, is used when a bottle of milk is given to a baby who has not yet been taught how to sip from a cup or a spoon.

Artificial nipples have been made of rubber or petroleum-based substances only since the mid-19th century. Prior to the invention of rubber, leather (cured animal skin) or the cured animal teat itself was used. In addition, some teats were made of cow or goat horn, wood, ivory, or metal. Most were difficult to impossible to clean; as a result, illness and death rates of "hand-fed" infants were extremely high. In most situations where the baby's own mother could not or would not breastfeed her infant, a wet nurse was usually found, for this was much safer than artificial feeding.

Modern-day artificial nipples are usually made of rubber or silicone. Their shape varies according to manufacturing specifications. For example, some artificial nipples are designed to be used by premature infants; they are constructed of very soft rubber that requires almost no pressure to compress. Nipples for healthy newborns are usually 15 to 25 percent smaller than those designed for older babies. Some artificial nipples have a single large hole at the end of the narrow nipple shaft, while others have a hole in the center of the rounded portion that is on the "top side" of the nipple, whose bottom side is flattened. Others are very short and are advertised to be "most like mother herself." Unfortunately, the very tiny artificial nipple forces the baby to purse his or her lips to maintain contact with the teat, which does not elongate in the baby's mouth, an action that is necessary neither on the human nipple nor on the longer artificial nipples currently on the market.

The artificial nipple remains continuously rigid and usually tops a slightly broader base. In some cases, when the artificial nipple may have a flattened lower portion and a rounder top, the manufacturers refer to their product as "orthodontic" or as an "exerciser," although no independently funded research studies have proven either claim.

Before artificial nipples are used, they should be boiled vigorously several times to remove the environmental contaminants the rubber contains. The most notable of these is nitrites, which leech out of the rubber when they are in contact with the saliva in the baby's mouth or with other fluids, such as milk, water, or juice. After each use, the artificial nipple requires careful cleaning to avoid contamination of later feeds with bacteria that grow in artificial milk and other fluids. If the baby develops thrush, a yeast infection in the mouth, all rubber objects on which the baby sucks or chews—including artificial nipples/teats and pacifiers (sometimes called "dummies") should be discarded and replaced with new ones that are sterilized after every use.

Because the artificial teat does not change its shape in response to the baby's sucking, it tends to drip continuously and to spurt a single large stream into the baby's mouth when pressure is applied anywhere along its shaft. This continuous dripping and an excessive amount of fluid, delivered to the front and center portions of the baby's mouth, increase the likelihood that the baby will choke when fed, particularly if the head is not raised above the level of his or her body and the neck is not flexed slightly forward.

To prevent choking, the newborn bottle-feeding baby must take defensive action by moving his or her tongue from the underside of the artificial teat to its end, where pressure from the tongue will slow the continuous flow of milk. Then the baby is able to swallow without choking, after which he or she takes a quick breath of air. Immediately thereafter, the baby must again hold his or her breath in order to avoid drawing milk into the larynx. As a result of the alternating swallows and quick breaths, many bottle-feeding babies seem to squeak when they are fed. This quick intake of air may be a stress reaction in response to the difficulty they have controlling the feed.

Recent research of healthy full-term newborns has found that oxygen deprivation occurs more frequently when babies are bottle-fed than when matched infants of the same age are breastfed. Researchers examining premature infants' responses while feeding have identified that a stress response, probably related to oxygen deprivation during the feeding, also occurs *after* the baby has finished bottle feeding. These same infants, when breastfed, show no such stress response during or after the feeding.

✱ KATHLEEN G. AUERBACH, Ph.D., IBCLC

See **Guide to Related Topics:** Infant Feeding

Resources

Fildes, V. (1986). *Breasts, Bottles and Babies: A History of Infant Feeding.* Edinburgh, Scotland: Edinburgh University Press.

Mathew, O.P. & Bhatia, J. (1989). "Sucking and Breathing Patterns during Breast- and Bottle-feeding in Term Neonates." *American Journal of Diseases of Childhood 143*: 588-92.

Meier, P. (1988). "Bottle- and Breast-feeding: Effects on Transcutaneous Oxygen Pressure and Temperature in Preterm Infants." *Nursing Research 37*: 36-41.

Meier, P. & Anderson, G.C. (1987). "Responses of Small Preterm Infants to Bottle- and Breast-feeding." *MCN 12*: 97-105.

NIPPLES, HUMAN

The human nipple is that portion of the human breast from which mother's milk flows. The nipple is surrounded by similar tissue of dark pigmentation called the areola. Most of the areola is drawn into the baby's mouth when breastfeeding, enabling the nipple to elongate as the baby's

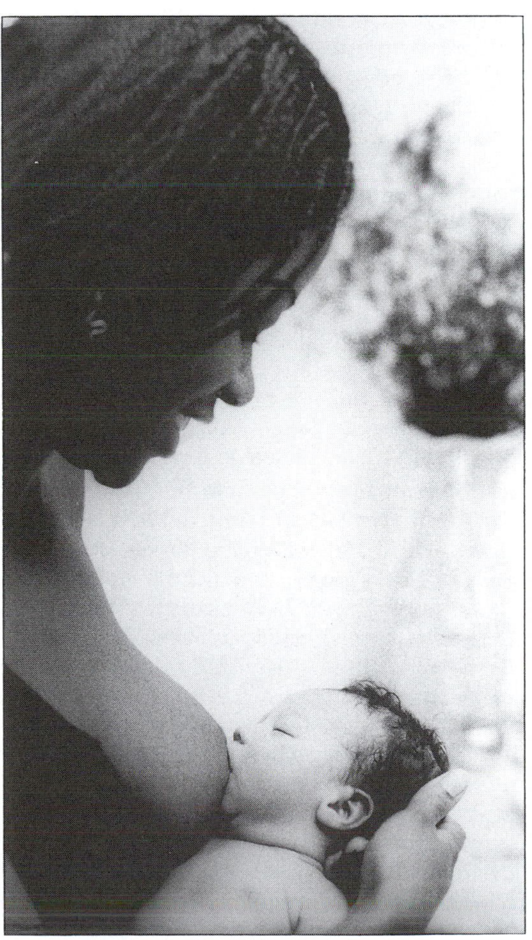

Note the position of the baby's mouth. Photo courtesy of Harriette Hartigan/Artemis.

tongue strokes the lower portion of the areola and nipple. As a result of the stroking action that occurs simultaneously with the baby's compression of the breast, nerve endings in the nipple and areola are stimulated, and milk is ejected in rhythmic spurts followed by brief pauses during which the mother's breast and nipple are not compressed.

When a baby is born, regardless of the gender, it will have two easily identified nipples. Under the skin on each side of the chest lies a breast bud (which feels a bit like a little pea) and the first few milk ducts, which do not develop until the onset of puberty, and then only in girls. The rise in estrogens and other female hormones during adolescence cause the breasts to begin to grow as fat is stored there, and milk glands, ducts, and sinuses develop and become more numerous. In adolescent girls and women, some growth of the milk glands and milk ducts occurs with each menstrual period, thus accounting for the nipple tenderness and generalized breast swelling that they sometimes notice. In addition, during pregnancy, the breasts prepare for breastfeeding by making milk. This preparation begins about three months into the pregnancy, and continues even for a short period after the baby's birth. Sometimes, because some of the mother's female hormones get into the baby through the placenta, a small amount of whitish fluid will be secreted by the baby's nipples; this is called "witches' milk." In nearly all infants, the breast tissue and the genitals appear to be swollen. This swelling goes away shortly after birth and is not a cause of concern.

The nipple does not store milk; rather it serves the same function as a faucet on a sink: It is a way for the milk to get from inside the mother's breast into the baby. Fifteen to 20 tiny pores spray milk—in different directions!—into the baby's mouth. Each of these pores is connected to a lactiferous sinus, which lies under the darker skin of the areola behind and all around the nipple. These sinuses are connected to milk ducts, which in turn connect the milk glands high in the breast to the lactiferous sinuses. The milk glands resemble many clusters of grapes. It is in these milk glands that the milk is made.

The nipple varies in size and shape from one woman to another and even from one breast to the other. The nipple that points outward is called everted; a variation is the inverted nipple, which disappears into the areola when stimulated. Some nipples appear to have dimpled areas so that the entire nipple does not evert, but neither does the entire nipple compress inward. Some nipples fold in on themselves, partially or completely, and some nipples look flat.

Sometimes women are told to "roll" their nipples to help make them stand out, in preparation for the baby's arrival. Such nipple rolling is not necessary, although it won't cause any harm—unless the mother-to-be is very rough. If what she is doing hurts, she should not continue the activity. Rubbing her tissue with a towel in the mistaken notion that this will "toughen" her nipples actually simply rubs off the top layer of skin and makes the nipples more, rather than less, sensitive. The only preparation needed is the usual cleaning that occurs in the shower or bath, with a minimum of soap, which can dry the skin.

While many nipples are rather thin, some are broad and rather flat. Lactation consultants sometimes refer to nipples as "dime-," "nickel-," or "quarter-sized." None of these size differences makes a difference to the baby, because when the nipple is drawn into the baby's mouth, its diameter narrows as it lengthens. All of these variations are part of the normal range and do not, by themselves, prevent the baby from suckling. While many women may appear to have inverted or flat nipples early in their pregnancy, most will find that by the end of the pregnancy, their nipples are standing out quite a bit more regardless of whether the mother wore breast shells (stiff protectors covering nipples) to encourage such action, rolled her nipples, or engaged in any other activity that is sometimes recommended to make the nipples evert. In fact, how the nipple looks before the baby begins nursing has little relationship to how the nipple looks when it is drawn into the baby's mouth. In the baby's mouth, the human nipple is pulled forward by the negative pressure that the baby's suckling action creates. The nipple, in response to the baby's suckling, stretches two to three times its "resting length," forming an elongated teat that rests against the top of the baby's mouth. When the mother lets down her milk, it sprays down the back of the baby's throat.

In all women, the nipple and areola tissue are darker than the skin color of the rest of her breast. During pregnancy, the nipple and areola tend to darken some more. In Caucasian women, the previously pink nipple appears beige or tan; in women of color, the nipple darkens to a deeper shade of brown or ebony.

✱ KATHLEEN G. AUERBACH, Ph.D., IBCLC

See also: Breastfeeding: Physiological and Cultural Aspects

See **Guide to Related Topics:** Infant Feeding

Resources

Huggins, K. (1991). *The Nursing Mother's Companion*. 2nd revised edition. Boston: Harvard Common Press.

Lawrence, R.A. (1989). *Breastfeeding: A Guide for the Medical Profession*. 3rd edition. St. Louis: C.V. Mosby.

Neville, M.C. & Neifert, M.R. (Eds.) (1983). *Lactation: Physiology, Nutrition and Breast-Feeding*. New York: Plenum Press.

Pryor, K. & Pryor, G. (1991). *The New Nursing Your Baby*. New York: Simon and Schuster.

Renfrew, M., Fisher, C., & Arms, S. (1990). *Breastfeeding: Getting Breastfeeding Right for You*. Berkeley, CA: Celestial Arts.

Riordan, J. & Auerbach, K.G. (forthcoming). *Breastfeeding and Human Milk*. New York: Jones and Bartlett Publishers, Inc.

NONSTRESS TESTS

Nonstress testing has become widely accepted as one method of evaluating fetal well-being. Developed in the mid-1970s, the nonstress test (NST) was so named to distinguish it from the contraction stress test (CST). The CST, developed in the early 1970s, evaluates the fetal heart as it responds to the stress of induced maternal uterine contractions. The NST involves external monitoring of fetal movements, fetal heart rate, and uterine activity, using a continuous fetal heart rate monitor, which prints a tracing of the fetal heart rate and maternal uterine activity on a paper strip.

There are many obstetrical and medical indications for which nonstress testing may be performed, including postdatism, intrauterine growth retardation (IUGR), chronic pregnancy-induced hypertension, diabetes mellitus, Rh isoimmunization, decreased or abrupt changes in fetal movement, pre-existing maternal conditions, premature rupture of membranes, and a maternal history of poor obstetric outcome.

When a healthy fetus moves, its heart rate accelerates in response, just as an adult's heart rate increases with physical exertion and returns to a baseline level at rest. Fetal heart rate accelerations, with or without perceived accompanying fetal movements, indicate the presence of adequate placental reserves for oxygenation (uteroplacental sufficiency) and an intact fetal central nervous system. The fetus, in response to chronic intrauterine hypoxia, will have reduced activity if the central nervous system becomes incapacitated by a lack of oxygen and the development of metabolic acidosis. As early as 26 to 28 weeks' gestation, a fetus considered to be at risk for uteroplacental insufficiency is a candidate for electronic fetal evaluation. The gestational age at which the testing is begun will depend upon the clinical circumstances surrounding the pregnancy.

Nonstress testing is usually performed by a nurse in a physician's office, a hospital, or a clinic setting. The pregnant woman being tested is placed in a Semi-Fowler's or a right or left lateral position. Two external monitoring transducers are applied to her abdomen and held in place by a special belt or stretchable "belly band." One transducer (toco) measures uterine activity and the other fetal heart rate. The nurse monitors maternal blood pressure for significant changes, such as hypotension, which may necessitate a position change. The usual testing time is 40 minutes. Test results are called either reactive, nonreactive, or equivocal.

The fetal heart rate tracing should demonstrate a baseline fetal heart rate range of 120 to 160 bpm (beats per minute). The definition of a reactive NST is heart rate accelerations, associated with fetal movements (two movements within 20 minutes), that exceed the baseline heart rate by 15 beats and last at least 15 seconds. All fetal movements perceived by the mother or the nurse are noted on the test strip. Most new fetal monitors are equipped with a cord that has a button the mother can push when she feels fetal movement. This produces a corresponding mark on the monitor tracing.

Nonreactive or equivocal tests demonstrate no acceleration of the fetal heart rate that fits the criteria. Because fetuses have been observed to have 40-minute sleep/wake cycles, testing may be continued up to 40 to 60 minutes. Before being called nonreactive, stimulation of the fetus may be employed by (1) changing maternal position, (2) introducing acoustic stimulation, (3) providing the mother with a cold drink, and (4) palpating the maternal abdomen. When follow-up or extended testing is necessary, the mother may be allowed to eat or get up and walk around before continuing, in an attempt to stimulate the fetus.

It may be difficult to obtain an adequate tracing due to the immature age of the fetus, maternal obesity, polyhydramnios, or extreme fetal activity. For example, it is not unusual, in premature fetuses less than 28 to 30 weeks' gestation, to produce strips in which there may be accelerations, with or without perceived movements, that do not exceed the baseline heart rate by 15 beats for 15 seconds.

Other observations that can be made during performance of NST include the frequency and duration of any uterine contractions that occur, and the presence of any fetal heart rate decelerations. These should be reported and follow-up initiated.

Data indicate that a reactive nonstress test is predictive of fetal well-being for one week from the date of testing. This "window of well-being" may be shortened in pregnancies deemed unstable and in which clinical conditions can change rapidly—such as in pregnancies complicated by insulin-dependent diabetes, gestational diabetes, postdatism, IUGR, chronic hypertension, oligohydramnios, or a maternal history of a previous stillborn.

While a reactive NST may be indicative of fetal well-being, a nonreactive or equivocal test result does not necessarily indicate fetal jeopardy. All equivocal or nonreactive tests should be followed up by a prolonged NST and/or additional testing such as ultrasound (biophysical profile), CST (also called OCT or oxytocin challenge test), or an intermittent maternal nipple stimulation test to induce uterine contractions. It is standard practice to use various measures to determine fetal and maternal status. If the NST continues to be nonreactive, the additional tests are not reassuring, and the clinical situation warrants, the patient is then evaluated for delivery. ✱ MARGARET R. PRIMEAU, R.N., M.B.A.

See also: Daily Fetal Movement Counting; Fetal Movement

See **Guide to Related Topics:** Prenatal Diagnosis and Screening

Resources

Afriat, Cydney I. (1989). *Electronic Fetal Monitoring.* Rockville, MD: Aspen Publications.

Huddleston, John F. & Freeman, Roger K. (1987). "Antepartum Fetal Surveillance." In Avroy A. Faranoff and Richard J. Martin (Eds.) *Neonatal Perinatal Medicine.* St. Louis: C.V. Mosby.

Mathews, D.D. (1973, Jun 9). "Fetal Movements and Fetal Well-Being." *Lancet 1* (815): 1315.

Parer, Julian T. (1983). *Handbook of Fetal Heart Rate Monitoring.* Philadelphia: W.B. Saunders Company.

Pearson, J.F. & Weaver, J.B. (1976, May 29). "Fetal Activity and Fetal Well-Being: An Evaluation." *British Medical Journal 1* (6021): 1305-07.

Sadovsky, Eliahu (1985, Apr). "Monitoring Fetal Movement: A Useful Screening Test." *Contemporary OB/GYN.* Reprint. Published by Medical Economics Company, Inc., Oradell, NJ 07649.

Sadovsky E., Yaffe, H., & Polishuk, W.Z. (1974). "Fetal Movement Monitoring in Normal and Pathological Pregnancy." *International Journal of Gynecology and Obstetrics 12* (3): 75-78.

Tucker, Susan M. (1978). *Fetal Monitoring and Fetal Assessment in High-Risk Pregnancy.* St. Louis: C.V. Mosby.

NORPLANT

Norplant is a scientifically effective new method of birth control. The first significantly innovative technology in contraception to be developed in 25 years, Norplant is surgically implanted under the skin in the upper or lower arm of a woman of childbearing age. The device, developed and marketed by the Population Council, is approved for use in 12 countries, and clinical trials with Norplant are being conducted in 37 other countries (Shoupe and Mishell, 1989). In December 1990, the Food and Drug Administration (FDA) approved Norplant for sale in the United States by Wyeth-Ayerst Laboratories, and the media hailed the implant as "revolutionary." The implant contraceptive has already been used by more than half a million women around the world since it was first introduced in Chile in 1968.

Perhaps most unique about Norplant is its promise of "hassle-free" contraception for up to five years. It is said to be more effective than sterilization. Norplant is reversible in that, after surgical removal by a trained professional, fertility is said to be restored immediately. To date, no data have been released that determine the safety of long-term use of Norplant or the effects of Norplant on blood coagulation, on levels of testosterone and rostenedione, or on blood pressure during the fourth and fifth year of use (UBINIG, 1988). Also unknown is the impact of Norplant use during pregnancy and lactation.

Norplant implants come in two forms or systems. The first system is composed of six plastic capsules containing a manufactured progestin hormone called levonorgesterol. Each capsule is made of a nonbiodegradable, silicone rubber tubing and together the capsules compose the 1.3-inch implant. From these capsules, 36 mg of the progestin hormone are slowly and steadily released into the blood for a period of about five years. The female hormone prevents pregnancy by stopping ovulation and also by thickening the mucus of the cervix to prevent sperm penetration. A suggested benefit of Norplant is that it does not use, and therefore does not have the ill effects of, estrogen, another female hormone used in oral contraception (the Pill). The other system is a second-generation development called Norplant-2, which works similarly. The newer device, however, is made up of only two tubes and contains 70 mg of levonorgesterol. There is no statistically significant difference in effectiveness or side effects between the two systems (The Population

Council, n.d.). Implantation and removal is said to be relatively easy and pain-free, but the cost of the initial procedure is high, approximately $300, which is to be paid at the time the capsules are inserted.

Although long-term effects of the Norplant systems are still unknown, shorter-term side effects have been reported. The manufacturer of Norplant states that changes in menstrual bleeding patterns, such as more frequent bleeding episodes, spotting between periods, or amenorrhea (absence of menstruation), are the most common effects of Norplant. The company's literature points out that even so, hemoglobin levels usually rise with the use of Norplant, so that the total blood lost by a woman is actually reduced by implant use (The Population Council, n.d.). The company also asserts that these bleeding irregularities frequently diminish after about three to six months of use, but this fact is disputed. Other side effects to be noted are headache, weight changes, depression, and acne. These, according to the Population Council, occur less often than is expected with the use of other hormonal contraceptives. Independent reports have found that up to 10 percent of Norplant users also developed benign but painful ovarian cysts, some of which have grown to 10 cm, and then resolved on their own within six weeks ("Hormonal Contraception," 1987). Other complaints include nervousness, mood swings, increased cramping, and hair growth (Darney et al., 1990). While some have argued that the side effects of Norplant are predictable, to many, they may be more discouraging than expected. Discontinuation rates in the U.S. have been close to 20 percent—mainly due to headaches and depression (Azim et al., 1990). Acceptability among women of bleeding irregularity is still unknown. Overall, tolerance of side effects is varied, though according to one study in the U.S., the effectiveness and convenience of Norplant outweighed the concerns of problems associated with it (Darney et al., 1990).

Other serious questions have arisen concerning the removal of Norplant and the foreseeable unethical uses of the device. Since removal of Norplant depends on the availability of trained professionals and is not completely within a woman's control, concern has been raised that women may not be able to obtain prompt removal of the device upon request. One study in Bangladesh, in fact, found that 75 percent of women requesting removal of Norplant were unable to get it removed on their first request, and on average, it took three requests and seven weeks for removal to be completed (Thapa, 1989). Because high-quality, responsive care can be difficult to access, Norplant may pose difficulties that counter its "hassle-free" promises. Also notable is the 7 percent local infection rate that occurred upon removal of Norplant in carefully conducted clinical trials and was associated with provider technique (Norsigian, 1989). The National Women's Health Network in the U.S., the Policy Research for Development Alternatives (UBINIG) in Bangladesh, and many women's health and rights organizations are concerned with the possible punitive use of the device against women's wills, or without their complete, informed consent. The fear is that Norplant will not be used to enhance reproductive freedom but instead to further abuse it, and in fact, all evidence points out that such reproductive abuse has already become the norm. For instance, just days after FDA approval in the U.S., the *Philadelphia Inquirer* published an editorial stating that readers should "think about" Norplant as a tool in the fight against black poverty. And in California, a judge ordered a woman, convicted of child abuse, to use Norplant as a part of her sentence. In Kansas, the legislature held hearings on a bill that would pay welfare mothers $500 to get the implant. The "incentive program" would also pay for the cost of implantation, plus a $50 check per year. A related proposal was introduced in Louisiana to provide a $100 incentive for women on public assistance to use the implant. In California, plans to make Norplant accessible to low-income teenagers and women of childbearing age who use drugs are in the works. The governor of the state reported that he and his staff had not yet decided whether or not to make Norplant mandatory for drug users. These legislative proposals and court decisions, formulated even before Norplant hit the market, indicate that the new technology may be an easy vehicle for forced sterilization.

In the meantime, research is being done on related progestrogen implants with a biodegradable carrier that gradually dissolves in body tissue. The carrier will not have to be removed, but cannot be removed once it has started to dissolve. Such scientific developments, plus the political and social realities surrounding women's reproduction, make implanted contraception a new and central issue for childbearing and reproductive choice in women's lives.

✱ MARY BETH CASCHETTA

See **Guide to Related Topics:** Contraception

Resources

Azim, T. et al. (1990, Jul). "Family Planning at the Cost of Women's Health." *Holiday* 27: 4-7.

Darney, P.D. et al. (1990, May-Jun). "Acceptance and Perceptions of Norplant among Users in San Francisco USA." *Studies in Family Planning 21* (3): 152-60.

"Hormonal Contraception: New Long-Acting Methods." (1987, Mar-Apr). *Population Reports Series K* (3).

Norsigian, J. (for the National Women's Health Network). (1989). Testimony at the Food and Drug Administration: Fertility and Maternal Health Drugs Advisory Committee, April 27.

The Population Council. (no date). "Facts about Norplant Implants." Summary.

Shoupe, D. & Mishell, D.R. (1989, May). "Norplant: Subdermal Implant System for Long-Term Contraception." *American Journal of Obstetrics and Gynecology 160*: 1286-92.

Thapa, S. (1989, Mar). "Discontinuation of Norplant Implants in Bangladesh." Paper presented at the Annual Meeting of the American Public Health Association.

UBINIG. (1988, Mar). "Norplant: The Five-Year Needle: An Investigation of the Bangladesh Trial." *Radical Journal of Health*: 101-08.

NURSE-MIDWIFERY: HISTORY IN THE UNITED STATES

> In France midwives were not nurses. In America nurses were not midwives. In England trained women were both nurses and midwives. After I had met British nurse-midwives, first in France and then on my visits to London, it grew upon me that nurse-midwifery was the logical response to the needs of the young child in rural America.
>
> Work for children should begin before they are born, should carry them through their greatest hazard which is childbirth, and should be most intensive during their first six years of life. These are the formative years—whether for their bodies, their minds or their loving hearts. (Breckinridge, 1952)

Thus the stage was set by Mary Breckinridge for American nurse-midwifery. Breckinridge, a woman from a prominent Kentucky family, had studied nursing at St. Luke's Hospital in New York and provided nursing care to children in devastated areas of France after World War I. She went back to Europe to study midwifery at the British Hospital for Mothers and Babies and eventually established the Frontier Nursing Service in the Appalachian Mountains of southeastern Kentucky in 1925.

But it was not easy to introduce the idea of reviving midwifery, even though a nursing prerequisite was instituted as a means of improving maternal and neonatal outcomes. According to Rooks:

> While obstetric leaders attacked and nearly effected the demise of midwifery, many other people were also concerned about the poor status of the nation's maternal and child health. As a result of this concern, three important institutions were started, each of which played important roles in introducing and supporting nurse-midwifery as a way to improve pregnancy and infant outcomes. (Rooks, 1990)

The three institutions were the Frontier Nursing Service, the Children's Bureau of the federal government, and the Maternity Center Association (MCA), a voluntary health agency based in New York.

While Breckinridge was struggling to improve the care available to poor rural families, in New York City the Maternity Center Association was working toward achieving the same goal on behalf of low-income urban families.

In 1917, the year that the Maternity Center Association was established as a program of the Women's City Club, the fledgling Children's Bureau recommended that public health nurses give prenatal instruction and care (Rooks, 1990). This in fact was MCA's first goal. Then in 1924 MCA attempted to affiliate with the Bellevue School for Midwives to respond further to the Children's Bureau's recommendation, but the plan was vetoed by the City Commissioner of Welfare. Finally, in 1931, after much exploration, disappointment, and persistence on the part of MCA, the Lobenstine Clinic opened and provided a home for midwifery education; it accepted as students public health nurses because of their orientation to prevention and teaching. From the outset, there was a university affiliation, initially with Teachers College, Columbia University.

The year 1939 saw the opening of the Frontier Nursing Service's School, the second in the country. By 1945, three more schools had opened: Tuskegee in Alabama and Flint-Goodridge Hospital and Dillard University in Louisiana, both designed to prepare black nurses in midwifery; and the Catholic Maternity Institute school in Santa Fe, New Mexico. The latter was to serve Spanish-speaking populations in New Mexico. All of these schools were motivated by the goal of reducing high rates of maternal and infant mortality among low-income families. By 1950, however, only three schools—the Maternity Center Association, the Frontier Nursing Service, and the Catholic Maternity Institute—survived (Hiestand, 1976).

During these years, program after program proved the effectiveness of nurse-midwifery services in fulfilling the expectation that they could improve care and outcomes (Thompson, 1986).

An important chapter in the ongoing history of nurse-midwifery began in 1955 with the establishment of the American College of Nurse-Mid-

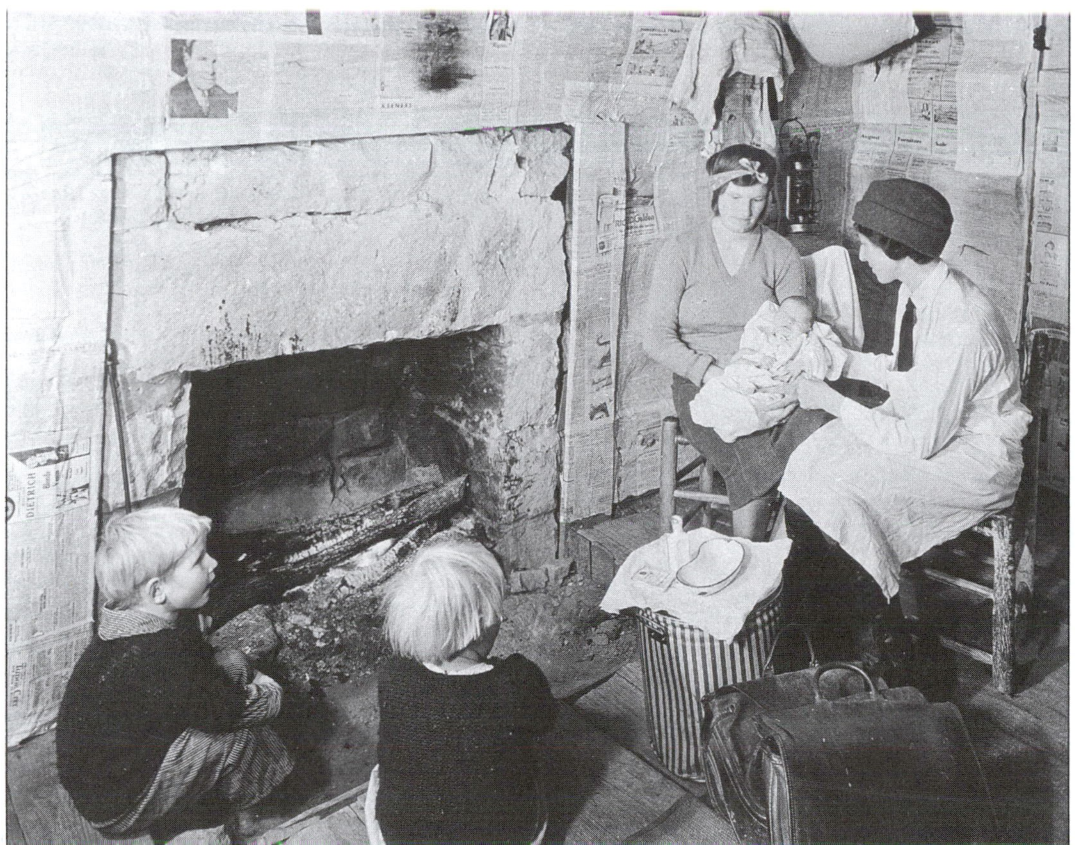

Early home visit, Frontier Nursing Service, 1932. Photo courtesy of Caufield and Shook. © 1932 by Frontier Nursing Service.

wifery (now Midwives). This professional organization took on the monumental task of ensuring a high quality of practice. Programs of school approval, certification of individuals, standards of practice, and continuing education were all established by the small membership on a volunteer basis. The ACNM also undertakes to inform the public and policymakers about the outstanding practice and experience of the profession in order to dilute the negative image surrounding midwifery.

In the 1980s, "several prestigious national bodies testified to the virtues of nurse-midwifery and recommended its support" (Rooks, 1990). Among those bodies are the Institute of Medicine (Institute of Medicine, 1988), the Office of Technology Assessment of the U.S. Congress (U.S. Congress, 1986), and the National Commission to Prevent Infant Mortality (The National Commission to Prevent Infant Mortality, 1988).

In 1982, Lubic noted that 23 percent of the schools that had opened in the preceding 50 years had failed (Lubic, 1982). She attributed the difficulties experienced by nurse-midwifery to a struggle between organized obstetrical groups and "others" with whom control of maternity care might have to be shared. Nurse-midwives are as small in number as they are in 1990—fewer than 4,300 have ever been certified—(Rooks, 1990) because of inability to obtain from medical educators the clinical experience necessary to round out a sound midwifery education.

Also in the 1980s, the free-standing birth center, a concept given new life in the United States by nurse-midwives, was adapted and adopted widely both nationally and internationally (Lubic and Ernst, 1978). Birth centers are showcases for the "with woman," noninterventionist practice, which is the heart of midwifery. The growing number of nurse-midwife-operated birth centers and other midwifery services are now making it possible for the education of greater numbers of students. A new community-based educational program developed by Case Western Reserve University's Frances Payne Bolton School of Nursing, the Frontier Nursing Service, the Maternity Center Association, and the National Association of Childbearing Centers is making it possible to prepare nurse-midwives in greater numbers. The very positive results of the intrapartum care of almost 12,000 women in the National Birth Center Study published in the *New England Journal of Medicine* in December 1989 (Rooks et al., 1989) further substantiate the responsibility of nurse-midwives and their sensitivity to families at all socioeconomic levels. As Litoff has put it:

> Over the past eight decades, American midwifery has endured in the face of overwhelming obstacles. Confronted by a predominantly hostile and powerful medical establishment, the midwife survived the early twentieth-century efforts to eradicate her. Although her numbers had been greatly reduced, she had not been defeated. Indeed, the seed had been planted for a new type of midwife: the professionally trained and certified nurse-midwife. (Litoff, 1986)

✱ RUTH WATSON LUBIC, C.N.M., Ed.D. FAAN

See also: Birth Centers; Midwife Licensing; Midwife-Attended Births; Midwifery: Overview; Midwifery and the Law

See **Guide to Related Topics:** Caregivers and Practitioners

Resources

Breckinridge, Mary. (1952). *Wide Neighborhoods*. New York: Harper and Brothers.

Hiestand, Wanda. (1976). "Midwife to Nurse-Midwife: A History of the Development of Nurse-Midwifery Education in the United States to 1965." Unpublished Ed.D. dissertation, Teachers College, New York.

Institute of Medicine. (1988). *Prenatal Care: Reaching Mothers, Reaching Infants*. Washington, DC: National Academy Press.

Levy, B.S., Wilkinson, F.S., & Marine, W.M. (1971). "Reducing Neonatal Mortality Rates with Nurse-Midwives." *American Journal of Obstetrics and Gynecology 109* (1): 50-58.

Litoff, Judy Barrett. (1986). *The American Midwife Debate: A Sourcebook on Its Modern Origins*. New York: Greenwood Press.

Lubic, Ruth. (1982). "Nurse-Midwifery Education—The Second Fifty Years." *Journal of Nurse-Midwifery 27* (5): 5-9.

Lubic, Ruth & Ernst, Eunice. (1978). "The Childbearing Center: An Alternative to Conventional Care." *Nursing Outlook 26* (12): 754-60.

Montgomery, Theodore A. (1969). "A Case for Nurse-Midwives." *American Journal of Obstetrics and Gynecology 105* (3): 309-13.

The National Commission to Prevent Infant Mortality. (1988, Aug). *Death Before Life: The Tragedy of Infant Mortality*. Washington, DC.

Rooks, Judith. (1990). "Nurse-Midwifery: Yesterday, Today and Tomorrow." *American Journal of Nursing 90* (10): 31-35.

Rooks, Judith et al. (1989). "Outcomes of Care in Birth Centers: The National Birth Center Study." *New England Journal of Medicine 321*: 1804-11.

Thompson, J.B. (1986). "Safety and Effectiveness of Nurse Midwifery Care: Research Review." In ACNM Foundation, *Nurse-Midwifery in America*. Washington, DC: ACNM Foundation, p. 40-44.

U.S. Congress, Office of Technology Assessment. (1986). *Nurse Practitioners, Physicians Assistants and Certified Nurse-Midwives: A Policy Analysis*. Washington, DC: U.S. Government Printing Office.

NURSING. *See instead* BREASTFEEDING

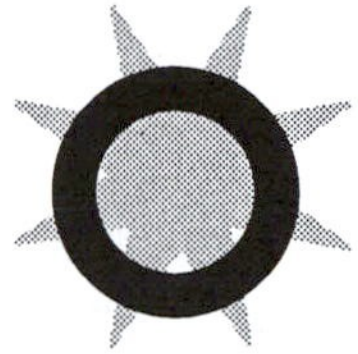

OBSTETRIC DRUGS: THEIR EFFECTS ON MOTHER AND INFANT*

Most women assume that the drugs offered them by their obstetricians during pregnancy, labor birth, and lactation have been approved by the U.S. Food and Drug Administration (FDA) as safe for use under those conditions. The fact is, there is no maternally administered drug that has been proven safe for the fetus. Nor is there any law or regulation that prohibits a physician from prescribing or administering to a childbearing woman a drug that has never been approved by the FDA as safe for such use.

Inherent Risks of Obstetric-Related Drugs. Seldom are pregnant women advised by their obstetricians that an unborn baby's central nervous system is rapidly forming throughout the latter months of pregnancy, the perinatal period and the first two years of life, and that during that time, the central nervous system is susceptible to permanent damage from drugs prescribed for or administered to the pregnant woman.

Changes in the placenta as pregnancy advances heighten the transfer to the fetal circulation of all drugs used in obstetric analgesia and anesthesia. As the time of birth grows near, the fetal brain is relatively large and the cerebral blood flow is high in comparison to the adult brain. In addition, the myelin content of the brain, the fatlike substance that protects the nerve fibers of the brain, is low when compared to the adult. The baby's brain and central nervous system, therefore, are more vulnerable to drugs administered to or taken by the mother during the perinatal period and during lactation.

Gestational age, previous and concomitant exposure to other drugs, relative hypoxia, and various pathological conditions can affect how a drug given to the mother will affect her unborn or newborn infant. The brain and heart of an about-to-be born or newly born infant are vessel-rich. Hypoxemia (low levels of oxygen of the blood) and a resulting build-up of lactic acid in the fetal blood during labor and birth can increase the uptake by the fetal brain and heart of drugs given to the mother.

Several studies have shown that drugs administered to the mother alter fetal brain function. Whether this dysfunction has implications for the child's future central nervous system development has not been the subject of a well-controlled scientific investigation. But many respected scientists are beginning to express their concern that drugs administered with the very best of intentions to the pregnant woman near or at term may limit the exposed offspring's ability to achieve his or her full potential in life.

Mothers-to-be are sometimes cautioned by their obstetrician or anesthesiologist that experiencing pain during labor can decrease the oxygen supply to the fetus but, in fact, no research has shown this to be true in the human fetus.

Drugs trapped in the infant's brain at birth have the potential to affect adversely the rapidly developing nerve circuitry of the brain and central nervous system by altering the following brain processes:

- The rate at which the nerve cells in the brain mature;

*Copyright © 1992 by Doris B. Haire.

- The process by which the brain cells develop individual characteristics and capacity to carry out specific functions;
- The process by which the brain cells are guided into their proper place within the brain and central nervous system;
- The interconnection of the branch-like nerve fibers as the circuitry of the brain is formed; and
- The forming of the insulating sheath of myelin (fatlike substance) around the nerve fibers, which helps to ensure that the nerve impulses—the messages to and from the brain—will travel their normal route at the normal rate of speed.

Dr. Joseph Altman, a neurobiologist at the University of Indiana, has pointed out that the development of the human brain appears to be programmed so that certain cells and nerve fibers must develop in synchrony, in order to make appropriate connections within the central nervous system. He has expressed concern that drug-induced alterations of the chemical components within the brain may interfere with the growth of the cells and nerve fibers, causing subtle or substantial misconnections within the developing brain.

To better understand this hypothesis, picture a technician preparing to connect hundreds of wires. The ends of each wire are color-coded to guide the electrician in connecting the wires properly. A chemical is spilled over the wires, removing the color. To meet his schedule the technician must continue to connect the wires, unable to be sure which wire to connect to another. The job is finished on schedule, the system functions, but it functions imperfectly.

Any alteration in the development of the intricately complex nerve circuitry of the brain has the potential for permanently altering the way the brain processes and responds to information. How much an individual fetus or newborn infant will be affected by a drug administered to the mother during pregnancy, childbirth, or lactation is unpredictable. Genetic susceptibility, which affects the final outcome, varies greatly, even among siblings. Well-controlled experiments in animals, for example, often produce varying results in the test animals, even among litter mates.

Most physicians and pharmaceutical manufacturers are quick to say that there is no drug on the market that is without risk. None of the drugs or chemicals used as medications or food additives, or in shampoo, hair coloring, underarm deodorants, skin treatments, and the like have been subjected to a well-controlled scientific investigation to determine what effect the drug or chemical has on the fetus. That doesn't mean that all of these drugs and chemicals are harmful. It just means it is not known if there are any adverse effects on the fetus and newborn.

FDA Status of Drugs. The United States Food and Drug Administration (FDA) never approves a drug for general or "universal" use, but only for specific indications and under certain conditions. Only if the words "pregnancy," "obstetrics," "labor," "delivery," or "lactation" appear in the *Indications* section of the drug's package insert (the FDA-approved information leaflet included in each carton of an approved drug) has the FDA approved the use of the drug for those conditions. If the conditions described above are discussed elsewhere in the package insert but are not specifically noted in the *Indications* section, the drug has not been approved by the FDA for such uses. If the package insert makes no mention that the use of the drug is contraindicated in pregnancy, labor, delivery, or lactation, one cannot assume that the drug is safe to be used at those times. The FDA, in general, does not require drug manufacturers to list contraindications to the use of a drug in the package insert.

FDA-Approved Drugs in Obstetrics. Two drugs approved by the FDA for use during pregnancy are a combination of doxylamine and pyridoxine (Bendectin) and ritodrine (Yutopar). Once prescribed as a remedy for morning sickness, Bendectin was taken off the market in 1983 because of the high costs incurred by the company in defending itself against lawsuits. Several lawsuits have been brought against the manufacturer of Bendectin by parents who contend that their children's birth defects resulted from prenatal exposure to the drug. Currently the litigation is lumbering through the courts, with both sides claiming victories. No one knows how many cases have been settled out of court, since in most such cases, the plaintiffs must swear to secrecy in order to receive the settlement.

The only other drug specifically approved by the FDA for use during pregnancy is ritodrine (Yutopar), a neurotransmitter prescribed or administered to pregnant women in order to halt preterm labor. Another drug, terbutaline, is also administered for the same purpose. However, the drug has not been approved by the FDA for that use.

Until fairly recently, some tranquilizers, such as diazepam (Valium), were frequently administered to women during labor to alleviate their anxiety. Because of their adverse effects on the newborn infant, the FDA no longer approves these drugs for such use. But as mentioned earlier, lack of FDA approval does not mean that a doctor is prohibited from prescribing a tranquilizer during labor.

Analgesics. The most frequently used drug in labor is a narcotic-like analgesic called meperidine (Demerol, Pethidine). The use of meperidine has largely replaced the use of morphine during labor. This drug is frequently offered to the laboring woman by the obstetrician, nurse, or midwife, accompanied by the standard remark, "This will help to take the edge off the contractions." Meperidine does not eradicate pain, but for many women, it makes the discomfort or pain of the contractions more tolerable. Other women find that meperidine causes them to lose control of their labor.

Meperidine is usually administered by injection, either intramuscularly (IM) or intravenously (IV), in doses of 50 mg, repeated every four hours if the health care provider so desires and the mother agrees. As with most pain-relieving drugs, meperidine can slow maternal respiration and circulation. When a narcotized mother breathes more slowly than normal and her blood flows more slowly than normal through her lung tissue, there is an increased possibility that the fetus will receive less than a normal supply of oxygen.

In a well-controlled investigation by John Morrison, an obstetrician at the University of Mississippi, one out of every four infants of mothers who received only 50 mg of meperidine during labor, within one to three hours before delivery, required resuscitation at birth. Unfortunately, it is difficult to insure that the baby will be born at a time when the effect of meperidine is minimal. For this reason, midwives often administer the drug in smaller doses, such as 25 mg or 12 mg, in order to ensure that the mother will feel in control of her labor and the baby will be ready to breathe on his or her own immediately after birth. After repeated administrations of the drug, even in smaller doses, meperidine and its metabolite, normeperidine, tend to accumulate in the fetal circulation.

Meperidine is not without side effects. They include sweating, dizziness, headache, nausea, vomiting, slowing of gastric function, agitation, tremor, uncoordinated muscle movement, transient hallucinations and disorientation, and visual disturbance. The more serious hazards of meperidine for the mother are respiratory depression, respiratory arrest, circulatory depression, shock, cardiac arrest, coma, and death. A less well-known fact about meperidine is that the drug can cause an increase in cerebral spinal fluid pressure. The implications of this effect on the mother and fetus, or newborn infant, however, have not been investigated. There is no way of knowing how frequently these adverse effects occur under normal clinical conditions because the law does not require physicians or midwives to report adverse drug reactions to the FDA, even if the patient dies.

The FDA has required the manufacturers of meperidine to provide in the drug's package insert only a minimum of information concerning the drug's adverse effects on the fetus and newborn infant. The insert acknowledges that the drug crosses the placenta and can depress the respiratory and the psychophysiologic functions of the newborn infant and can increase the likelihood that the newborn infant may require resuscitation. The insert does not make clear that meperidine given to the mother during labor can slow the fetal heart and impede the normal transfer of oxygen from the mother's circulation to that of her fetus.

Severe or prolonged oxygen depletion has been shown to cause the fetal brain to swell. Whether an increase in cerebral spinal fluid pressure in the presence of fetal hypoxia, ruptured membranes, and/or forceps extraction increases the likelihood of permanent brain dysfunction has yet to be investigated. There is some concern that the severely narcotized newborn infant may be more prone to aspirate or inhale its gastric fluids because the drug has blunted or paralyzed his or her protective gag reflex.

Other narcotic-like drugs approved by the FDA for use in labor are nalbuphine (Nubain), butorphanol (Stadol), and alphaprodine (Nisentil). Some drugs, namely hydromorphone (Dilaudid), fentanyl citrate (Sublimaze), and codeine, are also used in labor, but the FDA has not approved them for such use. Like meperidine, the delayed or long-term effects of drugs given during labor on the exposed fetus has not been adequately investigated. The little research that has been done on Nubain has shown the drug to concentrate more in the fetal circulation than in the mother's. Butorphanol is 40 times more powerful than meperidine and must be administered with extreme care to avoid an overdose. Hydroxyzine (Vistaril) is an anti-anxiety, anti-nausea drug sometimes administered to women during labor. The potentiating action of hydroxyzine must be considered when the drug is used in conjunction with other drugs that depress the central nervous system.

Narcotic Antagonist. Naloxone (Narcan) has been approved by the FDA for use in infants narcotized by drugs administered to the mother, but the FDA has not approved the use of naloxone during labor. In most cases, the sluggish, drugged infant becomes alert after receiving naloxone. However, once the short-acting naloxone has worn off, those infants given naloxone show no improvement over those infants who did not receive the drug. The infant receiving naloxone must be carefully and continuously observed because if the naloxone wears off before the effects of the meperidine have dissipated, the baby could be in jeopardy. Naloxone should not be administered to a depressed infant unless the infant is narcotized. If the newborn infant is hypoxic for reasons other than being narcotized, naloxone can actually deepen the hypoxic state of the infant.

Antiemetics. Meperidine is often administered in conjunction with a drug called promethazine (Phenergan) or in a combination called Mepergan. Promethazine relieves the nausea and vomiting caused by the administration of meperidine or other powerful pain relievers. Promethazine is thought to augment the effects of meperidine, allowing less of the latter drug to be used. Promethazine is not without risk, however. Research has shown that it can markedly impair platelet aggregation in the fetus and newborn, a condition that can cause bleeding within the brain of the fetus and newborn without a similar effect in the mother.

Antacids. Nausea and vomiting are common maternal side effects of the powerful pain-relieving drugs administered during labor. In an attempt to minimize the possibility of chemical pneumonia, which can occur if the heavily drugged or anesthetized mother vomits and aspirates the fluids or food from her stomach, women have been given various antacids during labor to reduce the acidity of the stomach's contents. This is done in the belief that, should the mother regurgitate in response to anesthesia, she is less likely to suffer chemical pneumonia. Antacids may improve the odds of a safe outcome, but they can not be relied upon to prevent maternal morbidity or mortality from aspiration. If aspiration occurs following the administration of an antacid, particles in the antacid itself can cause substantial maternal morbidity.

Although the FDA has not approved the drug for such use, a systemic antacid, sodium citrate and citric acid (Bicitra), is frequently administered to women during labor. The drug does cross the placenta and enter the fetus and its delayed, long-term effects on the exposed offspring have not been investigated. As with other antacids, the drug has not been approved by the FDA for use in obstetric care.

Regional Anesthesia. Drugs most commonly used in regional anesthesia to block pain impulses are bupivacaine (Marcaine, Sensorcaine), lidocaine (Xylocaine), mepivacaine (Carbocaine), and chloroprocaine (Nesacaine). Depending on the area to be anesthetized, they are administered as an epidural, spinal, caudal, saddle, or pudendal block, or as a local infiltration for episiotomy repair. The once popular paracervical block has been abandoned in most obstetric services because of its adverse effects on the fetus.

Epidural, spinal, and caudal anesthesia numb the woman from above her navel to her toes. All regional anesthetics reach the fetal circulation and, subsequently, the fetal brain within seconds or minutes of administration to the mother.

Each of these drugs has its own inherent risks. Because a health care provider is not required to report an adverse drug effect to the FDA, there is no way of knowing the exact incidence of such effects. The package insert of bupivacaine provided by the drug's manufacturer describes the potential problems. The package insert reads in part:

> Local anesthetics rapidly cross the placenta, and when used for epidural, caudal or pudendal block anesthesia, can cause varying degrees of maternal, fetal and neonatal toxicity. The incidence and degree of toxicity depend upon the procedure performed, the type and amount of drug used, and the technique of drug administration. Adverse reactions in the parturient, fetus and neonate involve alteration of the central nervous system, peripheral vascular tone, and cardiac function....
>
> Neurologic effects following epidural or caudal anesthesia may include spinal block of varying magnitude (including high or total spinal block); hypotension secondary to spinal block; urinary retention; fecal and urinary incontinence; loss of perineal sensation and sexual function; persistent anesthesia; paresthesia, weakness, paralysis of the lower extremities, and loss of sphincter control, all of which may have slow, incomplete or no recovery; headache; backache; septic meningitis; meningismus; slowing of labor; increased incidence of forceps delivery; cranial

nerve palsies due to traction on nerves from loss of cerebrospinal fluid.

Wide experience with the use of epidural blocks also indicates that epidural block (injection into the space between the spinal column and the dural membrane enveloping the spinal cord) is associated with significantly longer labors, increased use of oxytocin ("pit drip"), rotational forceps deliveries, and markedly more postpartum bladder catheterizations. It is well accepted that an episiotomy is almost unavoidable if regional anesthesia is in effect during delivery because the epidural block causes the mother to lose her ability to bear down effectively, unduly prolonging the expulsion of the baby.

Spinal Headache. The severe headache that some mothers experience for days, weeks, even months after having an epidural or spinal block is more likely to be due to the leakage of cerebral spinal fluid from the injection site than from the anesthetic itself. While a blood patch can be administered to stop the leakage, the procedure is not without risk, and there is no guarantee that it will be successful in quelling the headache.

The package insert for regional anesthetics provides little information as to the effect of the drugs on the immediate neurologic development of the exposed offspring and none on the delayed, long-term effects. Deborah Rosenblatt and her colleagues at St. Mary's Hospital in London found correlations between epidural anesthesia in childbirth and certain neurologic effects in the exposed offspring that persisted throughout a six-week testing period. The effect of adding fentanyl to the regional anesthetic used in epidurals is the subject of growing concern among lactation consultants.

Most obstetricians quietly agree that epidural block also increases the rate of cesarean section. An epidural block causes the pelvic musculature to become flaccid or limp. Therefore, the "trough" of pelvic muscles that normally rotates the baby into the proper position to move efficiently through the birth process dysfunctions.

Pudendal Block. Mothers who experience a drug-free birth often comment that one of the most rewarding sensations of giving birth is the feeling of power as they ease their babies out into the world. Yet, well-meaning obstetricians frequently take away this gratifying moment by administering a pudendal block to numb the mother's perineum just as she is about to give birth. A pudendal block is performed by injecting an anesthetic drug through the vagina into the pudendal nerve on either side of the vagina. The irony of this misguided kindness is that it can indirectly cause the mother's perineum to rupture. Why? Because the pudendal block blunts or obliterates the burning sensation that normally occurs as the baby's head distends the mother's perineum. This warning sensation, when intact, warns the mother to bear down with just enough force to ease her baby out but not enough to rupture her perineum.

The anesthetic used in a pudendal block reaches the infant's circulation in seconds or minutes and has the potential for having the same neurological effect on the fetus as an epidural injection of the same drug. Since a pudendal block is relatively short-lived, an additional anesthetic is usually administered to numb the perineum if sutures are required to repair an episiotomy or a rupture in the perineum.

General Anesthesia. General anesthesia is seldom used for vaginal birth today in the United States. It is used, however, for cesarean section if a rapid delivery is needed or if the mother is bleeding. It may also be used if there is a need or desire to provide absence of sensation and consciousness. Typically, for general anesthesia, an induction anesthetic, such as thiopental (Pentothal), is given by injection, rapidly followed by an injection of succinylcholine (Anectine). A few seconds later the mother drifts into unconsciousness, and pressure is applied to the cricoid cartilage, just below the larynx, to prevent aspiration while a laryngoscope is inserted into the mother's trachea. An endotracheal tube is inserted through the laryngoscope, and the cuff of the endotracheal tube is inflated to seal any space in the mother's trachea that the tube does not fill. The anesthetist or anesthesiologist listens to the mother's lungs with a stethoscope to be certain the endotracheal tube is in her airway and not in her esophagus. Once the seal is ensured, anesthesia is maintained with nitrous oxide and oxygen. A low concentration of a volatile agent such as halothane (Fluothane) is also given to provide amnesia. The endotracheal tube must not be removed until the mother is conscious enough to follow commands.

As with any type of anesthesia, general anesthesia must be given skillfully. Although women are often told not to eat if they think they may be in labor, there is no documented case of aspiration in a woman who was properly anesthetized according to today's standard of care, whether or not she ate.

The combination of nitrous oxide and oxygen can also be given by mask as analgesia, but it is seldom used in the United States. Sedatives and hypnotics such as barbiturates (Seconal, Luminal, Nembutal), chloral hydrate, and flurazepam (Dalmane) may sometimes be used in early labor, but the FDA has not approved their use in pregnancy or labor. These drugs may cause respiratory depression in the newborn.

Whether or not exposure to analgesic drugs during labor and birth contributes to the high rate of subtle difficulties in learning and behavior in children has yet to be adequately investigated.

Uterine Stimulants. Oxytocin (Pitocin, Syntocinon) is a powerful synthetic hormone administered to women in order to initiate and/or to stimulate labor. The drug is frequently the physician's preferred method of stimulating contractions and speeding up labor, even though it is well known that helping the mother to walk, stand, or sit during labor facilitates the normal progress of labor in the majority of women. Oxytocin is frequently necessary when epidural block alters the normal progress of labor.

The FDA has approved the use of oxytocin in labor and delivery when it is medically indicated. The FDA has not, however, approved the use of oxytocin for the elective stimulation of labor. Prostaglandin gel is also administered in some hospitals as a uterine stimulant or cervical "softener," but the FDA has not approved prostaglandin for such use.

The use of oxytocin in obstetrics, even if necessary, is not without risk. If the mother's membranes have ruptured, the augmentation of contractions can adversely affect the fetal brain by increasing compression of the fetal skull, increasing intracranial pressure, increasing the possibility of tears in the cerebral membranes, and inhibiting the normal transfer of oxygen from the mother's circulatory system to the fetal brain. During a normal contraction, the maternal blood vessels that carry oxygenated blood through the uterine wall to the placenta are constricted. During these periods of diminished blood flow, the oxygen in the mother's blood, which stores up in the placenta's intervillous space between contractions, maintains the fetal brain with a relatively constant supply of oxygen. Uterine stimulants that foreshorten these oxygen-replenishing intervals by making the contractions too long, too strong, or too close together increase the likelihood that brain cells will die. The situation is somewhat analogous to holding an infant under the surface of the water, allowing the infant to come to the surface to gasp for air, but not to breathe.

British scientific investigators have noted that the use of oxytocin to induce labor increases the incidence of jaundice in the newborn. Whether the frequent use of oxytocin in the United States to stimulate labor contributes to the high incidence of jaundice in the newborn period has yet to be investigated.

It would be wonderful to be able to provide the laboring woman with a magic remedy that would take away her pain, leave her with all her senses intact, and would be free of harm to her and her baby. Such a drug is not yet available. For now, each mother must be given the facts and allowed to make her own decisions as to what is right for her and her baby. ✱ DORIS B. HAIRE

See also: Epidural Anesthesia

See **Guide to Related Topics:** Childbirth Practices and Locations

Resources

Annas, G. (1989). *The Rights of Patients: The Basic ACLU Guide to Patient Rights.* 2nd edition. Carbondale, IL: Southern Illinois University Press, pp. 135-38.

Congressional Hearings on "Effects of Prescription Drugs during Pregnancy." Subcommittee on Investigations and Oversight of the Committee on Science and Technology, U.S. House of Representatives, Ninety-Seventh Congress, First Session. July 30, 1981 [No. 62]. U.S. Government Printing Office, 1981. Doris Haire, Principal Speaker.

Conway, E. & Brackbill, Y. (1970). "Delivery Medication and Infant Outcome: An Empirical Study." In W.A. Bowes et al. (Eds.) *Monographs of the Society for Research in Child Development 35*: 24-34.

Corby, D. & Schulman, I. (1971). "The Effects of Antenatal Drug Administration on Aggregation of Platelets of Newborn Infants." *Journal of Pediatrics 79* (2): 307-13.

Golding, J., Paterson, M., & Kinlen, L. (1990). "Factors Associated with Childhood Cancer in a National Cohort Study." *British Journal of Cancer 62*: 304-08.

Haire, D. (1985). "How the FDA Determines the 'Safety' of Drugs—Just How Safe is 'Safe'." National Women's Health Network.

———. (1987, Spring). "Drugs in Labor and Birth." *Childbirth Educator.*

Jacobson, B. et al. (1990). "Opiate Addiction in Adult Offspring through Possible Imprinting after Obstetric Treatment." *British Medical Journal 301*: 1067-70.

Kanto, I. & Erkkola, R. (1984). "Obstetric Analgesia, Pharmacokinetics and Its Relation to Neonatal Behavioral and Adaptive Functions." *Biological Research in Pregnancy 5*: 23-35.

Kuhnert, B. et al. (1985). "Disposition of Meperidine and Normeperidine following Multiple Doses during Labor: II Fetus and Neonate." *American Journal of Obstetrics and Gynecology 151*: 410-15.

MacArthur, C. et al. (1992). "Investigation of Long Term Problems after Obstetric Epidural Anaesthesia." *British Medical Journal 304*: 1279-82.

Morrison, J.C. et al. (1976). "Metabolites of Meperidine in the Fetal and Maternal Serum." *American Journal of Obstetrics and Gynecology 126*: 997-1002.

Nimmo, W., Wilson, J., & Prescott, L. (1975, Apr 19). "Narcotic Analgesics and Delayed Gastric Emptying during Labour." *Lancet*: 890-93.

Physician's Desk Reference. (1990). Oradell, NJ: Medical Economics Company, Inc.

Ralston, D. & Shnider, S. (1978). "The Fetal and Neonatal Effects of Regional Anesthesia in Obstetrics." *Anesthesiology 48*: 34-64.

Richard, L. and Alade, M. (1990). "Effect of Delivery Room Routines on Success of First Breast-Feed." *Lancet 336*: 1105-07.

Rosenblatt, D. et al. (1981). "The Influence of Maternal Analgesia on Neonatal Behavior: II Epidural Bupivacaine." *British Journal of Obstetrics and Gynecology 88*: 407-17.

Shnider, S. & Levinson, G. (1987). *Anesthesia for Obstetrics*. 2nd edition. Baltimore: Williams & Wilkens.

Studd, J. et al. (1980). "The Effect of Lumbar Epidural Anesthesia on the Rate of Cervical Dilatation and the Outcome of Labour of Spontaneous Outset." *British Journal of Obstetrics and Gynecology 87*: 1015-22.

Thorp, J. et al. (1989). "The Effect of Continuous Epidural Analgesia on Cesarean Section for Dystocia in Nulliparous Women." *American Journal of Obstetrics and Gynecology 161*: 670-75.

Zador, G., Lindmark, G., & Nielsson, B. (1974). "Pudendal Block in Normal Vaginal Deliveries." *Acta Gynecologic Obstetric Scandinavia Supplement 34*: 51-64.

OBSTETRICS, HISTORY OF

Medical customs differ from society to society because they are affected by the cultural context in which they develop. All societies have customs that guide labor and childbirth and that reflect, to some degree, the culturally patterned beliefs of the birth attendants (Eakins, 1986).

In the United States, birth has been defined as a medical-surgical event since the turn of the 20th century when male physicians (who, during the 18th and 19th centuries, were variously referred to as men-midwives, accoucheurs, and later, obstetricians) successfully gained control of childbirth from women-midwives. In so doing, physicians redefined childbirth from a natural state to a pathological condition requiring the intervention of surgeons and their instruments and set the pattern for modern aggressive obstetrical practices (Scully, 1980).

In the early 19th-century United States, the average woman gave birth at home attended by a woman-midwife. Organized medicine had little control over childbirth, although general practitioners, with little specific training, did conduct some home deliveries. Before about 1860, the time that anesthesia came into general use, women could obtain little relief for normal birth pain. In the small percentage of complicated deliveries (e.g., if the fetus lay in an abnormal position, obstructing birth, or if the pelvis was too narrow to permit passage of the fetus) childbirth could mean severe labor pain, even death, no matter who was in attendance. The cesarean section was not a solution for birth complications because the operation was fatal for women and therefore had been used for centuries as a method of delivering a child only after the death of the mother (Speert, 1973).

Seeking answers to such problems and focusing on the complications of childbirth, physicians were inventing and experimenting as early as the 18th-century with an array of instruments including perforators, used to reduce the size of the fetal head to allow passage through the pelvis; hooks and breaking and cutting devices, used to perform embryotomies in which the fetus was extracted in pieces (Gregory, 1974); and, later, the newly available Chamberlen forceps. The more surgery and instruments were used, the more necessary they seemed to become.

The encroachment of instrument-aided childbirth, referred to as "meddlesome midwifery," met with early resistance from such 18th-century midwives as Elizabeth Nihell, in her famous paper entitled, "A treatise on the Art of Midwifery, Setting Forth various Abuses therein, especially as to the Practice with Instruments, the whole serving to put all Rational Inquirers in a fair way of very safely forming their Own Judgement upon the Question which is best to employ in Cases of Pregnancy and Lying-In, a Man-Midwife or a Midwife" (Graham and Flack, 1960). Reflecting Victorian morality, some physicians also questioned male intervention in childbirth, believing that physical contact with female genitalia was an indiscretion both on the part of the physician and the woman who permitted it. Wertz and Wertz (1977) point out that the prohibition against exposure of the female body generated a number of unique modesty-preserving devices and retarded clinical training in obstetrics. Physicians' claims of improved care and better outcomes in complicated childbirth were also challenged. First, physicians possessed only crude skill with the newly developed obstetrical instruments, which frequently led to internal injuries, such as vesicovaginal fistula, or to death for the mother and fetus (Wertz and Wertz, 1977). Additionally, according to 18th- and 19th-century reports, instruments were often used unnecessarily for the sake of experimentation (Gregory, 1974).

By the turn of the 20th century, aggressive surgical techniques had become more acceptable as had the role of men in childbirth. However, the emerging profession had not yet demonstrated its ability to reduce maternal death. In fact, research revealed that the medical profession still lost at least as many women in childbirth as did women-midwives (Williams, 1912). Nonetheless, medical journals began to carry numerous articles charging that women-midwives were "hopelessly dirty, ignorant, and incompetent" (Edgar, 1911, p. 882) and were responsible for high rates of maternal death from puerperal sepsis (postpartum infection) (Korbin, 1966). Furthermore, many medical men believed that birth attendants had to be fully trained physicians and surgeons. As for female physicians: "It is needless to go on to prove this; it is obvious that we cannot instruct women as we do men, in the science of medicine" (Channing, 1947, p. 7).

It is ironic that physicians who were, at the time, incapable of reducing the mortality rate claimed that the elimination of women-midwives and the expansion of obstetrics constituted the solution to high infant mortality rates. Only a small faction believed the problem would be better handled by training and licensing women-midwives (Noyes, 1912). However, while the major impetus for the elimination of women-midwives was couched in terms of better care, the reason actually may have been economic (Emmons and Huntingdon, 1912). Not only was the volume of business for physicians decreased by women-midwives, but since midwives' clients were mostly poor and working-class women, the "material" with which to train new generations of obstetricians was diminished as well.

Part of the solution to the "midwife problem" was the establishment of large hospital-medical school complexes with obstetrics clinics and lying-in facilities. Early 20th-century hospitals were often overcrowded and intended largely for the poor and homeless. Although humanitarian concerns motivated some physicians, it was also true that hospitals for the poor provided a constant supply of clients who could be used for clinical observation, experimentation, and instruction. Thus, with one stroke, two objectives could be achieved. The need for women-midwives among the poor would be eliminated, and students would be provided with ample "material" on which to train (Korbin, 1966, p. 357).

Thus, as women-midwives were being systematically eliminated from the business of birth, childbirth was entering the machine age and the sterile, technologically oriented environment of American hospitals under the control of the medical profession. As middle-class women became persuaded that hospital deliveries were safer and less painful than home deliveries, birth came under the domination of new experts who not only perceived the process as problematic rather than natural, but who were also surgeons trained to intervene. Aggressive intervention became the norm in 20th-century obstetrics.

✱ DIANA SCULLY, Ph.D.

See also: Hospital Birth: An Anthropological Analysis of Ritual and Practice; Midwifery: Overview; Social Science Research on American Childbirth Practices

See **Guide to Related Topics:** Caregivers and Practitioners

Resources

Channing, Walter. (1974). "Remarks on the Employment of Females as Practitioners in Midwifery." (1820). In Charles Rosenberg and Carroll Smith-Rosenberg (Eds.) *The Male Mid-wife and the Female Doctor: The Gynecology Controversy in Nineteenth-Century America.* New York: Arno Press, pp. 3-22.

Eakins, Pamela. (1986). "The American Way of Birth." In Pamela Eakins (Ed.) *The American Way of Birth.* Philadelphia: Temple University Press, pp. 3-15.

Edgar, J. Clifton. (1911). "The Remedy for the Midwife Problem." *American Journal of Obstetrics 65*: 882.

Emmons, Arthur & Huntingdon, James. (1912). "The Midwife. Her Future in the United States." *American Journal of Obstetrics 65*: 393-403.

Graham, Harvey & Flack, Isaac. (1960). *Eternal Eve: The Mysteries of Birth and the Customs That Surround It.* London: Hulctinson Press.

Gregory, Samuel. (1974). "Man-midwifery Exposed and Corrected." (1848). In Charles Rosenberg and Carroll Smith-Rosenberg (Eds.) *The Male Mid-wife and the Female Doctor: The Gynecology Controversy in Nineteenth-Century America.* New York: Arno Press, pp. 7-50.

Korbin, Frances. (1966). "The American Midwife Controversy: A Crisis in Professionalization." *Bulletin of the History of Medicine 41*: 350-63.

Noyes, Clara. (1912). "Training of Midwives in Relation to the Prevention of Infant Mortality." *American Journal of Obstetrics 66*: 1056.

Scully, Diana. (1980). *Men Who Control Women's Health.* Boston: Houghton Mifflin Company.

Speert, Harold. (1973). *Iconographic Gyneatrica: A Pictorial History of Gynecology and Obstetrics.* Philadelphia: F.A. Davis.

Wertz, Richard W. & Wertz, Dorothy C. (1977). *Lying-in: A History of Childbirth in America.* New York: The Free Press.

Williams, J. Whitridge. (1912). "Medical Education and the Midwife Problem in the United States." *Journal of the American Medical Association 58*: 1-7.

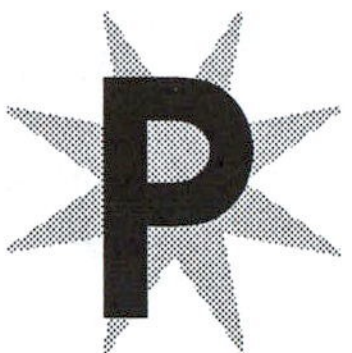

PAIN RELIEF IN LABOR: NONDRUG METHODS

Labor has always hurt, more or less. Throughout history women have employed many different methods to cope with labor pain. Even the stoic Greeks chewed willow bark (aspirin's predecessor) to ease the pain of birth. In pre-Victorian England, labor pain was considered the lot of womankind, a punishment for Eve's fall. British women suffered stoically through their labors until Queen Victoria set a new trend by getting whiffs of chloroform for the birth of her eighth child in 1853. Mothers in the Third World have traditionally employed various techniques to cope with labor pain. These methods range from native medicines to a host of nonpharmacologic aids.

In the early 20th century in the United States, a generation of educated women demanded and received twilight sleep. This medical concoction obliterated both labor pain and its memory, but drugged the babies as well as their mothers. The next generation of women sought out childbirth education to replace drugs during labor and promote active participation in the birth.

In its infancy, childbirth education emphasized primarily psychological methods of coping with labor pain—breathing and relaxation—and proclaimed that childbirth could or should be painless. For women who needed drugs or felt overwhelming pain, this approach induced needless guilt. Now, at middle age, childbirth education has finally begun to acknowledge the presence of pain in labor. At the same time, it has bolstered its traditional teachings with an array of auxiliary nonpharmacologic methods of pain relief. Derived from traditional birth practices, Oriental medicine, physical therapy, and generic pain management, these nondrug methods of coping with labor pain help minimize a woman's need for painkilling drugs during labor.

Nondrug methods of coping with labor can be divided into different categories, even though many of the methods work in more than one way to alleviate pain. Some techniques work primarily to alleviate fear of the unknown. That fear, according to Dr. Grantly Dick-Read (Dick-Read, 1944), produces the muscular tension that leads to labor pain. Other methods can actually alter a painful sensation. Practices such as massage work by substituting a different physical sensation for the sensation of pain. Techniques such as relaxation and patterned breathing restructure the message of pain psychologically by altering the brain's perception of pain.

Alleviating Fear of the Unknown. Learning about childbirth is the best way to combat fear. All over the world, women learn about childbirth by talking to women who have experienced it or by participating in home births. In the United States, where birth customarily takes place as a medical event in a hospital, many women supplement these discussions by reading books, watching movies, and attending childbirth classes.

Childbirth classes have been documented to result in less pain, less medication, a lower forceps rate, and a more positive attitude about birth among participants compared to nonparticipants (Cogan, 1980). Childbirth classes encourage the participation of a partner, usually the woman's husband, but sometimes a female friend, or "doula," in addition to or instead of the woman's mate. Research in Guatemala showed that women laboring with partners experienced shorter labors and significantly fewer complications such as fetal distress, oxytocin induction, and cesarean section (Sosa et al., 1980).

Altering the Sensation. One of the best methods to alter a painful sensation is to change positions, thereby altering relationships among gravity, the contractions, the baby, and the pelvis. Upright positions, standing, and walking all make labor more efficient and less painful. Indeed, a recent study showed that 80 women laboring in the hospital where they were free to move changed positions an average of 7.5 times during labor (Carlson et al., 1986).

However, freedom to change positions is frequently limited by typical obstetric procedures that require laboring women to be hooked up to IVs or electronic fetal monitors. A recent research report suggested that many such interventions, typically considered routine, cause stress and perhaps lead to unnecessary labor pain in a significant percentage of laboring mothers (Simkin, 1986). Reducing unnecessary medical interventions can contribute significantly to reducing labor pain.

Substituting a Different Physical Sensation. Massage, acupressure, transcutaneous electric nerve stimulation (TENS), water, warmth, or cold can all help to reduce labor pain by providing a competing sensation that blocks the perception of pain.

Different types of massage, from light fingertip stroking to firm kneading, activate touch receptors whose messages reach the brain more quickly than the message of pain. Firm pressure, especially against the low back, appears actually to reduce pain by slightly moving the sacrum. This counteracts the internal pressure from the baby's head.

Derived from traditional Oriental techniques, acupressure can be provided by the partner's or birth attendant's fingers at several key points to relieve pain or promote more efficient contractions. Acupressure points may also be stimulated by the application of transcutaneous electric nerve stimulation (TENS). TENS electrodes may be attached at the acupressure points to promote labor, or they can be placed on other points—usually in two pairs on either side of the spine at the waist and several inches below it. TENS provides a patient-controlled buzzing sensation that competes with labor pain. This relatively new method of pain relief has been employed by physical therapists to alleviate both chronic pain and acute postoperative pain (Mannheimer and Lampe, 1984).

In some hospitals, TENS may be offered to women who have had a cesarean section. A group of post-cesarean patients who used TENS needed significantly less Demerol and had shorter postpartum stays than the medicated control group (Hollinger, 1986). Although TENS is not yet widely used for labor in the United States, it is quite popular in Europe. TENS offers moderate to good pain relief for labor, produces no known side effects on the labor or the baby, and seems to be well accepted by mothers (Grim and Morey, 1985).

Water immersion for pain relief in labor became popular after the 1984 publication of Michel Odent's book, *Birth Reborn*. According to this French obstetrician, water diminishes the stress hormones, catecholamines, that slow labor down. Water may also permit a woman to enter a different, more instinctual, level of consciousness. Soaking in a tub or shower promotes relaxation and seems to make the contractions less painful.

Warmth, of course, has long been recognized as a simple, effective pain reliever, and it may be employed during labor in the form of baths, compresses, or heating pads. Some women prefer cold, which provides better relief for acute pain because it penetrates more deeply than heat. Ice packs can be used on the site of the pain, on the opposite side, or anywhere between pain and the brain.

Psychological Methods. Relaxation, breathing, biofeedback, imagery, and attention-focusing are all ways to change a pain message by altering one's response to it. Breathing and relaxation, of course, are the primary techniques learned in all prepared childbirth classes. Biofeedback, imagery, and attention-focusing can supplement and enhance the effects of breathing and relaxation.

Biofeedback—information about the body that can be used to improve health or comfort—may be learned using instruments such as an electrothermograph or electromyograph that register heat or muscle relaxation. A woman's birth partner may provide noninstrumental biofeedback in the form of verbal or touch cues that tell the woman whether or not she is relaxed (DiFranco, 1988).

Imagery can take the laboring woman's mind off pain or restructure the pain so that she perceives it positively. Or a woman may redirect her attention during labor by listening to music, chanting, looking at pictures, smelling a flower, or concentrating on breathing and relaxation (Lieberman, 1987).

Although pain exists in childbirth, many women prefer to cope with it by using their own resources, thereby minimizing reliance on pain-killing drugs. Combining several effective non-drug methods, a new mother can achieve the unique sense of mastery that comes from actively participating in the powerful experience of birth.

✱ ADRIENNE B. LIEBERMAN

See also: Bradley Method: Husband-Coached Childbirth; Breath Control in Labor; Epidural Anesthesia; Labor: Overview; Obstetric Drugs: Their Effects on Mother and Infant; Psychoprophylactic Method (Lamaze); Read Method: Natural Childbirth; Twilight Sleep

See **Guide to Related Topics:** Childbirth Practices and Locations

Resources

Carlson, Jerold M. et al. (1986). "Maternal Positioning during Parturition in Normal Labor." *Obstetrics and Gynecology 68*: 443.

Cogan, Rosemary. (1980). "Effects of Childbirth Preparation." *Clinical Obstetrics and Gynecology 23*: 1.

Dick-Read, Grantly. (1944). *Childbirth without Fear*. New York; London: Harper and Brothers.

DiFranco, Joyce. (1988). "Relaxation: Biofeedback." In Francine H. Nichols and Sharron Smith Humenick (Eds.) *Childbirth Education: Practice, Research, and Theory*. Philadelphia: W.B. Saunders Company, Chapter 9.

Grim, Louise C. & Morey, Susan H. (1985). "TENS for Relief of Parturition Pain: A Clinical Report." *Physical Therapy 65*: 1363.

Hollinger, Jan L. (1986). "Transcutaneous Electrical Nerve Stimulation After Cesarean Birth." *Physical Therapy 66*: 36.

Lieberman, Adrienne B. (1987). *Easing Labor Pain*. New York: Doubleday.

Mannheimer, Jeffrey S. & Lampe, Gerald N. (1984). *Clinical Transcutaneous Electric Nerve Stimulation*. Philadelphia: F.A. Davis Company.

Odent, Michel. (1984). *Birth Reborn*. New York: Random House.

Simkin, Penny. (1986). "Pain, Stress, and Catecholamines in Labor." *Birth 15*: 227.

Sosa, Roberto et al. (1980). "The Effect of a Supportive Companion on Perinatal Problems, Length of Labor, and Mother-Infant Interaction." *New England Journal of Medicine 303*: 597.

PATRESCENCE. *See instead* MATRESCENCE AND PATRESCENCE

PEDIATRICS, HISTORY OF

Although the ancient Greeks coined the word "pediatrics" to mean "child," their benign and devalued attitudes toward children reflected those of all classical antiquity, and this attitude continued through to the mid-19th century. For 14 centuries the specification of knowledge and techniques for the care and cure of the child in an organized manner in medicine did not exist.

The cultural idea and ideal of "the child" at any particular point in history had much to do with the acceptability and legitimacy of treating or caring for the child, especially the sick child. Thus, the sociocultural and physical care of children in the English colonies in the early 17th century parodied the European fatalism and the devaluation of the child as noted in European medical literature (Ruhrah, 1925). It was not until the end of the 18th century that the value of children began to be appreciated. Because of the European roots of American pediatrics, much of the embryonic American pediatrics paralleled a variety of remedies and anecdotal treatments used in Europe against the formidable diseases of infancy and childhood (Caulfield, 1951). The scarcity of physicians in the New World resulted in the care of children left primarily and traditionally in the hands of parents, midwives, and wet nurses. Part-time pediatrics was practiced by the clergy and political leaders. Governor John Winthrop, Jr., of Connecticut practiced extensively through colonial mails, describing such problems as rashes, jaundice, seizures, and diarrhea, and was the first to document a description of child abuse. However, most healers, including nonphysicians as well as European-trained physicians, were poorly prepared to deal with the pediatric ailments of the time:

> In addition to diphtheria, dysentery, measles and scarlet fever, smallpox influenza and tuberculosis should certainly be included in the list of common diseases of colonial children. A surprisingly large proportion of them had worms. Death from falls, burns, and poisonings were frequent. It seems a little surprising that any of them survived. (Caulfield, 1951)

Despite the formation of medical schools in the United States as early as 1765, little, if any teaching of the diseases of children took place. The earliest "professor" who published and lectured on children's diseases, including spasmodic asthma, diphtheria, and diseases of the mind, and who coined the term *cholera infantum*, was Dr. Benjamin Rush. In addition to acting as a signer of the Declaration of Independence, he practiced massive and frequent phlebotomy or "bleedings" as his major treatment.

The first formal textbook of pediatrics, *A Treatise on the Physical and Medical Treatment of Children*, was written by Dr. William Potts Dewees and published in 1825. For 40 years, between 1813 and 1852, Dr. Eli Ives of Yale Medical School lectured and received the first faculty appointment in pediatrics in the country. Although Dr. Ives used phlebotomy "sparingly" (Buford, 1991) he subscribed to Dr. Benjamin Rush's theories that all diseases were "fevers" and had to be treated by "depletion therapies" (bloodletting, vomiting, or purging).

Very few documented remedies specifically addressing the diseases of infancy and childhood existed, and high mortality rates, especially among infants, were accepted as universal both in Europe and the United States. Between 1820 and 1900 the mortality rates in the United States were as high as one quarter (25 percent) of all children under five years of age. These mortality rates and high rates of intestinal infections and infectious diseases were attributed to the Industrial Revolution, with its dire living and working conditions, especially for children. It was common knowledge that infants in particular had a predisposition to illness, and for some, disease was considered part of a process of moral regeneration.

Public concern and an age of reformism followed as a reaction to the inhumane conditions of rapid urbanization and industrialization. On its coattails came an intense activism, and beginning unionism, which created the "child saving movement." It was this movement that was responsible for child labor laws; compulsory education; and health, welfare, and criminal reforms.

The mid-19th century also signaled the growth of pediatrics as a specialty. The number of physicians primarily treating children grew from an initial 50 in 1850 to over 1,700 in 1934. The Children's Hospital of Pennsylvania, opened in 1855, was the first in the United States, followed by the Boston Children's Hospital in 1869. Dr. Abraham Jacobi, the "Father of American Pediatrics," established a number of children's clinics in New York hospitals in the 1860s and held the first academic appointment in the United States. Soon medical schools established curricula in pediatrics and hospitals offered residencies. Other factors in establishing the specialty of pediatrics included the formation of a number of pediatric medical societies, the first being the American Medical Association's (AMA) Section of Diseases of Children in 1879, and followed by The American Pediatric Society in 1888.

The height of consolidation of pediatrics as a specialty took place between 1880 and 1935 with more associations formed, wider inclusion of pediatrics in medical school education, and an increase in physicians practicing pediatrics as a specialty. However, as pediatrics grew during this period, the irony is that the children needing pediatric care dwindled. Infant and child mortality rates dropped dramatically through the positive effect of the successful child and labor reform movements, improved living conditions, and the public health movement (including sanitation reform, and in particular, attention to removing the cause of polluted water and contaminated food and milk). Another major factor was that immunology as a field was established by Pasteur; from that research, many vaccines for child-killing diseases were made available. Concurrently, work on nutrition research (with the discovery of vitamins in 1912) and more focus on maternal nutrition and health contributed to the all-around eradication of many of the diseases brought on by the poor conditions of the Industrial Revolution.

Pediatric physicians tended to support these types of social and health reforms but primarily concentrated on single pragmatic issues such as the question of artificial feeding for infants. Up to 90 percent of childhood deaths due to intestinal infections occurred among bottle-fed children, for up until the 1930s the relationship between milk and disease remained unclear. Pediatricians worked so frequently with adjusting formulas on complicated mathematical schemes that they became known as "baby feeders."

With success in pasteurization of milk and cleaner methods of transporting, packaging, marketing, and handling milk, the infant and child mortality and disease rate dropped and the demand for pediatric specialists decreased. The major competitor of the pediatrician became the primary care practitioner. In order to maintain an adequate market share in light of scarce resources (sick children) and tough competition (primary care physicians), pediatricians set out to redefine their market. Their focus on the sick child widened to the total well-being, growth, and development (both physically and behaviorally) of the child. In this way the pediatrician's role in assisting the child to reach optimum capacity and full potential, and even to help plan for unmet needs, was legitimized. An arena called the "new pediatrics" emerged with up to 85 percent of pediatricians' practices focused on preventive psychological or emotional care.

Questions for the future remain as to the nature of pediatrics as a specialty due to changing sociocultural conditions favoring primary and managed care from allied health personnel and primary care physicians.

✱ MARGARETE YARD, R.N., M.P.H.

See also: Baby Diaries: The History of Child Development; Breastfeeding: Historical Aspects; Infant Feeding and Care: Nineteenth and Twentieth Centuries, United States; Spock, Dr. Benjamin

See **Guide to Related Topics:** Baby Care; Caregivers and Practitioners

Resources

Buford, Nichols. (1991). *History of Pediatrics.* New York: Raven Press, p. 59.

Caulfield, E. (1951). "Some Common Diseases of Colonial Children." Translation. *Colonial Society of Massachusetts 35*: 4-13.

Ruhrah, J. (1925). *Pediatrics of the Past: An Anthology.* New York: Hoeber.

PELVIC INFLAMMATORY DISEASE

The leading cause of infertility and ectopic pregnancy, pelvic inflammatory disease (PID) is inflammation of the internal pelvic organs—uterus, Fallopian tubes, ovaries, and/or pelvic cavity. One episode of PID raises, by 15 percent, the chance of infertility; three episodes raises it by 75 percent. Symptoms include fever, cramps, thick cervical discharges, and/or abdominal pain or tenderness. Yet PID is usually difficult to diagnose and may even cause infertility without any overt symptoms.

Chlamydia bacteria cause most PID infections; gonorrhea bacteria can also cause this infection. Staphylococcus and streptococcus infections are sometimes involved. Bacteria enter the pelvic organs from the vagina, via the cervix, and may be carried on sperm, on an IUD, or may be introduced during an intrauterine procedure such as a D&C, an abortion, or an infertility diagnosis and treatment procedure. The scars after PID may prevent a uterus from holding a fetus, Fallopian tubes from allowing smooth passage to a fertilized egg, or an ovary from releasing eggs. Although the correct antibiotic can kill the offending bacteria, it cannot repair the scars. The extent of scarring can often be determined by laparoscopy; some repair can be done via the laparoscope.

To prevent PID, women should avoid using IUDs; a condom will protect against chlamydia and gonorrhea. A woman who has had pelvic surgery, an abortion, or an intrauterine diagnostic test should be tested for bacterial infection three months later. ✷ HELEN BEQUAERT HOLMES, Ph.D.

See also: Ectopic Pregnancy; Sexually Transmitted Diseases

See **Guide to Related Topics:** Infertility

Resources

Bellina, Joseph H. & Wilson, Josleen. (1985). *You Can Have a Baby: Everything You Need to Know about Fertility.* New York: Crown Publishers, Inc.

Berger, Gary S., Goldstein, Marc, & Fuerst, Mark. (1989). *The Couple's Guide to Fertility: How New Medical Advances Can Help You Have a Baby.* New York: Doubleday.

PELVIC MUSCLES

The pelvic muscles are a group of muscles that support the uterus, vaginal, urethral, and rectal structures and, like other muscles, have the capacity for contraction and relaxation. During childbirth these muscles aid the movement of the baby downward and forward along the birth canal (Oxorn, 1986). These muscles may be stressed during childbirth beyond their limit, resulting in genital prolapse. Genital prolapse may manifest itself in uterine prolapse (descension of the uterus), cystocele (prolapse of the anterior vaginal wall and bladder into the vagina), and rectocele (herniation of the rectum and posterior vaginal wall into the vagina). Any of these conditions are found in varying degrees of severity and combinations (Zacharin, 1985). The symptoms associated with genital prolapse are stress urinary incontinence (SUI), pelvic heaviness, backache, a bearing-down sensation, and pain with intercourse.

Despite the controversy that surrounds its efficacy as a prophylactic measure in prevention of prolapse (Thorp and Bowes, 1989; Cosner, Dougherty, and Bishop, 1991), episiotomy became a routine procedure in the 1920s (DeLee, 1920; Gainey, 1943, 1955) and continues to be a routine procedure today. Beynon (1957) proposed that pelvic relaxation may be prevented if women were allowed to push during second-stage labor as they felt the urge rather than when commanded. This would result in less stress on the structures that support the pelvic organs. Beynon used the analogy of a coat sleeve that is lined loosely. If one puts the coat on rapidly, the lining will slip out with the arm, but if the arm is put in slowly, the lining will have less tendency to roll out. Her research supported the claim that forced pushing was also associated with greater perineal trauma.

Kegel (1948) addressed pelvic muscle relaxation and included women who had never been pregnant and some who had delivered by cesarean section. Instructions for the "kegel exercise," which involves contraction of the pelvic muscles, have been altered (Sampselle and Brink, 1990) and are recommended to all women to prevent and improve prolapse and SUI and to enhance sexual sensations. The pelvic muscle exercise consists of contracting the pelvic muscles for five to 10 seconds at a time and working up to 80 tightenings a day.

Prolapse and SUI may be attributed to childbirth, but one cannot ignore the existence of multiple factors (Schrag, 1979). Prenatal muscle function, genetic maternal tissue, nutrition, exercise, and such obstetrical factors as baby weight, length of second-stage labor, maternal positions during labor and delivery, pushing technique, episiotomy, and perineal outcome must all be considered. Postpartum exercise may enhance pelvic muscle function (Henderson, 1983; Gordon and Logue, 1985; Dougherty et al., 1988).

The goals of obstetricians and midwives include the implementation of practices that research has demonstrated to prevent or improve genital prolapse and the avoidance of practices that research has indicated may aggravate this condition. However, this subject continues to be controversial in obstetrics today, and more research is needed to clarify the causes, prevention, and correction of genital prolapse.

✷ KAREN COSNER, M.S.N., C.N.M.

See also: Bodywork; Episiotomy

See **Guide to Related Topics:** Pregnancy, Physical Aspects

Resources

Beynon, C. (1957). "The Normal Second Stage of Labor: A Plea for Reform in Its Conduct." *Journal of Obstetrics and Gynecology of the British Empire* 64: 815-20.

Cosner, K.R., Dougherty, M., & Bishop, K.R. (1991). "The Dynamic Characteristics of the Circumvaginal Muscles (CVM) during Pregnancy and the Postpartum." *Journal of Nurse-Midwifery 36*: 4.

DeLee, J.B. (1920). "The Prophylactic Forceps Operation." *American Journal of Obstetrics and Gynecology 1*: 34-44.

Dougherty, M.C. et al. (1988). "The Effect of Exercise on the Circumvaginal Muscles (CVM) in Postpartum Women." *Journal of Nurse-Midwifery 34* (1): 8-14.

Gainey, H.L. (1943). "Postpartum Observation of Pelvic Tissue Damage." *American Journal of Obstetrics and Gynecology 45*: 457-66.

———. (1955). "Postpartum Observation of Pelvic Tissue Damage: Further Studies." *American Journal of Obstetrics and Gynecology 70*: 800-09.

Gordon, H. & Logue, M. (1985). "Perineal Muscle Function after Childbirth." *Lancet:* 123-25.

Henderson, J.A. (1983). "Effects of a Prenatal Teaching Program on Postpartum Regeneration of the Pubococcygeus Muscle." *Journal of Obstetric, Gynecologic and Neonatal Nursing* 12: 403-08.

Kegel, A.H. (1948). "Progressive Resistance Exercise in the Functional Restoration of the Perineal Muscles." *American Journal of Obstetrics and Gynecology 56*: 238-48.

Oxorn, H. (1986). *Human Labor and Birth.* 5th edition. Norwalk, CT: Appleton-Century-Croft.

Sampselle, C.M. & Brink, C.A. (1990). "Pelvic Muscle Relaxation Assessment and Management." *Journal of Nurse-Midwifery 35*: 127-32.

Schrag, K. (1979). "Maintenance of Pelvic Floor Integrity during Childbirth." *Journal of Nurse-Midwifery 24*: 26-31.

Thorp, J.M. & Bowes, W.A. (1989). "Episiotomy: Can Its Routine Use Be Defended?" *American Journal of Obstetrics and Gynecology 160* (1): 1027-30.

Zacharin, R.F. (1985). *Pelvic Floor Anatomy and the Surgery of Pulsion Enterocele.* New York: Springor-Verlag.

THE PERFECT BABY

The "perfect baby" has become a popular catchword. It reflects growing scientific and technological capabilities to locate genetic or other conditions before birth, and to select and possibly alter the embryo or fetus. Several hundred conditions—with numbers growing rapidly—can be detected through carrier screening and prenatal diagnosis. When chosen, selective abortion can prevent the birth of an "imperfect" baby. Fetal surgery, still rare and limited to life-threatening situations, can correct conditions prior to birth. The fastest growing area of research, which also affects prenatal diagnosis, is DNA analysis to locate genes for single-gene disorders. When combined with projects to map and sequence all human genes, DNA research, applied to human embryos or gametes, could provide the means to select or alter the genetic makeup at the early or pre-embryo stage.

Discussion arises over whether the elements are in place for creating the perfect baby. The idea of human perfectibility has a long history in Western thought. It found secular and scientific expression in the perfectibility of man of the Enlightenment, in the ideology of progress, and finally in the racist, selective breeding programs of the eugenics movement. Even though eugenicist excesses were discredited, belief in human progress and improvement, to be achieved through science, remains an article of faith. By the mid-20th century, urban middle-class parents had come to see their children as an "emotional investment," cultural values and economics combining to sharply reduce family size. The recent trend in delayed childbearing has further upped the value of that "investment." In the medical profession, preventive medicine and response to demands for patient autonomy have become integral to the broader medical goals of treating disease and alleviating suffering. The social climate in which parents and medical professionals make decisions finds the birth of a disabled child a "terrible burden," even a "tragedy," although disabled persons are increasingly challenging this climate. The social and political economy puts a premium on the productive, the beautiful, and the successful, sustaining the idea of the child as an "improved product." Popularization of DNA research heightens attention to genes—"good" and "bad"—putting a further premium on inheritance.

Such factors serve to underwrite and support the new reproductive technologies and the perfect baby ideal. Concerns grow over a "new eugenics" or the custom-designing of a child. Since most human traits are caused by multiple factors or genes in constantly changing environments at every stage of development, that level of genetic manipulation may be a long way off. More immediate are the possible consequences from selective access to and use of these new technologies, especially of prenatal diagnosis. Among white middle-class parents—who are the highest users of such technologies—most abort when the test result is positive (Rothman, 1986). Many poorer parents, of those who do undergo testing, do not abort. As the number of "imperfect" babies declines among the privileged classes and clusters among the poor and families of color, a new health hierarchy of birth may emerge. Stigma for such children might increase, social services and facilities will be further reduced, and the association of poverty and minority race with mental and physical disability will be reinforced. The perfect baby becomes white, middle-class, male if firstborn, gifted and intelligent, and as defect-free as medicine and the ability to pay can provide.

As these class, race, and disability issues are raised, reproductive rights come under attack. While supporting every woman's right to choose, feminists show how choices are structured, questioning the perfect baby ideal itself, its social context, and its consequences.

✱ JOAN ROTHSCHILD, Ph.D.

See also: Amniocentesis, History of; Eugenics; Genetics; Genome Mapping; Selective Abortion; Wrongful Birth and Wrongful Life

***See* Guide to Related Topics:** Prenatal Diagnosis and Screening

Resources

Arditti, Rita, Klein, Renate Duelli, & Minden, Shelley. (Eds.) (1984). *Test-tube Women: What Future for Motherhood?* Boston: Pandora Press.

Holmes, Helen B., Hoskins, Betty B., & Gross, Michael. (Eds.) (1981). *The Custom-made Child? Women-centered Perspectives.* Clifton, NJ: Humana Press.

Hubbard, Ruth. (1986). "Eugenics and Prenatal Testing." *International Journal of Health Services 16* (2): 227-42.

Kevles, Daniel J. (1985). *In the Name of Eugenics.* New York: Alfred A. Knopf.

Rothman, Barbara Katz. (1986). *The Tentative Pregnancy.* New York: Viking.

Rothschild, Joan. (1989). "Engineering Birth: Toward the Perfectibility of *Man?*" In Steven L. Goldman (Ed.) *Science, Technology, and Social Progress.* Bethlehem, PA: Lehigh University Press, pp. 93-120.

———. (1992). *Engineering Birth.* Bloomington, IN: Indiana University Press.

Wertz, Richard W. & Wertz, Dorothy C. (1989). *Lying-in: A History of Childbirth in America.* Expanded edition. New Haven, CT: Yale University Press, Chapter 8.

PERINEAL MASSAGE, PRENATAL

Prenatal perineal massage is a procedure taught by some childbirth caregivers and considered a method to help stretch the woman's vagina and condition the perineum (area between the vagina and the rectum) prior to vaginal birth. It is thought to soften the tissues around the vagina, increase perineal elasticity, and help relax the pelvic floor muscles against pressure during vaginal birth. This massage is practiced daily for five minutes during the last six weeks of pregnancy. Evidence suggests that improved perineal tissue conditioning may reduce the need for episiotomy and laceration incidence (Avery and Burket, 1986; Avery and Van Arsdale, 1987; Mynaugh, 1988). The necessity of episiotomy is even now being questioned (Thorp and Bowes, 1989).

The massage technique involves the woman inserting her thumbs into her vagina and pressing downward to the rectum and then moving her thumbs up and out to the sides. The woman stretches this tissue for a couple of minutes. Then, with one thumb in the vagina, she presses down to the rectum and squeezes, massages, or kneads the tissue in the perineal area between her thumb (inside) and her index finger (outside). This is also done for a couple of minutes. The combined massage time takes five minutes. The woman's partner may perform the massage by inserting both index fingers into her vagina up to the second knuckle and performing the massage just as she did. A vegetable oil or vitamin E oil on the fingers or thumbs provides lubrication for the woman's tissues.

Brendsel, Peterson, and Mehl (1979, 1980), Schrag (1979), Stiles (1980), and Stewart and Clark (1982) advocated perineal massage in the professional literature as preparation for vaginal birth. Avery and Burket (1986) and Avery and Van Arsdale (1987) reported that women delivered by nurse-midwives had statistically significant lower episiotomy and laceration rates when they massaged than did women who had not massaged.

In Mynaugh (1988), results show significantly lower rates of perineal lacerations in massagers (p = .037) than in nonmassagers. The decision for episiotomy for vaginal birth was left to the physicians of the women under study, so assessment of massage effects on episiotomy rates could not be done here. There was also evidence to suggest that perineal massage decreases the chances of combined episiotomy and lacerations in massagers compared with nonmassagers ($p = .036$). Risk factor analysis demonstrated that women who do not practice perineal massage have almost two-and-a-half times the risk for developing perineal lacerations than do massagers. With the research presented above, the data suggest that prenatal perineal massage significantly reduces trauma to the tissues during vaginal birth.

✱ PATRICIA MYNAUGH, R.N., Ph.D.

See also: Episiotomy

See **Guide to Related Topics:** Pregnancy, Physical Aspects

Resources

Avery, Melissa D. & Burket, Barbara A. (1986). "Effect of Perineal Massage on the Incidence of Episiotomy and Perineal Laceration in a Nurse-Midwifery Service." *Journal of Nurse-Midwifery 31* (3): 128-34.

Avery, Melissa D. & Van Arsdale, Laura. (1987). "Perineal Massage: Effect on the Incidence of Episiotomy and Laceration in a Nulliparous Population." *Journal of Nurse-Midwifery 32* (3): 181-84.

Brendsel, Carol, Peterson, Gail, & Mehl, Lewis E. (1979). "Episiotomy: Facts, Fictions, Figures, and Alternatives." In D. Stewart and L. Stewart (Eds.) *Compulsory Hospitalization or Freedom of Choice in Childbirth?* Marble Hill, MO: NAPSAC Reproductions, pp. 169-75.

———. (1980). "Routine Episiotomy and Pelvic Symptomatology." *Women & Health 5* (4): 49-60.

Mynaugh, Patricia A. (1988). "The Effectiveness of Prenatal Health Practices and Two Instructional Educational Methods on Labor and Delivery: A Case Study of Perineal Massage." *Dissertation Abstracts International*, #8902979. Ann Arbor, MI: University Microfilms Inc.

Schrag, Kathryn. (1979). "Maintenance of Pelvic Floor Integrity during Childbirth." *Journal of Nurse-Midwifery 24* (6): 26-31.

Stewart, Richard B. & Clark, Linda. (1982). "Nurse-Midwifery Practice in an In-Hospital Birthing Center: 2050." *Journal of Nurse-Midwifery 27* (3): 21-26.

Stiles, Donna. (1980). "Techniques for Reducing the Need for an Episiotomy." *Issues in Health Care of Women 2*: 105-11.

Thorp, John M., Jr. & Bowes, Watson A., Jr. (1989). "Episiotomy: Can Its Routine Use Be Defended?" *American Journal of Obstetrics & Gynecology 160:* 1027-30.

PHOTOGRAPHY AND BIRTH

The ancient drama of women giving birth and babies being born is the profound experience by which every human being comes into this world. Images of this primal reality are among the earliest of artwork. Details of pregnancy, labor, and birth have been inscribed on cave walls, sculptured in bowls and ceremonial objects, woven within fabric, and carved on stone and clay since the beginning of human history. This art is both descriptive and reverent of birth.

Photography is a present-day clay tablet, a means to record what people want to see, know, and remember. The process of childbirth in its beauty, mystery, and power is a natural focus for camera and film.

> "That's me! That's me!" a three-year-old girl says excitedly as she points to her head in a photograph, coming out of her mother's body.
>
> "I can't wait to see the photographs! When will they be ready?" a mother asks, holding her baby, newly born and moist from birth. "I want to see what I did, what I was like."
>
> "I fell in love with my husband all over again when I saw him in the photographs caring for me during labor."

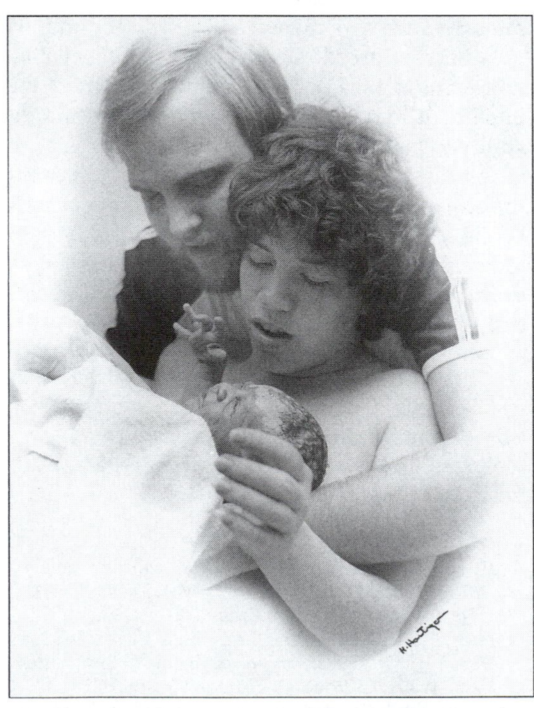

Birth portrait. Photo courtesy of Harriette Hartigan/ Artemis.

"I've changed so much already," a new mother sighs softly and with awe as she looks at the photographs of herself in labor and birth a few weeks earlier.

"I look at the pictures of my son's birth every day," a woman says months after her son's birth day.

"My friends all had tears in their eyes after looking at my birth photographs."

Photographs give witness. They make visible the details and nuances of what is lived. They attest to and authenticate, Roland Barthes wrote, what actually existed (Barthes, 1981). Photographs are visual memory, continuing beyond the experiences photographed.

Childbirth is a vast and passionate effort. Physically it requires one human being to open her body to another. Emotionally, great courage, strength, and compassion are demanded. Spiritually, woman becomes the very passage for human life to come to earth. For each of us,the journey from womb to the world is the intimate process of our own being.

A woman's body is sculptured in pregnancy by the alchemy of matter and spirit forming new life.

A mother's expression is intense with bravery as contraction after contraction pressures her body.

Looking into the eyes of the loved one, a mate gives reassurance as labor continues on for hours.

Children, open and curious to the ways of their own births, share in the family experience of a sibling being born.

The midwife's touch reaches deep into the birthing woman's back, bringing comfort for the pain that marks movement of the baby into the birth canal.

Still edged between eternity and birth, the baby's head is born and the body is as yet embraced by the woman's own body.

The faces of newborns are each of us entering this life with the masks of birth. Our color has no equivalent, the stillness is deep.

A mother embraces her child for the first time outside her body. The baby searches the mother's face with eyes so seeing they look from the beginning.

Holding his child's fresh soft body against his own flesh, a father cries with love beyond words.

Grandparents feel the continuity of time and generations as they snuggle their grandchild close to their hearts.

This is the realm of birth photography.

The experience of giving birth and being born creates the language's deepest metaphors. The emotional efforts and physical work demand the far reaches of human potential. Awareness of death and mortality is an archetypal presence. The very intimacy of personal relationship is embodied in two lives, woman and fetus, together yet separate. First breath, required of each new life, is the imperative of existence. Such riches of human reality are visible through the lens.

But camera and lens cannot see these dimensions. It is the consciousness of the human heart and spirit that brings the nature of birth to film. As a process, childbirth is a continuing flow of many moments. The vision of insight seeks and searches the moments to photograph.

Photographing is an act of relationship. Photographing childbirth is a personal and intimate relationship with birthing mother and babe, and often other family members and attendants. Each birth is unique. There is a responsibility to be accurate. The original Latin meaning of the word "accurate" is "to take care." Photographing accurately encompasses caring for those with whom one is in relationship, and for the images created. Sensitive attention to the emotions and needs of the people being photographed and to the details of the birthing experience is essential. There are moments when not photographing is the best of care.

Birth photographs have personal value and social significance. Women and their families look again and again, remembering and understanding more fully what they have lived. Birth, even when labor is long, is over quickly, often too quickly to integrate the massive amount of emotions and sensations. Photographs confirm what was experienced. They hold a moment of time still so one may look and feel back to what was. Susan Sontag has written, "Each still photograph is a privileged moment, turned into a slim object that one can keep and look at again" (Sontag, 1977). Images that give viewers a sense of themselves in relation to the moments photographed have meaning beyond the information revealed.

Birth photographs are part of the visual vocabulary of a culture, personal as well as public.

According to the dictionary, public means "belonging to or concerning the people as a whole." Such is birth, the public experience that each one who has been born shares. Photography makes birth visible to the public eye.

"There was a child went forth," said Walt Whitman. What he or she saw, "these things became part of that child." Birth photography shows the love and courage of women giving birth, emotions of fathers deeply caring, and the joy of families celebrating new life. Adults and children see themselves in the eyes of a babe's first sight, the newborns they once were. Keeping birth in sight is as significant for people today as it was for their earliest ancestors. ✱ HARRIETTE HARTIGAN

See **Guide to Related Topics:** Literature and the Arts

Resources

Arms, Suzanne. (1978). *Five Women/Five Births*. Ann Arbor, MI: IH/IBP.

Barthes, Roland. (1981). *Camera Lucida*. New York: Hill and Wang.

Hartigan, Harriette. (1986). "Photographing Birth." *International Journal of Childbirth Education* 1 (3): 16.

———. (1989). *The Birth Disc: A Visual Experience*. Stamford, CT: Artemis.

Sontag, Susan. (1977). *On Photography*. New York: Farrar, Straus and Giroux.

Whitman, Walt. (1924). *Leaves of Grass*. Garden City, NY: Doubleday & Company, Inc.

PHOTOTHERAPY. *See instead* JAUNDICE, NEWBORN

PID. *See instead* PELVIC INFLAMMATORY DISEASE

THE PILL

The Pill was a brainchild of Margaret Sanger, founder of Planned Parenthood, popularizer of the diaphragm, and an indomitable fighter for women's rights. In 1950, when she was nearing 90, Sanger raised some $150,000 for research on a "universal" contraceptive.

Oral contraceptives were not originally intended for educated women in developed countries who, in fact, became the principal users. This is evidenced in a fundraising letter by Sanger who, for all her great works, was a bit of an elitist:

> I consider that the world and almost all our civilization for the next 25 years is going to depend upon a simple, cheap, safe contraceptive to be used in poverty-stricken slums and jungles, and among the most ignorant people... I believe that now, immediately, there should be national sterilization for certain dysgenic types of our population who are being encouraged to breed and would die out were the government not feeding them. (Vaughan, 1970)

This concern for controlling world population allowed the Pill (and the IUD) to enjoy a "diplomatic immunity" from careful scientific scrutiny of potential short- or long-term side effects for their first decade of widespread use.

When Enovid®, manufactured by the G.D. Searle pharmaceutical company, was approved as a contraceptive in 1960, the public was led to believe it had been tested on thousands of women in Puerto Rico. In truth, as a Senate investigation revealed in 1963, the U.S. Food and Drug Administration's decision to approve Enovid was based on clinical studies of only 132 women who had taken it continuously for a year or longer. Three young women died but no autopsies were conducted, leaving unanswered many questions about the Pill's safety.

Proponents of the Pill argued that any drug must be in widespread use before all of the possible side effects can be tallied. While these arguments have merit, the Pill was nevertheless a special case for several reasons:

- With the contraceptive Pill, for the first time in pharmaceutical history a powerful drug was being recommended for normal, healthy women.
- The Pill was for continuous, long-term use, not just for a few days or weeks, like most such potent medicines.
- Estrogen was known to be carcinogenic, so the original researchers sought to use only progestin. Soon, however, estrogen was discovered to be necessary for adequate contraception. When it was incorporated into the Pill, the issue of carcinogenicity was suddenly dropped.
- The questions of pituitary suppression and metabolic effects from ingesting sex hormones were of grave concern to reproductive scientists, many of whom demanded more research and clinical trials before allowing widespread public use. Unlike most drugs, which have narrower effects, contraceptive steroids alter every organ and system in the body.

Thus, of all new drugs, the Pill should have been *more* thoroughly pretested than others, but it was not. So crude were the initial trials that appropriate dosage was not even established. It was discovered only after millions of women had taken Enovid that the amount of estrogen in the Pill was 10 times as high as is usually necessary for contraception. The dosages today are a great deal lower—a fraction of what they were—but discomforts and dangerous side effects still remain a concern.

The Pill and Liberation. Writer Clare Booth Luce made a fine metaphoric point when, in 1969, she stated that with the Pill, "modern woman is at last free, as a man is free, to dispose of her own body, to earn her living, to pursue the improvement of her mind, to try a successful career." Like many liberal Catholics, Luce hoped the Pope would give his blessing to the Pill because it was "natural" and "physiologic." He did not. Certainly the idea or ideal of the Pill encouraged countless women to aspire toward personal and sexual liberation. Alas, the reality of the Pill fell short and continues to fall short as two women out of three experience side effects that lead them to discontinue using it within two years. Most ironic, the present epidemic of sexually transmitted diseases (STDs) and consequent pelvic inflammatory disease (PID) inspired the Centers for Disease Control of the U.S. Department of Health and Human Services to issue a new recommendation in 1991: "Use barrier methods. Use condoms, diaphragms, and/or vaginal spermicides for protection against STD, even if contraception is not needed." (One million U.S. women experience PID each year; 50 percent become sterile after three episodes, 12 percent after just one.) Thus, Pill users who wish to preserve their pelvic health and their fertility are now advised by public health authorities to employ barriers *in addition to* oral contraceptives. And so, while the Pill had the positive effect of increasing women's aspirations, the overpromotion of it as safe, simple, and suitable for all women led men to abandon the condom, clinics to stop stocking barriers, and STDs to revive and spread.

For almost a decade, the frequent and sometimes-lethal side effects of the initial high-dose birth control pills were generally swept under the carpet and denied. Manufacturers and eminent physicians, including the Pill's co-developer, Dr. John Rock of Harvard, repeatedly insisted that the contraceptive was natural, physiologic, and safe. The publication in 1969 of two books by science writers whose 'beat' had included the Pill (Morton Mintz at the *Washington Post* and this author, then a columnist and contributing editor at *Ladies Home Journal*), triggered a Senate investigation conducted by Gaylord Nelson of Wisconsin and his staff assistant Ben Gordon. The investigation sparked repeated media-attracting feminist demonstrations organized by Alice Wolfson (a founder of the National Women's Health Network). Only these events embarrassed the FDA and manufacturers into getting serious about (a) warning consumers, and (b) lowering dosages to make the Pill less toxic. In 1991 and 1992, Americans witnessed an eerie kind of replay of the 1969 to 1970 birth control pill scandal in the form of a feminist campaign to expose the dangers of silicone breast implants. In this case the key consumer advocate/journalist was Esther Rome, a member of the National Women's Health Network and co-author of *Our Bodies Ourselves*. The key ally in Congress was Representative Ted Weiss of Manhattan. Both times, the laziness and greed of some physicians provided a major obstacle to ferreting out the truth.

The Pill is far easier to prescribe (one need only push a piece of paper across a desk) than the diaphragm or cervical cap are to fit properly, and the silicone implants are easier for the busy surgeon to work with and shape than are the apparently safer saline equivalents. The testing and marketing of products for women appears more slipshod, cavalier, and cynical than that for products which are also used by men. This disparity is most notable with products that concern female sexual availability or allure,—i.e., the Pill and breast implants. Readers of this article who wish to get up-to-date objective, conservative information about the safety of medical products for women are urged to contact the National Women's Health Network, which remains the only national public-interest organization devoted solely to women and health. (See Appendix for address.)

Side Effects. The new Pills, containing 100 micrograms or less of estrogen, appear to be less dangerous than the older formulations. However, they have their own drawbacks, including more frequent complaints of breakthrough bleeding and depression, as well as complicated new dose schedules and instructions. Statistics on the number of side effects are not being well kept, but there appear to be fewer blood clots, strokes, and other disorders requiring hospitalization than there were in the past. Both patients and prescribers are becoming more selective, due in part to the patient package inserts (PPIs) that now accompany every Pill prescription. High-risk women are less likely than in the past to use oral contraceptives, and if they start to get sick while taking this medication, they can check their symptoms against the PPI to find out if they need to discontinue use. The PPIs were suggested and lobbied for by health feminists in the late 1960s and 1970s. They were opposed by both the pharmaceutical industry and organized medicine but were finally mandated by the U.S. Food and Drug Administration (FDA) in 1975.

Women should not take the Pill if they smoke, and especially if they smoke and are over 35 years of age. Women should not take it if they are pregnant or suspect that they are, or if they have any of the following conditions:

- A history of heart attack, stroke, or blood clots
- Known or suspected cancer
- Chest pain
- Unexplained vaginal bleeding
- Jaundice or liver disorders

They should exercise substantial caution in taking the Pill if they have, or have had:

- Breast nodules, fibrocystic disease, or an abnormal mammogram
- Diabetes
- Elevated cholesterol or triglycerides
- High blood pressure
- Migraine or other headaches or epilepsy
- Mental depression
- Gallbladder, heart, or kidney disease
- History of scanty or irregular periods
- Fibroid tumors

Women should not take the Pill if they are breastfeeding, if they plan to have surgery within one month, or if they have recently had surgery. Women who take antibiotics, sedatives, or certain other medications can expect them to reduce the effectiveness of the Pill; additional contraception should be used when these medications are taken.

The most serious side effects of the Pill include blood clots, heart attacks and strokes, gallbladder disease, liver tumors, high blood pressure, chemical diabetes and carbohydrate intolerance, depression, and infertility. The link between the Pill and female cancers, particularly of the breast and cervix, is still unclear, but estrogens are well known to promote some cancers, so much so that anti-estrogens are now used as a cancer treatment. The National Women's Health Network concludes that "there is growing evidence of an association between breast cancer and oral contraceptives. Women who appear at highest risk include: those who use oral contraceptives before the age of 25 and who continue for some years before having a baby; those who have a family history of breast cancer" (Seaman, 1989).

More than 100 different side effects have been reported from the Pill. Some of these seem trivial to doctors, but not necessarily to users. For example, some reported side effects, in addition to the now very common breakthrough bleeding, include loss of scalp hair, or the growth of hair in unwanted places; acne or melasma (a spotty darkening of the skin on the face); allergic rashes; spider veins; intolerance to contact lenses; nausea, vomiting, abdominal cramps, bloating, and water retention; headaches and dizziness; increased risk of chlamydia and candidasis (vaginal infections); changes in weight; changes in cervical erosion and secretion; changes in sex drive; and folic acid deficiency. Not all of these symptoms are reversible. Some women feel fine using oral contraceptives, but over time a majority do not. The Pill must be considered in connection with almost any symptom that a user develops while she is taking it. The "health benefits" of the Pill were promoted as part of a deliberate drug company campaign to resell the Pill in the early 1980s, when use had dropped sharply as awareness of its drawbacks spread. However, since the Pill suppresses normal menstruation—substituting "withdrawal bleeding" in its place—it does decrease the incidence of menstrual pain and remains useful as a medical treatment for this condition.

It has long been known that certain other medications interact unfavorably with the Pill, sometimes creating a greater danger of side effects, and sometimes making the Pill less effective, leading to what are called breakthrough pregnancies. These interactions, although quite well established, are not ordinarily included in the consumer labeling, nor discussed with patients by most prescribing physicians. Here is a summary of some of the most common interacting pharmaceuticals, stimulants, and vitamins:

1. Anti-anxiety drugs called benzodiazepines. Danger: Increased risk of drowsiness, loss of muscle coordination, alertness. Some brand names: Xanax, Halcion, Librium, Valium, Dalmane.

   The names of three benzodiazepine products which may be safer in that they appear not to interact with the Pill: Serax, Ativan, Restoril.
2. Caffeine. Danger: The stimulant effect of caffeine may be increased leading to nervousness, headache, agitation, irritability, insomnia.

3. Theophyllines are used for asthma and bronchospasm. Danger: Theophylline toxicity, including rapid or irregular heartbeat, nausea, dizziness, possible seizures. Some brand names: Somophylline, Choledyl, Aerolate, Bronkodyl, Bronkaid, Primatene.
4. Anti-fungal agents called grisofulvin used to treat ringworm and some bacterial infections. Danger: Decreased effectiveness of the Pill. Breakthrough bleeding and possible pregnancy. Some brand names: Fulvicin, Grisfulvin.
5. Antibiotics including the penicillins, the tetracyclines, and the rifampins. Danger: These all may decrease the effectiveness of the Pill leading to breakthrough bleeding and/or breakthrough pregnancies.

   Penicillins, which have dozens of brand names and generic variants, are used for microbial infections.

   Tetracyclines, used for microbial infections, also have many brand and generic names.

   Rifampins, a specialized antibiotic used for tuberculosis and for meningitis carriers bear such brand names as Rifadin, Rifamate, and Rimactane.

   Alternative methods of contraception should be used while taking any of the above groups of antibiotics.
6. Anti-seizure medications in the phenytoin or Dilantin family. Danger: They also decrease the effectiveness of the Pill, increasing the risks of pregnancy. Here, too, an alternative contraceptive should be used.
7. Troleandomycin or Tao, an antibiotic used for microbial infections. Danger: In combination with the Pill can cause cholestatic jaundice, with symptoms such as yellow discoloration of the skin and eyes, fatigue, itching, and loss of appetite.
8. Vitamin C, also called ascorbic acid. Danger: High levels of ascorbic acid have a complex and curious interaction with estrogens. Dosages of 1000 mg or more daily may increase the risk of pregnancy *when the vitamin is withdrawn* due to a resultant lowering of the blood levels of the hormones. While high doses of the vitamin are being taken the estrogen-associated side effects of the Pill may become more pronounced.

   Women using the Pill should probably not take more than 250 to 500 daily mg of vitamin C.
9. Cigarette smoking is well known to increase the risk of adverse cardiovascular effects from the Pill such as heart attacks and blood clots. The interaction is more pronounced in women over 35 and those smoking more than 15 cigarettes a day.

   Moderate and heavy smokers should probably not use the Pill and vice versa.

It is odd that most doctors warn their patients about the interaction between smoking and the Pill, but not about the contraceptive's equally serious interactions with other prescription drugs. Perhaps the pharmaceutical companies are still failing in their duty to warn physicians, or perhaps some of the physicians know but fear lawsuits. (If a woman smokes and takes the Pill she increases her own risks. If her doctor prescribes a medication that interacts dangerously with the Pill, she may have a good case against the doctor if she falls ill.) After three decades of widespread use the Pill can still be called experimental as new brands with new dosages and even some new chemical progestins are now entering the market. The most prudent choice for the health of most women remains with the barrier methods, carefully and consistently applied.

✱ BARBARA SEAMAN

See **Guide to Related Topics:** Contraception

Resources

Harkness, Richard. (1991). *Drug Interactions Guide Book.* Englewood Cliffs, NJ: Prentice Hall.

Mintz, M. (1970). *The Pill: An Alarming Report.* Boston: Beacon Press.

Seaman, Barbara. (1969). *The Doctors' Case against the Pill.* New York: Peter H. Wyden.

———. (1972). *Free and Female.* New York: Coward McCann.

———. (1984). "Contraception, 1984." In Kay Weiss (Ed.) *Women's Health Care: A Guide to Alternatives.* Reston, VA: Reston Publishing Company, Inc.

———. (1989). "Testimony on Breast Cancer and the Pill." Presented to the U.S. Food and Drug Administration, Fertility and Maternal Health Drugs Advisory Committee, for the National Women's Health Network, January 5.

Seaman, Barbara & Seaman, Gideon. (1977). *Women and the Crisis in Sex Hormones.* New York: Rawson.

U.S. Department of Health and Human Services, Centers for Disease Control. (1991). "PID: Guideline for Prevention and Management." *Morbidity and Mortality Weekly Report,* April, 26. Atlanta, Georgia.

Vaughan, P. (1970). *The Pill on Trial.* New York: Coward-McCann.

PLACENTA

The placenta is a vascular organ developed within the uterus during gestation. Its name is derived from a Latin word which means "flatcake," since it is disk-shaped in appearance.

The placenta develops from a process called implantation, which begins about three to four days after the fertilized ovum enters the uterus. The fertilized ovum develops fingerlike projections, called chorionic villi, which embed into the uterine wall. A thin layer of the uterine wall, called the endometrium, clings to these branching projections, and together they make up the placenta. It continues to grow, and by the 10th week of gestation, the placenta covers one-third of the uterine wall.

The placenta is the organ through which oxygen and nutrients are received from, and wastes of the fetus are eliminated into, the circulatory system of the mother. This diffusion back and forth occurs through the process of osmosis. Oxygen is diffused from the maternal blood stream, since the lungs of the fetus do not serve this function *in utero*. Nourishment such as glucose, calcium, amino acids, fatty acids, phosphorus, and iron also diffuse through the placenta to the fetus. Fetal waste products diffuse in the opposite direction, from the fetus to the placenta.

Pregnant women should be aware that any substance traveling through the blood stream can be passed to the fetus by way of the placenta. Avoiding exposure to chemicals and certain infections is advisable. All mothers should also think about any harm that certain medications may cause. It is important that she consult with her health care provider before taking any medications, either prescription or those purchased over-the-counter.

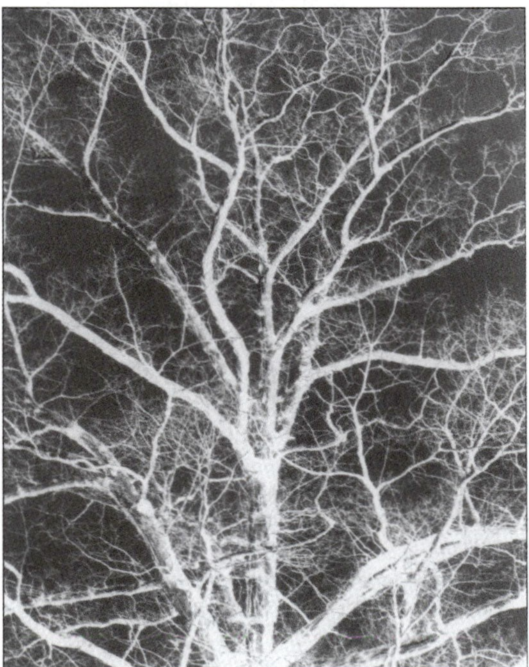

Tree of life within: The circulatory system of the placenta. Photo courtesy of Harriette Hartigan/Artemis.

The fetus is connected to the placenta by the umbilical cord. The umbilical cord is about 20 inches in length and three-quarters of an inch in diameter. It contains two arteries that transport nutrients and oxygen to the fetus, and one large vein that transports waste from the fetus.

In addition to being the life-support system to the fetus, the placenta secretes hormones necessary to sustain the pregnancy. At least five hormones are known to be secreted by the placenta. The placenta secretes estrogen and progesterone and becomes the major source of these hormones after two months' gestation. These hormones are thought to be responsible for growth of the uterus and the preparation of the mother's breasts for lactation.

The placenta is separated and expelled after the birth of the baby in what is referred to as the third stage of labor. Its expulsion is caused by uterine contraction and intra-abdominal pressure. The woman can facilitate the expulsion of the placenta by bearing down. At term, the placenta weighs about one to one-and-a-half pounds. The fetal surface is smooth and glistening, and the maternal surface is red and fleshlike.

Placenta Previa. Placenta previa is the most common cause of bleeding during the late months of pregnancy. Placenta previa is characterized by painless uterine bleeding, usually occurring after the seventh month. The bleeding may be intermittent, in gushes, or, more rarely, continuous. Placenta previa occurs about once in every 200 deliveries and occurs less often in first pregnancies.

Rather than being attached higher up on the uterine wall, the placenta is attached to the lower uterine segment and either wholly or partly covers the region of the cervix. The bleeding is caused by the separation of the placenta from the uterine wall as a result of changes that take place in the lower segment of the uterus during the later months of pregnancy. There are three types of placenta previa: total placenta previa, in which the placenta completely covers the internal os of the cervix; partial placenta previa, in which the os is partially covered; and low implantation of the placenta, in which the placenta encroaches upon the region of the os but does not extend beyond the margin of the internal os.

The management of placenta previa will depend on the type, the gestational age of the fetus, and any risks to the mother or fetus. If the bleeding is not excessive and the fetus is premature, this condition can be managed by bedrest. If possible, delivery is postponed until after the 36th week of pregnancy.

Placenta Abruptio. Placenta abruptio is a complication of the last half of pregnancy in which the normally located placenta separates from the uterine attachment. The precise cause is unknown; however, it is often associated with toxemia. In placenta abruptio the mother may or may not have external bleeding, depending on the location of the separation. Marginal separation of the placenta will cause drainage of blood behind the membranes, down through the cervix. The woman will experience painless, external bleeding or hemorrhage. Central separation of the placenta causes blood to trap behind the placenta. The uterus enlarges and becomes tender and exceedingly firm. With central separation there is no external evidence of bleeding. The woman experiences severe uterine pain, backache, and regional tenderness. All of the above symptoms indicate that the health care provider be contacted.

A woman may experience some light vaginal bleeding when the cervix begins to dilate. This is often nothing to be concerned about. It usually means that labor has begun.

✱ DIANE D'ALESSANDRO, R.N.

See also: Umbilical Cord

See **Guide to Related Topics:** Pregnancy, Physical Aspects

Resources

Creasy, Robert K. & Resnik, Robert. (1984). *Maternal-Fetal Medicine Principles and Practice*. Philadelphia: W.B. Saunders Co.

Jensen, Margaret Duncan & Bobak, Irene M. (1980). *Handbook of Maternity Care. A Guide for Nursing Practice.* St. Louis: The C.V. Mosby Company.

Reeder, Sharon R. et al. (1976). *Maternity Nursing*. 13th edition. New York: J.B. Lippincott Company.

POPULATION CONTROL. *See instead* CONTRACEPTION: DEFINING TERMS

POSTPARTUM EMOTIONAL DISORDERS

It is generally acknowledged that there are three distinct postpartum disorders, each with its own incidence rate, symptom description, etiological theories, treatment, course, and prognosis. Any consideration of illnesses occurring during the postnatal period must take into account the fact that, as a life event, birth causes more disruptions of the woman's life space than any other event. There are changes in the woman's body shape, health, and biochemistry, her self-image, her social role, her marital and family relationships, her independence, her sexuality, her occupation and career course, her economic status, and living arrangements, among others. Her illness must be examined within this complex matrix of change.

The Postpartum (Baby) Blues. The blues usually begin on the third day after birth, with the greatest severity of symptoms occurring between the fifth and 10th days. The blues affect between 50 and 80 percent of birthing women and are so frequent as to be thought of as "normal" (Yalom et al., 1968; Butts, 1969; Colman, 1969; Brown, 1981; Steiner, 1990). The most common symptoms are depression, elation, emotional instability, insomnia, headaches, poor concentration, tearfulness, fatigue, and confusion. The episode usually disappears without treatment after two weeks. The mother usually feels better with help at home and support from her partner and other women. Prenatal education about the stresses of this period is very helpful. The etiology (or cause) of the blues is unknown. However, a hormonal "vulnerability" is a likely partial explanation as the blues affect so many women within the same period after the birth. No direct correlation has been found with specific hormone levels, however. The relationship of the blues to PMS and menstrual irregularities is still under investigation. Research has indicated that the blues are not related to being hospitalized for the birth, to parity, sex of the infant, labor/delivery variables, social class, or marital variables (Treadway et al., 1969; Dalton, 1971; Nott et al., 1976; Endicott et al., 1981).

The Postpartum Depression. Postpartum depression usually starts gradually. For some women it starts with the baby blues; other women are asymptomatic until the onset of the episode. This occurs from between two weeks to several months after the birth. It affects from 7 to 10 percent (Pitt, 1973) to 10 to 20 percent of new mothers (Brown, 1981). The usual symptoms are sustained depressed mood, heightened concern about her own and the baby's health, anxiety, somatic preoccupation, indecisiveness, fatigue, irritability, and sleep disturbance. Disturbed sleep occurs even in the absence of being woken up by the baby; sleep monitoring has documented altered sleep cycles that persist as long as four months after the birth of the baby (Kane, 1985). Severe feelings of poor self-esteem and inadequacy may be present; the mother may feel that she is a terrible parent and have no confidence in her mothering abilities. Suicide is a possibility. Psychotic symptoms (delusions and hallucinations) are never present.

Treatment is imperative. Psychotherapy and medication are usually necessary. Standard antidepressants are usually used, with the choice being determined by whether a sedating or energizing effect is desired. Hospitalization may be necessary if the mother is suicidal. Environmental support is very important; the mother needs a lot of help at home, both to help her through this demanding period and to help model appropriate mothering behavior. Two-thirds of the affected women recover within a year. For others, there may be long-term depression and marital/parenting problems.

Research into the causes of postpartum depression has focused on several areas: genetics, hormonal changes, environmental stresses and sociodemographic status or change, marital support, psychodynamics, psychiatric history, and PMS (Gise, 1985; Kane, 1985; Steiner, 1990). None of these areas has, however, yielded a complete explanation of the occurrence of postpartum depression.

While specific childbirth events, or the use of certain medical procedures (such as the cesarean) have not been connected with postpartum mood change, the experience of feeling helpless during childbirth has been associated with increased depression afterwards (Greene, 1990). It is also known that if women have had prior episodes of depression, they are likely to have one after birth. Many women are also depressed during pregnancy, and this mood change is the single best predictor of depression afterwards. Having a supportive partner is the best "protective" factor. Prenatal education designed to anticipate and prepare for such mood changes is also helpful.

The Postpartum Psychosis. The psychosis usually begins slowly. The woman may be asymptomatic for between 2 to 3 weeks after the birth, to as long as 6 to 12 months. It affects between one out of 400 (Gordon, 1957) to one out of 1,000 new mothers (Brown, 1981). The symptoms partially resemble those of postpartum depression, with sleep disturbance, fatigue, depression, headache, indecisiveness, irritability, and emotional lability. In addition, however, there may also be confusion, a dreamy state, complaints of poor memory, and finally, the hallmark psychotic symptoms. The woman may have somatic delusions concerning what was done to her body during birth or delusions regarding her identity, the identity of the baby, the fidelity of her husband, or the special powers she believes her baby has. Frequently these false ideas have a religious connotation. The mother may believe that she is the Virgin Mary or that her baby is Jesus or the devil. The distortions of reality may be profound and may lead the mother to kill herself and/or her baby. She may also have obsessive thoughts about hurting the baby, and she may engage in repetitive or ritualistic behaviors to protect the baby or control its thoughts.

Treatment is imperative because of the danger to the mother and baby. Hospitalization is usually required, along with the administration of appropriate antipsychotic medication. The chances of recovery are good, but the mother must remain on medication for a long time. Women with a prior psychotic or schizophrenic episode have nearly a 50 percent chance of having an episode after birth. Research into the causes has followed the lines of research into schizophrenia.

Manic-depressive women can also become psychotic during an episode of illness. Lithium, an extremely effective medication for this condition, can be started prophylactically immediately after birth. Bipolar women have a 50 percent chance of having a postpartum episode of their illness.

✱ KAREN GREENE, Ph.D.

See also: Doula; Emotional Recovery Following Obstetric Interraction; Matrescence and Patrescence

See **Guide to Related Topics:** Pregnancy, Psychological Aspects

Resources

Brown, W.A. (1981). "Psychiatric Problems during the Postpartum Period." In W.A. Brown (Ed.) *Psychological Care during Pregnancy and the Postpartum Period.* New York: Raven Press.

Butts, H. (1969). "Postpartum Psychiatric Problems." *Journal of the National Medical Association 51*: 136-204.

Colman, A.D. (1969). "Psychological State during the First Pregnancy." *American Journal of Orthopsychiatry 39*: 787-97.

Dalton, K. (1971). "Prospective Study into Postpartum Depression." *British Journal of Psychiatry 118*: 689-92.

Endicott, J. et al. (1981). "Premenstrual Changes and Affective Disorders." *Psychosomatic Medicine 43*: 519-29.

Gise, L. (1985). "Psychiatric Implications of Pregnancy." In S.H. Cherry, R.L. Berkowitz, & N.G. Kase (Eds.) *Rovinsky and Guttmacher's Medical, Surgical and Gynecological Complications of Pregnancy.* 3rd edition. Baltimore: Williams and Wilkins.

Gordon, R. (1957). "Emotional Disorders of Pregnancy and Childbearing." *Journal of the Medical Society of New Jersey 54*: 16-23.
Greene, K. (1990). "Postpartum Disorders." *The New York State Psychologist 41*: 24-27.
Kane, F.J. (1985). "Postpartum Disorders." In H.I. Kaplan & B.J. Sadock (Eds.) *Comprehensive Textbook of Psychiatry*. Baltimore: Williams and Wilkins.
Nott, P.N. et al. (1976). "Hormonal Change and Mood in the Puerperium." *British Journal of Psychiatry 12*: 379-83.
O'Hara, M.W., Neunsher, D.J., & Zekoski, E.M. (1984). "Prospective Study of Postpartum Depression: Prevalence Course, and Predictive Factors." *Journal of Abnormal Psychology 93*: 158-71.
Pitt, B. (1973). "Maternity Blues." *British Journal of Psychiatry 122*: 431-33.
Steiner, M. (1990). "Postpartum Psychiatric Disorders." *Canadian Journal of Psychiatry 35*: 89-95.
Treadway, C.R. et al. (1969). "A Psychoendocrine Study of Pregnancy and the Puerperium." *American Journal of Psychiatry 125*: 1380.
Yalom, I. et al. (1968). "'Postpartum Blues' Syndrome." *Archives of General Psychiatry 18*: 17-27.

POSTURE FOR LABOR AND BIRTH

Throughout history, in cultures around the world, women have typically walked about during labor and given birth in upright postures, including sitting, standing, and squatting (Atwood, 1976; Russell, 1982). Women have supported themselves in these positions either by hanging onto a stake, bar, or suspended rope; by resting on a low stool or stone; or commonly by leaning back against the chest of a companion (Figure 1).

As the place of birth has shifted to institutions during the past 60 years, most Western women have been required to lie on their backs during both labor and delivery. The supine position is more convenient for the birth attendant and facilitates the use of drugs and instrumental delivery. But recent evidence indicates that the upright posture is more beneficial for mother and baby. In recent years, many hospitals have revised their policies to allow women to walk and assume whatever positions they find comfortable during labor and delivery.

Historical Concerns about Posture. The supine posture first came into use in Europe about 400 years ago. At first, the "lithotomy" posture (back flat, knees drawn up, legs spread apart) was used only for complicated births requiring forceps or some other form of *accouchement forcé*. The supine posture came to be used more and more for normal deliveries, however, until by the turn of the century in the United States, virtually all women giving birth under the supervision of a physician were required to lie on their backs in bed during labor and to assume a lithotomy position on a delivery table for birth.

In 1882, American physician George J. Engelmann published *Labor among Primitive Peoples*, which describes his investigation into the birth postures used by Native American people. Through correspondence with ethnologists and physicians working with native people, Engelmann discovered that most so-called "primitive" people gave birth in an upright posture. Having noted in his own practice that labor in the supine posture could be more painful and slow, Engelmann described the "civilized" practice as irrational. He wrote: "I deem it a great mistake that we in this age of culture, should follow custom or fashion so completely, to the exclusion of reason and instinct, in a mechanical act which so nearly concerns our animal nature as the delivery of the pregnant female" (Engelmann, 1882). But influential physicians during the early part of the 20th century maintained that the lithotomy posture, along with the routine use of forceps, was essen-

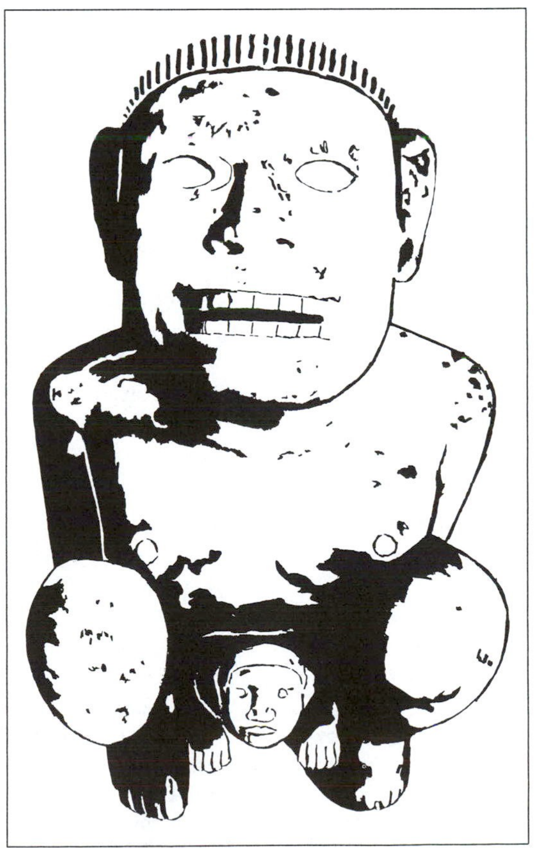

Tlazolteotl, the Aztec goddess of childbirth, gives birth in a squatting position. Drawing by Janet Isaacs Ashford after a piece in the Dunbarton Oaks Collection, Washington, DC. © by Janet Isaacs Ashford.

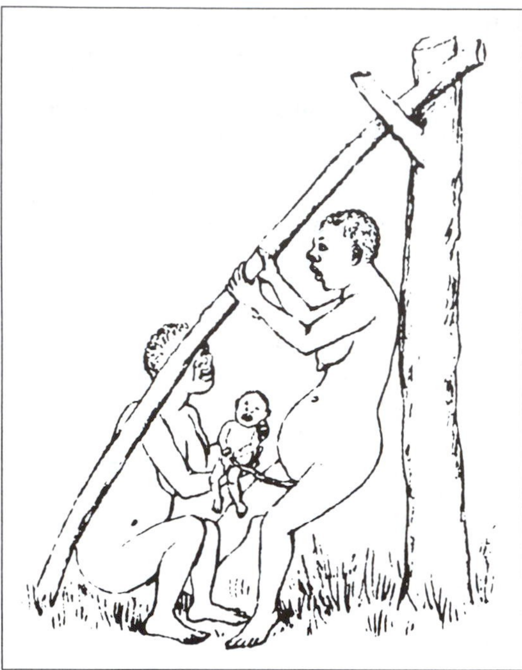

Birth custom of the Longo people of central Africa. The mother gives birth standing up, using a tree and slanted pole for support. From "Notes on Labor in Central Africa" by Robert W. Felkin, *Edinburgh Medical Journal*, April 1984. © by Janet Isaacs Ashford.

tial for safety (DeLee, 1920). Until recently, there have been few well-designed studies to investigate the effects of labor posture.

A recently published comprehensive review of the effects of medical care on pregnancy and birth looks at the effects of labor posture. Echoing Engelmann's concerns, the editors state: "At the present time recumbency continues to be a policy in many maternity units, and is required by many of the professionals who provide care during labour. The available data cast doubt on the wisdom of this policy" (Enkin, Keirse, and Chalmers, 1989).

Effects of Posture during Labor. According to the controlled clinical trials surveyed by Enkin, Keirse, and Chalmers, lying down on the back and sitting during labor are associated with reduced blood flow to the uterus, resulting in contractions that are less effective and more frequent. Lying on the side or standing up improves blood flow and the efficiency of contractions. In addition, women who are upright or lying on their sides have shorter labors and use less narcotic analgesia, epidural anesthesia, and oxytocin augmentation than those who are supine (Roberts, 1989). Many hospitals now allow women to walk and assume comfortable positions during labor, though the use of continuous electronic fetal monitoring can restrict the mother's mobility.

Effects of Posture during Birth. Enkin, Keirse, and Chalmers also found that use of an upright posture when the mother is pushing shortens the length of second-stage labor. They found no clear evidence indicating that posture affects the rate of instrumental delivery or the incidence of trauma to the perineum (Sleep, Roberts, and Chalmers, 1989). However, use of a molded birth chair that restricts the mother's freedom of movement has been associated with perineal edema, resulting in significant postpartum hemorrhage if perineal lacerations occur (Goodlin and Frederick, 1983; Cottrell and Shannahan, 1986). Babies born to women in upright postures have fewer abnormal heart rate patterns and less chance of low Apgar scores (Sleep, Roberts, and Chalmers, 1989). Women prefer the upright posture for birth and report less pain and backache than in the supine posture (Schneider-Affeld and Martin, 1982; Marttila, Kajanoja, and Ylikorkala, 1983; Stewart, Hillan, and Calder, 1983; Liddell and Fisher, 1985).

The use of a squatting posture for birth has been shown to increase intra-abdominal pressure and also increase the sagittal diameter of the pelvic outlet (Davies and Renning, 1964; Borell and Fernstrom, 1967; Russell, 1982). Both factors can contribute to a shorter, more effective labor. However, researchers note that Western women are not accustomed to assuming a squatting posture (for defecation or resting, for example) and may find it difficult to assume this position for birth.

Conventional maternity wards are often equipped with labor beds and delivery tables that encourage or enforce the supine posture. However, the use of upright postures can be facilitated by providing a clean sheet on the floor for the mother to squat upon, using a bed with pillows or an adjustable back support, using a low stool or chair, or providing helpers to support the mother in a standing position (Romond and Baker, 1986). The mother's ability to freely change position as prompted by her own feelings of comfort may be as important as the position adopted (Roberts, 1989).

✱ JANET ISAACS ASHFORD

See also: Labor: Overview

See **Guide to Related Topics:** Childbirth Practices and Locations

Resources

Atwood, R.F. (1976). "Parturitional Posture and Related Birth Behavior." *ACTA Obstetrica et Gynecologica Scandinavica* (Supplement 57).

Borell, U. & Fernstrom, I. (1967). "The Mechanisms of Labor." *Radiology Clinics of North America 5*: 73-85.

Cottrell, B.H. & Shannahan, M.D. (1986). "Effect of the Birth Chair on Duration of Second Stage Labor and Maternal Outcome." *Nursing Research 35*: 364-67.

Davies, J.W. & Renning, E.L. (1964). "The Birth Canal—Practical Applications." *Medical Times 92*: 75-86.

DeLee, J.B. (1920). "The Prophylactic Forceps Operation." *American Journal of Obstetrics and Gynecology 1*: 34-44.

Engelmann, G.J. (1882). *Labor among Primitive Peoples*. St. Louis: J.H. Chambers & Co. (Reprinted in 1977 by AMS Press, New York.)

Enkin, M., Keirse, M.J.N.C., & Chalmers, I. (1989). *A Guide to Effective Care in Pregnancy and Childbirth*. New York: Oxford University Press.

Goodlin, R.C. & Frederick, I.B. (1983). "Postpartum Vulvar Edema Associated with the Birthing Chair." *American Journal of Obstetrics and Gynecology 146*: 334.

Liddell, H.S. & Fisher, P.R. (1985). "The Birthing Chair in the Second Stage of Labour." *Australian and New Zealand Journal of Obstetrics an Gynaecology 25*: 65-68.

Marttila, M., Kajanoja, P., & Ylikorkala, O. (1983). "Maternal Half-sitting Position in the Second Stage of Labor." *Journal of Perinatal Medicine 11*: 286-91.

Roberts, J. (1989). "Maternal Position during the First Stage of Labour." In I. Chalmers, M. Enkin, & M.J.N.C. Keirse (Eds.) *Effective Care in Pregnancy and Childbirth*. Volume 2. New York: Oxford University Press, pp. 883-92.

Romond, J.L. & Baker, I.T. (1986, Sept/Oct). "Squatting in Childbirth: A New Look at an Old Tradition." *Journal of Obstetric, Gynecological and Neonatal Nursing*: 406-11.

Russell, J.G.B. (1982, Sept). "The Rationale of Primitive Delivery Positions." *British Journal of Obstetrics and Gynecology 89*: 712-15.

Schneider-Affeld, F. & Martin, K. (1982). "Delivery from a Sitting Position." *Journal of Perinatal Medicine 10* (Supplement 2): 70-71.

Sleep, J., Roberts, J., & Chalmers, I. (1989). "Care during the Second Stage of Labour." In I. Chalmers, M. Enkin, & M.J.N.C. Keirse (Eds.) *Effective Care in Pregnancy and Childbirth*. Volume 2. New York: Oxford University Press, pp. 1129-44.

Stewart, P., Hillan, E., & Calder, A.A. (1983). "A Randomised Trial to Evaluate the Use of a Birth Chair for Delivery." *Lancet 1*: 1296-98.

PRECONCEPTION HEALTH: WHOLISTIC APPROACHES

Optimum preconception health is essential in minimizing the chances of infertility, miscarriage, and birth defects. Hazards abound in today's highly technological society and exert their influence long before a couple begins trying to become pregnant. Even though heredity plays a role in an individual's reproductive health, preconception health can be maximized by knowing how to avoid hazards and by taking steps to counteract them.

In recent years, the focus has been on the woman giving up bad habits once she is pregnant. Motivation is then high to give up smoking, alcohol, drugs, coffee, and the like. However, increased medical and alternative research, spurred on by the infertility epidemic, shows that the focus on health must begin earlier, and must include *men* as well as women.

Preconception health in the medical view means routine gynecology checkups, infertility "work ups" for couples if pregnancy doesn't take place after a specified age-appropriate time, and high-tech diagnostic and treatment techniques. A "low-tech" approach, however, is more wholistic. The major focus here is on preventing reproductive health problems throughout life. The emphasis is on self-reliant, noninvasive, and low-cost modalities. Growing numbers of scientists and doctors are concerned about long-term effects of fertility drugs such as Clomid and Pergonal, and routine use of sonograms. Increasing numbers of couples are going against the norm by using natural approaches and successfully reversing reproductive problems, including infertility. They are improving nutrition, minimizing environmental hazards, and reducing emotional stresses. Also, adjusting to these changes in habit in advance of conception makes it easier to sustain them throughout a pregnancy and beyond.

Of course, neither high- nor low-tech approaches to good health can prevent or cure all instances of infertility. Still, many infertility factors, such as blocked oviducts, early stages of endometriosis, endocrine disorders, and low-quality sperm and semen, have improved and been reversed through wholistic means. Contrary to popular belief, the origin of many birth defects is not mysterious but a result of nutritional deficiencies and/or environmental hazards preconception (men and women) and *in utero* that can be controlled.

Some preconception health factors that can be enhanced with the proper knowledge, motivation, and support are these:

Non-Food Intake: Avoid (or eliminate) use of hard drugs, alcohol, cigarettes, caffeine, etc.

Nutrition: Ideally, a non-junk food, completely vegetarian (organic if possible) diet will prevent intake of growth-stimulating hormones, antibiotics, and other detrimental chemicals found in flesh foods, eggs, and dairy products. These excessively high protein, high acid-forming foods are implicated in fibroids, ovarian cysts, and poor-quality mucus and sperm.

Health Care: Minimize x-rays.

Birth Control: Learn fertility awareness methods to avoid or reduce hazards of artificial methods, especially of the Pill and IUD. Fertility awareness methods are also important in pinpointing the fertile time and becoming aware of possible problems.

Water: Avoid contaminants in tap water (fluoride, chlorine, industrial and farming chemical run-off) known to cause birth defects by using other water sources.

Occupational Hazards: Use safety equipment and procedures to minimize exposure to factory chemicals, radiation, etc. Prepare for job or occupation change if hazards are unavoidable.

Personal Hygiene: Use toothpaste, deodorants, make-up, etc., that do not contain harmful additives.

Home Environment: Use nontoxic cleaners, paints, and furnishings.

Detoxification: Learn about fasting and cleansing diets to eliminate stored toxins.

Physical Condition: Exercise helps detoxify the body and improves nutrient absorption, circulation, etc.

Emotional/Psychological: Reduce stress through yoga, meditation, breathing, and relaxation techniques. Plan fun times. Discuss problems with trusted friends, relatives, or professionals.

Environment: Personally minimize pollution to air, water, and food by practicing and supporting recycling, organic farming, and other growing efforts toward planetary health and peace.

✱ BARBARA FELDMAN

See also: Infertility Prevention

Resources

The American Vegan Society, 501 Old Harding Highway, Malaga, NJ 08328.

DeCava, Judith A. (1988, Jan). "Perils of Pregnancy, Part I-V." *The Journal of the National Academy of Research Biochemists.*

Edwards, Margot. (Ed.) (1989). *A Stairstep Approach to Fertility.* Crossing Press.

Jansen, Erik. *Birth Defect Prevention News.* Newsletter of National Network to Prevent Birth Defects, Box 15309, Southeast Station, Washington, DC 20003.

New York State Coalition Opposed to Fluoridation, Inc., P.O. Box 263, Old Bethpage, NY 11804-0263.

Nissim, Rina. (1986). *Natural Healing in Gynecology.* London: Pandora Press.

Robbins, John. (1987). *Diet for a New America.* Wallpole, NH: Stillpoint Publishing.

Women's Occupational Health Resource Center, 117 St. Johns Place, Brooklyn, NY 11217.

PREGNANCY AFTER PREGNANCY LOSS

For most of those couples who experience a pregnancy loss, whether it is a first-trimester miscarriage or the death of a newborn, the idea of trying again usually comes up very quickly. Reactions vary from wanting to try immediately to being terrified at the thought of trying again. It is not until after the initial acute phase of the grief process has passed that rational decisions can be made.

The length of time that is advisable before attempting another pregnancy varies. Emotional as well as physical factors must be taken into account. Most doctors recommend a minimum wait of three months for physical reasons; however, it should be kept in mind that the risk of premature labor is higher if the interval between full-term or close-to-full-term pregnancies is less than a year. This is an important consideration for couples who have lost a baby due to premature birth.

Sometimes more important than the physical factors are the emotional ones. Parents are advised to thoroughly mourn their loss before conceiving again. The length of time this takes is individual and may be clouded by other issues, such as the woman's age and her "biological clock." The characteristics of the grief process are similar for all types of pregnancy loss, but it is likely that it will take longer to heal from a stillbirth or infant death than from an early miscarriage. The average length of time is usually considered to be one year.

The importance of allowing enough time for mourning has to do with avoiding what is known as the replacement child syndrome. In the early stages of grief, parents want another baby to replace the one who died. They need time to accept the fact that replacing another human being is not possible and that the child they will be creating is an individual in its own right. If the new baby is meant as a replacement, this can lead to disappointment, confusion, and a problematic relationship with the subsequent child. A child who does not live very long tends to be idealized, creating an image that no real child can live up to.

In successful grief work, there comes a time for resolution. If resolution is sought in the form of another pregnancy, the parent(s) are likely to find that rather than having completed their grief work, they have entered a new phase of it. This subsequent pregnancy becomes a part of the grief process and thus is a substantially different experience from most other pregnancies.

Anxiety is paramount and can reach rather high levels. The level of anxiety will depend, in part, on how much is known and understood about the reasons for the prior loss, whether it is likely to recur, and whether or not measures can be taken to prevent its recurrence. Thorough understanding of the causes and / or the likelihood of recurrence is helpful in lessening anxiety but not eliminating it. Even in the best of cases, there will be levels of fear that are not usually seen even in first pregnancies. This fear or anxiety usually peaks around the time in the pregnancy that corresponds to when the prior loss occurred. The innocence, naiveté, and romantic images often seen in first-time parents are nonexistent.

Dealing with the anxiety and keeping it manageable ought to be an integral part of the prenatal care. Bereavement groups designed for pregnancy loss may be inappropriate as there are often new participants with recent losses and very fresh grief that can be difficult for the pregnant woman and her partner or family to deal with. While they may have succeeded in reassuring themselves that the causes of their baby's death are unlikely to be repeated, they are constantly being exposed to all of the other things that sometimes go wrong, and this feeds their insecurity.

Groups and childbirth preparation classes designed specifically for subsequent pregnancies are helpful, but hard to find. Health care professionals can help by putting couples in touch with each other for mutual support. The only people who truly understand the experience are those who have been or are going through it themselves.

One of the most frustrating experiences for these parents is dealing with the well-meaning advice of others, professionals as well as friends and family. Outsiders tend to minimize or negate the emotions the couple is experiencing and make remarks such as, "What are you worried about? It couldn't possibly happen again!" More helpful would be to offer concrete suggestions to ease anxiety and promote a sense of well-being. For caregivers, this might mean scheduling more frequent prenatal visits to hear the baby's heartbeat and taking time to talk to the parent(s) about feelings. It could mean checking up on the mother's nutrition, making sure she's getting enough nutrients both to sustain the pregnancy and compensate for the additional stress. Relaxation training, massage, or a prenatal exercise class if not medically contraindicated can also be helpful.

The assumption that a woman who has experienced a prior pregnancy loss is automatically at high risk of future losses is incorrect. Most of these women might be considered "emotionally high risk" and warrant extra care as described above, but actual medical risk factors are handled on a case-by-case basis. If the cause is unlikely to recur, there is no reason why a woman can't proceed with a noninterventive, natural approach to her pregnancy, labor, and delivery. Alternative birthing centers and home births are still options for the healthy woman with no risk factors other than the previous loss.

Once the new baby is born, the parents may experience some difficulty bonding with the new baby, even if a sufficient length of time has passed between pregnancies. Reluctance to attach to the infant or an overprotective attitude are not uncommon. With patience and support from friends, family, and health care providers, these difficulties will be overcome. The child who died will not be forgotten but will assume an appropriate position in the emotional life of the family as parents and children move on to have a normal family life.

✱ JUDI LOWENBURG FORMAN, C.C.E.

See also: Support Groups for Infant Loss

See **Guide to Related Topics:** Pregnancy Loss and Infant Mortality

Resources

Forman, Michael & Forman, Judi. (1988, Aug). "After a Baby Dies." *Parents Magazine* 63 (8): 114-87.

Schwiebert, Pat & Kirk, Paul. (1986). *Still to Be Born.* Portland, OR: Perinatal Loss.

PREGNANCY AND SOCIAL CONTROL*

The U.S. Supreme Court recently decided that women who are fertile can work in jobs that may pose a risk to a fetus, and that employers may not deny them good employment in the name of "fetal safety" (*International Union, UAW v. Johnson Controls,* 1991). The employer's policy was purportedly designed to protect fetal health, but it also threatened women's access to "more than 20 million jobs" (Easterbrook, 1989, p. 914).

The case shares fundamental characteristics with a series of recent cases: prosecutions of women who use drugs or alcohol during pregnancy; removal of newborns from their mothers' custody on the basis of a positive drug toxicology test or a blood alcohol test; and mass drug screen-

* An earlier version of this article appeared in the March 1991 issue of *Biolaw*, vol. II, no. 48. Special thanks to Laurie Beck, Peggy Chase, Ellen Silbergeld, Jeanne Stellman, Ana Taras, Nadine Taab, and Liz Werky for valuable assistance on preparing this article.

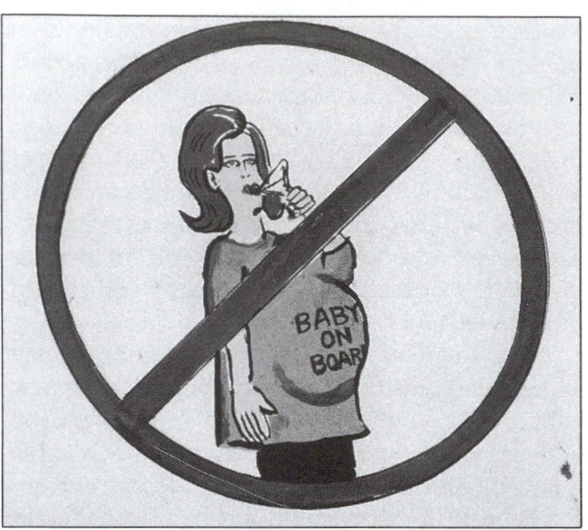

"Baby on Board," a hand-made sign found in a bar in Brooklyn. Posters warning against drinking during pregnancy are appearing all over the country. Photo courtesy of Claudia Mann.

ing of pregnant women and newborns, with mandatory reporting to government authorities of positive test results. These and other proposals attempt to define the legal and moral limits of women's conduct during pregnancy, purportedly to maximize fetal health. Many of these efforts, like the one considered by the Supreme Court, would extract a high price from women in the name of fetal well-being.

The Supreme Court has recognized that women are entitled to make their own decisions about the possible effects of their employment on the health of a potential or actual fetus, holding that "[i]t is no more appropriate for the courts than it is for individual employers to decide whether a woman's reproductive role is more important to herself and her family than her economic role." While the question of women's *legal* right to make their own employment-related decisions has been answered, discussion about the moral and legal obligations of these and other women, who are characterized as advancing their own interests at the expense of fetal interests, remains contentious.

The popular press portrays a "maternal-fetal conflict" in which protection of fetuses inevitably conflicts with "women's rights," implying that women don't care about inflicting harm on their fetuses. In fact, most pregnant women, like everyone else, want to promote fetal health, but the task is complicated and the goal is elusive, as the experiences of women reveal. Proposals that ignore the complexities and dilemmas of women's lives may do more harm than good. In fact, simplistic attempts to protect fetuses, at the expense of the women who bear them, may undermine the health of current and future children.

Women and Work. Imagine a young woman, with a child, an unstable marriage, and financial responsibility for her family. She has a high school education and has worked as a checker in a convenience store. Now she has a job working at a chemical plant. The pay and benefits are great, including sick leave and health care. Her family is relatively financially secure for the first time, but her employer says the job may be hazardous to a fetus. She can only continue working if she gets sterilized. Does this policy "protect" anyone? It ignores the health and financial consequences of unemployment, and it extracts a high price to eliminate a risk of undefined probability and severity. In addition, it requires women workers, instead of their employers, to bear the burden of avoiding potential risks associated with hazardous workplace conditions.

The women (and men) who work in hazardous workplaces do not work there *because* of the hazards but in spite of them. Presumably, they are not thoughtless or selfish people who ignore the well-being of their children. Most accept the risks of employment, over which they have little or no control, precisely because the employment enables them to provide for their families. The work is often strenuous, and there are other obstacles as well. In predominantly male workplaces where the pay is highest (Norwood, 1986, pp. 29-30, Table 4), women often complain of isolation and sexual harassment (*Christman, et al. v. American Cyanamid Co.*, 1980). For unskilled women especially, no other employment provides comparable income and benefits (Bertin, 1989).

Many women make a judgment that this is the best way to provide for their current and future children. That judgment may well be correct, when the options are fully evaluated. At issue is more than the right of women to work; it is also their decision-making capacity. Thomas Murray, a medical ethicist, compares the fertile woman working in a battery plant to the farmer who loses his farm and decides to move to an industrial area where employment opportunities are better.

> Taking the job means a low, but genuine threat of cancer to his children. It also means better food, housing, clothing and health care, as well as greater peace of mind for him. Would he be morally wrong in taking the job—and the risk it entails . . . ? Or is he making a reasonable judgment? (Murray, 1990)

As Murray notes, corporate "fetal protectionism" that restricts fertile women from certain work derives from a legitimate concern for fetal safety but is misguided because it "sentimentalizes women and oversimplifies their moral choices . . . as if their only important moral attribute were pregnancy or pregnancy potential."

"Lifestyle" Decisions. Employment has greater redeeming value than the use of drugs or alcohol, but the response to these problems in women reflects the same sort of sentimentalizing and oversimplification apparent in the employment context. It's easy to condemn the woman who engages in such "selfish" behavior, potentially destructive to herself and others, but that response is inadequate and ineffectual. According to a recent report of the American Medical Association, female substance abusers "have high levels of depression, anxiety, sense of powerlessness, and low levels of self-esteem and self-confidence." Their drug use is not "a failure of individual willpower," and it is not "meant to harm the fetus but to satisfy an acute psychological and physical need . . ." (American Medical Association, 1990, p. 13). Condemnatory responses are unlikely to promote fetal health; only treatment can do that.

Yet addiction treatment services fall far behind the demand for them, and women are especially underserved. The National Association of State Alcohol and Drug Abuse Directors ("NASADAD") reported that, in 1989, approximately 4 million women needed treatment, but only about 550,000 received it. Of those needing treatment, 250,000 were pregnant, and only 30,000 received it (National Association of State Alcohol and Drug Abuse Directors, 1990). Many of the women who have been prosecuted for some form of criminal "fetal abuse" had unsuccessfully sought treatment for their drug addiction.[1]

Sentimentalizing women facilitates blaming those who stray from the ideal and makes it possible to forget that the principal victim of addiction is the woman herself. A recently published study reports the prevalence of violence against pregnant women (4 to 8 percent), as well as associations between male substance abuse, violence against pregnant women, and subsequent substance abuse by physically abused women:

> Among men who batter their female partners, substance abuse has been found to frequently accompany battering. . . . [M]ultiple drug use among male partners is independently associated with over a two-fold increase in women's experience of violence during pregnancy. (Amaro et al., 1990)

The study also noted that "women who are abused may self-medicate with alcohol, illicit drugs, and prescription medication in order to cope with the violence. [In one study] increased alcohol and drug use followed the first incident of abuse" (Amaro et al., 1990, p. 578).

The typical response to pregnant women's drug abuse—report the mother, sometimes to the prosecutor, and take custody of the child—drives away the women who most need medical intervention (American Medical Association, 1990). Punitive responses disproportionately afflict poor and minority communities (Chasnoff et al., 1990). The children are placed in foster care, in congregate care facilities, or, if lucky, with a relative. Many are moved constantly, some suffer abuse or neglect in their institutional or foster homes, many do not receive even minimally acceptable medical care, and some die (Wexler, 1990).

The Dangers of Oversimplifying and Sentimentalizing Motherhood. Oversimplification of the pregnancy health issue in the employment context ignores the significance of women's employment to healthy pregnancies and the maintenance of families. The very jobs at issue in the recent Supreme Court case are the ones most likely to provide decent wages and health insurance benefits. The same process is also apparent in the assessment of "lifestyle" factors. For example, socioeconomic factors that are often beyond individual women's control are critical to pregnancy outcome and family welfare but are often ignored in the simplistic equation that defines maternal rights and responsibilities.

A recent study compared upper-middle-class *alcoholic* women with lower-class *alcoholic* women and found that the incidence of fetal alcohol syndrome among their children was highly correlated with socioeconomic factors: The incidence was 70.9 percent for lower-class mothers and 4.5 percent for upper-middle-class mothers (Bingol et al., 1987). Another study examined the effects of more moderate prenatal alcohol consumption on childhood IQ at age four. Among the women (47 subjects) who drank more than three drinks a day, a statistically significant effect was seen, but it was not as influential as maternal and paternal education (strong socioeconomic indicators) and various other factors, including birth order (Streissguth et al., 1989).

The impulse to control women's conduct to promote fetal and childhood health obscures critically important messages including the significance of socioeconomic factors such as parental education and the overriding importance of post-natal influences. Greater attention to such factors might fuel efforts to improve nutrition, education, and economic conditions for infants and parents and would be a more effective way to promote fetal health and early childhood development. Instead, women are warned not to drink at all when they are pregnant.[2] The message is directed not only at women with a dependency they may be unable to control without treatment, which may or may not be available, but also at healthy, well-nourished pregnant women who have an occasional drink or glass of wine, a habit that poses no documented risk (Abel and Sokol, 1990; Alpert and Zuckerman, 1991; Knupfer, 1991). While individual women might elect to err on the side of caution, an entirely different message is conveyed by governmentally compelled warnings instructing all women to avoid conduct that poses no significant risk for many.

Similarly, regression analyses in a study of the effects of cocaine on pregnancy outcome revealed that one significant effect (reduction in head circumference) was about the same for women who tested positive for cocaine as for women who smoked one pack of cigarettes a day (Zuckerman et al., 1989). While both cigarettes and cocaine are undoubtedly risk factors in pregnancy, these data suggest that cocaine may not be responsible for all the adverse pregnancy-related effects that have been attributed to it; other factors, including socioeconomic factors, may significantly influence pregnancy outcome in cocaine-using women (Weston et al., 1989).

Social disapproval of certain maternal conduct plainly influences how risks are evaluated, as evidenced by a study comparing the publication rate for positive and negative studies on the prenatal effects of cocaine:

> Of 9 negative abstracts (showing no adverse effect) only 1 (11%) was accepted, whereas 28 of the 49 positive abstracts were accepted (57%). This difference was significant. Negative studies tended to verify cocaine use more often and to have more cocaine and control cases. . . . This bias against the null hypothesis may lead to distorted estimation of the teratogenic risk of cocaine. . . . (Koren et al., 1989, p. 1440)

The authors concluded that "most negative studies were not rejected because of scientific flaws, but rather because of bias against their non-adverse message" (Koren et al., 1989, p. 1441).

The focus on maternal responsibility and conduct also deflects attention from the significant biological role males play in reproduction and the well-being of children. Male exposures to chemicals, drugs, alcohol, and other substances can influence the course of pregnancy and potentially the health of a future child, because of the potential for toxic agents to alter genetic material or damage sperm in other ways (Paul, 1988). Paternal preconception exposures have been associated with childhood cancers (e.g., Wilkins and Koutras, 1988; Gardner et al., 1990), reduced birth weights (Little and Sing, 1987), and other adverse pregnancy outcomes (Savitz et al., 1989). The risk of adverse pregnancy outcome may be increased when both parents are exposed to certain chemicals (Hemminki et al., 1983).

In studies of children with fetal alcohol syndrome, "[a] possible risk factor that has received relatively little attention thus far is paternal alcohol consumption" (Abel and Lee, 1988, p. 349). Notwithstanding evidence that male exposure to alcohol may affect pregnancy outcome (Little and Sing, 1987; Abel and Lee, 1988), the Department of Agriculture and the Department of Health and Human Services recently issued dietary guidelines in which they confine their recommendations about the effects of alcohol on reproduction to pregnant women (Dietary Guidelines Advisory Committee, 1990). The selective concern about women's conduct is apparent in the report's reference to a study on the effects of alcohol on lactation (Little et al., 1989), while omitting mention of a study *by the same author* reporting an association between father's preconception drinking and reduced birth weight (Little and Sing, 1987).

Leaving aside reproductive effects, the other direct effects of toxic exposures on males are profoundly important to their families' well-being. If, for example, an occupational exposure poses a risk to the fetus and increases the chances of cardiovascular disease in adult males, does it help families (even if that's the only focus of concern) if Dad has a heart attack or high blood pressure? Similarly, women (whether or not pregnant) and children may all suffer enormously from the addiction or substance abuse of a male family member. Physical violence, unemployment, and other destructive outcomes often accompany male substance abuse, to the detriment of the entire family.

These examples demonstrate how the incantation of "fetal protection" can trigger simplistic responses directed at women that actually fail to foster maternal, fetal, or child health. Such responses often reflect an implicit assumption that fetuses and children are best protected in a "traditional" setting, with a stay-at-home mother. The picture is reminiscent of 19th-century medical advice given to women that their "natural" role was to be nurturing and unselfish, devote themselves to others, and eschew education and other forms of self-advancement (Newman, 1985).

Life for most women is not, and probably never was, so simple. The "traditional" household, with a working father and stay-at-home mother, never defined life for most people and has become a rarity even in this country (Norwood, 1986, pp. 8-9). Women bear heavy financial and other responsibilities, often providing care for children and other dependents unassisted. Many have personal goals and aspirations to participate in, and contribute to, the community. In sum, any attempt to press women into a homogenized, idealized maternal mold "simultaneously makes both women and their children worse off" (Easterbrook, 1989, p. 918).

Controlling Women: Retribution for Reproductive Autonomy?. Drug abuse has tremendous destructive potential. Whole communities are afflicted, but pregnant women are especially singled out, as if they alone are special culprits. Similarly, the problems associated with the hazardous workplace—the risks to all workers, community residents, and consumers from the massive creation, use, transport, and disposal of toxic substances—are all obscured by the focus on the fetus, as if the problems would simply melt away if women didn't work. Perhaps it is because these problems are so daunting that the simplistic response has such appeal. As a result, however, women once again are held to a higher duty of care and to conformity with social ideals from which men may routinely stray.

Ironically, the idealized maternal role model has gained unexpected power from the very event that has liberated so many women, the ability to control pregnancy. The fact that procreation is now deemed voluntary has created an expectation that childbearing should be done only under optimal circumstances. Now that women have a choice, some contend that any woman who elects to carry a pregnancy to term should ensure the best possible fetal environment (Robertson, 1983; Dershowitz, 1989; Shaw, 1989). The imposition of a "duty of care" on pregnant women, however, becomes a penalty on the right to procreate—a form of retribution for women's control over the reproductive process.

Indeed, many women do not have a choice, because abortion is not available to many poor women and others would not terminate an unwanted pregnancy for personal or religious reasons. Other women are not able to control other elements of their lives so as to create the perfect fetal environment. Some women who work in hazardous environments would prefer not to work during pregnancy, but cannot afford it. Others would prefer not to be addicted to drugs, but cannot obtain treatment.

Proponents of the "duty of care" theory, like some employers, oversimplify women's choices and blur an important distinction between moral and legal duties. While parents of both sexes may have a moral obligation to maximize opportunities for their children, there is no basis for singling out pregnant women and imposing "maternal behavior codes," potentially enforceable by state officials, with the additional threat of tort liability against women who do not conform or who make poor judgments.[3] Social tolerance for the choices that men routinely make, even when they advance their own interests at the expense of their children or partners, reveals respect for male decision making and autonomy, even the right to make mistakes.[4] Fathers can be human; mothers must be perfect.

Conclusion. Much of the popular press suggests that women who work at hazardous jobs, and women who take (any) drugs or drink when they are pregnant, demonstrate the existence of a so-called "maternal-fetal conflict." But the term is a fabrication of the sound-bite society. Indeed, in almost every case, the interests of prospective mothers and their future children are aligned: The well-being of the fetus cannot be promoted without attending to the needs of the woman in whose body it resides, even if that means improving working conditions or providing appropriate drug treatment services.

When women are held to an idealized maternal image, they are deprived of their humanity; their children and families are deprived of concrete benefits that result when women's opportunities are expanded and when social responsibility for the welfare of the next generation is more equitably and realistically allocated.

✱ JOAN E. BERTIN, J.D.

See also: Childbearing in Prison; Fetal Alcohol Syndrome; Pregnancy and Work; Pregnant Addicts, Treatment of

See **Guide to Related Topics:** Legal Issues

Notes

1. Jennifer Johnson, who was prosecuted in Florida for delivering drugs to a minor, based on the theory that cocaine metabolites passed through the umbilical cord in the moments after birth, but before the cord was severed, presents such a case. Appellant's In-

itial Brief, pp. 1-5, *Johnson v. State of Florida*, No. 89-1765 (Dist. Ct. App., 5th Dist., 1990). The unavailability of drug and alcohol treatment services to pregnant women has been widely documented (Chavkin, 1990). A lawsuit pending in New York City alleges that the refusal to provide such services to pregnant women violates that state's anti-discrimination laws. *Elaine W. v. North General Hospital, et al.*, No. 6230-90 (N.Y.Co. Supreme Court, 1990).

2. Local ordinances around the country require bars, restaurants, and liquor stores to post signs warning that "alcohol causes birth defects" and that pregnant women should abstain from drinking alcoholic beverages. The problem lies in the failure to communicate *accurate* information. It is misleading to say that "alcohol causes birth defects," since that implies that any amount may do so, while the evidence supports such an effect only at high doses. It would be accurate to advise women that moderate drinking may be a risk factor during pregnancy, but that the nature and extent of the risk is not yet understood.

3. For example, in *Grodin v. Grodin*, 301 N.W.2d 869 (Mich. App. 1981), a Michigan intermediate appellate court allowed a child to sue his mother, alleging that her negligent conduct during pregnancy caused him injury. That case involved the mother's use of the prescription antibiotic tetracycline that, if used in pregnancy, may cause tooth staining in the later born child. The same court has limited application of this case in other challenges to the doctrine of parental immunity *not* involving pregnant women. See *Thelen v. Thelen*, 435 N.W.2d 495 (Mich. App. 1989). It remains to be seen whether that court will carve out exceptions from the parental immunity doctrine for acts of pregnant women. The Illinois Supreme Court has rejected such a result. *Stallman v. Youngquist*, 531 N.E.2d 355 (Ill. 1988).

   Some prosecutors have relied on case law holding third parties responsible for injuries to a viable fetus, resulting from acts done to the pregnant woman, to justify prosecutions of women for taking drugs or driving while intoxicated during pregnancy. This theory was recently rejected by a Massachusetts trial court in *Commonwealth v. Pellegrini* (Commonwealth of Mass., Plymouth Co., Superior Court No. 87970), which, like the *Stallman* decision, recognized the important distinction between acts done by an outside agent inflicting harm on a pregnant woman and acts undertaken by the woman herself. Recent news reports of prosecutions of parents whose children have been injured in automobile accidents and who had failed to use seat belts, if successful, may indicate a trend towards imposing additional criminal liability on parents of either sex for unlawful or unwise conduct.

4. For example, parents are not legally required to donate an organ or bone marrow, even if it would cause them no significant harm and would save their child's life, although they might be morally obligated to do so. The only situations in which a competent adult person has been forcibly subjected to physically invasive procedures in order to serve the interests of another involve pregnant women, as the forced cesarean cases demonstrate. See Kolder, Veronica et al. (1987). "Court-Ordered Obstetrical Interventions." *New England Journal of Medicine 316*: 1192-96.

Resources

Abel, Ernest L. & Lee, Julia A. (1988). "Paternal Alcohol Exposure Affects Offspring Behavior but not Body or Organ Weights in Mice." *Alcoholism: Clinical and Experimental Research 12* (3): 349-55.

Abel, Ernest L. & Sokol, Robert J. (1990). "Is Occasional Light Drinking during Pregnancy Harmful?" In R. Engs (Ed.) *Controversies in the Addiction Field*. 158-64.

Alpert, Joel J. & Zuckerman, Barry. (1991). "Alcohol Use during Pregnancy: What Is the Risk?" *Pediatrics in Review*.

Amaro, Hortensia et al. (1990). "Violence during Pregnancy and Substance Use." *American Journal of Public Health 80* (5): 575-79.

American Medical Association. (1990). Report of the Board of Trustees, Legal Interventions during Pregnancy: Court-Ordered Medical Treatments and Legal Penalties for Potentially Harmful Behavior by Pregnant Women, Report: 00 (A-90).

Bertin, Joan E. (1989). "Women's Health and Women's Rights: Reproductive Health Hazards in the Workplace." In K.S. Ratcliffe et al. (Eds.) *Healing Technology: Feminist Perspectives*. Ann Arbor, MI: University of Michigan Press, pp. 289-303.

Bingol, Nesrin et al. (1987). "The Influence of Socioeconomic Factors on the Occurrence of Fetal Alcohol Syndrome." *Advances in Alcohol and Substance Abuse*, pp. 105-18.

Chasnoff, Ira et al. (1990). "The Prevalence of Illicit-Drug or Alcohol Use during Pregnancy and Discrepancies in Mandatory Reporting in Pinellas County, Florida." *New England Journal of Medicine 322* (17): 1202-06.

Chavkin, Wendy. (1990). "Drug Addiction and Pregnancy: Policy Crossroads." *American Journal of Public Health 80* (4): 483-87.

Christman, et al. v. American Cyanamid Co., Civ. Action No. 80-0024P (N.D.W.Va.) Second Amended Complaint (1980).

Dershowitz, Alan. (1989, May 14). "Drawing the Line on Prenatal Rights." *Los Angeles Times*.

Dietary Guidelines Advisory Committee. (1990). Report on the Dietary Guidelines for Americans to the Secretary of Agriculture and the Secretary of Health and Human Services.

Easterbrook, Frank. (1989). Dissenting Opinion. *International Union, UAW v. Johnson Controls*, 886 F.2d 871, 908-21 (7th Cir. 1989) (*en banc*), rev'd U.S., 59 U.S.L.W. 4209 (U.S. No. 89-1215, Mar 20, 1991).

Gardner, Martin J. et al. (1990). "Results of Case-Control Study of Leukaemia and Lymphoma among Young People near Sellafield Nuclear Plant in West Cumbria." *British Medical Journal 300*: 423-29.

Hemminki, Kari et al. (1983). "Spontaneous Abortions in an Industrialized Community in Finland." *American Journal of Public Health 73* (1): 32-37.

International Union, UAW v. Johnson Controls, U.S., 59 U.S.L.W. 4209 (U.S. No. 89-1215, Mar. 20, 1991).

Knupfer, Genevieve. (1991). "Abstaining for Foetal Health: The Fiction That Even Light Drinking Is Dangerous." *British Medical Journal of Addiction*.

Koren, G. et al. (1989). "Bias against the Null Hypothesis: The Reproductive Hazards of Cocaine." *Lancet 2* (8677): 1440-42.

Little, Ruth E. et al. (1989). "Maternal Alcohol Use during Breastfeeding and Mental and Motor Development at One Year." *New England Journal of Medicine 321*: 425-30.

Little, Ruth E. & Sing, Charles F. (1987). "Father's Drinking and Infant Birth Weight: Report of an Association." *Teratology 36*: 59-65.

Murray, Thomas. (1990). "Are Fetal Protection Policies Ethical?" *Health and Environment Digest 4* (6): 6.

National Association of State Alcohol and Drug Abuse Directors. (1990). "Highlights of Results from Recent NASADAD Survey on State Alcohol and Drug Agency Use of FY 1989 Federal and State Funds."

Newman, Louise Michelle. (1985). *Men's Ideas/Women's Realities: Popular Science, 1870-1915*. New York: Pergamon Press.

Norwood, Janet L. (1986). Hearing before the Select Committee on Children, Youth, and Families, "Work in America, Implications for Families." U.S. House of Representatives, 99th Cong., 2d Sess., April 17, 1986. Committee Reprint 5-59.

Paul, Maureen. (1988). "Reproductive Fitness and Risk." *Occupational Medicine: State of the Art Reviews 3* (2): 323-40.

Robertson, John. (1983). "Procreative Liberty and the Control of Conception, Pregnancy and Childbirth." *University of Virginia Law Review* 69: 405.

Savitz, David A. et al. (1989). "Effects of Parents' Occupational Exposures on Risk of Stillbirth, Preterm Delivery, and Small-for-Gestational-Age Infants." *American Journal of Epidemiology 129* (6): 1201-18.

Shaw, Margery. (1989). "Conditional Prospective Rights of the Fetus." 5 *Journal of Legal Medicine* 63.

Streissguth, Ann P. et al. (1989). "IQ at Age 4 in Relation to Maternal Alcohol Use and Smoking during Pregnancy." *Developmental Psychology 25* (1): 3-11.

Weston, Donna R. et al. (1989). "Drug Exposed Babies: Research and Clinical Issues." *Zero to Three: Bulletin of the National Center for Clinical Infant Programs 9* (5): 1-7.

Wexler, Richard. (1990). *Wounded Innocents: The Real Victims of the War Against Child Abuse*. Buffalo, NY: Prometheus Books.

Wilkins, John R. & Koutras, Ruth A. (1988). "Paternal Occupation and Brain Cancer in Offspring: A Mortality-Based Case-Control Study." *American Journal of Industrial Medicine 14*: 299-318.

Zuckerman, Barry et al. (1989). "Effects of Maternal Marijuana and Cocaine Use on Fetal Growth." *New England Journal of Medicine 320*: 762-68.

PREGNANCY AND WORK

Prior to the Industrial Revolution, adults and children worked together in the home. However, since the 19th century, "home" and "job" have been considered to be separate, and women (at least middle-class women) have been expected to manage the former, and, until recently, have no interest in the latter.

Some women today have choices about whether or not they will seek employment, and the type of job they will consider. Factors that affect those choices include race, class, education, physical and mental fitness, economic status, ability, and the status of women in their community. Today, 53 percent of all women are employed, and over 70 percent of those women are employed full-time (Kessler-Harris, 1985). Until recently, when women did work outside the home, pregnancy signaled the end of their paid employment. Now most women who are employed at the start of their pregnancy will continue working throughout the pregnancy—some until the onset of labor (Brown, 1987).

Occupational health and safety during pregnancy have been studied and three categories of reproductive hazards in the workplace have been identified: (1) physical hazards, such as noise, radiation, vibration, physical activity, and materials handling; (2) biological hazards, such as viruses, fungi, spores, and bacteria; and (3) chemical hazards, such as anesthetic gases, pesticides, lead, mercury, and organic solvents (Bernhardt, 1990). There is a potential for these hazards to affect a worker's ability to have healthy children by causing damage to genetic material of the fetal cells (mutagenesis), abnormal embryonic or fetal growth (teratogenesis), and/or cancer in children that occurs because of parental exposure. Although many studies have been conducted to explore these hazards, there are conflicting reports about their effects on reproduction. Rosenberg, Feldblum, and Marshall (1987) suggested that weaknesses in the way the studies were conducted may be responsible for the inability to clearly determine the extent to which occupational influences affect reproduction. They cite the following problems: too few participants, poor response rates, selection of only those women with a specific poor pregnancy outcome, unclear definitions about what constitutes an "exposure" to a particular hazard, and failure to account for factors outside of the employment environment that might confound the results.

Most of the occupational research into reproductive outcome to date has focused on women, although there is an emerging focus of study about the effect of exposure to occupational hazards on the quality of men's semen as well (Schenker et al., 1988). It is interesting to observe that when a negative effect on the developing fetus is postulated, and men (or at least semen quality) are perceived to be at risk, changes in the workplace environment are proposed. However, when women are involved, the solution generally has been to exclude the pregnant women from the workplace, even though federal, state, and local pregnancy discrimination statutes exist to protect women from job discrimination when they are pregnant (Postol, 1988). The debate continues about the rights of the woman to be employed in certain jobs and the rights of the fetus to be protected from potential harm (Michael, 1990).

In addition to issues of occupational health and safety, there has been some research conducted to explore the effect of pregnancy on the capability of the pregnant woman to perform her assigned tasks. For example, Masten and Smith (1988) studied pregnant and nonpregnant women's reaction times and strength and reported that they found no significant differences. In a review of the epidemiological literature, Saurel-Cubizolles and Kaminski (1978) demonstrated that concern about the effect of women's employment on perinatal outcome has persisted since the turn of the century. However, in general, when researchers have studied birth *outcomes* for the mother or baby, they have found no differences in those outcomes between employed and nonemployed pregnant women (Marbury et al., 1984; Zuckerman et al., 1986).

Pregnant women's work encompasses more than their activities in their employment roles. Hall (1986) described housework as a common example of an activity that has all the necessary elements of "work" but is not often described as such in government statistics or scholarly writing. To date, there has been a lack of systematic study about the effects of housework on pregnancy. In addition to home management, most women are still responsible for the care of the family, whether or not they actually perform the tasks involved in that care (Glazer, 1984; Blau and Ferber, 1985).

A woman may work in many roles during pregnancy but becoming a parent is the central work of pregnancy. Rubin (1975) was one of the first researchers to describe the "tasks" or "work" of pregnancy. She reported that women worked to ensure the safe passage and social acceptance for themselves and their children to identify their children and themselves in relation to their children, and to explore the meaning of giving/receiving. Other tasks during pregnancy have also been noted: transition from woman-without-child to woman-and-child; reevaluation of relationships with the woman's partner and her own mother; and the experience of shifting patterns of dependence and nurturance (Grossman et al., 1980; Lederman, 1984; Tilden, 1984; Hees-Strauthamer, 1985; Mercer, 1986).

Little definitive information is available on the consequences of women's work in each/all of their roles during pregnancy, either for themselves or the babies they are carrying. However, women can learn what *is* known about the hazards specific to their work in order to make decisions about where and/or if they will work during pregnancy (American College of Obstetricians and Gynecologists, 1977; American Medical Association, 1984a, 1984b, 1985; U.S. Congress, 1985).

✱ JEANNE F. DEJOSEPH, Ph.D.

Resources

American College of Obstetricians and Gynecologists. (1977). *Guidelines on Pregnancy and Work.* Washington, DC: National Institute for Occupational Safety and Health, p. 12.

American Medical Association, Council on Scientific Affairs. (1984a). "Effects of Physical Force on the Reproductive Cycle." *Journal of American Medical Association 251*: 247-50.

———. (1984b). "Effects of Pregnancy on Work Performance." *Journal of American Medical Association 251*: 1997.

———. (1985). "Effects of Toxic Chemicals on the Reproductive System." *Journal of American Medical Association 253*: 3431-37.

Bernhardt, Judy Hayes. (1990). "Potential Workplace Hazards to Reproductive Health." *Journal of Obstetrical and Gynecological Nursing 19* (1): 53-62.

Blau, F.D. & Ferber, M.A. (1985). "Women in the Labor Market: The Last Twenty Years." In L. Larwood, A.H. Stromberg & B.A. Gutek (Eds.) *Women and Work.* Newbury Park, CA: Sage Publications, pp. 19-49.

Brown, Marie Annette. (1987). "Employment during Pregnancy: Influences on Women's Health and Social Support." *Health Care for Women International 8* (2-3): 151-67.

Glazer, Nola. (1984). "Paid and Unpaid Work: Contradictions in American Women's Lives Today." In K.M. Borman, D. Quarm, & S. Gideouse (Eds.) *Women in the Workplace: Effects on Families.* Norwald, NJ: Ablex Publishers, pp. 169-85.

Grossman, F.K. et al. (1980). *Pregnancy, Birth, and Parenthood.* San Francisco: Jossey-Bass Publishers.

Hall, Richard. (1986). *Dimensions of Work.* Beverly Hills, CA: Sage Publications.

Hees-Strauthamer, J.C. (1985). *The First Pregnancy: An Integrating Principle in Female Psychology.* Ann Arbor, MI: UMI Research Press.

Kessler-Harris, Alice. (1985). "The Debate over Equality for Women in the Work Place: Recognizing Differences." In L. Larwood, A. Stromberg, & B. Gutek (Eds.) *Women and Work.* Newbury Park, CA: Sage Publications, pp. 141-61.

Lederman, Regina. (1984). *Psychosocial Adaptation in Pregnancy.* Englewood Cliffs, NJ: Prentice Hall.

Marbury, Marian et al. (1984). "Work and Pregnancy." *Journal of Occupational Medicine 26* (6): 415-21.

Masten, W. Yondell & Smith, James L. (1988). "Reaction Time and Strength in Pregnant and Nonpregnant Employed Women." *Journal of Occupational Medicine 30* (5): 451-56.

Mercer, Ramona. (1986). "The Relationship of Developmental Behaviors to Maternal Behavior." *Research in Nursing and Health 11* (2): 83-95.

Michael, Suzanne E. (1990, Jul). "U.S. Supreme Court Agrees to Hear Fetal Protection Employment Policy." *Occupational Health and Safety*: 40-41.

Postol, Lawrence P. (1988). "Handicap Discrimination Considerations in Treating the Impaired Worker: Drugs, Alcohol, Pregnancy, and AIDS in the Workplace." *Journal of Occupational Medicine 30* (4): 321-27.

Rosenberg, Michael J., Feldblum, Paul J., & Marshall, Elizabeth G. (1987). "Occupational Influences on Reproduction: A Review of Recent Literature." *Journal of Occupational Medicine 29* (7): 584-91.

Rubin, Reva. (1975). "Maternal Tasks in Pregnancy." *Maternal-Child Nursing Journal 4*: 143-53.

Saurel-Cubizolles, M.J. & Kaminski, M. (1978). "Work in Pregnancy: Its Evolving Relationship with Perinatal Outcome (A Review)." *Social Science in Medicine 22* (4): 431-42.

Schenker, Marc B. et al. (1988). "Prospective Surveillance of Semen Quality in the Workplace." *Journal of Occupational Medicine 30* (4): 336-44.

Tilden, Virginia. (1984). "The Relation of Selected Psychosocial Variables to Single Status of Adult Women during Pregnancy." *Nursing Research 36* (4): 239-43.

U.S. Congress, Office of Technology Assessment. (1985). *Reproductive Health Hazards in the Workplace.* Washington, DC: U.S. Government Printing Office.

Zuckerman, Barry et al. (1986). "Impact of Maternal Work outside the Home during Pregnancy on Neonatal Outcome." *Pediatrics 77* (4): 459-64.

PREGNANCY LOSS: FAMILY RESPONSE

> Our hearts are broken. Our world seems like it has ended. Our dreams, our hopes and our future with this child are over. Our precious baby has died. (Ilse, 1990)

This quote by a mother whose baby died epitomizes the pain and anguish felt by many families after the death of their child through stillbirth or early infant death. Much to many people's surprise, these feelings are also shared by a majority of the millions of families who suffer a miscarriage (Limbo and Wheeler, 1986).

Although most would agree that babies are not supposed to die, given the current technology and advances in medicine, it does happen. Well over one million losses occur in the United States each year, resulting from miscarriage (1 in 3 pregnancies), stillbirth (1 in 100 births), neonatal death (9 to 10 in 1,000 births), and SIDS (Sudden Infant Death Syndrome or Crib Death) (5 in 1,000 babies) (Borg and Lasker, 1989). Miscarriage is the unintended ending of a pregnancy before the time the fetus could survive outside the mother. This is usually considered by most states to be the 20th week of pregnancy. A neonatal death usually occurs in the first 28 days after birth, even if the baby is born at 21+ weeks and then dies.

When parents experience the unexpected death of a baby, it is natural for them to feel a wide range of emotions, ranging from disbelief and anger to intense sorrow. There is usually a profound sense of disappointment and loss when a baby dies. Plans for bringing the baby home, watching the child grow, and changing family lifestyles have been dashed. Of course, not all parents feel the loss in an intense and profound way. Everyone is unique and should be allowed the expression of personal feelings without judgment.

According to a recent study, parents experiencing perinatal loss are strongly attached to their babies, and it is important for them to have contact with them (Ransohoff-Adler and Berger, 1990). It has become common practice throughout the United States, and in some parts of the world, to encourage families to spend time with their tiny babies who have died. The purpose of this difficult, but important, time is to say "hello" and try to make the dream more of a reality, before rushing to say "goodbye." Time spent with the baby, along with pictures, footprints, handprints, a lock of hair, a bracelet, the blanket and gown the baby wore, and ceremonies such as baptism or a commendation ceremony, provide memories that sustain bereaved families in the days and years that follow the death. Throughout time, bathing, dressing, and openly mourning the dead, including tiny infants, was a common practice. Today, hospitals and other care providers are being encouraged by bereaved families everywhere to return to these very humane and loving rituals (Ilse, 1990).

Men and women experience the loss of the baby differently because of such things as sex differences, societal expectations, and family history. Some typical reactions mothers have after such losses include extreme loss of control; sensations of the baby kicking; wide emotional swings (often partially due to hormonal changes); inability to eat or sleep; a change in priorities; an intense feeling of emptiness as if a part of their heart had been ripped away; anguish; sorrow; a tightness in the chest; continual sighing; and much more. Fathers may feel many of the same emotions in addition to such feelings as vulnerability and helplessness; concern for their partner; a confusion about their role; mixed emotions that may not be able to be expressed but are felt inside; anger; distress; or a calmness in the early hours and days while decisions need to be made and their partner needs their strength. Many men often comment that the family and community's concern is focused on the woman, with few people asking how the father is. This lack of concern for the father makes it more difficult to legitimately express the feelings of grief. Men tend to look for physical outlets rather than verbal opportunities. Both men and women commonly have feelings of guilt, shame, and blame, which are more difficult to express, but are very real.

Children are often forgotten mourners who need extra attention and need to be included in this process. Their baby brother or sister has died and they, too, are forever changed. They have less of an adult understanding about how to cope with this unexpected and upsetting event. Depending on their age, many children feel some sense of blame and guilt: Maybe they didn't want to share their room or their parent's attention, or maybe they accidentally bumped their mother's belly. Talking openly with children and seeking help from school counselors, clergy, and medical care providers might be considered standard care. Other family members, such as grandparents, are also affected in significant ways. They suffer the loss of a grandchild and the inability to protect their children from suffering. A pregnancy loss is a family loss, affecting each member in some manner.

Most parents feel isolated and lonely in their loss because the intangible and often unexplainable loss of dreams, hopes, and future is rarely understood by others who haven't gone through a similar experience. Pregnancy loss and infant death haven't been openly discussed until rather recently; thus, misunderstandings and myths abound. Much of the population believes that "having another baby" will make everything better, as if replacing one person with another will make the grief go away. Others try to offer advice such as "It's not as if you knew them," or "It was nature's way; there must have been something wrong." These well-meaning, but inappropriate, comments only serve to invalidate the normal feelings the parents are experiencing, causing them to question their sanity and their right to have such feelings. There are some behaviors that seem to make the situation worse for parents/families: offering advice, trying to minimize or take the pain away, comparing the loss with other situations, and ignoring the loss by not discussing it.

Yet, there are many things that can be done to support the bereaved family. Experts on pregnancy loss and bereaved parents agree that some of the supportive measures relatives and friends can offer are to listen and share time and concern. A few concrete ideas that might help are: remembering the baby by saying its name, sending a card or plant, and talking openly about the child and the parent's dreams. Due dates, anniversaries, and holidays such as Mother's Day and Father's Day are usually difficult times for families when support is often needed.

Many support organizations and groups have been created since the early 1980s to meet the needs of the bereaved families and to sensitize the caregiving professionals. Services provided range from frequent support meetings, to parent-to-parent support networks, referrals to counselors, extensive literature and newsletters, and educational programs for the community and professionals. Key organizations that can refer people to groups in their area are to be found in the appendix. ✱ SHEROKEE ILSE

See also: Infant Funerals: Contemporary Practices; Pregnancy after Pregnancy Loss; Support Groups for Infant Loss

See **Guide to Related Topics:** Pregnancy Loss and Infant Mortality

Resources

Berezin, Nancy. (1982). *After a Loss in Pregnancy: Help for Families Affected by a Miscarriage, a Stillbirth or the Loss of a Newborn.* New York: Simon and Schuster.

Borg, Susan & Lasker, Judith. (1989). *When Pregnancy Fails.* New York: Bantam.

Davis, Deborah. (1990). *Empty Cradle, Broken Heart: Surviving the Death of Your Baby.* Goldon, CO: Fulcrum Publishing.

DeFrain, John. (1986). *Stillborn: The Invisible Death.* New York: Lexington Books.

Erling, Jake. (1986). *Our Baby Died. Why?* Minneapolis, MN: Pregnancy and Infant Loss Center.

Fritz, Julie with Ilse, Sherokee. (1988). *The Anguish of Loss.* Maple Plain, MN: Wintergreen Press.

Ilse, Sherokee. (1990). *Empty Arms: Coping with Miscarriage, Stillbirth and Infant Death.* Maple Plain, MN: Wintergreen Press.

Ilse, Sherokee & Burns, Linda Hammer. (1985). *Miscarriage: A Shattered Dream.* Maple Plain, MN: Wintergreen Press.

———. (1985). *Sibling Grief.* Minneapolis, MN: Pregnancy and Infant Loss Center.

Ilse, Sherokee & Leininger, Lori. (1986). *Grieving Grandparents.* Minneapolis, MN: Pregnancy and Infant Loss Center.

Limbo, Rana and Wheeler, Sara. (1986). *When a Baby Dies.* Resolve Through Sharing.

Rando, Therese. (1986). *Parental Loss of a Child.* Chicago: Research Press Company.

Rank, Maureen. (1988). *Free to Grieve.* Minneapolis, MN: Bethany House Publishing.

Ransohoff-Adler, Martha & Berger, Candyce S. (1990). "When Newborns Die: Do We Practice What We Preach?" *Journal of Perinatology IX* (3).

Schaefer, Dan & Lyons, Christine. (1986). *How Do We Tell the Children? A Parent's Guide to Helping Children Understand and Cope When Someone Dies.* New York: Newmarket Press.

Woods, James & Esposito, Jennifer. (1987). *Pregnancy Loss: Medical Therapeutics and Practical Considerations.* Baltimore: Williams & Williams.

PREGNANCY TESTING

From time immemorial women and their care providers have sought objective means for determining pregnancy, in part because of the almost universal ambivalence regarding the reality of pregnancy during the early weeks, regardless of how wanted the baby may be. When pregnancy is unwanted, women seek to know as soon as possible so that a decision can be made regarding early termination. Care providers have also sought this knowledge for various clinical and political reasons—among them, control over women and their knowledge of and confidence in their bodies.

A variety of pregnancy tests using urine have been performed throughout the centuries. Since these tests have a wide margin of error, a woman's knowledge of her body and the changes that she experienced were the primary means of determining pregnancy for thousands of years (Oakley, 1986). It wasn't until 1925 that laboratory diagnosis of pregnancy became possible with the advent of modern testing (Oakley, 1986). This innovation was a significant hallmark in the transition from community-based, woman-centered care in the home to the institutionalization of childbirth in the hospital under the care of medical experts.

As the medical profession increased its efforts to establish itself as the source of maternity care for the middle class, popular childbirth books throughout the 1930s and 1940s discouraged women from listening to the "old wives' tales" of their mothers and friends and encouraged them to depend on the doctor as their sole source of information. An integral part of this process was to encourage women to value scientific procedure in all aspects of life. In obstetrics, this began with the determination of pregnancy taking place in the laboratory, bringing young women into the privacy of the doctor's office early in gestation where he could influence her perceptions. This undermining process has been so successful that today many women rely completely upon test results to answer pregnancy-related questions. This laboratory focus removed a woman-centered perspective and replaced it with a system that demands women to petition the expertise and authority of their care providers. The medical profession and medical tests then become an interface between the woman and knowledge of her own body.

All pregnancy tests are based upon the detection of human chorionic gonadotropin (HCG), a placental hormone that rises dramatically in the blood and urine during the early weeks of pregnancy. Although the normal range varies widely from woman to woman, the rate of elevation is fairly constant from day to day during the early weeks and peaks 9 to 10 weeks after the first day of the last menstrual period.

Urine tests are available that offer qualitative results—that is, they detect the presence of HCG. The various lab and at-home tests are all based on the same principle: detecting chemical changes brought about by sufficient levels of HCG in the urine (Hacinli, 1989).

The key word is *sufficient.* Although many urine tests claim 98 to 99 percent accuracy as early as the first day of a missed menstrual period, many women will not be excreting enough HCG at that point to show a positive result. Many others will have marginal levels, which may yield an equivocal result. To increase the likelihood of an accurate test, waiting a week or so and using the first morning urine (which is the most concentrated), regardless of what the instructions suggest, will help.

A number of over-the-counter urine tests are available in pharmacies. Such tests put laboratory methods in the hands of women (a controversial issue among medical doctors when these tests were first proposed). Home pregnancy tests vary widely in the number of steps needed to perform the test and the ease of determining results. Tests that require the mixing of liquids tend to be more time-critical (and more vulnerable to error), as well as being more difficult to interpret. "Dipstick" methods involve fewer steps. Most tests promise results within one to 16 minutes. Many kits now include two tests. If the first test is negative or equivocal, the second test can be performed one week later (Gurin, 1988; Hacinli, 1989). If a week goes by and the result is still negative without the onset of menstruation, a care provider should be consulted. A number of factors (including stress) could be upsetting the hormonal balance and confusing the result. There are a few women who never show a positive urinary HCG test, yet go on to have perfectly normal pregnancies.

Blood test (referred to as Beta-pregnancy tests) determine serum levels of HCG and are only available through a laboratory. This means the test must be ordered by a recognized care provider in the area (who may legally order such tests varies from state to state, but those receiving care cannot order them, period). Making laboratory analysis unavailable to the public is one way the medical profession attempts to ensure that medical advisors of some sort are involved in a person's health care.

Blood tests are accurate when administered four days after the expected onset of menstruation. Although these tests can also be false negative in the early weeks, this is less likely than with a urine test. Blood tests are also more useful when monitoring problems because they can detect either the presence of HCG or the actual amount of HCG (quantitative testing) in the blood stream at a given point. This information can help determine the number of weeks' gestation or fetal viability if a threatened miscarriage has occurred. This makes serial blood tests the most noninvasive clinical means of determining if a fetus is still alive (Frye, 1990).

Laboratory tests, when used appropriately, can empower women and offer valuable information to confirm a woman's own sense of what is happening in her body. Blood tests in particular can help clarify the situation when signs and symptoms are confusing. However, tests and technology should never be used in such a way that a woman's self-confidence in her body is undermined or devalued. (For example, one-third of the time tests are false negative in ectopic pregnancy.) With these thoughts in mind, women can begin to investigate potential care providers and the attitudes that will affect their view of pregnancy, labor, and birth. ✱ ANNE FRYE

See also: Fetus, Maternal Experience of

See **Guide to Related Topics:** Pregnancy, Physical Aspects

Resources

Frye, Anne. (1990). *Understanding Lab Work in the Childbearing Year.* New Haven, CT: Labrys Press. (Available from Moonflower Birthing Supply, P.O. Box 128, Louisville, CO 80027; 1-800-747-8996).

Gurin, Joel. (1988, Sept). "Home Medical Tests: What Works, What Doesn't, What's Right for You." *Glamour*: 142-45.

Hacinli, Cynthia. (1989, Mar). "All Pregnancy Tests Are Not Equal." *Mademoiselle*: 142.

Oakley, Ann. (1986). *The Captured Womb: A History of the Medical Care of Pregnant Women.* London: Basil Blackwell, Ltd.

PREGNANT ADDICTS, TREATMENT OF

In 1903, a letter to the *Journal of the American Medical Association* described the case of a female morphine addict who had given birth. Noting apparent withdrawal symptoms in the newborn, the writer asked "[I]s it possible for a fetus to contract the morphine habit . . .?" The letter was one of the first references in the medical literature to a pregnant addict. Since then, the question of how to treat such women and their newborns has become a major sociomedical problem. The history of the field covers a number of distinct eras.

Pre-1945. Until prohibited in the early 1900s by federal law, notably the 1914 Harrison Act, opium and its derivatives—laudanum, morphine, and heroin—were available without prescription, often as ingredients of patent medicine. Their use, frequently by women, had become widespread by the late 1800s.

Despite the law, addiction to morphine and heroin became prevalent in many large cities after World War I. About one-fifth of the addicts were women, and a mid-1920s survey of 570 New York State physicians found that 51 had observed cases of "congenital narcotic addiction." No programs for pregnant addicts existed; any care was given individually, doctor to patient. Such care became increasingly rare as Supreme Court decisions from 1919 to 1922 in effect barred physicians from treating addicts. The creation of the Federal Bureau of Narcotics in 1930 made opiate addiction almost wholly a law enforcement matter.

Later, as the nation's attention focused first on the Depression and then on World War II, opiate addiction became less visible. Addict births undoubtedly continued to occur, but as the medical profession now had little contact with addicts, virtually nothing about them appeared in the medical literature.

1945-1965. After World War II, the present heroin epidemic began, mainly in the poorer sections of the nation's large cities. Females made up the minority of the addict population, but almost all were of childbearing age. By the mid-1950s, reports appeared from various hospitals on groups of addict births. They noted that the mothers usually lacked prenatal care and often suffered obstetrical complications, and that the newborns were often premature, of low birth weight, and showed signs of withdrawal. Apart from withdrawal, it was not clear whether the other problems were due solely to the mother's heroin use or due in part to lack of prenatal care, poor nutrition, and so on.

By the early 1960s, at the urging of the American Bar Association, the American Medical Association, and the 1963 Presidential Commission on Narcotic and Drug Abuse, medical treatment of addiction began to regain favor. New Supreme Court decisions, federal legislation, and a reorganization of relevant federal agencies made it possible for the medical profession to treat addicts. However, medicine could not yet offer pregnant addicts anything to counteract the lure of heroin and thus bring them into treatment.

1965-1980. Methadone is an oral synthetic opiate. In 1965, in New York City, the first experimental methadone maintenance program opened. By giving methadone daily to addicts, the program allowed them to avoid withdrawal and the craving for heroin. They could thus function normally. By the late 1960s, thousands of addicts were on methadone. It was this lure that brought many pregnant addicts into treatment. At a number of hospitals around the country, informal programs began, which provided, in addition to methadone, prenatal obstetrical care to the pregnant addict and pediatric care to her newborn.

In 1974, a federal agency, the National Institute on Drug Abuse (NIDA), made funds available for a limited time to set up such programs on a formal basis at hospitals in Detroit, Houston, New York City, Philadelphia, San Francisco, and Washington, DC. These six programs offered medical care, addiction treatment, counseling, and parent education. NIDA also funded a residential facility in New York City for addicts who had given birth and their infants. In addition to providing care, the programs researched treatment results, generally finding that the well-being of the programs' mothers and babies was much improved over those who lacked such care. By 1980, NIDA funding ended. Some programs survived; others did not. Despite the knowledge that had been gained, many pregnant addicts—like many other poor women—continued to go without care.

1980-1990. Cocaine emerged as a major problem in the 1980s; among the urban poor the smokeable form, "crack," was prevalent. By 1988, the rate of births to cocaine users in New York City, for example, had increased 20 times over the 1980 rate, from 1.0 to 21.1 per 1,000 live births. (Births to heroin addicts also increased, from 2.3 per 1,000 to 4.3 per 1,000.) Studies of prenatal cocaine use found it was associated with low birth weight, prematurity, and neurological problems. But whether these conditions were attributable just to cocaine use, or to other substances the mother may have used prenatally, or to such poverty-related factors as lack of prenatal care, was not clear. It *was* clear that the treatment system had few programs for pregnant cocaine or crack users, even those who wanted care. Moreover, there was no methadone analog to cocaine to draw into treatment those who otherwise would not have come.

While the cocaine epidemic was spreading, so, too, was AIDS. Drug-abusing women were at high risk of infection with HIV (the human immunodeficiency virus, which causes AIDS). They could get it by sharing needles with IV (intravenous) drug users or by having sex with an infected man, who was usually an IV user. And once infected, a pregnant addict could transmit HIV to her fetus.

The multiplicity of problems—heroin, cocaine, AIDS—often compounded by such other problems as homelessness and domestic violence, led, by 1990, to a renewed public concern for pregnant addicts. But while federal funds again became available for new programs, in many states women, usually poor or of minority group background, were prosecuted for drug abuse during pregnancy. Which way the pendulum will ultimately swing—toward prosecution or treatment—remains to be seen.

✱ FREDERIC SUFFET, M.A.

See also: HIV and Pregnancy; Pregnancy and Social Control; Violence against Pregnant Women

***See* Guide to Related Topics:** Pregnancy Complications

Resources

Beschner, George M. & Brotman, Richard. (Eds.) (1977). *Comprehensive Health Care for Addicted Families and Their Children.* Washington, DC: U.S. Government Printing Office.

Finnegan, Loretta P. (Ed.) (1970). *Drug Dependence in Pregnancy: Clinical Management of Mother and Child.* Washington, DC: U.S. Government Printing Office.

Hoffman, Jan. (1990, Aug 19). "Pregnant, Addicted—and Guilty?" *New York Times Magazine.*

Kay, Katherine et al. (1989, May). "Birth Outcomes for Infants of Drug Abusing Mothers." *New York State Journal of Medicine 89*: 256-61.

Musto, David F. (1973). *The American Disease: Origins of Narcotic Control.* New Haven, CT: Yale University Press.

National Research Council. (1989). *AIDS: Sexual Behavior and Intravenous Drug Use.* Washington, DC: National Academy Press.

New York City Health Department. (1989). "Maternal Drug Abuse—New York City." *City Health Information 8* (8): 1-4.

Queries and Minor Notes. (1903). "Fetal Morphine Addiction." *Journal of the American Medical Association 40:* 1092.

Terry, Charles E. & Pellens, Mildred. (1928). *The Opium Problem.* New York: Committee on Drug Addictions.

THE PREGNANT THERAPIST

The psychotherapist's pregnancy is a unique, time-limited experience that creates new and special problems, as well as opportunities, for the therapist-client relationship. For the client, this event may raise feelings of abandonment and loss, anger, sadness, anxiety, and envy. For the therapist, it may elicit feelings such as sadness and guilt about causing premature ending of the relationship, greater than usual self-involvement, as well as concerns about how to effectively handle issues such as self-disclosure.

To the client, the therapist's pregnancy indicates an inevitable interruption or termination of therapy. If the therapist takes a temporary maternity leave, or ends the treatment altogether, the client must deal with feelings of separation and loss. Many of these feelings, such as sadness and loss associated with past events, are quite similar to those felt during the normal termination process. However, they take on a different meaning when the client is coping with the therapist's pregnancy. For example, female clients may experience memories related to previous abortions, the death of a child, a child given up for adoption, or perhaps the sadness associated with children never conceived (Nadelson et al., 1974). Clients of both sexes may feel envy based on their own unfulfilled expectations and desires to have a home and family. They may also idealize the life they perceive the therapist as having. The pregnancy may elicit feelings about the therapist as a sexual being. Perhaps it will intensify issues related to the client's mother, such as maternal love and care, as well as neglect and sibling rivalry. Knowledge of each client's history of losses can assist the therapist in anticipating her clients' individual reactions. This may be a time for the client to mourn unresolved grief at the same time that he or she is grieving the loss of the therapist.

Often, impending termination of therapy causes the client to temporarily regress to earlier behaviors and problems. Crises may develop as last-resort attempts to maintain contact with the therapist, dissuade her from leaving, or to reestablish contact following termination. No matter how the crises present themselves, they can usually be interpreted as the client saying, "Please don't leave me! How can I make it without you?" Crises that are specific to the therapist's pregnancy might involve an increasing dependence on the therapist and a specific desire to be mothered (Rubin, 1980).

In order for the therapist to help prevent crises from developing, she should develop some type of intermittent plan for the client involving previously planned phone calls or letters, emergency back-up and coverage during the maternity leave, or transfer to another therapist if the termination is permanent and the client chooses to continue treatment.

The therapist may very likely experience intense feelings and concerns that may directly affect the therapeutic relationship. This is known as counter-transference. While pregnant, the therapist will probably be more self-involved than usual. She will most likely be thinking about the physical changes in her body as well as the overall changes in her life. This self-involvement may diminish her ability to "give" to the client, and as a result, she may experience feelings of guilt. It is crucial for the therapist to assess her own new feelings as they arise and examine how they may affect the therapy.

Because the therapist's pregnancy is physically obvious, she is forced to disclose more about herself than she might normally choose. While opinions vary, most schools of therapy agree that self-disclosure by the therapist may be beneficial in helping the client to discuss his or her own feelings about the therapist's pregnancy. The challenge to the therapist is to use this self-disclosure in a way that will be most helpful to the client.

✷ JILL STANZLER-KATZ, M.S.W.

See **Guide to Related Topics:** Pregnancy, Psychological Aspects

Resources

Benedek, Elissa P. (1973). "The Fourth World of the Pregnant Therapist." *Journal of the American Medical Women's Association 28* (7): 365-68.

Bridges, Nancy & Smith, Janna. (1988). "The Pregnant Therapist and the Seriously Disturbed Patient: Managing Long Term Psychotherapeutic Treatment." *Psychiatry 51*(1): 104-09.

Fenster, Sheri, Phillips, Suzanne B., & Rapoport, Estelle R.G. (1986). *The Therapist's Pregnancy: Intrusion in the Analytic Space.* Hillsdale, NJ: The Analytic Press.

Nadelson, Carol et al. (1974). "The Pregnant Therapist." *American Journal of Psychiatry 131* (10): 1107-11.

Rubin, Carol. (1980, May). "Notes from a Pregnant Therapist." *Social Work*: 210-15.

Underwood, Maureen M. & Underwood, Edwin D. (1976, Nov). "Clinical Observations of a Pregnant Therapist." *Social Work*: 512-14.

PREIMPLANTATION DIAGNOSIS

Preimplantation diagnosis describes a variety of methods to screen ova (eggs) and early embryos before they are implanted in the uterus. The goal is to identify the presence of recessive genes for a lengthy list of hereditary and genetic conditions.

Most preimplantation diagnosis currently being developed uses *in vitro* fertilization (the so-called test tube baby method) to obtain the eggs and embryos. For *in vitro* fertilization, the woman is given strong hormones that stimulate her reproductive system to produce multiple eggs, rather than the single egg normally produced each month. Multiple eggs are desired because of the belief that the more eggs or embryos produced, the greater the chance that abnormalities will not be present in all of the gametes. Replacing multiple embryos is also believed to increase the chance of a pregnancy when *in vitro* fertilization is used. The eggs that are obtained are individually screened, or fertilized with the partner's sperm in the lab. The resulting embryos are then screened.

Up to now, the main focus of *in vitro* fertilization has been in the treatment of infertility. Preimplantation diagnosis of embryos and ova has moved reproductive technology in a new direction, extending *in vitro* fertilization to fertile couples. Most couples who are candidates for preimplantation diagnosis are fertile; however, all of them have a family history of hereditary and genetic diseases and are at risk of passing on one of these conditions to any children they might have.

Currently two methods of preimplantation diagnosis are in use. The most common form of preimplantation diagnosis involves screening of the embryo. At a very early stage of embryo growth (two to three days after fertilization), one or two cells are removed from the embryo. The remaining embryo is left to continue to grow or can be frozen for later implantation. Although removing cells at this early stage does not appear to interfere with the embryo's ability to continue to grow, scientists are still not certain if this procedure may result in any later problems. The DNA of the cell that has been removed from the embryo is then analyzed. To do this, scientists use a technique called polymerase chain reaction, which duplicates enough copies of the DNA to allow for analysis.

One method of embryo diagnosis currently in use in England uses the polymerase chain reaction to determine the sex of the embryo. The couples in this trial have a family history of Lesch-Nyhan disease, a rare but devastating neurological disorder that causes an obsessive desire for self-mutilation. Because the disease only occurs in males, only female embryos are reimplanted.

Other centers are developing methods to screen embryos for specific conditions like cystic fibrosis, hemophilia, and some muscular dystrophies. A Chicago center is screening ova (eggs) for genetic and hereditary conditions even before the embryo is fertilized. The women whose eggs will be screened also receive drugs to produce multiple eggs. The goal is to collect six or seven viable eggs to assay.

All human cells contain 46 chromosomes, but female eggs need only 23 chromosomes because the additional 23 will be supplied by sperm. (In this way humans inherit characteristics from each parent.) Eggs start off with 46 chromosomes but jettison the extra set of 23 before fertilization. This second set of cells is referred to as the polar body. The Chicago scientists remove the polar body from the egg for analysis. They believe that by examining the polar body to determine whether or not it contains abnormal genes, they can determine if the egg is normal; if an abnormality occurs in genes in the polar body, it means that all the genetic material in the remaining egg is normal. On the other hand, if no recessive genes are found for specific conditions in the polar body, then it is likely that an abnormality exists in the egg. Only eggs believed free of abnormalities are fertilized. Normally, abnormal genes from both parents are needed for carriers of genetic and hereditary diseases to pass these conditions to offspring.

Preimplantation diagnostic techniques are being developed as an alternative to prenatal screening methods currently in use—amniocentesis and chorionic villus sampling—which are used only after a pregnancy has been established. With these prenatal screening techniques, abortion is the only option for couples who want to terminate a pregnancy. The physicians and scientists developing preimplantation diagnosis believe it is a more suitable option for couples who are opposed to abortion or who may have difficulty deciding to terminate a pregnancy where the fetus may be at risk.

Preimplantation diagnosis is a highly controversial technique. One area of controversy is the accuracy of current techniques. The egg screening method, for example, has been highly criticized by some scientists who believe it is possible for both the polar body and the egg to contain abnormal genes. Other scientists have expressed concern that the cells removed for embryo screening may not provide an accurate picture of the make-up of the remaining cells in the embryo, and that current screening methods may give a false picture of the embryo.

Currently preimplantation techniques are used to identify the risk of diseases only inherited by males. But because all preimplantation techniques identify the sex of the embryo, preimplantation diagnosis opens the possibility of sex selection. Even where these techniques are designed to be used solely to screen embryos for medical reasons, the possibility exists that preimplantation diagnosis could be used as a new form of eugenics. Preimplantation diagnosis can only indicate the presence of a recessive gene; it cannot determine with any certainty how severe the condition might be in any resulting child, or even, in some disorders, when it might appear. Many people with these conditions have mild forms of the disease and lead relatively normal lives.

But even now, developers of preimplantation diagnosis have said that they believe it could become the method of choice for all couples, both fertile and infertile, to be used as a kind of quality control to produce so-called "better" babies.

✷ ANN PAPPERT

See also: Egg Retrieval; Eugenics; Genetics; Prenatal Diagnosis: Overview; Sex Selection, Preconception

See **Guide to Related Topics:** New Procreative Technologies; Prenatal Diagnosis and Screening

Resources

"Abstracts of the First International Symposium on Preimplantation Genetics." (1990, Aug). *Journal of In Vitro Fertilization and Embryo Transfer 7* (4): 84-211.

Handyside, A. et al. (1989, Feb 18). "Biopsy of Human Preimplantation Embryos and Sexing by DNA Amplification. *Lancet.*

Handyside, A. et al. (1990). "Pregnancies from Biopsied Human Preimplantation Embryos Sexed by Y-Specific DNA Amplification." *Nature 344*: 768.

PREMATURE BIRTH: PREVENTION

Premature birth interrupts approximately 10 percent of pregnancies in the U.S. each year and is responsible for the majority of infant deaths; a troublesome array of diseases, disabilities, and neurological disorders; school failure; and devastating financial cost (Committee to Study the Prevention of Low Birthweight, 1985) (See Table 1). Increasingly aggressive neonatal intensive care has reduced mortality for premature infants but raises concerns regarding the quality of life for survivors, especially very low birth-weight infants (Hack and Fanaroff, 1989).

The preterm birth rate for blacks is approximately double that for whites (12 percent versus 6 percent). Problems related to poverty—lack of prenatal care, substance abuse, and others—have been implicated as factors that contribute to preterm birth (Committee to Study the Prevention of Low Birthweight, 1985). Although the problems of poverty are obstacles to the prevention of prematurity, known interventions have been successfully applied to poor populations (Papiernik, 1984; Mueller-Heubach et al., 1989; Morrison et al., 1990), and according to Iams (1989), "prematurity is not a social disease beyond the reach of medical care."

Traditionally, preterm labor has been treated with tocolytic drugs, which can inhibit labor and prolong pregnancy. But despite advances in the use of tocolytics, the prematurity rate has not declined. This lack of decline has been attributed mainly to the fact that therapy is usually initiated too late, when cervical dilation and preterm labor are already too far advanced for tocolytics to be effective. Only about one-third of women who arrive at the hospital in preterm labor can be treated with tocolytic therapy, and among those treated, the failure rate is 40 percent (Huszar and Naftolin, 1984).

Modern approaches to prematurity prevention attempt to be more anticipatory by detecting preterm labor at its earliest, thereby giving tocolytic therapy a better chance at success. These approaches began with Papiernik's publication of a method for identifying women at risk for preterm labor (Papiernik-Berkhauer, 1969). In 1971, the French government made reducing the incidence of premature birth a national goal and has since funded prevention efforts. Papiernik's program includes risk assessment, patient and prenatal care provider education, stress and physical work reduction and financial and social support for pregnant women, changes in risk-associated behaviors of pregnant women, cervical examination, and medical interventions. Employing this approach, the French have succeeded in reducing the prematurity rate from 8.2 percent in 1973 to 5.3 percent in 1982 (Committee to Study the Prevention of Low Birthweight, 1985). An even greater decrease was demonstrated for very low birthweight babies (<1,500 g) in the largest of the French studies (Papiernik et al, 1985).

Meis et al. (1987) note that in instances where individuals (patients and doctors) were asked to change their attitudes and behavior, there was a time lag of several years before improvements were seen in the statistics, suggesting the need for long-term trial programs and highlighting the importance of attitude and commitment in achieving success (Iams, Peaceman, and Creasy, 1988; Mueller-Heubach, 1989).

In the U.S., there has been resistance on the part of obstetricians to the idea of prematurity prevention. Iams (1988) attributes it to, among others, these traditional beliefs: Eastman's 1947 dictum that only when the causes of prematurity are clearly understood can any intelligent attempt at prevention be made; to wait too long to diagnose preterm labor is to guarantee failure, while to treat too quickly is to treat too many; the problem is social, not obstetric; the progress made in neonatal intensive care justifies a passive approach to prematurity; and much time and effort must go into prevention, without additional economic return.

Table 1. Risk Factors for Premature Birth

Multiple gestation	Vaginal spotting or bleeding
Previous preterm delivery	Vaginal or urinary infection (can by asymptomatic)
Previous preterm labor, term delivery	History of infertility
Abdominal surgery during pregnancy	Fetal abnormalities
DES exposure	Poor nutrition
Excess amniotic fluid	Inadequate prenatal care
Uterine abnormality	Smoking, drinking, drug abuse
Uterine fibroids	Strenuous or stressful work
History of cone biopsy	Long commute, more than 3 flights of stairs
Uterine irritability	Under 18 years old or older than 40
More than one second trimester abortion	Low socioeconomic status
Cervical dilation	Low education attainment
Cervical effacement	Unmarried

Adapted from Papiernik, 1984; Gonik and Creasy, 1986; Main, 1988; Holbrook, Laros, and Creasy, 1989; and Semchyshyn and Colman, 1989.

Iams concludes that if obstetricians gave up these beliefs, made "a profound change in [their] collective attitude toward prematurity," and made prematurity prevention the number one focus of their care, great progress would be made, as it has been with other not completely understood conditions, such as preeclampsia.

A growing body of medical literature devoted to prematurity prevention now exists. Researchers are investigating the effects of various interventions and combinations of interventions. Efforts to discover the actual causes of preterm labor are also underway.

Thorough education of the medical community to techniques of prevention (including elicitation of and responsiveness to patient complaints) and methods of treatment is a vital component of prematurity prevention (Papiernik, 1984; Committee to Study the Prevention of Low Birthweight, 1985; Iams, Johnson, and O'Shaughnessy, 1988). Intensive patient education regarding early signs and symptoms of preterm labor, self-detection of contractions, awareness of events that trigger contractions, and the importance of immediate reporting of symptoms is also critical (Table 2). Although the symptoms of preterm labor can occur in normal pregnancy, women who go on to develop preterm labor experience those symptoms more frequently than women who give birth at term, leading Iams et al. (1990) and Iams, Johnson, and Hamer (1990) to conclude that women who report such symptoms should be assessed for cervical status and uterine activity.

Risk assessment has been found to be an important tool for identifying women at risk for preterm labor and for planning interventions based on individual needs. Reassessment of low-risk mothers throughout the pregnancy is suggested, since at present, assessment instruments can predict only about half the women who will experience preterm labor (Iams, Peaceman, and Creasy, 1988). The predictive ability of assessment tools varies with the population assessed.

Additional medical strategies that contribute to the prevention of preterm delivery include individualization of care, increased attention to genito-urinary infection (which can be asymptomatic), and frequent assessment of cervical status. Cervical examination is not a part of routine prenatal care in the U.S. but is a component of many successful prevention programs. Cervical exam at each prenatal visit, with accompanying protocol for infection prevention, can detect cervical changes known to precede preterm labor (Leveno, Cox, and Roark, 1986; Papiernik et al., 1986). Under study are the association of progesterone deficiency and inadequate plasma volume expansion with preterm labor.

Other promising methods for prevention include the use of a subcutaneous terbutaline pump for long-term tocolysis, in which lower doses of medications are needed and successful prolongation of pregnancy can result (Lam et al., 1988) and home uterine activity monitoring, which allows observation of the increased uterine activity that can occur before actual preterm labor. Monitoring devices can detect preterm labor at its earliest,

Table 2. Symptoms of Preterm Labor

- Contractions
- Backache
- Mucous or watery vaginal discharge
- Vaginal spotting or bleeding
- Pelvic pressure
- Menstrual-like cramps
- Abdominal cramps
- Diarrhea

even before women report perceiving contractions, allowing prompt, effective treatment with tocolytics. Morrison et al. (1990) report a preterm delivery rate due to failed tocolysis or advanced cervical dilation of less than 10 percent in monitored women.

Home monitoring involves close (frequently daily) contact between the pregnant woman and a nurse specially trained in prematurity prevention. Even when monitor data were not used in patient care, a significant decrease in preterm deliveries resulted (Porto et al., 1987), leading Iams, Peaceman, and Creasy (1988) to the interpretation that "frequent provider initiated contact, offering support, education and symptom recognition may be as effective as home contraction monitoring in reducing the frequency of preterm delivery in high risk women." ✱ CAROL J. CASTELLANO

See also: Low Birth Weight: United States; Newborn Intensive Care; Prenatal Care in the United States

Resources

Committee to Study the Prevention of Low Birthweight. (1985). *Preventing Low Birthweight.* Washington, DC: National Academy Press.

Gonik, B. & Creasy, R.K. (1986). "Preterm Labor: Its Diagnosis and Management." *American Journal of Obstetrics and Gynecology 154*: 3-8.

Hack, M. & Fanaroff, A.A. (1989). "Outcomes of Extremely-Low-Birthweight Infants between 1982 and 1988." *The New England Journal of Medicine 321*: 1642-47.

Holbrook, R.H., Laros, R.K., & Creasy, R.K. (1989). "Evaluation of a Risk Scoring System for Prediction of Preterm Labor." *American Journal of Perinatology 6*: 62-68.

Huszar, G. & Naftolin, F. (1984). "The Myometrium and Uterine Cervix in Normal and Preterm Labor." *The New England Journal of Medicine 311*: 571-81.

Iams, J.D. (1988). "Obstetric Inertia: An Obstacle to the Prevention of Prematurity." *American Journal of Obstetrics and Gynecology 159*: 796-99.

———. (1989). "Current Status of Prematurity Prevention." *Journal of the American Medical Association 262*: 265-66.

Iams, J.D. et al. (1990). "Symptoms that Precede Preterm Labor and Preterm Premature Rupture of the Membranes." *American Journal of Obstetrics and Gynecology 162*: 486-90.

Iams, J.D., Johnson, F.F., & Hamer, C. (1990). "Uterine Activity and Symptoms as Predictors of Preterm Labor." *Obstetrics and Gynecology 76*: 42S-46S.

Iams, J.D., Johnson, F.F., & O'Shaughnessy, R.W. (1988). "A Prospective Random Trial of Home Uterine Activity Monitoring in Pregnancies at Increased Risk of Preterm Labor. Part II." *American Journal of Obstetrics and Gynecology 159*: 595-603.

Iams, J.D., Peaceman, A.M., & Creasy, R.K. (1988). "Prevention of Prematurity." *Seminars in Perinatology 12*(4): 280-91.

Lam, F. et al. (1988). "Use of the Subcutaneous Terbutaline Pump for Long-term Tocolysis." *Obstetrics and Gynecology 72*: 8810-13.

Leveno, K.J., Cox, K., & Roark, M.L. (1986). "Cervical Dilation and Prematurity Revisited." *Obstetrics and Gynecology 68*: 434-35.

Main, D.M. (1988). "The Epidemiology of Preterm Birth." *Clinical Obstetrics and Gynecology 31*: 521-32.

Meis, P.J. et al. (1987). "Regional Program for Prevention of Premature Birth in Northwestern North Carolina." *American Journal of Obstetrics and Gynecology 157*: 550-56.

Morrison, J.C. et al. (1990). "Cost/Health Effectiveness of Home Uterine Activity Monitoring in a Medicaid Population." *Obstetrics and Gynecology 76*: 76S-81S.

Mueller-Heubach, E. et al. (1989). "Preterm Birth Prevention: Evaluation of a Prospective Controlled Randomized Trial." *American Journal of Obstetrics and Gynecology 160*: 1172-78.

Papiernik, E. (1984). "Proposals for a Programmed Prevention Policy of Preterm Birth." *Clinical Obstetrics and Gynecology 27*: 614-35.

Papiernik, E. et al. (1985). "Prevention of Preterm Births: A Perinatal Study in Haguenau, France." *Pediatrics 76*: 154-58.

Papiernik, E. et al. (1986). "Precocious Cervical Ripening and Preterm Labor." *Obstetrics and Gynecology 67*: 238-42.

Papiernik-Berkhauer, E. (1969). "Coeffecient de risque d'Accouchement Premature." [Coefficients of the Risk of Premature Birth.] *La Presse Medicale 77*: 793-94.

Porto, M. et al. (1987). "The Role of Home Uterine Activity Monitoring in the Prevention of Preterm Birth (abstract no. 96)." Seventh Annual Meeting of the Society of Perinatal Obstetricians, Feb. 6, 1987, Orlando, Florida.

Semchyshyn, S. & Colman, C. (1989). *How to Prevent Miscarriage and Other Crises of Pregnancy.* New York: Macmillan.

PREMATURITY AND LOW BIRTH WEIGHT: AN ALTERNATIVE MANAGEMENT

Neonatal intensive care units are generally believed to be of enormous importance in saving the lives of infants born prematurely. Since this is the belief, it is generally considered unethical to run an experiment testing the hypothesis by assigning some prematurely born babies to hospital care, and some to home care. Thus, this article explores the issue of prematurity and low birth-weight management by looking at historical data, available from Nottingham, United Kingdom, of premature births between 1952 and 1966.

Place of Birth: Selection and Management. Although women who were defined as being "in need" of hospital confinement for medical, obstetrical, or social reasons were referred for National Health Service hospital booking, not all were accepted during this time due to bed shortages. Births were managed in one large and three small NHS hospitals. Those who had no medical need but simply wanted a hospital birth could only ensure one by booking early or paying privately.

In Nottingham between 1952 and 1966, there were 85,027 births, of which 43,173 occurred in a hospital and 41,854 at home. In keeping with the rest of the country, the ratio of home to hospital births diminished over time; in 1962, home births represented 50.2 percent of all births occurring in the city; by 1966, this had been reduced to 42 percent. Today, the number is less than 1 percent.

Of the total 85,027 births, 6,586 resulted in babies weighing less than 5 pounds 8 ounces, and it is the care of these babies that is considered in this article. Of these births of babies under 5 pounds 8 ounces, 2,051 took place at home and 4,535 in hospital. The British Perinatal Survey of 1958 (Butler and Bonham, 1963) showed that there was a bias toward higher social classes in women booked for hospital birth and toward the lower social classes for women booked at home. Low birth weight is known to be associated with social deprivation. This statistical skew toward premature births taking place at home is countered by the screening of women "in need" of hospital birth being more likely to be accepted for hospitalization. However, because many women resisted hospital birth, and others were referred back from the hospital without a bed, up to 50 percent of women who delivered at home in Nottingham fell outside of today's criteria for a home birth.

Women who were booked for home birth were cared for by a district midwife responsible for a geographical "patch" of the city. Each midwife was well known in the neighborhood, attending women in the home and holding weekly prenatal and mothercraft clinics.

Care and Assessment of Small Babies. All babies weighing less than 5 pounds 8 ounces were described as premature, although different care was implemented according to whether the infant was preterm or growth-retarded. In the hospital, small babies were given care in a nursery on the ward, or transferred to a special care baby unit. At home, the district midwife decided either to seek the assistance of a specially trained "premature baby midwife," who would visit the home as many as four times a day, or to transfer the baby to hospital if she believed its needs were beyond her capabilities.

Sometimes the very sickest babies whose deaths were inevitable were kept at home. There were two reasons: first, special care facilities were believed to be wasted on babies for whom there was no hope; and second, it was generally accepted that the mother would wish to nurse her baby within the loving confines of the family and home.

Outcomes. Table 1 shows the mortality outcome of low birth-weight babies born in Nottingham by place of birth between 1952 and 1966. Some of those babies born at home were born to women who were booked for hospital birth but failed to get there because of precipitate labor; that

Table 1. Mortality Outcome of Low Birth-Weight Babies Born in Nottingham, U.K., 1952-66, by Place of Birth

Weight	Born at Home	Referred to Hospital	Died	%	Nursed at Home	Died	%	Born at Hospital	Died	%
Up to 3 pounds 4 ounces	115	94	51	54.3	21	15	71.4	641	455	71.0
4 pounds 6 ounces	268	219	34	15.5	49	3	6.1	937	162	17.3
4 pounds 15 ounces	378	106	16	16.0	272	4	1.5	931	70	7.5
5 pounds 8 ounces	1290	103	27	26.2	1187	27	2.3	2026	91	4.5
TOTALS	2051	522	128	24.5	1529	49	3.2	4535	778	17.2
				SUMMARY						
HOME	2051		128		+	49 =			177	8.6
HOSPITAL								4535	778	17.2

is, the fast and early labor resulting in prematurity made for unintended home births. Other women, although screened for and booked for hospital birth, nonetheless avoided going to hospital and birthed at home. The home birth numbers also include unexpected home births to women who had concealed their pregnancy, had no prenatal care, and only summoned aid when the birth was in progress. Thus, this group is not comparable to the carefully screened home birth populations more commonly found today, and this explains the much higher rates of low birth weight and prematurity. Among those born in the hospital, some had been booked for home birth but transferred either during pregnancy or labor when a premature labor or growth-retarded infant was anticipated.

Of babies weighing less than 5 pounds 8 ounces who were born at home, whether or not it was their intended place of birth, 8.6 percent died, whether or not they were transferred to the hospital. Of those small babies born in hospital, 17.2 percent died. Babies of all weights survived at a greater rate if delivered at home, except the very smallest babies, whose chances for survival were the same whether they remained at home or transferred to the hospital (Tew, 1990).

Discussion. A clear question arises: Why did small babies have a better chance of survival if born at home? This is a particularly interesting question since many of the families of babies born at home were socially deprived. It can be argued that the factor that played the most significant part is lack of stress to the babies. Unlike those babies born in the hospital who were immediately separated from their mother and nursed in a brightly lit area by a number of different staff, babies born at home were nursed by their mother, with the family's love and support and the midwife's encouragement. Those mothers gained a sense of ownership and control and allowed for early bonding, which is beneficial to the newborn.

✱ JULIA ALLISON

See also: Newborn Intensive Care; Premature Birth: Prevention

See **Guide to Related Topics:** Special Needs Infants

Resources

Butler, N.R. & Bonham, D.G. (1963). *Perinatal Mortality: The First Report of the 1956 Perinatal Mortality Survey.* Edinburgh; London: E & S Livinstone Ltd.

Chamberlain, R. et al. (1975). *British Births.* Volume 1. London: S. Heinemann.

Crosse, V.M. (1957). *The Premature Baby.* London: J & A Churchill Ltd.

Tew, Marjorie. (1990). *Safer Childbirth.* London: Chapman and Hall.

PRENATAL CARE IN THE UNITED STATES

Medical experts regard early prenatal care as critical to infant and maternal health. Although it often cannot be explained why mothers who enter the prenatal health care system early in pregnancy have improved pregnancy and newborn outcomes, many studies have linked early receipt of prenatal care with a decreased risk of low birth weight and preterm delivery (Institute of Medicine, 1985; Public Health Service Expert Panel, 1989; Singh, Forrest, and Torres, 1989; Taffel, 1989).

Because of concern to reduce high-risk births, the Public Health Service included among its *Healthy People 2000* infant health objectives a goal that 90 percent of pregnant women in each racial and ethnic group obtain prenatal care within the first trimester of pregnancy (Public Health Service, 1990). In 1988, only 79 percent of white mothers and 61 percent of black mothers began care in the first trimester. Moreover, in 1988, 5 percent of white mothers and 11 percent of black mothers delayed care until the last trimester or received no care at all (Tables 1 and 2).

Data from the birth certificates of the 50 states and the District of Columbia provide further demographic information on those women who are most likely to initiate care in the first trimester and those who tend to delay care until the third trimester or do not receive any care at all. Mothers receiving care in the first trimester are more likely to be white, older, married, more educated, and pregnant with a first-order baby than their counterparts who initiate care later. Mothers who begin care late or receive no care at all are most likely to be black, teenaged, unmarried, with less than 12 years of education, and pregnant with a fourth- or higher-order baby (Table 1).

Timing of care affects birth outcome. For example, early care is associated with a reduced incidence of low birth weight. In 1988, among white mothers who had full-term births, 2.2 percent who initiated care in the first trimester, 3.4 percent who initiated care in the second trimester, 3.9 percent who initiated care in the third trimester, and 7.8 percent who received no care at all had a low birth-weight baby. The respective proportions for black mothers who had full-term births of low birth weight were: 5.2 percent, 6.3 percent, 6.6 percent, and 13.3 percent. The greatest differences

Table 1. Timing of the Initiation of Prenatal Care by Selected Characteristics: United States, 1988

Selected Characteristics	Total	Trimester of Pregnancy Prenatal Care Began		
		1st	2nd	3rd
	Percent			
Race of child				
White	100.0	79.4	15.6	5.0
Black	100.0	61.1	28.0	10.9
Age of mother				
Under 20 years	100.0	53.1	34.0	12.9
30 years or more	100.0	84.8	11.7	3.5
Marital status of mother				
Married	100.0	82.9	13.4	3.7
Unmarried	100.0	55.4	31.3	13.3
Years of school completed by mother 1/				
Less than 12 years	100.0	56.2	31.1	12.7
16 years or more	100.0	92.2	6.5	1.2
Birth order of child				
First order	100.0	77.7	17.3	5.1
Fourth or higher order	100.0	62.7	25.3	12.0

1/ Excludes data for California, Texas, and New York State (not including New York City) which did not require reporting of educational attainment of mother.

in the risk of a low birth-weight outcome are for mothers receiving some care versus those receiving no care. Chances of a low birth-weight baby are substantially lower for mothers receiving care, regardless of when they initiate care, compared with mothers receiving no care at all. These patterns persist for all educational attainment groups with the low birth-weight percent improving, if only marginally, with increased educational attainment (Figure 1).

For the period 1970 to 1980, there were yearly increases in the percent of mothers obtaining early care. Yet, since 1980, there has been virtually no improvement in the proportion of mothers receiving early care (Table 2). Examination of different subgroups of mothers by race, age, marital status, and educational attainment indicates that race and marital status have been the most important factors contributing to the lack of improvement in receipt of timely care in the 1980s.

The proportion of both married and unmarried white mothers receiving care in the first trimester increased during the period 1980 to 1988 (Table 3); the increase was more pronounced for unmarried white mothers. In 1988, 57 percent of unmarried white mothers began care in the first trimester compared to 53 percent in 1980. Despite these increases, the overall proportion of white mothers beginning care in the first trimester remained at 79 percent, because the proportion of births to unmarried mothers increased from 11 percent to 18 percent.

Among black mothers there was little change in the proportions of married and unmarried mothers beginning care in the first trimester. Yet, the overall proportion of black mothers receiving care in the first trimester declined from 63 percent to 61 percent between 1980 and 1988. Again, this decline is due to the increasing proportion of births to unmarried mothers, which rose from 55 percent to 63 percent.

The proportions of both black and white women receiving late or no prenatal care declined from 1970 to 1980; since 1980 the proportions have increased for both groups (Table 2). The proportion of married and unmarried white women receiving late or no care changed little during the period 1980 to 1988. However, among all white mothers, the proportion receiving late or no care increased from 4 percent to 5 percent, due to the

Table 2. Percent Distribution of Live Births by Month of Pregnancy Prenatal Care Began, According to Race: United States, 1970, 1975, and 1980-88

Race	Total	Trimester of Pregnancy Prenatal Care Began			
		1st	2nd	3rd	No Prenatal Care
All races 1/					
1988	100.0	75.9	18.0	4.2	1.9
1987	100.0	76.0	17.9	4.1	2.0
1986	100.0	75.9	18.1	4.1	1.9
1985	100.0	76.2	18.1	4.0	1.7
1984	100.0	76.5	17.9	3.9	1.7
1983	100.0	76.2	18.3	3.9	1.6
1982	100.0	76.1	18.5	3.9	1.5
1981	100.0	76.3	18.5	3.8	1.4
1980	100.0	76.3	18.6	3.8	1.3
1975	100.0	72.4	21.6	4.7	1.3
1970	100.0	68.0	24.1	6.2	1.7
White					
1988	100.0	79.4	15.6	3.5	1.5
1987	100.0	79.4	15.6	3.5	1.5
1986	100.0	79.2	15.9	3.5	1.5
1985	100.0	79.4	15.8	3.4	1.3
1984	100.0	79.6	15.7	3.3	1.3
1983	100.0	79.4	16.0	3.3	1.3
1982	100.0	79.3	16.2	3.3	1.2
1981	100.0	79.4	16.3	3.2	1.1
1980	100.0	79.3	16.4	3.2	1.0
1975	100.0	75.9	19.1	3.9	1.0
1970	100.0	72.4	21.4	5.0	1.2
Black					
1988	100.0	61.1	28.0	6.8	4.1
1987	100.0	61.1	27.8	6.8	4.3
1986	100.0	61.6	27.9	6.6	4.0
1985	100.0	61.8	28.2	6.7	3.4
1984	100.0	62.2	28.2	6.4	3.3
1983	100.0	61.5	28.7	6.5	3.3
1982	100.0	61.5	29.0	6.4	3.1
1981	100.0	62.4	28.5	6.2	2.8
1980	100.0	62.7	28.5	6.1	2.7
1975	100.0	55.8	33.7	7.8	2.7
1970	100.0	44.4	39.1	12.2	4.4

1/ Includes races other than white and black.

Figure 1. Births of Low Birth-weight Babies, 1988

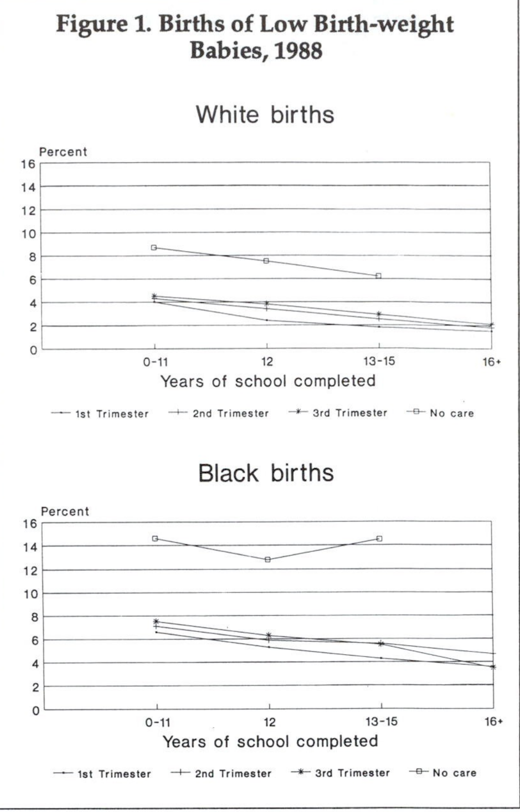

Note: Refers only to full-term births, i.e., births of 37 weeks or more gestation.

increasing proportion of births to unmarried mothers.

The proportion of black women receiving late or no care rose from 9 percent to 11 percent between 1980 and 1988. Some of this rise can be attributed to the increasing proportion of births to unmarried women. However, there also were increases in the proportions of both married and unmarried mothers receiving late or no care. This rise was most pronounced for unmarried mothers, with an increase from 11 percent to 14 percent. Although the timing of the first prenatal visit is often used as a measure of the adequacy of prenatal care received, its usefulness is limited because early care does not always mean continuous care. The Kessner Index provides an alternative, multicomponent measure that examines when prenatal care began in light of the number of prenatal visits made by the mother and the gestational age of the baby (Kessner et al., 1973). Care is defined as "adequate," "intermediate," and "inadequate." In 1988, 69 percent of all mothers received adequate care, 23 percent received intermediate care, and 8 percent received inadequate care. The substantial racial disparity noted with regard to initiation of

Table 3. Percent Distribution of Live Births by Trimester of Pregnancy Prenatal Care Began, According to Marital Status of Mother and Race of Child: United States and the District of Columbia, 1980 and 1988

Marital Status of Mother and Race of Child	Total	Trimester of Pregnancy Prenatal Care Began: 1st	2nd	3rd	No Pre-natal Care
	Percent				
All races 1/					
Married					
1980	100.0	81.3	15.2	2.7	0.8
1988	100.0	82.9	13.4	2.7	1.0
Unmarried					
1980	100.0	53.8	33.7	8.7	3.8
1988	100.0	55.4	31.3	8.5	4.7
White					
Married					
1980	100.0	82.6	14.3	2.5	0.7
1988	100.0	84.1	12.5	2.5	0.9
Unmarried					
1980	100.0	52.9	33.7	9.5	3.9
1988	100.0	57.1	30.2	8.5	4.2
Black					
Married					
1980	100.0	72.3	22.0	4.2	1.5
1988	100.0	74.0	20.2	4.1	1.7
Unmarried					
1980	100.0	54.9	33.8	7.6	3.7
1988	100.0	53.5	32.6	8.4	5.5

1/ Includes races other than white and black.

care also is apparent for adequacy of care. In 1988, 73 percent of white mothers and only 51 percent of black mothers received adequate care (Figure 2). Likewise, 6 percent of white mothers and 16 percent of black mothers received inadequate care.

In order to reach the Public Health Service's goal for prenatal care for the year 2000, increases in the percent of mothers initiating care in the first trimester are needed for all subgroups. However, prenatal care promotion needs to focus specifically on reaching black women and unmarried women having babies. ✱ CAROLINE T. LEWIS, M.A.

See also: Low Birth Weight: United States; Premature Birth: Prevention

Resources

Institute of Medicine. (1985). *Preventing Low Birthweight.* Washington, DC: National Academy Press.

Kessner, D.M. et al. (1973). "Infant Death: An Analysis by Maternal Risk and Health Care." *Contrasts in Health Status.* Volume I. Institute of Medicine. Washington, DC: National Academy of Sciences.

Lewis, C.T. (1989, Oct 24). "Prenatal Care in the 1980's." Paper presented at the annual meeting of the American Public Health Association, Chicago.

Public Health Service. (1990). *Healthy People 2000: National Health Promotion and Disease Prevention Objectives.* Washington, DC: U.S. Department of Health and Human Services.

Figure 2. Adequacy of Care, 1988

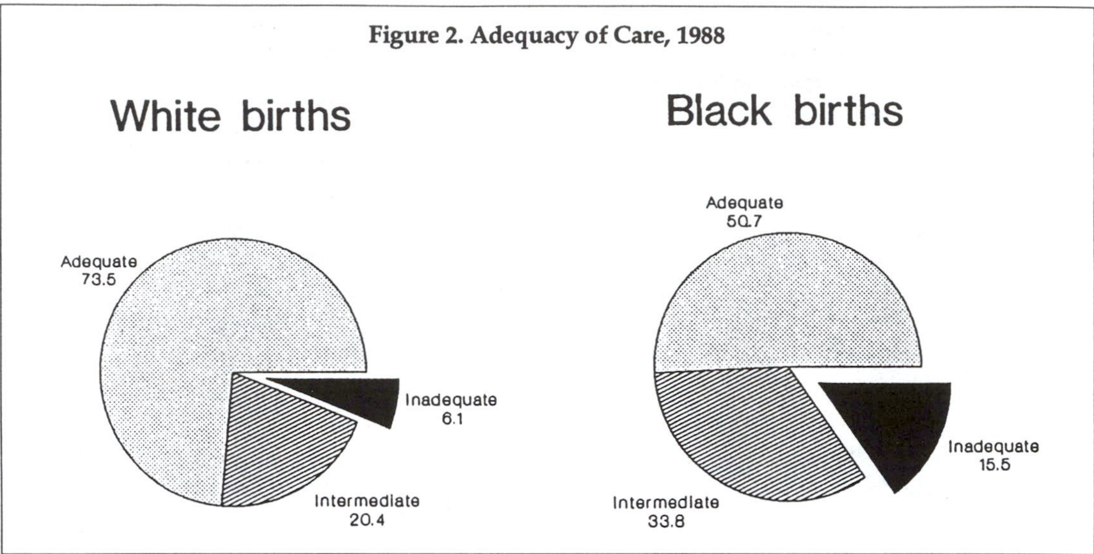

Note: Adequacy of care is defined by the Kessner Index.

Table 4. Percent of Full-term Births of Low Birth Weight by Trimester of Pregnancy Prenatal Care Began, Educational Attainment of Mother, and Race of Child: 1988

Educational Attainment and Race	Trimester of Pregnancy Prenatal Care Began			
	1st	2nd	3rd	No Care
White				
0-11	4.0	4.3	4.5	8.7
12	2.4	3.4	3.8	7.5
13-15	1.8	2.5	2.9	6.2
16+	1.5	1.8	2.1	*
Black				
0-11	6.6	7.1	7.5	14.6
12	5.3	5.9	6.3	12.8
13-15	4.3	5.6	5.5	14.5
16+	3.6	4.7	3.5	*

* Figure does not meet standard of reliability.

Public Health Service Expert Panel on the Content of Prenatal Care. (1989). *Caring for Our Future: The Content of Prenatal Care.* Washington, DC: U.S. Government Printing Office.

Singh, S., Forrest, J.D., & Torres, A. (1989). *Prenatal Care in the United States: A State and County Inventory.* New York: The Alan Guttmacher Institute.

Singh, S., Torres, A., & Forrest, J.D. (1985). "The Need for Prenatal Care in the United States: Evidence from the 1980 National Natality Survey." *Family Planning Perspectives 17* (3): 118-24.

Taffel, S.M. (1989). "Trends in Low Birth Weight: United States, 1975-85." National Center for Health Statistics. *Vital Health Statistics 21* (48): 16-18.

U.S. Surgeon General. (1980). *Promoting Health/Preventing Disease—Objectives for the Nation.* Washington, DC: U.S. Government Printing Office.

PRENATAL DIAGNOSIS: OVERVIEW

The medical-industrial complex has succeeded in changing the pregnancy experience. Nowhere is this more evident than in the area of prenatal genetic testing. The commercialization of clinical genetic research has resulted in the development of numerous prenatal screening and diagnostic tests that include maternal serum alpha-fetoprotein (MSAFP) screening, fetal ultrasound (sonography), amniocentesis, chorionic villus sampling (CVS), percutaneous umbilical blood sampling (PUBS), and DNA testing. Each of these are medical and/or surgical procedures performed on a pregnant woman to provide information, with varying degrees of accuracy, on the health of the fetus. The psychological sequelae associated with prenatal genetic testing has been well documented (Hubbard, 1984; Rothman, 1986; Blatt, 1988).

Prenatal genetic diagnosis is the term frequently used to describe amniocentesis. The application of amniocentesis in the diagnosis of genetic disease became acceptable medical practice in the 1960s after documentation of its ability to obtain amniotic fluid for cytogenetic analysis. The other prenatal genetic technologies accepted today as safe and justifiable for use in pregnancy have been developed only within the past decade.

Amniocentesis (often referred to as an "amnio" or "tap") is a surgical procedure. It is performed by an obstetrician and requires special training and expertise in genetics and laboratory medicine. It is usually performed in an office setting between 16 and 18 weeks of pregnancy, counting from the first day of the last menstrual period (LMP). Early amniocentesis, performed at 12 to 14 weeks' gestation, is currently being investigated as an alternative to amniocentesis at 16 to 18 weeks or to chorionic villus sampling at 9 to 12 weeks.

Amniocentesis involves insertion of a needle into the uterus to remove a sample of amniotic fluid. The amniotic fluid contains cells and substances shed by the fetus that can be analyzed in a specialized laboratory to determine the genetic make-up of the fetus. Specific cytogenetic, biochemical, or molecular tests may be done to determine the presence of chromosome disorders and metabolic and biochemical conditions, as well as DNA-based diseases. Prenatal diagnosis can also be used for fetal sex determination.

Amniocentesis is performed under constant transabdominal or transvaginal ultrasound guidance in order to avoid harm to the fetus or placenta. It can be performed in the presence of multiple births (twins); however, it poses additional challenges.

Failure to obtain sufficient amniotic fluid can occur in the presence of uterine cramping, tightening of the amniotic membranes, fibroids, and other conditions. It is not unusual for an obstetrician to insert the needle into the uterus more than once. Complications may increase with additional needle insertions. Rescheduling the procedure is sometimes indicated. Possible complications of amniocentesis include infection, leakage of fluid, vaginal bleeding, isoimmunization, fetal injury, and pregnancy loss (miscarriage). Risks of the procedure are estimated to be approximately 0.5 percent. The conclusions of the National Institute of Child Health and Human Development Amniocentesis Registry Study (NICHD National Registry for Amniocentesis Study Group, 1976) and the Medical Research Council of Canada's Working Group Report on Prenatal Diagnosis (Medical Research Council, 1977) are often used to support the safety and accuracy of prenatal diagnosis.

Results of amniocentesis usually take two to three weeks and are considered highly accurate when performed in a reputable laboratory. The majority of prenatal genetic tests will reveal a healthy fetus. Contrary to popular belief, however, a normal prenatal test result cannot *guarantee* a perfect baby at birth. It can only indicate whether the fetus has the particular condition(s) for which it is being tested. If prenatal diagnosis reveals the presence of a fetal disability, a woman has a number of options, including continuing the pregnancy and planning for special care at the time of delivery, relinquishing the child for adoption at birth, or terminating the pregnancy.

Routine application of prenatal genetic tests stems from a variety of medical, social, political, legal, and economic factors. While originally designed for use with "high-risk" women, prenatal diagnosis is increasingly offered to pregnant women regardless of age and family history as a follow-up to their tests or to calm maternal anxiety. New obstetrical classification systems that place all pregnancies into a risk category have increased the number of women eligible for testing. Other reasons for its increased use include the postponement of pregnancy until a later age, desire for the perfect baby, fear and superstition surrounding disabilities based mostly on unfounded stereotypes, expanded media coverage about "breakthroughs" in research on birth defects and genetic disorders, physician liability and fear of malpractice, and economic reward.

Prior to the initiation of prenatal genetic tests, comprehensive and nondirective genetic counseling for the expectant parent(s) to assist in decision making is recommended. An explanation of the test, up-to-date information about the disabilities able to be identified, and the risks and benefits of the test to both mother and fetus need to be provided to the parent(s) for informed decision making. A thorough early prenatal genetic assessment of maternal and paternal age; ethnic background; medical and family history; and reproductive, social, environmental, occupational, and nutritional history can be useful when evaluated by a knowledgeable practitioner in order to determine individual risk status. However, much more than the communication of risk figures for a particular disorder is necessary to make a decision about whether to undergo prenatal diagnosis. Understanding and insight into the disabilities that can be detected, the emotional impact of this choice, and the potential sequelae are necessary.

Widespread application of genetic screening and diagnostic tests raises serious questions about interference with the natural process of pregnancy, experimentation on women, disability rights, and who the patient is—pregnant woman or fetus? Other issues of concern include access to linguistically and culturally appropriate educational materials and counseling, financial and geographic access to services, informed choice, reproductive autonomy, respect for individual decisions and confidentiality of genetic information. As research in prenatal genetics continues, new techniques will expand the number of genetic disorders that can be diagnosed and treated *in utero* as well as the ethical issues inherent in the prenatal genetic screening and diagnostic process. The modern medicalization of pregnancy and the exportation of prenatal genetic tests is occurring worldwide. Other Western countries reveal patterns of usage similar to the U.S.; however, prenatal genetic disease detection remains less of a priority in developing countries.

✷ ROBIN J.R. BLATT, M.P.H.

See also: Amniocentesis, History of; Childkeeping and Childbearing; Chorionic Villus Sampling; Eugenics; Genetic Counseling; Genetics; Genome Mapping; Imaging Techniques; Maternal Serum Alpha-Fetoprotein Screening; The Perfect Baby; Preimplantation Diagnosis; Risking; Selective Abortion; Wrongful Birth and Wrongful Life

See **Guide to Related Topics:** New Procreative Technologies; Prenatal Diagnosis and Screening

Resources

Arditti, R., Kelin, R.D., & Minden, S. (1984). *Test-tube Women: What Future for Motherhood?* Boston: Pandora Press.

Astbury, J. & Walters, W.A.W. (1979). "Amniocentesis in the Early Second Trimester of Pregnancy and Maternal Anxiety." *Australian Family Physician 8*: 595-99.

Blatt, Robin J.R. (1988). *Prenatal Tests: What They Are, Their Benefit and Risks and How to Decide Whether to Have Them or Not.* New York: Vintage Books.

Fava, G.A. et al. (1982). "Psychological Reactions to Amniocentesis: A Controlled Study." *American Journal of Obstetrics and Gynecology 143*: 509-13.

Hubbard, R. (1984). "Prenatal Courage Is Not Enough: Some Hazards of Childbearing in the 80s." *Test-tube Women: What Future for Motherhood?* Boston: Pandora Press.

Kaiser, I.H. (1982). "Amniocentesis." *Women and Health* 7: 29-38.

Medical Research Council. (1977). *Diagnosis of Genetic Disease by Amniocentesis during the Second Trimester of Pregnancy.* Ottawa, Canada.

Neilsen, C.C. (1981). "An Encounter with Modern Medical Technology: Women's Experiences with Amniocentesis." *Women and Health* (6): 109-29.

NICHD National Registry for Amniocentesis Study Group. (1976). "Mid-trimester Amniocentesis for Prenatal Diagnosis Safety and Accuracy." *Journal of the American Medical Association* (236): 1471-76.

President's Commission for the Study of Ethical Problems in Medicine and Biomedical and Behavioral Research (1983). *Screening and Counseling for Genetic Conditions.* Washington, DC: U.S. Government Printing Office.

Rapp, R. (1984, Apr). "The Ethics of Choice: After My Abortion Mike and I Faced the Toughest Decision of Our Lives." *Ms.* (12): 97.

Rothman, Barbara Katz. (1986). *Tentative Pregnancy: Prenatal Diagnosis and the Future of Motherhood.* New York: Viking Press.

Silvestre, D. & Fresco, N. (1980). "Reactions to Prenatal Diagnosis: An Analysis of 87 Interviews." *American Journal of Orthopsychiatry 50*: 610-17.

Verjaal, M., Leschot, N.J., & Treffers, P.E. (1982). "Women's Experiences with Second Trimester Prenatal Diagnosis." *Prenatal Diagnosis* 2: 195-209.

PROBLEM PREGNANCY COUNSELING

Women are sometimes faced with unintended pregnancies or pregnancies that were planned but which subsequently seem undesirable to carry to term; for example, when there is known fetal abnormality (*see* "Prenatal Diagnosis Overview") or when relationships or life circumstances change unexpectedly. In such cases, the woman may seek counseling from a health or social service agency or a therapist. A pregnant woman has only three choices: bearing a child and keeping it, bearing a child and putting it up for adoption, or seeking an abortion. When none of these options seems attractive or feasible, as is often the case with an unintended or unwanted pregnancy, the woman may have difficulty in making a timely decision, dealing with her feelings, and handling the practical aspects of the pregnancy, such as financial cost or other related issues that surface at this time.

The goals of problem pregnancy counseling are (1) to help the woman face the need for decision; (2) to provide her information about each of the options and about the decision-making process; (3) to help her examine her feelings and values so that her decision can be consonant with them; (4) to assist her in anticipating the impact the consequences of her decision will have on herself and relevant others; and (5) to provide her a referral to appropriate services so she can implement her decision or obtain additional counseling if needed.

Because decisions about a problem pregnancy involve life, death, and sexuality, most women feel ambivalent; they have mixed feelings about each of the alternatives. Finding the most appropriate course of action is often a painful process, and the woman will likely continue to have some difficult feelings regardless of which option she chooses, though most women are able to manage those feelings and take action successfully after a brief counseling intervention. The most common outcome of a pregnancy counseling session is a choice for abortion because it is usually the woman who feels strongly that she cannot continue her pregnancy but has not yet been able to work through her mixed feelings who seeks pregnancy counseling; however, some women will decide to continue the pregnancy. A very small number select adoption, which is perceived by most women as the most emotionally difficult of the three choices.

The first nationwide organized problem pregnancy counseling service in the U.S. was begun by the Rev. Howard Moody in New York City in the mid-1960s under the name Clergy Consultation Service. This group of ministers, whose purpose was to assist women of limited resources in making decisions about unwanted pregnancy and to find physicians who would perform safe and low-cost abortions, rapidly expanded, so that by the end of the 1960s, there were Clergy Consultation Services in most major cities in the U.S. Because of the restrictive legislation at that time, the CCS groups were obliged to operate underground. After the legalization of abortion in 1973, pregnancy counseling services were added to the reproductive health services provided by Planned Parenthood and other health department and community social service agencies. During the 1980s, a new kind of problem pregnancy counseling clinic was devised by groups opposed to abortion and run by them. At these clinics the goal is to promote childbearing and discourage abortion. Many abortion clinics now also offer pregnancy counseling as part of their standard service in order to ensure that abortions are done only for women who are certain they want them and who have given fully informed consent. In 1991 federal regulations were enacted to prohibit abortion counseling in federally funded Title X clinics. Many clinics, particularly those of Planned Parenthood, have chosen to refuse federal funds to subsidize family planning care for poor women rather than comply with the so-called "gag rule."

✱ TERRY BERESFORD

See also: Abortion Counseling; Adoption, Closed; Adoption, Open; Birthmothers; Selective Abortion

See **Guide to Related Topics:** Abortion; Adoption

Resources

Baker, Anne. (1985). *The Complete Book of Problem Pregnancy Counseling.* Granite City, IL: The Hope Clinic for Women.

Beresford, Terry. (1988). *Short Term Relationship Counseling: A Self-Instructional Manual for Family Planning Clinics.* Baltimore: Planned Parenthood of Maryland.

Saltzman, Lori et al. (1988). *Pregnancy Counseling.* San Francisco: Planned Parenthood of San Francisco/Alameda, San Francisco.

PROLAPSE. *See instead* PELVIC MUSCLES

PSYCHOPROPHYLACTIC METHOD (LAMAZE)

The psychoprophylactic method, or PPM, of "painless childbirth" was developed in 1949 in the Soviet Union by a team of Kharkov medical researchers including two neuropsychiatrists, I. Velvovsky and K. Platonov, and two obstetricians, V. Ploticher and E. Shugom (Chertok, 1959, p. 98). For many years, Russian researchers had been studying the use of hypnosis in producing "painless" childbirth. The first woman trained by Platonov in hypnosis for childbirth gave birth in 1923, and in 1925, Platonov and Velvovsky started to publish work in this area (Chertok, 1959, p. 32). The PPM arose out of the failure of hypnosis in childbirth (Chertok, 1959, p. 95; Velvovsky et al., 1960, p. 93). Russian workers shared with Grantly Dick-Read the understanding that fear and tension lead to pain, and they believed that education, exercise and relaxation techniques, and a sympathetic hospital environment could do a great deal to reduce the pain of labor (Velvovsky et al., 1960, p. 392). But they were critical of Read's encouraging what they viewed as a passive role, preferring what they called an active role for the laboring woman. The woman's task in pregnancy is to practice deep-breathing techniques in response to the signal of the beginning of uterine contractions, so that by the time labor begins, the breathing techniques will be so well learned that they have become a conditioned reflex. The breathing gives the birthing woman something to do to distract her from the pain of the contraction, so that she will either not notice the contraction or will not focus on the discomfort it causes. In addition, the woman is trained to massage her abdomen ("effleurage") during the later stages of labor to send a competing, pleasurable message to the brain, thus inhibiting the pain message the uterus would otherwise be sending. This "gate-control theory" suggests that the brain can receive only one message from a particular part of the body at a time. Herein lies the major difference between the PPM and Read's, or other, relaxation models of childbirth training: The woman using PPM is trained to *do* something. The "something" she is doing is not only relaxing, but taking her mind away from the activity of the uterus (Vellay, 1960, p. 25).

Lamaze Brings PPM to the West. The PPM was publicized and adopted nationwide in the Soviet Union with the issuance of a Ministry of Health directive in February 1951 (Chertok, 1959, p. 92). In that same year an international symposium on the method was held in the Soviet Union to which a French obstetrician, Fernand Lamaze (1890-1957), head of the maternity hospital of the metallurgists' union, was invited. Lamaze, who at that time had been practicing obstetrics for 30 years, was amazed at the method, which he not only heard about but saw firsthand. He determined to bring the method to France on a large scale. Lamaze altered the method somewhat. Instead of relying solely on deep breathing as the Russians had, he added two additional types of shallower breathing to be used as the contractions get more intense. These complicated breathing patterns involve more effort on the part of the laboring woman and are therefore said to be more effective in distracting her from the discomfort of stronger contractions (Lamaze, 1965, pp. 14-15).

Lamaze returned to the Soviet Union in 1955, where his former teachers congratulated him on having actually established the method in France (Vellay, 1960, p. 16). The second country outside the Soviet Union to adopt the psychoprophylactic method was China; a large study (Ch'en Wen-chan, 1957) reports the successful use of the method in a Beijing hospital. How widely it was adopted and how much it continues in use today are not clear, however; a tour of China by American childbirth educators showed widespread emphasis on prenatal education about nutrition and the anatomy and physiology of pregnancy and childbirth, but no PPM training (Shearer, 1983).

Karmel Brings PPM to the United States. Lamaze had little success in trying to introduce the PPM in the United States in the early 1950s. Arms (1975, pp. 288-89) attributes this poor reception to the political climate of the McCarthy period, in which Lamaze was seen as a foreigner who worked at a "communist" union hospital and had adopted a Russian childbirth method. When the method was praised by Pope Pius XII in 1956 as a "benefit for the mother in childbirth" that "fully conforms to the will of the Creator" (Vellay, 1960, p. 17; Karmel, 1965, p. 13), some of the political stigma previously attached to it was removed. It was finally introduced in the United States in 1959 by Marjorie Karmel, an American who had given birth to her first child at Lamaze's hospital in France and wanted to use the method in the United States for the birth of her second child. Her book (Karmel, 1965) was the first work published in this country about the PPM, which she referred to as the "Pavlov method" (Karmel, 1965, p. 172). With physical therapist Elisabeth Bing, Karmel founded the American Society for Psychoprophylaxis in Obstetrics, and the method rapidly gained popularity—to some extent because the founders of ASPO worked very hard to involve obstetricians in their organization, reassuring them that their authority was in no way being challenged.

At the time the psychoprophylactic method was introduced into American obstetrics, the dominant childbirth technique being practiced was still twilight sleep. The impact of the Lamaze method has been to allow the mother to be "awake and aware" of the birth of her child, as the title of the first book on the subject by an American obstetrician indicates (Chabon, 1966). The experience of being present at the birth of one's child makes an enormous psychological difference to women. Many women whose children were born before 1960 feel that they missed out on the birth of their children, often expressing envy of the younger generation of women, who get to "be there" when their babies are born. Another profound change wrought by the use of the Lamaze method in American hospitals is the acceptance of the presence and active participation of the father, which has coincided perfectly with the increased emphasis given shared parenting by the women's movement in recent years. The image of the father-to-be pacing the floor nervously outside the labor and delivery suite has been supplanted by the image of father-as-coach (and indeed, some Lamaze-trained men wear "coach" t-shirts to the hospital).

There are also great advantages for babies whose mothers have taken less medication during labor and delivery. So great has the impact of "awake and aware" childbirth been that nowadays women who *haven't* taken childbirth preparation classes are given smaller doses of medication than were many women who *had* taken Lamaze classes when the method was first introduced (Charles et al., 1978, p. 50).

In recent years, there has been much criticism of the Lamaze method as it is currently practiced in American hospitals. Many feel that the method has become so popular from the standpoint of doctors and hospital staff because the Lamaze-trained laboring woman is in fact in control only of her own behavior, not of the situation or the medical decisions that are being made about how to conduct her labor (Rothman, 1982). Instead of grunting, crying, hollering, or otherwise making a nuisance of herself, the Lamaze-trained woman pants and puffs politely with each contraction, saying, in effect, "I'll behave myself if you'll please let me stay awake and watch the birth of my baby." Hospital staff are trained to do something for women who make noise, as they are for patients whose illnesses cause them to be in pain; if women keep quiet and control themselves with breathing techniques, the hospital staff will not intervene. Thus the Lamaze method's interventionist philosophy meshes with American medicine's own interventionism more easily than a relaxation method such as Grantly Dick-Read's, in which women aren't doing anything—except having babies. ✷ MARTHA LIVINGSTON, Ph.D.

See also: Breath Control in Labor; Hypnosis for Childbirth; Labor: Overview; Pain Relief in Labor: Nondrug Methods; Read Method: Natural Childbirth

***See* Guide to Related Topics:** Childbirth Practices and Locations

Resources

Arms, S. (1975). *Immaculate Deception: A New Look at Women and Childbirth.* New York: Bantam Books.

Chabon, I. (1966). *Awake and Aware: Participating in Childbirth through Psychoprophylaxis.* New York: Dell.

Charles, A.G. et al. (1978). "Obstetric and Psychological Effects of Psychoprophylactic Preparation for Childbirth." *American Journal of Obstetrics and Gynecology 131*: 44-52.

Ch'en Wen-chan. (1957). "A Clinical Analysis of 8063 Cases of Painless Labor by the Psychoprophylactic Method." *Chinese Medical Journal 75*: 337-43.

Chertok, L. (1959). *Psychosomatic Methods in Painless Childbirth: History, Theory and Practice.* New York: Pergamon Press.

Karmel, M. (1965). *Thank You, Dr. Lamaze.* Garden City, NY: Doubleday.

Lamaze, F. (1965). *Painless Childbirth.* New York: Pocket Books.

Rothman, B.K. (1982). *In Labor: Women and Power in the Birthplace.* New York: W.W. Norton & Co.

Shearer, B.C. (1983). "Childbirth in China." *C/Sec Newsletter 9*: 1.

Vellay, P. (1960). *Childbirth without Pain.* New York: E.P. Dutton.

Velvovsky, I. et al. (1960). *Painless Childbirth through Psychoprophylaxis.* Moscow: Foreign Languages Publishing House.

PUERPERAL FEVER

Puerperal sepsis, better known as childbed fever, was a much feared cause of death, particularly among women giving birth in hospitals. Epidemics of childbed fever would sweep through hospitals, killing women in great numbers. Prior to the development of germ theory, and the consequent development of "sterile technique," physicians moved from autopsy to delivery, unknowingly spreading the disease with unwashed hands and blood- and pus-stained clothing. The physician Semmelweiss met with great opposition when he identified the physicians themselves as spreading the disease.

Puerperal fever, while it did occur in people's homes, took the form of small, very localized epidemics until maternity wards came to be common in hospitals and the fever became a national scourge. Epidemiologically, the fever was abating in virulence—or widespread resistance was developing, or both—*before* the first antibiotic came on the market.

In 1936, hospital maternal mortality rates, which had consistently been far above those of the home, began to drop sharply. In the same year, researchers in Great Britain began working with a new drug, which they called "prontosil." It was the first version of the antibiotic "sulfanilamide," a relatively weak antibiotic now used mainly for bladder infections.

Because of the conjunction of the dramatic drop in mortality and the discovery of the first antibiotic, it has since been widely accepted that the drop in maternal mortality, when it finally came, was *caused* by the discovery of antibiotics. There was a time lag, however, between the discovery of the drug and its release for general use. By the time prontosil came on the market, deaths from puerperal sepsis had fallen from 800 a year in Great Britain in 1934 to half that figure—347—in 1937. By 1946, when penicillin became available in Great Britain, the number of deaths from puerperal sepsis had already dropped to 53 a year.

Observers from the time felt that some factor outside of anything they were doing was responsible for the drop. Many physicians had not had any experience using sulfonamides. Initial research on prontosil appeared to show dramatic results where it was used, because the "controls" for the patients treated with the drug were simply the mortality statistics of previous years.

Although many physicians had been promoting the value of modern obstetrics in safeguarding the mother for decades, when the actual improvement came, they initially responded with disbelief and caution, lest this turn out to be a slight blip before the rate were to return to its previous high. And in fact, in Ontario, the hospital rates did increase again in 1940, although not nearly as much as previously had been the case. And then the curve went down again.

It took about 10 years before it became accepted wisdom that modern medicine had "caused" this change, and another decade before the reasons became universally enshrined: Improvement in the safety of childbirth was caused by three things:

(1) the discovery of sulfonamides, (2) the use of blood transfusions, and (3) the increase in hospital birth. The even more dramatic drop in the following decade was explained by the "further increase in the use of hospitals" and the "general availability of antibiotics after the war." These explanations passed into the categories of common sense and are still with us today. ✱ JUTTA MASON, Ph.D.

Resource

Oakley, Ann. (1984). *The Captured Womb: A History of the Medical Care of Pregnant Women*. London: Basil Blackwell Publisher, Ltd.

QUICKENING. *See instead* FETUS, MATERNAL EXPERIENCE OF

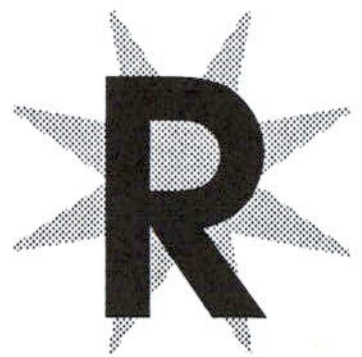

READ METHOD: NATURAL CHILDBIRTH

Grantly Dick-Read (1890-1959), an English doctor, was the earliest proponent of "natural childbirth," which was the title of his first book (Dick-Read, 1933). Dick-Read believed that women's most important reason for being was to bear children, and saw childbearing as the "perfection of womanhood" (Dick-Read, 1972, p. xxi). From a religious standpoint, he could not understand why God would have made this most perfect example of his love painful. Dick-Read viewed misinterpretations from the Bible as the source of some of the anxiety with which women were taught to view birth, and he sought to rewrite some of the prayers women were taught to say in relation to childbirth to eliminate references to pain and death. Dick-Read may not have been a feminist, but he approached laboring women with respect and awe, leading Rothman (1982, p. 86) to comment that "while [this view] may not do much for women's place in the larger society, it is not necessarily a bad perspective with which to approach a laboring woman."

As Dick-Read tells it, his awakening came when, as a young doctor, he attended a very poor woman in labor in a Whitechapel, London, slum. When it came time for the baby to be born, he handed her a chloroform mask, which she refused. He later asked why she had refused the chloroform, and she said, "It didn't hurt. It wasn't meant to, was it, Doctor?" (Dick-Read, 1944, p. 2). This and similar experiences, as well as a profound experience he himself had while recovering from a major injury in World War I, persuaded him that the pain of what he later called "cultural childbirth" was not a natural state, but was brought on by a combination of fear and tension, which were caused by ignorance of the birth process, by the isolation in which women were left during labor, and by the unsympathetic care they received in hospital labor and delivery suites.

The woman who has been led to believe that childbirth is a painful experience will interpret the novel sensation of uterine contraction as pain; this interpretation will lead her to tense the round muscles in the lower uterine segment which, in the "natural" state, would be flaccid, allowing for the passage of the baby. This actual holding back of the baby contrary to the normal physiology of labor leads to real pain, which, however, was caused entirely by culturally induced fear. Dick-Read dubbed this the fear-tension-pain syndrome.

Dick-Read distinguished among three kinds of childbirth: natural childbirth, cultural childbirth, and abnormal childbirth. In natural childbirth, the body performs its physiological task unencumbered by fearful expectation. Not only is natural birth seen as not painful, but the moment of birth is described in the most blissful language. In cultural childbirth, the physiology is tampered with by the cultural expectation that birth will be a harrowing, painful experience; reeducation and sympathetic birth attendants can transform this birth into a natural birth, but untrained women in this condition are likely to need, and should be given, some medication to alleviate the albeit culturally caused pain they experience. In the third condition, abnormal or surgical delivery, anesthesia is, of course, necessary. Unlike some later proponents of various forms of natural and prepared childbirth, Dick-Read did not blame the victim: He saw the culture in general, not women, as responsible for laboring women's fears.

Dick-Read's natural childbirth method consisted of educating women about the anatomy and physiology of labor, and training them in progressive relaxation techniques. Relaxation, as he saw it, would lessen the tension that gave rise to pain in labor and would reduce fatigue, which magnified the subjective experience of the pain of labor. Dick-Read was also well aware of other psychological principles and their relation to pregnancy and childbirth, writing about autosuggestion, imagery, and the conditioned reflex. Dick-Read's method asked both more (patience) and less (intervention) of obstetricians and medical attendants, and was not well received. Doctors saw themselves as providing the pain relief that was essential and inevitable in every labor, though it meant rendering women unconscious for the birth of their babies. They also claimed that the amount of time spent with laboring women by doctors using Dick-Read's method was excessive.

Dick-Read's method was imported into the United States in the 1940s, but was never widely used. Those women who tried to use it here were confronted with trying to accomplish natural childbirth in an unnatural, hospital environment, often rooming with women who had been given twilight sleep and were disoriented and screaming, and with little or no encouragement from labor and delivery room staff. Although Dick-Read claimed that nine out of 10 of his patients required no medication, a study done at Yale (Rothman, 1982, p. 88) showed that five out of 10 women required medication there. One widely held misinterpretation of Dick-Read's method, which he stoutly refuted, was that he withheld pain medication from women who wanted it:

> If, in spite of all, there is pain, it should be immediately overcome. Painless labor is the greatest gift that our profession can make to humanity, but if painless labor is obtained at the cost of the integrity of the function, it becomes a choice between two evils. (Dick-Read, 1972, p. xxi)

Dick-Read's method did not become the dominant method of childbirth preparation in the United States, but it does remain the scientific and philosophical underpinning for much of what came later. For example, recent studies show that higher circulating levels of catecholamines (adrenaline and noradrenaline, the "fight or flight" hormones) in anxious laboring women render their uterine contractions less effective, leading to prolongation of labor and a reduced supply of oxygen to the fetus (Levinson and Shnider, 1979). The description of anxiety leading to less effective uterine contractions exactly parallels Dick-Read's work of nearly 40 years ago, and all of the later methods of prepared childbirth have built on Dick-Read's understanding of education, relaxation, and support during labor as major components of uncomplicated, unmedicated birth.

✱ MARTHA LIVINGSTON, Ph.D.

See also: Labor: Overview

See **Guide to Related Topics:** Childbirth Practices and Locations

Resources

Dick-Read, G. (1933). *Natural Childbirth.* London: Heinemann.

———. (1944). *Childbirth without Fear.* New York; London: Harper and Brothers.

———. (1972). *Childbirth without Fear.* 4th edition. New York: Harper & Row.

Levinson, G. & Shnider, S.M. (1979). "Catecholamines: The Effects of Maternal Fear and Its Treatment on Uterine Function and Circulation." *Birth and the Family Journal* 6: 167-78.

Rothman, B.K. (1982). *In Labor: Women and Power in the Birthplace.* New York; London: W.W. Norton.

REBIRTH

Rebirthing is the process of reexperiencing one's birth. The purpose of rebirthing is to complete, gain insights, or consciously reevaluate perceptions originating in response to events surrounding birth. Perceptions surrounding birth are pre-language and often are unable to be addressed verbally. It is believed that perceptions create belief systems or rules by which peoples' lives are guided. As in verbal therapy, one of the precepts of rebirthing is that perceptions of an earlier experience can trigger conscience reevaluation, clearer understanding, or a new imprint. When this occurs, it may reduce undesirable influences of erroneous perceptions that may have been influencing that person's life.

Rebirthing can be a totally nonverbal process, or the nonverbal experience can lead to verbal processing. Nonverbal techniques used to stimulate perceptions of birth or prenatal or postnatal events may include: compressing the person's body from their feet; matching and amplifying certain body rhythms; using birth pictures, images, music, or breathing to stimulate recall and reenactment of the birth; holding or stroking a person's head or face, inducing a trancelike state; or visualizing cellular fetal or birthing images.

Rebirthing is a new field. There are many different approaches. Leaders in the field include Elizabeth Noble, Sondra Ray, Graham Farrant, Stanislav Grof, and Bonnie Bainbridge Cohen.

Spontaneous Rebirth. For years, observations have been made by many body workers and dance or movement therapists of clients experiencing spontaneous rebirths during sessions.

A person's own perinatal experiences, whether or not they are remembered, may determine deep and basic beliefs called birth-engendered beliefs. Beliefs are not just abstract thoughts; they are psychophysical realities. Everybody knows that tension interferes with breathing and efficient muscle functions. What is not common knowledge is that unresolved perinatal conflicts can initiate tension patterns that tend to live on throughout a person's whole life on a nonverbal and nonconscious level. These tensions live in the body's memory: the musculature, the fascia, and the cells of the body. Birth-engendered beliefs are anchored in the body in breathing and movement patterns, which condition perception and the interpretation of experience. They affect behavior and relationships throughout life, as Stanislav Grof (1985), Arthur Janov (1983), and Sondra Ray and Bob Mandel (1987) have shown.

Birth-engendered beliefs can also help or hinder a woman's experience of giving birth by functioning as nonconscious imperatives that must be obeyed. Patterns of unresolved conflict tend to repeat themselves. It may be that when a prospective mother experiences spontaneous rebirthing, an opportunity is being presented to complete some important learning about her own birth that might otherwise interfere with her giving birth.

Research has centered on what stimulates spontaneous rebirth, how to facilitate it when it presents itself, and how to help carry it to completion, particularly for pregnant women.

Living in the body as they do, patterns of tension and their accompanying beliefs are accessible to receptive, noninvasive touch administered with an attitude of respect for the purpose motivating the spontaneous rebirth experience.

Spontaneous rebirthing is not a blanket prescription for everyone. People sometimes go into spontaneous rebirth experiences during bodywork sessions when they are encouraged to pay attention to sensations, feelings, and movement impulses. For example, a body therapist might gently move a pregnant woman's head and neck with the intention of showing her how to release tension, which would be helpful to her throughout her pregnancy and in giving birth. Releasing tension might also upset habitual holding patterns that may be covering early traumatic conflict, and stimulate spontaneous rebirth experiences.

A person's movement during a dance or movement therapy session in which he or she is allowed to follow body impulses into movement might also lead to an unresolved traumatic event (such as reexperiencing being a baby who is ready to come out and being held back until the doctor arrives). If there is something about the person's own birth experience that needs to be completed, the body seems to want to go back and finally resolve it.

If, during a bodywork or dance or movement therapy session, a person is moving, and his or her head starts to press into the therapist's hands or some object, there's a good chance that a spontaneous rebirth experience is about to present itself. The therapist can offer his or her hands to push into and "listen" with the hands for any response. The therapist matches the person's response, offering resistance that equals the push of the head and diminishing pressure when the head does so. He or she follows the lead of the "baby" as it actively births itself with his or her partnership.

Infants also exhibit spontaneous rebirthing behavior. Behavioral clues that a baby is beginning this process may include the baby spontaneously pushing or making searching movements with the head, pushing with the feet, or having unexplained periodic bouts of alternating crying and/or flexing and pausing. When this spontaneous rebirthing has proceeded to completion, there may be a profound change in physiological response such as eye contact that had not occurred before, or just a deep relaxation, or a cessation of rebirthing behavioral cues.

When a pregnant woman reexperiences her own birth, sounds, smells, or feelings of memories may spontaneously arise, leading to realizations about the human relationships that existed at the time. The therapist plays the role of Mother Nature, midwife, and mother, helping the "baby" discover that it can take an active role in its own birth and can succeed in doing something difficult in cooperation with another person.

This physical experience can be the foundation of the woman's new beliefs about childbirth, deactivating lifelong, birth-engendered beliefs that have controlled her behavior without her conscious awareness. Her new perspective on birth may enable her to fulfill her role in giving birth more effectively and happily.

✱ AILEEN CROW and SANDRA JAMROG, C.C.E., R.M.T.

See **Guide to Related Topics:** Pregnancy, Psychological Aspects

Resources

Grof, Stanislav. (1985). *Beyond the Brain.* Albany, NY: State University of New York Press.

Janov, Arthur. (1983). *Imprints.* New York: Coward-McCann, Inc.

Noble, Elizabeth. (1991). *Inside Experiences.* New York: Simon and Schuster.

Pre and Peri-Natal Psychology Journal. Carlton University, Human Science Press, Inc., 233 Spring Street, New York, NY 10013-1578.

Ray, Sondra & Mandel, Bob. (1987). *Birth and Relationships.* Berkeley, CA: Celestial Arts.

REFUGEE WOMEN*

The refugee experience can affect many of the processes surrounding women's childbearing and childrearing. Of the problems, emotional and physical, that may emerge as a result of women giving birth as refugees, the most basic are those that stem from the sometimes highly unsanitary conditions surrounding childbirth in refugee camps.

In one camp of Afghan refugees in Pakistan, for example, a woman about to give birth holds on to ropes hung from the roof beam or top of the tent and squats over a hole dug into the dirt floor into which the baby is delivered. The midwife in attendance has no sterilized instruments, so she cuts the umbilical cord with whatever instrument is available. The baby is removed from the hole in the floor, and the afterbirth is buried in the same hole. Gynecological problems may result from these kinds of conditions and, because of the lack of female doctors and the practices of *purdah*, often go untreated. However, the circumstances of childbirth were in some cases not much healthier in the home countries of refugees.

It is the combination of unsanitary conditions with other factors specific to refugees, however, that can make the experience of childbirth so traumatic for refugee women. They give birth in a refugee camp or in an alien community, outside the context of their traditional culture and without the support of extended family. Their children are born lacking the foundation in society with which they themselves and their ancestors had started life. Their identities and futures will not be secured by the community in the same way; although in some cases they may have a wider range of opportunities than their parents did, their situation is grounds for a good deal of worry by refugee mothers.

According to a study done of Vietnamese women who gave birth in Great Britain, refugee mothers encounter a great many problems because of contrasting and even clashing beliefs about the best way to care for a mother and child prior to, during, and just after birth. Many Vietnamese refugees have a strong prejudice against giving birth in hospitals; the sterilized atmosphere is quite different from the atmosphere of family and communal support during childbirth in the home country. Traditionally, a midwife or older woman trusted by the community acts as birth assistant. The Western doctors or midwives who assist at a birth are inevitably less trusted by the mother and, because of this, may contribute to greater difficulties, both psychological and physical, during the course of the birth. The Vietnamese believe that the Western custom of having a shower after birth causes weakness and fainting spells in the mother. They believe that ice-chewing during labor may contribute to certain diseases that are thought to arise from an imbalance of the elements of hot and cold in the body. After a traditional birthing the umbilical cord is kept covered in order to prevent the entrance of evil spirits into the baby's body; the absence of such practices in Western hospitals may cause additional anxiety in the mother. Some traditional customs, as a result, have been observed to continue, both in reception centers and after resettlement in British society.

Despite the difficulties involved, however, many refugee women decide to have children in order to affirm the continuity and joy of life in the face of the hardship they have undergone. Childbirth for them is an expression of hope and strength and refusal of despair.

Breastfeeding. The cultural unfamiliarity of countries of asylum and resettlement may cause problems for refugee mothers in childbirth and during their infants' first months, but sometimes it is very concrete changes in the refugees' physical environments that challenge women to adapt themselves. Traditional African practices, like some of those surrounding breastfeeding, which rely on concoctions made of herbs only available around the home community, may be altered as a result of the move; often the ability to adapt such practices to the new circumstances is a great asset, but some adapted methods prove problematical.

Many Northern Ethiopian mothers, for example, traditionally apply the juice from a bitter plant to their breasts in order to encourage weaning. Because this plant is not available in Eastern Sudanese refugee camps, some mothers have been known to use bitter-tasting antibiotic drugs as a substitute. The practice is dangerous because it

*Copyright © 1992 by World Council of Churches, Refugee Service, P.O. Box 2100, 1211 Geneva 2, Switzerland.

could lead to immunity to the antibiotics in the children concerned.

Children and Society. Various dynamics develop between refugee mothers and their children as a result of the tension, within and among refugees, between maintaining ties to the home culture and integrating into the new society. Refugee children often adapt more easily and quickly than their mothers to the new cultures in which they find themselves. They may learn the language more quickly. They are less isolated, especially if they are able to attend school. Refugee women who are lonely or confused may as a result become dependant on their children to act as both linguistic and cultural interpreters for them. A disturbing kind of reversal of roles between mothers and children sometimes becomes even more explicit when older children become wage-earners for the first time in the new country and their mothers are financially as well as otherwise dependent on them. Women's dependence is increased when they need most of all to acquire a sense of control in their lives, while children are deprived of the steady guidance many of them have been accustomed to rely upon in their mothers.

Older Southeast Asian women refugees often wish to maintain their traditionally close relationships with their adult and even married sons. Some follow those who move to different areas of their countries of resettlement to find employment, and even leave their own husbands in order to do this. While their children may want to break away and follow the customs of the new country, mothers may feel deeply hurt and confused by the sense that both they as people and the traditional ways they have brought with them have been rejected by their children.

Many Southeast Asian refugee mothers in France, it was found, feel torn between happiness because of the relatively easy adaptation of their children and a desire, which they feel powerless to fulfill, that their children may maintain some sort of contact with their own language and culture. Such women feel themselves to be losing their hold on a role essential to them and one that gave them a sense of function and validity in their home countries: the traditional role of teacher and guide for their children. ✷ SHARON KRUMMEL

See **Guide to Related Topics:** Pregnancy Complications

Resources

Kelley, Ninette. (1988). *Working with Refugee Women.* Geneva, Switzerland: NGO Working Group on Refugee Women.

Krummel, Sharon. (1988). "Refugee Women and the Experience of Cultural Uprooting." *Refugees.* (Prepared by the Refugee Service of the Commission on Interchurch Aid, Refugee and World Service, World Council on Churches, Geneva.)

RELACTATION

Relactation is the reestablishment of a milk supply in a woman who has lactated at any time in the past (Riordan, 1983). In practice it is used to refer to restimulating a milk supply that has been significantly reduced or has ceased following a recent (no more than a few months) birth or weaning (Anderson, 1986).

A woman may choose to relactate if:

- breastfeeding has been delayed because of illness in her baby or herself;
- the baby develops a medical condition or serious formula intolerance, making it imperative to produce mother's milk;
- weaning has been untimely or the mother has simply changed her mind about bottle feeding;
- she wants to nurse a baby adopted within a short time after she has lost or weaned a previous baby.

In the course of a normal pregnancy, estrogen, progesterone, prolactin, and the adrenal corticol steroids cause the alveoli and ducts in the breast to increase in both size and number (Riordan, 1983). Following the birth and expulsion of the placenta, the hormonal balance shifts. Estrogen and progesterone go down and prolactin goes up, signaling the alveoli to produce milk (Hormann, 1989). The baby's sucking stimulates continued prolactin secretion (Riordan, 1983). As long as the baby sucks, the breasts will continue to make milk. When sucking slows down—or stops—so does milk production. Renewed sucking, on the other hand, starts the process again. Particularly if only a brief time has elapsed since lactation ceased, frequent, regular breast stimulation can bring in an abundant milk supply. If it has been some time since the woman lactated or if she is relactating following weaning of an older baby or toddler, alveoli and milk ducts will have involuted (Riordan, 1983) and it may take considerable time to establish even a modest milk supply. Biologically, such a woman resembles a nulliparous woman inducing lactation.

Relactation depends not only on stimulation, but also on the mother's motivation, her perseverance, and the baby's cooperation. Most young infants can be taught to suck at the breast even after a period of bottle feeding, but considerable patience may be required until the baby's initial resistance is overcome. Relactating women should be prepared for this resistance and should be reassured that a bottle-trained baby balking at the breast is not rejecting his or her mother any more than a breastfed baby is rejecting his or her mother when refusing a bottle. Babies need time to learn new skills and resistance in the learning period is not unusual.

A relactating woman can expect a considerable investment of her time and energy until her milk is reestablished. The baby needs to be offered every possible chance to nurse—at least every two hours in the daytime and through the night. The breast should be offered to comfort as well as to feed. As much as possible, pacifiers and bottles should be avoided to minimize nipple confusion and provide an incentive for the baby to suck at the breast. Formula feeding is frequently necessary in the early days of relactation to ensure that the baby has an adequate intake of fluid and calories. Ideally, supplements should be given by spoon, cup, eyedropper, or via a specially designed nursing supplementer system that delivers the milk at the mother's breast. Relactating women need a great deal of practical and emotional support while they are reestablishing their milk supplies. Usually this is best accomplished with a referral to a mother support group such as La Leche League or a breastfeeding counselor with experience in helping women relactate.

Goals for relactation vary, depending on the situation. When relactation is undertaken for reasons of health, establishing an abundant milk supply is usually a primary goal and a reasonable one if the baby is under two (Riordan, 1983) or three (Hormann, 1977) months. With older or adopted babies—or babies without health problems—establishing a nursing relationship may be the first priority, with milk supply a secondary consideration.

There are various measures of success in relactation. Duration of nursing is one such measure. In a study of 366 North American women relactating following the birth of a premature or low birth-weight baby, hospitalization of mother or infant, or untimely weaning (Auerbach and Avery, 1980), two-thirds of the babies were nursed for at least six months. Half of them nursed into the second half of the first year, and 17 percent nursed beyond a year. In a society in which only 54.1 percent of mothers begin breastfeeding, with a modest 21 percent still nursing at six months (Lawrence, 1989), these figures are remarkable by any standard.

Milk supply is another measure of breastfeeding success. In the population at large, 58 percent of women who wean in the first four months give inadequate milk supply as a reason (Lawrence, 1989). Among the relactating mothers, by contrast, 57 percent were fully breastfeeding within four weeks. Another quarter took longer than four weeks, but were able, eventually, to breastfeed without supplements. Most striking were the 174 mothers (48 percent of the women in the study) who had weaned their babies prematurely—many of them because they thought they had too little milk; 75 percent of them were ultimately able to breastfeed exclusively. This suggests that the level of information and support available to the breastfeeding mother plays a decisive role in her perception of milk sufficiency.

Self-evaluation is the ultimate measure of success for relactation since subjective satisfaction plays such a central role. In the Auerbach study 75 percent of the mothers evaluated the experience positively. Self-evaluation—both positive and negative—was unrelated to milk supply and length of nursing. This confirms other research indicating a high degree of satisfaction in women who undertake relactation (Hormann, 1977).

✱ ELIZABETH HORMANN

See also: Breastfeeding beyond Infancy; Lactation, Induced; Weaning

See **Guide to Related Topics:** Infant Feeding

Resources

Anderson, Kathryn. (1986). *Breastfeeding Your Adopted Baby*. Franklin Park, IL: La Leche League Information Sheet #55.

Auerbach, K.G. & Avery, J.L. (1980). "Relactation: A Study of 366 Cases." *Pediatrics 65*: 236.

———. (1981). "Induced Lactation: A Study of Adoptive Nursing by 240 Women." *American Journal of Disabled Children 135*: 340.

Fleiss, Paul. (1988). "Herbal Remedies for the Breastfeeding Mother." *Mothering 48*.

Hormann, Elizabeth. (1977). "Breastfeeding the Adopted Baby." *Birth and Family Journal 4* (4).

———. (1987). *After the Adoption*. Old Tappan, NJ: Revell.

———. (1989). *When You Nurse Your Adopted Baby*. Cologne, Germany.

Jelliffe, D. & Jelliffe, E.F.P. (1978). *Human Milk in the Modern World*. New York: Oxford University Press.

Lawrence, Ruth. (1989). *Breastfeeding: A Guide for the Medical Profession*. St. Louis: Mosby.

Phillips, Virginia. (1971). "Non-Puerperal Lactation Among Australian Aboriginal Women." *New Zealand Parents' Centres Bulletin*.

Riordan, Jan. (1983). *A Practical Guide to Breastfeeding*. St. Louis: Mosby.

U.S. Department of Health and Human Services. (1984). Report of the Surgeon General's Workshop on Breastfeeding and Human Lactation. Washington, DC.

Waletzky, L.R. & Herman, E.C. (1976). "Relactation." *American Family Practice* 14: 69.

THE REPRODUCTION OF MOTHERING*

In spite of the apparently close tie between women's capacities for childbearing and lactation on the one hand and their responsibilities for child care on the other, and in spite of the probable prehistoric convenience (and perhaps survival necessity) of a sexual division of labor in which women mothered, biology and instinct do not provide adequate explanations for how women come to mother.

Women's mothering as a feature of social structure requires an explanation in terms of social structure. Conventional feminist and social psychological explanations for the genesis of gender roles—girls and boys are "taught" appropriate behaviors and "learn" appropriate feelings—are insufficient, both empirically and methodologically, to account for how women become mothers.

Women's mothering includes the capacity for its own reproduction. This reproduction consists in the production of women with, and men without, the particular psychological capacities and stance that go into primary parenting. Psychoanalytic theory provides a theory of social reproduction that explains major features of personality development and the development of psychic structure, and the differential development of gender personality in particular. Psychoanalysts argue that personality both results from and consists of the ways a child appropriates, internalizes, and organizes early experiences in his or her family—from the fantasies children have, the defenses they use, the ways they channel and redirect drives in this object-relational context. A person subsequently imposes this intrapsychic structure, and the fantasies, defenses, and relational modes and preoccupations that go with it, onto external social situations. This reexternalization (or mutual reexternalization) is a major constituting feature of social and interpersonal situations themselves.

Psychoanalysis, however, has not had an adequate theory of the reproduction of mothering. Because of the teleological assumption that anatomy is destiny, and that women's destiny includes primary parenting, the ontogenesis of women's mothering has been largely ignored, even while the genesis of a wide variety of related disturbances and problems has been accorded widespread clinical attention. Most psychoanalysts agree that the basis for parenting is laid for both genders in the early relationship to a primary caretaker. Beyond that, in order to explain why women mother, they tend to rely on vague notions of a girl's subsequent identification with her mother, which makes her and not her brother a primary parent, or on an unspecified and uninvestigated innate femaleness in girls, or on logical leaps from lactation or early vaginal sensations to caretaking abilities and commitments.

The psychoanalytic account of male and female development, when reinterpreted, provides a developmental theory of the reproduction of women's mothering. Women's mothering reproduces itself through differing object-relational experiences and differing psychic outcomes in women and men. As a result of having been parented by a woman, women are more likely than men to seek to be mothers, that is, to relocate themselves in a primary mother-child relationship, to get gratification from the mothering relationship, and to have psychological and relational capacities for mothering.

The early relation to a primary caretaker provides in children of both genders the basic capacity to participate in relationship with the features of the early parent-child one, and the desire to create this intimacy. However, because women mother, the early experience and preoedipal relationship differ for boys and girls. Girls retain more concern with early childhood issues in relation to their mother and a sense of self involved with these issues. Their attachments therefore retain more preoedipal aspects. The greater length and different nature of their preoedipal experience, and their continuing preoccupation with the issues of this period, mean that women's sense of self is continuous with others and that they retain capacities for primary identification, both of which enable them to experience the empathy and lack of reality sense needed by a cared-for infant. In men, these qualities have been curtailed, both because they are treated early in life as an opposite by their mother and because their later attachment to her must be repressed. The relational basis for mothering is thus extended in women, and inhibited in men, who experience themselves as more separate and distinct from others.

*Reprinted with permission from Nancy Chodorow, *Reproduction of Mothering: Psychoanalysis and the Sociology of Gender*, pages 205-09. Copyright © 1978 by The Regents of the University of California.

The different structure of the feminine and masculine oedipal experience that results from women's mothering contributes further to gender personality differentiation and the reproduction of women's mothering. As a result of this experience, women's inner object world and the affects and issues associated with it are more actively sustained and more complex than men's. This means that women define and experience themselves relationally. Their heterosexual orientation is always in internal dialog with both oedipal and preoedipal mother-child relational issues. Thus, women's heterosexuality is triangular and requires a third person—a child—for its structural and emotional completion. For men, in contrast, the heterosexual relationship alone recreates the early bond to their mother; a child interrupts it. Men, moreover, do not define themselves in relationships and have come to suppress relational capacities and needs. Such repression prepares them to participate in the affect-denying world of alienated work, but not to fulfill women's needs for intimacy and primary relationships.

The oedipus complex, as it emerges from the asymmetrical organization of parenting, secures a psychological taboo on parent-child incest and pushes boys and girls in the direction of extrafamiliar heterosexual relationships. This is one step toward the reproduction of parenting. The creation and maintenance of the incest taboo and of heterosexuality in girls and boys are different, however; for boys, superego formation and identification with their father, rewarded by the superiority of masculinity, maintains the taboo on incest with their mother, while heterosexual orientation continues from their earliest love relationship with her. For girls, the heterosexual orientation they have from birth maintains the taboo. However, women's heterosexuality is not as exclusive as men's, making it easier for them to accept or seek a male substitute for their fathers. At the same time, in a male-dominant society, women's exclusive emotional heterosexuality is not so necessary, nor is her repression of love for her father. Men are more likely to initiate relationships, and women's economic dependence on men pushes them anyway into heterosexual marriage.

Male dominance in heterosexual relationships and marriages solves the problem of women's lack of heterosexual commitment and lack of satisfaction by making women more reactive in the sexual bonding process. At the same time, contradictions in heterosexuality help to perpetuate families and parenting by ensuring that women will seek relationships with children, not finding heterosexual relationships alone satisfactory. Thus, men's lack of emotional availability and women's less exclusive heterosexual commitment help ensure women's mothering.

Women's mothering, then, produces psychological self-definition and capacities appropriate to mothering in women, and curtails and inhibits these capacities and this self-definition in men. The early experience of being cared for by a woman produces a fundamental structure of expectations in women and men concerning mothers' lack of separate interests from their infants and total concern for their infants' welfare. Daughters grow up identifying with these mothers, about whom they have such expectations. This set of expectations is generalized to the assumption that women naturally take care of children of all ages and the belief that women's "maternal" qualities can and should be extended to the nonmothering work that they do. All of these results of women's mothering have ensured that women will mother infants and will take continuing responsibility for children.

The reproduction of women's mothering is the basis for the reproduction of women's location and responsibilities in the domestic sphere. This mothering, and its generalization to women's structural location in the domestic sphere, links the contemporary social organization of gender and social organization of production and contributes to the reproduction of each. That women mother is a fundamental organizational feature of the sex-gender system: It is basic to the sexual division of labor and generates a psychology and ideology of male dominance as well as an ideology about women's capacities and nature. Women, as wives and mothers, contribute as well to the daily and generational reproduction, both physical and psychological, of male workers and thus to the reproduction of capitalist production.

Women's mothering also reproduces the family as it is constituted in male-dominant society. The sexual and familial division of labor in which women mother creates a sexual division of psychic organization and orientation. It produces socially gendered women and men who enter into asymmetrical heterosexual relationships; it produces men who react to, fear, and act superior to women, and who put most of their energies into the nonfamilial work world and do not parent. Finally, it produces women who turn their energies toward nurturing and caring for children physically, psychologically, and emotionally. They thus contribute to the perpetuation of their own social roles and position in the hierarchy of gender.

Institutionalized features of family structure and the social relations of production reproduce themselves. A psychoanalytic investigation shows that women's mothering capacities and commitments, and the general psychological capacities and wants that are the basis of women's emotional work, are built developmentally into feminine personality. Because women are themselves mothered by women, they grow up with the relational capacities and needs, and psychological definition of self-in-relationship, which commits them to mothering. Men, because they are mothered by women, do not. Women mother daughters who, when they become women, mother. ✷ NANCY J. CHODOROW, Ph.D.

See **Guide to Related Topics:** Pregnancy, Psychological Aspects

Resources

Chodorow, Nancy. (1978). *The Reproduction of Mothering: Psychoanalysis and the Sociology of Gender*. Berkeley, CA: University of California Press.

———. (1989). *Feminism and Psychoanalytic Theory.* Berkeley, CA: University of California Press.

Chodorow, Nancy & Contratto, Susan. (1982). "Fantasy of the Perfect Mother." In Barrie Thorne (Ed.) *Rethinking the Family: Some Feminist Questions.* New York: Longman.

Kestenberg, Judith. "Regression and Reintegration in Pregnancy." *Psychoanalytic Inquiry.* (Special issue on pregnancy.)

RESEARCH ISSUES IN CHILDBIRTH

Women want, and caregivers aim to provide, the forms and elements of care in childbirth that they think are the best available. What is perceived as "best," however, varies widely from time to time, from place to place, and from person to person. The alternatives chosen may reflect differences in goals or priorities on the part of either women or their caregivers, and sometimes choices are limited by lack of facilities. But most often, the varied opinions reflect a disagreement as to what is most likely to be effective, safe, and satisfying.

Each woman has the right to choose, and each caregiver has the duty to recommend, those elements of care that they believe to be best. But the choice, to be a real choice, should be based on valid information; a poorly informed choice is as bad as no choice at all. A woman's autonomy in childbirth, thus, is a function of the accuracy of the information on which she makes her choices.

Sometimes that information may be an informal impression, based on a woman's (or a clinician's) own observations or those of her friends, family, colleagues, or social network. Sometimes an impression of what will be best is based on theoretical reasoning, authoritarian doctrine, or locally accepted practices. Often these impressions prove to be correct. Equally often, however, even widely and strongly held beliefs prove to be wrong when formally tested.

There were good theoretical grounds, for example, to believe that the synthetic hormone diethylstilbestrol (DES) might prevent miscarriage, premature labor, and toxemia of pregnancy. Several large observational studies appeared to confirm the expected benefit. Not surprisingly, doctors tended to prescribe, and women to request, a treatment that might prevent these serious problems. DES was prescribed for over two million pregnant American women between 1950 and 1970. Randomized trials, however, showed the drug to be totally ineffective, and it was later shown to have caused serious adverse effects on children exposed to it during their mother's pregnancy. Had the trials been carried out before the drug came into widespread use, these tragedies could have been avoided.

On the other hand, the observation that the use of corticosteroids for mothers in preterm labor seemed to prevent respiratory distress syndrome and often death in premature babies was tested in a series of randomized trials and found to be highly effective. This hormone can now be used with confidence that it can prevent needless suffering and death.

Uncontrolled observations about the effects of care practices leave many questions unanswered concerning what might have happened with a different form of care. To determine the effects of a particular element of care, comparisons must be made between what happens to women who receive that form of care and what happens to women who have received a different form of care (or no care at all). Moreover, such comparisons must be able to demonstrate whether any differences observed were due to differences in the care received or to differences in the women who received the care. The only form of study that can accomplish this is a randomized controlled trial. Unless these trials are carried out, effective forms of care will not be recognized as such and brought into use as promptly as possible; ineffective or harmful forms of care will not be detected efficiently and may, therefore, do harm on a wider scale than necessary.

Women have the right to effective care during pregnancy and childbirth. With that right, however, comes the responsibility to help determine what constitutes effective care, and that does not come easily. The first essential is to give up the comforting fiction that the doctor always knows best and accept that much of what constitutes effective care is not known; the second essential is to collectively demand that proper controlled research into the questions that are important to women be carried out; and the third essential is to participate in that research.

Childbearing women themselves must make the decision as to whether, when the advantages and disadvantages of particular elements of care are unknown or unclear, their interests are protected more effectively by controlled experimentation than by the uncontrolled experimentation that characterizes much of obstetric care today. Although the power of the professionals in the perinatal field may appear to be overwhelming, the collective exercise of choice and pressures by women has influenced perinatal care in the past, and can continue to exert its powerful influence today.

When the most effective form of care is not known, the woman who participates in a randomized trial is not a "guinea pig." By her participation, she reduces by half the likelihood that she personally will receive the inferior form of care, and at the same time she improves the likelihood that all women in the future will receive the better form of care. ✷ MURRAY W. ENKIN, M.D., FRCS(C)

See also: DES: Diethylstilbestrol; Informed Consent in Labor; Women's Health Movement

Resources

Bryce, R. & Enkin, M.W. (1985). "Six Myths about Controlled Trials in Perinatal Medicine." *American Journal of Obstetrics and Gynecology 151*: 707-10.

Chalmers, I. (1986). "Minimizing Harm and Maximizing Benefit during Innovation in Health Care: Controlled or Uncontrolled Experimentation?" *Birth 13* (3): 155-64.

Enkin, M.W., Keirse, M.J.N.C., & Chalmers, I. (Eds.) (1989). *A Guide to Effective Care in Pregnancy and Childbirth.* Oxford: Oxford University Press.

RETINOPATHY OF PREMATURITY AND RETROLENTAL FIBROPLASIA

Retinopathy of prematurity (ROP) is a disease of the retina characterized by avascularity in the peripheral regions of the retina, hemorrhage in the vitreoretinal interface, and fibrosis of the retinal tissue.

The retina is the inner layer of the eyeball. It occupies about four-fifths of the inner surface towards the back of the eye. Nerve fibers from all parts of the retina come together at the rear of the eye to form the optic nerve. The optic nerve is the medium through which messages are passed from the eye to the brain. When light hits the healthy retina the nerve fibers transmit, via the optic nerve, signals to the brain. These signals represent what a person "sees." The formation of the retina begins at around 10 weeks of gestational age. It proceeds anteriorly from the optic nerve, completing in approximately the 36th week. In the preterm infant, retinal formation is not complete, i.e., the preterm infant lacks blood vessels in the peripheral of the retina. The incomplete vascular system may result in several possible destructive processes, leaving the retina partially or totally dysfunctional.

The severity of ROP is inversely proportional to gestational age. It is believed to be connected with the administration of hyperbaric (amounts greater than that found in the atmosphere) oxygen given to premature infants to support underdeveloped breathing mechanisms (lungs) and to support conditions that interfere with normal oxygen consumption, e.g., apnea. There is, however, disagreement about the cause of ROP. Some physicians and researchers make a distinction between ROP and retrolental fibroplasia (RLF), specifying that dosages of concentrated oxygen are responsible for the latter condition but not necessarily the former (Sardegna and Paul, 1990, p. 193). The precise cause or causes of both ROP and RLF are unspecified; however, both are associated with vascularization of the retina in premature infants.

The incidence of ROP/RLF is estimated at 65 percent of infants with birth weight less than 1,500 g (3.3 lb.) and up to 77 percent of infants weighing less than 1,000 g (2.2 lb.). About 500 cases are reported in the United States annually (Vaughan, Asbury, and Tabbara, 1990, p. 172).

The disease progresses through several phases, including fibrosis at the vitreoretinal interface. At worst this results in vitreous hemorrhage and/or detached retina. However, 80 to 90 percent of infants diagnosed with ROP/RLF undergo spontaneous regression with no significant clinical consequences (Vaughan, Asbury, and Tabbara, 1990, p. 172). About 15 percent of the cases progress to mild ROP/RLF, with approximately 5 percent developing severe ROP/RLF with accompanying retinal detachment and other severe consequences (Sardegna and Paul, 1990, p. 194).

Diagnosis and Treatment. Ophthalmological examination takes place in premature infants born at 32 weeks or less, especially those who have been administered hyperbaric oxygen. This examination will determine the existence of

ROP/RLF as well as the location and extent of the condition. Treatments range from cryotherapy to vitamin E dietary supplement to invasive surgery, depending on the extent of disease.

Prevention. Modern medical technology has made it possible to deliver smaller and smaller infants. Because of this, the incidence of ROP/RLF is on the increase, despite well-managed neonatal care. The condition is found in 40 to 77 percent of infants weighing less than 1,000 g (2.2 lb.). Thus, premature infants should be administered only that amount of oxygen *necessary* for survival. For a discussion of the history of ROP/RLF as a case study of introducing new technologies with insufficient research and potentially disastrous consequences, see William A. Silverman's *Retrolental Fibroplasia: A Modern Parable* (1980).

✱ ALLEN G. KLEIMAN

See **Guide to Related Topics:** Special Needs Infants

Resources

Sardegna, Jill & Paul, T. Otis. (1990). *The Encyclopedia of Blindness and Vision Impairment*. New York: Facts on File, Inc.

Silverman, William A. (1980). *Retrolental Fibroplasia: A Modern Parable*. New York: Grune and Stratton.

Vaughan, Daniel, Asbury, Taylor, & Tabbara, Khalid F. (1990). *General Ophthalmology 1989*. 12th edition. Norwalk, CT: Appleton & Lange.

Rh INCOMPATIBILITY

Approximately 85 percent of all people have a protein substance called the Rh factor that coats the surface of their red blood cells. Having this factor means the person is Rh positive (Rh+). The remainder of the population lacks this substance and is said to be Rh negative (Rh-). The presence or absence of the Rh factor has absolutely no effect on a person's health and is only of importance during pregnancy and when typing blood for transfusion.

Rh incompatibility may occur when an Rh-negative woman has a child with an Rh-positive man and the baby inherits Rh-positive blood from its father. If blood from the Rh-negative mother mixes with the blood of the Rh-positive fetus, the mother's blood will become sensitized to the foreign substance in her baby's blood and begin to form antibodies to destroy it. This destruction of the fetus's red blood cells is called Rh hemolytic disease and can cause anemia, severe jaundice, heart failure, brain damage, and death.

Affected babies can sometimes be treated with complete blood transfusions while still in the womb. Others may require premature induction of labor or cesarean section so they can receive immediate treatment outside their mother's bodies. Each of these procedures involves risk for both mother and baby.

First babies (in birth order) are usually not affected since maternal and fetal blood supplies rarely mix until birth. However, if the child is Rh positive, the mother's blood can become sensitized at that time. Subsequent pregnancies would then be at risk for Rh hemolytic disease. There are no problems if the baby is Rh negative, or if both mother and father are Rh negative. An Rh-positive mother can carry an Rh-negative fetus without fear of incompatibility.

Fortunately, Rh hemolytic disease has become increasingly rare since the introduction in 1968 of RhoGAM (Rh immune globulin), which prevents the formation of Rh antibodies. Pregnant Rh-negative women who are at risk for bearing an Rh-positive child should receive RhoGAM at 28 weeks' gestation and again within 72 hours of giving birth to an Rh-positive child (Semchyshyn and Colman, 1989). Women who have already become sensitized must be closely monitored throughout pregnancy for signs of disease.

All women of childbearing age need to know their Rh factor so they can safeguard themselves against sensitization. Rh-negative women should have a RhoGAM injection following every miscarriage, abortion, amniocentesis, or any other circumstance in which maternal and fetal blood could be exchanged. Blood transfusions are also a cause of Rh sensitization (Myles, 1985). Although RhoGAM has almost made Rh incompatibility a problem of the past, women must be sure they receive the medication when they need it. They should also be aware that occasionally a woman will become sensitized even with the use of RhoGAM (Rothman, 1982). ✱ CASSIE LUHRS, C.C.E.

See **Guide to Related Topics:** Pregnancy Complications

Resources

Baldwin, Rahima. (1986). *Special Delivery*. Berkeley, CA: Celestial Arts.

Gaskin, Ina May. (1977). *Spiritual Midwifery*. Summertown, TN: The Book Publishing Company.

Myles, Margaret F. (1985). *Textbook for Midwives*. New York: Churchill Livingstone.

Rothman, Barbara Katz. (1982). *In Labor: Women and Power in the Birthplace*. New York: W.W. Norton.

Semchyshyn, Stefan & Colman, Carol. (1989). *How to Avoid Miscarriage and Other Crises of Pregnancy*. New York: Macmillan Publishing Company.

RIGHTS OF THE PREGNANT PATIENT*

Most pregnant women are not fully aware of their rights to informed consent or the obstetrician's legal obligation to obtain informed consent for treatment. Almost 20 years ago the American College of Obstetricians and Gynecologists recognized the pregnant patient's right of informed consent in the following excerpt from its 1974 *Standards for Obstetric-Gynecologic Services*:

> it is important to note the distinction between "consent" and "informed consent." Many physicians, because they do not realize there is a difference, believe they are free from liability if the patient consents. In addition, the usual consent obtained by a hospital does not in any way release the physician from his legal duty of obtaining an informed consent from his patient.
>
> Most courts consider that the patient is "informed" if the following information is given:
>
> ✱ The processes contemplated by the physician as treatment, including whether the treatment is new or unusual.
> ✱ The risks and hazards of the treatment.
> ✱ The chances for recovery after treatment.
> ✱ The feasibility of alternative methods of treatment.
>
> One point on which courts do agree is that explanations must be given in such a way that the patient understands them. A physician cannot claim as a defense that he explained the procedure to the patient when he knew the patient did not understand. The physician has a duty to act with due care under the circumstances: this means he must be sure the patient understands what she is told.
>
> It should be emphasized that the following reasons are not sufficient to justify failure to inform:
>
> 1. That the patient may prefer not to be told the unpleasant possibilities regarding the treatment.
> 2. That full disclosure might suggest infinite dangers to a patient with an active imagination, thereby causing her to refuse treatment.
> 3. That the patient, on learning the risks involved, might rationally decline treatment. The right to decline is the specific fundamental right protected by the informed consent doctrine.

Any physician caring for a pregnant patient has a legal obligation to obtain that patient's informed consent to treatment unless there is a clear cut medical emergency that prevents her participation or her next of kin from participating in the decision making process. In addition to the right set forth in the American Hospital Association's "Patient's Bill of Rights," the pregnant patient, because she represents *two* patients rather than one, should be recognized as having the additional rights listed below.

The pregnant patient has the right, prior to the administration of any proposed therapy, whether drug or procedure, to be informed by the health professional caring for her:

- Of any potential direct or indirect effects, risks or hazards to herself or her unborn or newborn infant which may result from the use of a drug or procedure prescribed for or administered to her during pregnancy, labor, birth or lactation.
- Of available alternative therapy, such as childbirth education classes which could help to prepare the Pregnant Patient to cope with the discomfort or stress of childbirth and thereby reduce or eliminate her need for drugs and obstetric intervention.
- That any drug she receives during pregnancy, labor and birth, and lactation, no matter how or when the drug is taken or administered, may adversely affect her baby, directly or indirectly, and that there is no drug or chemical which has been proven safe for the unborn child.
- Of the brand name and generic name of the proposed drug, in order that she may advise the health professional of any past adverse reaction to the drug.
- That if a cesarean birth is anticipated, minimizing her intake of non-essential pre-operative drugs will benefit her baby.
- That there are areas of uncertainty regarding the safety of obstetric related drugs and procedures because NONE has been subjected to a properly controlled follow-up investigation to evaluate the delayed, long-term effects of the drugs and procedures on the physiological, mental and neurological development of the infant exposed in utero (or during lactation).

The Pregnant Patient has the right to be informed, prior to the administration of any drug or procedure, by the health professional caring for her:

*Copyright © 1992 by Doris B. Haire.

- To determine for herself, without pressure from her attendant, whether she will accept the risks inherent in the proposed therapy or refuse a drug or procedure.
- To know the name and qualification (student, resident, attending physician) of the individual administering a drug or procedure to her during labor or birth.
- Whether the procedure is being administered to her for her or her baby's benefits (medically indicated) or as an elective procedure (for convenience, teaching purposes or research).

The Pregnant Patient has the right:

- To be accompanied during the stress of labor and birth by someone she cares for, and to whom she looks for emotional comfort and encouragement.
- To choose a position for labor and birth, if there are no medical contraindications, that is least stressful to her baby and to herself.
- To have her baby cared for at her bedside if her baby is normal.
- To feed her baby according to her baby's needs rather than according to the hospital regimen.
- To be informed in writing of the name of the person who actually delivered her baby, the professional qualifications of that person, and whether that information also appears in the birth certificate.
- To be informed if there is any known or indicated aspect of her or her baby's care or condition which may cause her or her baby later difficulty or problems.
- To have her and her baby's hospital medical records complete, accurate and legible and to have their records, including nursing notes, retained by the hospital until the child reaches at least the age of majority, or alternatively, to have the records offered to her before they are destroyed.
- To have access, both during and after her hospital stay, to her complete hospital medical records, including nursing notes, and to receive a copy upon payment of a reasonable fee and without incurring the expense of retaining an attorney.

It is the obstetric patient and her baby, not the health professional, who must sustain any trauma or injury resulting from the use of a drug or obstetric procedure. The observation of the rights listed above not only will permit the obstetric patient to participate in the decisions involving her and her baby's health care, but will help to protect the health professional and the hospital against litigation arising from resentment or misunderstanding on the part of the mother.

Author's Note: The above is a slightly abbreviated version of "The Pregnant Patient's Bill of Rights," published by the International Childbirth Education Association. The complete version can be found in the book *The Rights of Hospital Patients* by Dr. George Annas. He points out that while the full document is primarily aimed at helping to encourage change in obstetric practices and at empowering pregnant women, almost all of its provisions have at least some support in the law.

✷ DORIS B. HAIRE

See also: Informed Consent in Labor

***See* Guide to Related Topics:** Legal Issues

RISKING

Health care providers use the term "risk" to refer to the likelihood that problematic situations, such as preterm birth, will occur. The provider's definition is based on an assessment of standardized, weighted factors that give a mathematical probability of the occurrence of a pregnancy complication (Creasy, Gummer, and Liggins, 1980; Gaziano, Freemon, and Allen, 1981; Papiernik, 1984). These factors are based on the patient's reproductive history and on clinical assessment of her current pregnancy status. While the patient's history is screened once early in pregnancy, clinical assessment for problematic changes continues throughout the pregnancy. Therefore, medical risk is defined as the mathematical probability that a problem will occur.

Pregnant women define risk as some degree of shift from certainty to uncertainty, from expected to unexpected, which is then verified by their social network of family and friends. Women define certainty as the expectation, projection, or anticipation of a pregnancy outcome based on knowledge of past similar outcomes and on shared experiences of present outcomes (Shalin, 1986; Patterson, 1990). This definition is based on culturally bound knowledge of biophysical and social norms pertaining to pregnancy. Woman-identified risk, then, is defined as a situation where women experience uncertainty and are unable to determine the outcome of pregnancy because of an unexpected shift in events.

✷ KATHRYN A. PATTERSON, Ph.D., C.N.M.

***See* Guide to Related Topics:** Prenatal Diagnosis and Screening

Resources

Creasy, R.K., Gummer, B.A., & Liggins, G.C. (1980). "System for Predicting Spontaneous Preterm Birth." *Obstetrics and Gynecology 55* (6): 692-95.

Gaziano, E.P., Freeman, D.W., & Allen, T.E. (1981). "Antenatal Prediction of Women at Increased Risk for Infants with Low Birthweights." *American Journal of Obstetrics and Gynecology 140* (1): 99-107.

Papiernik, E. (1984). "Predication of the Preterm Baby." *Clinics of Obstetrics and Gynecology 11* (2): 315-36.

Patterson, K. (1990). *The Social Construction of the Pregnancy Experience by Black Women at Risk for Preterm Birth.* Ann Arbor, MI: University Microfilms International.

Shalin, D.N. (1986, Feb). "Pragmatism and Social Interactionism." *American Sociological Review 51*: 9-29.

ROE v. WADE

On January 22, 1973, the Supreme Court of the United States decided the landmark abortion case *Roe v. Wade,* which guaranteed women the right to choose to terminate a pregnancy free from governmental interference. Prior to the Supreme Court decision, most states had very restrictive abortion laws, making the procedure a crime unless performed to save a woman's life. Women facing unwanted pregnancies were forced to obtain illegal abortions, often performed in back alleys by boatyard workers, automotive mechanics, and real-estate salesmen (Jaffe, Lindheim, and Philip, 1981).

In *Roe v. Wade,* a single pregnant woman argued that a Texas law that allowed only those abortions necessary to save a woman's life was invalid under the United States Constitution. The Supreme Court agreed, finding that the law violated a woman's right to privacy. The Court stated that the right to decide whether to terminate a pregnancy was a fundamental right, and therefore, the government could not interfere. The Court recognized that forcing a woman to carry her pregnancy to term could result in physical, emotional, and social harm to the woman (*Roe v. Wade,* 1973).

Roe v. Wade did not give women an absolute or unlimited right to have an abortion. Justice Blackmun, who wrote the opinion in the case, attempted to balance the woman's right to terminate her pregnancy with the state's interest in maternal health and the potential life of the fetus. He created a framework for deciding when states could regulate abortions, based on the stages of pregnancy. During the first trimester, the abortion decision must be left to the woman and her attending physician, without state regulation. During the second trimester, states may regulate the abortion procedure in ways that are reasonably related to protecting the woman's health. During the third trimester, states can prohibit abortions except when necessary to protect the woman's life or health (*Roe v. Wade,* 1973). Under the *Roe v. Wade* trimester framework, abortion laws in at least 49 states and the District of Columbia were invalid (Tribe, 1990).

Roe v. Wade affected women's lives in very important ways. First, *Roe v. Wade* protected women's health and lives by giving them access to legal abortions. Prior to the legalization of abortion, significant numbers of women died or were seriously harmed by illegal abortionists or self-induced abortions. According to one source, there were 320 such deaths recorded in 1961. Since 1974, an average of fewer than five women a year have died from illegal abortions (Jaffe, Lindheim, and Philip, 1981).

Second, *Roe v. Wade* helped equalize access to safe, legal abortions. Prior to the Supreme Court's decision, only those women who were educated and economically secure had access to safe, legal abortions. Uneducated and poor women had neither the knowledge nor the economic means to travel to states or countries where abortion was safe and legal. These women were left with only two choices: give birth to an unwanted child or risk their lives in back-alley abortions (Jaffe, Lindheim, and Philip, 1981). *Roe v. Wade* gave all women, especially poor women, a real choice: Women could now choose to terminate unwanted pregnancies through safe, legal abortions.

✱ CAROL WRIGHT NAPIER, J.D.

See also: Abortion, Politics of; Webster v. Reproductive Health Services

See **Guide to Related Topics:** Abortion; Legal Issues

Resources

Faux, Marian. (1988). *Roe v. Wade: The Untold Story of the Landmark Supreme Court Decision That Made Abortion Legal.* New York: Macmillan Publishing Co.

Jaffe, Frederick, Lindheim, Barbara, & Philip, Lee. (1981). *Abortion Politics, Private Morality and Public Policy.* New York: McGraw-Hill Book Co.

Roe v. Wade, 410 U.S. 113 (1973).

Rubin, Eva. (1982). *Abortion, Politics, and the Courts: Roe v. Wade and Its Aftermath.* Westport, CT: Greenwood Press.

Tribe, Laurence. (1990). *Abortion: The Clash of Absolutes.* New York: W.W. Norton and Co.

ROOMING-IN

"Rooming-in" is a hospital practice in which the newborn infant stays with the mother after birth and during the postpartum period, giving parents and infant the opportunity to get to know each other through extended and reciprocal interaction and contact. It is the cornerstone of a program of family-centered maternity care (International Childbirth Education Association, 1978; Interprofessional Task Force, 1978). Rooming-in programs, preferably using nurses assigned to mother-baby couples, may include continuous 24-hour rooming-in, modified rooming-in with the baby returning to the nursery at night, or some other arrangement based on the mother's needs (Haire and Haire, 1970; Young, 1982; McKay and Phillips, 1984).

Rooming-in was introduced in the 1940s and 1950s in response to concern over the adverse psychological effects on hospitalized children who were separated from their mothers (Spitz, 1945; Bowlby, 1958) and on the maternal-newborn relationship resulting from rigid hospital postpartum routines that separated mothers and babies (Moloney, 1949). The severe outbreaks of staphylococcal infections in hospital nurseries further stimulated implementation of rooming-in (Farer et al., 1959; Montgomery et al., 1959). Yale-New Haven Medical Center (formerly Grace-New Haven Community Hospital) (Jackson et al., 1948), followed by Duke Hospital (McBryde, 1951), introduced the earliest rooming-in programs in the United States.

Studies comparing infection rates in mothers and newborns who stayed in a central nursery with those mothers and newborns who had a rooming-in arrangement demonstrated greatly reduced rates of colonization and infection in rooming-in infants (McBryde, 1951; Farrer et al., 1959; Montgomery et al., 1959) and of maternal infections (Farrer et al., 1959). Recognition that cross-infection of newborn infants was caused by nursery staff led to endorsement of rooming-in by medical organizations (American Academy of Pediatrics, 1977; American Medical Association, 1977).

A majority of over 25 studies comparing the effects of restricted and extended early mother-infant postpartum contact demonstrated increased maternal affectionate and attachment behavior among mothers who had extended contact (Klaus et al., 1972; Klaus and Kennell, 1982; Young, 1982; Thomson and Westreich, 1989). Fathers who had extended early contact with their newborns also demonstrated increased attachment behaviors and involvement and interest in their babies (Greenberg and Morris, 1974; Parke and Sawin, 1976; Rodholm and Larsson, 1979). Studies of newborns have shown a wide range of responses to environmental stimuli, encouraging reciprocal parent-infant interaction during the postpartum period (Macfarlane, 1977; Brazelton, 1980).

Ten studies showed that women who had extended mother-infant contact through rooming-in breastfed longer (Klaus and Kennell, 1982; Thomson and Westreich, 1989). Also associated with rooming-in are higher maternal confidence and competence in infant caretaking (McBryde, 1951; Greenberg, Rosenberg, and Lind, 1973; Seashore et al., 1973), less infant crying (McBryde, 1951; de Chateau and Wiberg, 1977a, 1977b; Keefe, 1987), more quiet infant sleep patterns (Keefe, 1987), and absence of maternal sleep disruptions (Keefe, 1988). Rooming-in allows maternity staff to advise and instruct parents in infant care and development.

No research has indicated advantages or justification for routinely restricting postpartum contact between mothers and babies: in fact, such separation appears to have adverse consequences (Klaus and Kennell, 1982; Young, 1982; Thomson and Westreich, 1989). ✱ DIONY YOUNG

See also: Breastfeeding: Physiological and Cultural Aspects; The Family Bed; Family-Centered Maternity Care

See **Guide to Related Topics:** Baby Care

Resources

American Academy of Pediatrics (AAP). (1977). *Standards and Recommendations for Hospital Care of Newborn Infants.* Evanston, IL: American Academy of Pediatrics.

American Medical Association (AMA). (1977). "Statement on Parent and Newborn Interaction." Proceedings of House of Delegates, 31st Interim Meeting, Chicago, IL, Dec. 4-7.

Bowlby, J. (1958). "The Nature of a Child's Tie to His Mother." *International Journal of Psychoanalysis 39*: 350-73.

Brazelton, T.B. (1980). "Behavioral Competence of the Newborn." In P.M. Taylor (Ed.) *Parent-Infant Relationships.* New York: Grune & Stratton, Inc.

de Chateau, P. & Wiberg, B. (1977a). "Long-term Effect of Mother-Infant Behaviour of Extra Contact during the First Hour Post Partum: First Observations at 36 Hours." *Acta Pediatrica Scandinavica 66*: 137-44.

———. (1977b). "Long-term Effect of Mother-Infant Behaviour of Extra Contact during the First Hour Post Partum: A Follow-up at Three Months. *Acta Pediatrica Scandinavica 66*: 145-51.

Farrer, S.M. et al. (1959). "Surveillance and Control of Staphylococcic Infections in a Maternity Unit." *Journal of the American Medical Association 171* (8): 1072-79.

Greenberg, M. & Morris, N. (1974). "Engrossment: The Newborn's Impact upon the Father. *American Journal of Orthopsychiatry 44*: 520-31.

Greenberg, M., Rosenberg, I., & Lind, J. (1973). "First Mothers Rooming-in with their Newborns: Its Impact upon the Mother. *American Journal of Orthopsychiatry 43*: 783-88.

Haire, D. & Haire, J. (1970). *Implementing Family-Centered Maternity Care with a Central Nursery.* Minneapolis, MN: International Childbirth Education Association.

International Childbirth Education Association (ICEA). (1978). *Position Paper on Planning Comprehensive Maternal and Newborn Services.* Minneapolis, MN: International Childbirth Education Association.

Interprofessional Task Force on Health Care of Women and Children. (1978). *Joint Position Statement on the Development of Family-Centered Maternity/Newborn Care in Hospitals.* Washington, DC: American College of Obstetricians and Gynecologists.

Jackson, E.B. et al. (1948). "A Hospital Rooming-in Unit for Four Newborn Infants and Their Mothers. *Pediatrics 1*: 28-43.

Keefe, M.R. (1987). "Comparison of Neonatal Nighttime Sleep-Wake Patterns in Nursery versus Rooming-in Environments." *Nursing Research 36* (3): 140-44.

———. (1988). "The Impact of Infant Rooming-in on Maternal Sleep at Night." *Journal of Obstetric and Gynecologic Nursing 17* (2): 122-26.

Klaus, M.H. et al. (1972). "Maternal Attachment: Importance of the First Post-partum Days." *New England Journal of Medicine 286*: 460-63.

Klaus, M.H. & Kennell, J.H. (1982). *Parent-Infant Bonding* 2nd Edition. St. Louis: C.V. Mosby Co.

Macfarlane, A. (1977). *The Psychology of Childbirth.* Cambridge, MA: Harvard University Press.

McBryde, A. (1951). "Compulsory Rooming-in and Private Newborn Service." *Journal of American Medical Association 145* (9): 625-28.

McKay, S. & Phillips, C.R. (1984). *Family-Centered Maternity Care: Implementation Strategies.* Rockville, MD: Aspen Systems Corp.

Moloney, J.C. (1949). "The Cornelian Corner and Its Rationale, abstracted." *American Journal of Diseases in Childhood 78*: 465.

Montgomery, T.L. et al. (1959). "A Study of Staphylococcic Colonization of Postpartum Mothers and Newborn Infants: Comparison of Central Care and Rooming-in." *American Journal of Obstetrics and Gynecology 78* (6): 1227-33.

O'Connor, S. et al. "Reduced Incidence of Parenting Inadequacy Following Rooming-in." *Pediatrics 66*: 176-82.

Parke, R.D. & Sawin, D.B. (1976). "The Father's Role in Infancy: An Evaluation." *Family Coordinator 25*: 365-71.

Rodholm, M. & Larsson, K. (1979). "Father-Infant Interaction at the First Contact after Delivery." *Early Human Development 3*: 21-27.

Seashore, M.J. et al. (1973). "The Effects of Denial of Early Mother-Infant Interaction on Maternal Self-confidence." *Journal of Personality and Social Psychology 26* (3): 369-78.

Spitz, R. (1945). "Hospitalism: An Inquiry into the Genesis of Psychiatric Conditions in Early Childhood." *Psychoanalyitic Study of Childhood 1*: 53.

Thomson, M. & Westreich, R. (1989). "Restriction of Mother-Infant Contact in the Immediate Postpartum Period." In I. Chalmers et al. (Eds.) *Effective Care in Pregnancy and Childbirth.* Vol. 2. New York: Oxford University Press.

Young, D. (1982). *Changing Childbirth: Family Birth in the Hospital.* Rochester, NY: Childbirth Graphics, Ltd.

RU486

RU486 (Mifepristone), known as the "abortion pill," is a 19-norsteroid that has the ability to inhibit progesterone binding competitively at the receptor level. The result is that it can be used to interrupt early pregnancy by preventing implantation of the fertilized egg. The pregnancy termination is characterized by a heavy menstrual bleed.

RU486 is available in France during the first 49 days of amenorrhea (absence of the menstrual period) for the purpose of terminating a pregnancy, provided that: (1) it is taken under a physician's supervision and in conjunction with a follow-up dose of prostaglandin derivative; (2) there is no contraindication to mifepristone (adrenal insufficiency, long-term administration of glucocorticoids, clotting disorders) or to prostaglandins (asthma, severe hypertension); and (3) it is taken in accordance with French abortion law, which requires a one-week waiting period between the request for an abortion and the procedure.

Pregnancy terminations reach 98.7 percent effectiveness when 600 mg of mifepristone is followed three days later with a 0.5 mg intramuscular injection of the prostaglandin analogue sulprostone. Side effects are minimal. Of 2,115 French women using the drug in 1988, in various dosages of prostaglandin analogues, failures included persisting pregnancies (1.0 percent), incomplete expulsions (2.1 percent), and the need for hemostatic procedure (0.9 percent). The average time for expulsion ranged from 4.5 hours to 22.7 hours, depending upon the dose of prostaglandin, and on average, uterine bleeding continued for 8.9 days (range, 1 to 35). Use of the drug was characterized by transient abdominal bleeding after receiving prostaglandin, but few other side effects. One woman of the 2,115 received a blood transfusion. Incomplete abortions were completed by suction technique.

The availability of RU486 in the United States has been blocked by religious fundamentalists and anti-choice activists. In the mid-1980s, these groups formed the RCR Alliance, which spearheaded a campaign against the drug's French manufacturer, Roussel-Uclaf, and its parent company, Hoechst A.G. of the Federal Republic of Germany. RCR Alliance identified Hoechst's major corporate investors and threatened to organize a boycott against them unless they sold their stock in Hoechst or persuaded Hoechst to restrain

Roussel-Uclaf from further RU486 sales. It also identified those international brokerage houses large enough to handle a possible sale of Roussel-Uclaf and notified them that they too would be the target of a public relations campaign should they help Hoechst to sell the troublesome subsidiary. RCR Alliance then retained legal counsel in Paris to be ready to bring product liability suits against Roussel-Uclaf and Hoechst should there be any women who suffer serious side effects, and placed its religious affiliates in developing countries on alert to look for such women should RU486 be tested in their area.

Finally, the group threatened to join with the group Operation Rescue to picket Roussel-Uclaf and Hoechst offices and to advertise the fact that Hoechst A.G. was a descendent company of I.G. Farben, a company notorious for manufacturing the Zyklon B gas used in the gas chambers in Nazi concentration camps. RCR Alliance and the National Right to Life Committee characterized RU486 as a drug that "turns wombs into death ovens."

These threats, combined with anonymous threats to the physical safety of Roussel-Uclaf executives and general concerns about the commercial consequences of investing in a politically controversial drug, led Roussel-Uclaf in October 1988 to withdraw RU486 from the French market only weeks after its approval by the French Ministry of Health. The French government, as minority shareholder in the company, exercised a provision of French law that allowed it to force the company to put the drug back on the market on pain of losing the patent rights. Justifying this action, Minister of Health Claude Evin said there was no excuse for denying women access to a safer form of a legally protected medical procedure, and he called RU486 the "moral property of women."

Although the drug was once again available in France, Roussel-Uclaf dropped plans for rapid expansion into other European markets. As of early 1992, the drug has not been licensed to any company outside of France and Great Britain, and the company has announced that it will not allow introduction of the drug into any country where the government and public is not supportive of abortion rights.

The U.S. government has taken a particularly hostile stance toward the drug via the U.S. Food and Drug Administration (FDA). The FDA has classified RU486 as unreasonably dangerous and, therefore, not eligible for private importation under supervision of an American physician, as are most other drugs not yet approved for U.S. marketing. The American Medical Association, however, has recommended that RU486 be tested for use in the United States, and numerous feminist and professional groups have organized to persuade Roussel-Uclaf to release the drug to U.S. companies.

Despite the potential of RU486 for providing abortion alternatives and treatment for endometriosis, breast cancer, and prolonged labor, anti-abortion groups as well as a very small number of women's health advocates have claimed the drug dangerous, particularly in combination with prostaglandins. Major scientific and health associations disagree.

Groups calling for United States trials of RU486 include the American Association for Advancement of Science, the American Association of Physicians for Human Rights, American Institute of Biological Sciences, American Public Health Association, The Association of Reproductive Healthcare Professionals, and the National Women's Health Network. A coalition of major cities and several state legislatures have also called for testing, as has a congressional resolution introduced by Ron Wydes, Democrat, of Oregon.

Should RU486 become available in the United States, it would make even early abortions safer and approximately 50 percent less expensive—of particular importance to poor women, who are routinely denied Medicaid coverage for abortions. It would also make it possible for any physician to administer the drug during an office visit, reducing the need for abortion clinics. These clinics have become the highly visible targets of pickets and bombs by Operation Rescue as well as of state legislative attempts to render them uneconomic. The chances remain very low that RU486 will be available to women in the United States before the end of the century.

✷ R. ALTA CHARO, J.D.

See **Guide to Related Topics:** Abortion; Contraception

Resources

Avrech, O. et al. (1991). "Mifepristone (RU486) Alone or in Combination with a Prostaglandin Analog for Termination of Early Pregnancy: A Review." *Fertility and Sterility 56* (3): 385-93.

Baulieu, E. "RU 486 as an Antiprogesterone Steroid: From Receptor to Contragestin." *Journal of American Medical Association 26* (13): 1808-14.

Bygdeman, M. & Van Look, P.F. (1989). "The Use of Prostaglandin and Antiprogestins for Pregnancy Termination." *International Journal of Gynecology and Obstetrics 29* (2): 5-12.

Charo, R. Alta. (1990). "A Case History of RU-486." In Kathi Hanna (Ed.) *Biomedical Decisionmaking in a Pluralistic Society.* Washington, DC: National Academy Press.

Cook, R. (1989). "Antiprogestin Drugs: Medical and Legal Issues." *Family Planning Perspectives 21* (6): 267-72.

Cossey, M. & Tearse, S. (1990, Aug). "The French Experience with RU-486 and the Outlook for Great Britain." A report to the Reproductive Technologies Project, 1601 Connecticut Avenue, N.W., Suite 801, Washington, DC 20009, (202) 328-2200.

Djerassi, C. (1989, Jul). "The Bitter Pill." *Science 245*: 256-61.

Greenhouse, J. (1989, Feb 12). "A New Pill, A New Battle." *New York Times Magazine*: 23.

Grimes, D. et al. (1990). "Predictors of Failed Attempted Abortion with the Antiprogestin Mifepristone (RU486)." *American Journal of Obstetrics and Gynecology 162* (4): 910-17.

Gruhier, R. (1988, Nov). "Adventures de la Pillules RU486." (Adventures of the RU486 Pill.) *Le Nouvel Observateur*. 1252: 3-9.

Hodges, G. (1991). "Antiprogestins: The Political Chemistry of RU486." *Sterility and Fertility 56* (3): 394-95.

Klitsch, M. (1989). "RU-486: The Science and the Politics." Washington, DC: Alan Guttmacher Institute.

Silvestre, L. et al. (1990). "Voluntary Interruption of Pregnancy with Mifepristone (RU 486) and a Prostaglandin Analogue: A Large Scale French Experience." *New England Journal of Medicine 322* (10): 645-48.

Ullman, A., Teutsch, G. & Phillbert, Z. (1990). "RU486." *Scientific American 262* (6): 42-48.

Urquhart, R. et al. (1990, Jun). "The Efficacy and Tolerance of Mifepristone and Prostaglandin in First Trimester Termination of Pregnancy: U.K. Multicentre Trial." *British Journal of Obstetrics and Gynecology 97*: 480-86.

RUBELLA. *See instead* TORCH SYNDROME

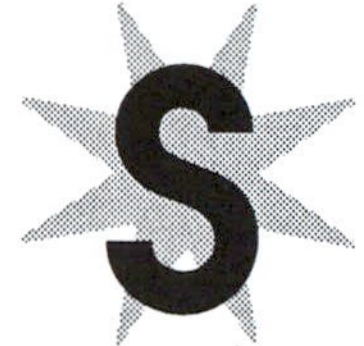

SANGER, MARGARET

Margaret Sanger was born in 1879 in Corning, New York, the sixth of 11 children in the poverty-stricken Higgens family. She received nurse's training, and her work among the poor in New York City was pivotal in the genesis of her life crusade: making every child a wanted child. For poor women of her time, there was no relief from unchecked fertility. Contraception was a guarded secret of upper-class women. All other women were compelled to bear children excessively; septic self-induced abortions were exceedingly common. In addition, the infant-maternal mortality-morbidity rates worldwide were very high, concurrent with poor living standards. Information, and, indeed, methodology, for fertility control was illegal following the notorious Comstock Act of 1873. This federal statute made it a criminal offense not only to import, mail, or transport in interstate commerce any article for the prevention of conception but made it equally criminal to transport obscene literature, with no differentiation between the two.

In 1912 Sanger began educating women on their reproductive options through her writings and speeches. In 1916 she and her sister opened the first birth control clinic outside of the Netherlands, in Brownsville, New York, for which they were jailed. She ultimately was jailed eight times but remained undeterred by either legal or religious opposition to her cause. The Catholic Church and its highly organized hierarchy were among her most powerful and strident opponents, often precipitating legal action against her. Clearly, however, the time had come for her movement to achieve fruition. She experienced tremendous success in awakening first the populace, then the medical profession, to the need for birth control, a term which she coined.

In 1921 Sanger organized the American Birth Control League and served as its president until 1928. She organized the World Population Conference in Geneva in 1927 and the International Conference for Doctors and Scientists in 1930. At this time, little was known about the physiology of the human reproductive system. The few birth control methods available were unsophisticated, marginally reliable, and difficult for most women to obtain. This 1930 conference was a catalyst for

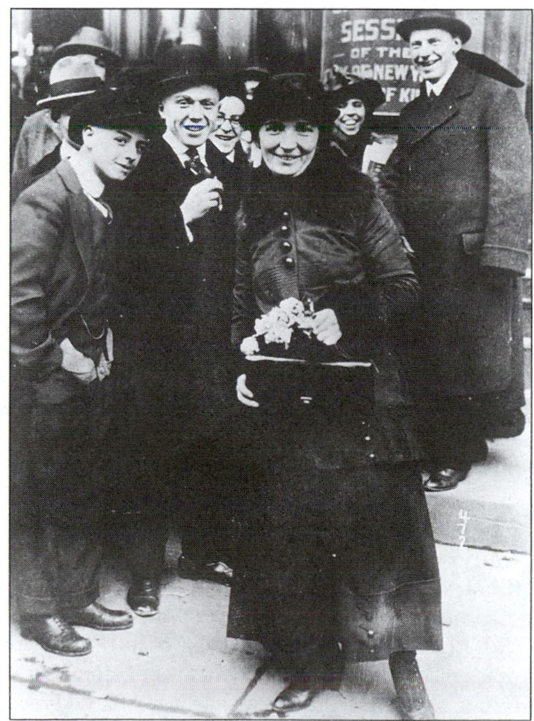

Margaret Sanger. Photo courtesy of Planned Parenthood of New York City.

research into effective, reliable birth control. Indeed, Sanger was instrumental in facilitating the development of the modern diaphragm, spermicide, and oral contraceptive pill. She helped to educate the medical profession in the United States by engaging a full-time lecturer to speak nationwide at state and local associations. With Sanger's organizational support, Dr. Helen Stone headed up the Medical Research Bureau, which would eventually document 100,000 case histories demonstrating the necessity of child spacing and assessing current techniques for doing so. This constituted the first organized birth control research.

Simultaneous with the espousal and development of contraceptive information and methods, Sanger worked relentlessly to change the laws that prevented women from obtaining and using birth control. In 1936 birth control under medical direction became legal in the United States when the Comstock Act was struck down. Although individual states continued to attempt to criminalize birth control into the 1960s, the inevitability of universal availability of birth control was established in 1936.

Sanger worked tirelessly to spread the doctrine and practice of population control worldwide, especially in Japan and the Far East. She engaged in extensive international speaking tours until she was 80 years old, despite lifelong chronic health problems, including tuberculosis. In 1953, at age 73, she organized the International Planned Parenthood Federation and was its president for six years. At that time 27 countries participated. The Planned Parenthood Federation is her enduring legacy, the ensurance that her life's work would be continued on the local, national, and international levels.

Margaret Sanger was a woman of the world. She had many close friends and intimates worldwide. She married twice and had three children. Her involvements included the Progressive Labor Movement; early socialist groups; and the European Free Love Movement, which stressed a single sexual standard for women as well as men. Her life and work emphasized teaching people to accept their sexuality and to have rational responses to it. She encouraged women to choose consciously when and how many children they would bear and to develop themselves into fulfilled, self-realized human beings.

Sanger identified unchecked population growth as the most important deterrent to the mass of humanity enjoying a decent standard of living and the fruits of technology, as well as a major cause of war. Her work has saved the lives of uncounted women, as well as helping to improve the lives of people worldwide who practice contraception. ✱ JOANNA VARADI, C.N.M.

See also: The Pill

See **Guide to Related Topics:** Contraception

Resources

Douglas, Emily Taft. (1970). *Margaret Sanger: Pioneer of the Future.* New York: Holt, Rinehart and Winston.

Hardin, Garrett. (1969). *Population, Evolution and Birth Control.* San Francisco: Freeman and Co.

National Commission on Federal Legislation for Birth Control. (1937). *A New Day Dawns for Birth Control.* New York: National Commission on Federal Legislation for Birth Control, Inc.

Sanger, Margaret. (1920). *Woman and the New Race.* New York: Truth Publishing Co.

———. (1938). *An Autobiography.* New York: W.W. Norton.

SELECTIVE ABORTION

Abortions following prenatal diagnosis are called "selective" abortions because in such cases a particular fetus is selected for abortion. Such a selective abortion stands in contrast to the far more common abortion, in which the woman needs to end the pregnancy regardless of any particular characteristics of the fetus.

Although some people have discussed the value of being forewarned of genetic or other diseases even in a pregnancy a woman intends to carry to term, abortion is an integral part of the technology of prenatal diagnosis. Fetal treatments do not exist for the conditions to be diagnosed. The overwhelming majority of people who are told of serious disease or damage in the fetus do abort. These abortions to prevent the birth of a handicapped or disabled child are among the most socially acceptable of abortions. In the United States, more than 80 percent of people surveyed approved of the use of abortion in this situation. Because these abortions are socially acceptable, many people have assumed that they are psychologically more acceptable than are abortions for what is called "less reason," abortions because the woman does not want to be pregnant. That is not true. The psychological acceptability of an abortion lies in the meaning of the abortion for the woman who is having it.

Women's willingness to use abortion for unwanted pregnancies has been perceived as a devaluing of motherhood. On the contrary, it is because women continue to take motherhood so very seriously that abortion is necessary. Women understand that motherhood will change their lives and involve a deep and permanent condition. If women did not take motherhood seriously, other options for managing an unwanted pregnancy would be available, from simple abandonment to selling the babies.

In a sense, the motherhood-abortion paradox parallels the marriage-divorce paradox. The divorce rate is highest when expectations for marriage are highest. If marriage were considered less important, divorce would be less common. Thus the paradox is that the high divorce rate demonstrates not a devaluing of marriage, but a commitment to the importance of the marriage relationship; abortion as a solution to an unwanted pregnancy demonstrates the importance to women of the mother-child relationship.

Abortions to prevent the birth of a disabled child may be more socially acceptable, but they are not in any sense easier for the woman. They present a deeper, more fundamental challenge for both the woman and society at large. These selective abortions introduce conditionality into the development of mother love: Mothers are asked to "hold off" on thinking of their future babies as babies until the medical all-clear has been sounded. This sets up a difficult contradiction of demands for women in pregnancy: They have to do everything they can to take care of the baby they hope to have, while being prepared to abort the particular fetus they may be carrying. And this contradiction continues, in the case of amniocentesis, for as long as, or even longer than, 20 weeks—half the length of pregnancy.

These late abortions are themselves very difficult, both physically and emotionally. Most American women having late abortions experience a labor and deliver a dead fetus. A drug, prostaglandin, can be used to start the labor. A second approach is to inject saline solution or urea into the amniotic fluid, which kills the fetus. Labor then starts after the fetus has died. The third, less common, procedure is a "D & E," dilation and evacuation, in which the cervix is dilated painlessly over a period of several days, with the woman unconscious or heavily sedated and the fetus removed in pieces. This procedure is viewed as more difficult for the medical personnel, because it is they who must dismember and remove the fetus. While the medical literature often says that this procedure is easier for the woman because she need not labor or go through the harrowing experience of delivering a dead fetus, not all women agree that a D & E is easier. Because these are not unwanted pregnancies, the woman may have a very real image of the *baby* that she carries.

The conditions under which late abortions are performed most often make the dreadful situation even worse. Many women are left to labor and abort on maternity floors, surrounded by newborn nurseries and new mothers. Others use abortion facilities, where the women around them are experiencing far more relief to be out of an unwanted pregnancy than the kind of grief that women experience when a wanted pregnancy is lost.

There have been some attempts to establish support groups for women who have terminated pregnancies following prenatal diagnosis, but because of the relative rarity of the problem, among other reasons, very few such support groups have been established.

Reactions following the abortion of a pregnancy after prenatal diagnosis more closely resemble those following miscarriage than those following other abortions, with the added burden of responsibility for the "choice." For the individual woman, the particular condition of the fetus that she carried, or the lack of services that that fetus would have needed had it gone on to become a child, may take away all meaningful choice. Yet she is still left with the responsibility, and with the grief. ✷ BARBARA KATZ ROTHMAN, Ph.D.

See also: Amniocentesis, History of; Childkeeping and Childbearing; Chorionic Villus Sampling; Eugenics; Prenatal Diagnosis: Overview; Wrongful Birth and Wrongful Life

See **Guide to Related Topics:** Abortion; Prenatal Diagnosis and Screening

Resources

Luker, Kristen. (1984). *Abortion and the Politics of Motherhood.* Berkeley, CA: University of California Press.

President's Commission for the Study of Ethical Problems in Medicine and Biomedical and Behavioral Research. (1983). *Screening and Counseling for Genetic Conditions: The Ethical, Social and Legal Implications of Genetic Screening, Counseling and Educational Programs.* Washington, DC: U.S. Government Printing Office.

Rothman, Barbara Katz. (1986). *The Tentative Pregnancy: Prenatal Diagnosis and the Future of Motherhood.* New York: Viking.

SEX SELECTION, PRECONCEPTION

In humans, sex is determined when a sperm merges with an egg: A sperm carrying a Y chromosome determines a male; one with an X, a female. Behaviors during sexual intercourse that purportedly favor one or the other sperm type result in sex determination ratios scarcely better than chance. Such behaviors include timing of intercourse or of orgasm, position during intercourse, depth of penetration, level of acidity in the vagina, and amount of salt in the diet. Because the Y chromosome is smaller than the X chromosome, theories claim that the Y chromosome swims faster: In one unproven timing theory for conceiving a boy, intercourse should occur when the supposedly faster Y sperm can reach the egg as it moves down the fallopian tube. ProCare of Colorado marketed its Gender Choice kit based on such a theory ("Deception Charged," 1987). However, no hard data support any timing hypotheses, some of which disagree with each other (James, 1983; Hoskins and Holmes, 1984; Holmes, 1985).

Also tried have been laboratory manipulations of semen to separate the two kinds of sperm for sex selection through artificial insemination. Apparatus used includes centrifuges, columns of albumen for sperm to swim up, columns of gel beads for sperm to swim down, and electric fields. The "Ericsson method," available in several U.S. clinics, uses the albumen column and purports to produce over 75 percent boy babies; however, tests of the separated sperm reveal ratios close to 50-50 (Ericsson and Beernink, 1987; Gledhill, 1988; Carson, 1988). Methods that check the sex of separated sperm are not completely accurate and can also kill sperm or use them up (e.g., one test used them to fertilize hamster eggs). Animal scientists using various laboratory methods to separate Y- and X-sperm of livestock also have had little success (Gledhill, 1988). Despite over 30 years' failure with livestock and human semen, Gledhill is optimistic that separation techniques will shortly be successful.

Ethical Issues. Persons who would not abort a human fetus of the "wrong" sex might nevertheless be willing to select sex before conception. ProCare sold 50,000 kits in four months in 1986. Reasons to select sex in Western countries include "balancing" families, having a son inherit, sharing a sex-typed hobby or sport, and pleasing husband or wife. However, anyone planning sex selection is subtly, if not explicitly, sexist. The parent desires a child because of specific genderized behavioral or character traits that, in a given society, are tightly linked to sex. Harm may come to the selected child who believes he or she is being loved for stereotypical traits, not as a person in his or her own right, especially if the child fails to fit the stereotype and then is punished. Harm may also come to selection failures or children of the opposite sex in such a family, when those children realize that a basic trait of theirs (sex) was unsatisfactory to their parents.

Proponents of sex selection for the benefit of society point to the problem of overpopulation. They argue that, with a preferred mix of children of chosen sex, a family will be smaller; furthermore, with fewer females in a society, population will decrease because fewer wombs produce fewer babies. However, when females are in short supply, they may be forced to reproduce frequently. Data from all over the world have shown that population reduction often occurs when women are educated and valued and can postpone age of first pregnancy. Furthermore, gains made towards equal treatment of, and equal opportunities for, the sexes are set back when people act in any way on sex prejudices.

✱ HELEN BEQUAERT HOLMES, Ph.D.

See also: Preimplantation Diagnosis

See **Guide to Related Topics:** New Procreative Technologies

Resources

Bennett, Neil G. (Ed.) (1983). *Sex Selection of Children.* New York: Academic Press.

Carson, Sandra Ann. (1988). "Sex Selection: The Ultimate in Family Planning." *Fertility and Sterility 50*: 16-17.

"Deception Charged on Choosing Sex of Babies." (1987, Feb 1). *The New York Times*: 26.

Ericsson, Ronald J. & Beernink, Ferdinand. (1987). "Sex Chromosome Ratios in Human Sperm." *Fertility and Sterility* 47 (3): 531-32.

Gledhill, Barton L. (1988). "Selection and Separation of X- and Y-Chromosome-bearing Mammalian Sperm." *Gamete Research 20*: 377-95.

Holmes, Helen B. (1985). "Sex Preselection: Eugenics for Everyone?" In J. Humber & R. Almeder (Eds.) *Biomedical Ethics Reviews—1985.* Clifton, NJ: The Humana Press, pp. 39-71.

Hoskins, Betty B. & Holmes, Helen B. (1984). "Technology and Prenatal Femicide." In R. Arditti, R.D. Klein, & S. Minden (Eds.) *Test-Tube Women: What Future for Motherhood?* London: Pandora Press, pp. 237-55.

James, William H. (1983). "Timing of Fertilization and Sex Ratio of Offspring." In N.G. Bennett (Ed.) *Sex Selection of Children.* New York: Academic Press.

Raymond, Janice. "Sex Selection." In H.B. Holms, B.B. Hoskins, & M. Gross (Eds.) *The Custom-made Child? Women-centered Perspectives.* Clifton, NJ: The Humana Press, pp. 177-224.

SEXUALITY IN PREGNANCY

Sexuality encompasses all an individual is, thinks, feels, and does in his or her life span that relates to being male or female, masculine or feminine. Sexual behavior is the broad, outward expression of the male or female's positive or negative feelings and attitudes. These include the manner in which they dress, walk, communicate (verbal and nonverbal), and the various forms of touch, hugging, body massage, stroking, breast caressing, kissing, licking, sucking, self-pleasuring, mutual masturbation, oral and anal sex, and sexual intercourse or coitus. In past literature, sexuality was incorrectly equated solely with intercourse, and empirical research, including that concerning pregnancy, centered around coital desire, frequency, satisfaction, and orgasm.

Cultural mores, socially reinforced myths, religious taboos, and social learning all affect sexual perceptions and expressions in everyday living. Negative feelings about their own bodies, especially the genitals, are often reinforced within the family, so that young women are often given messages to avoid looking at or touching their genitals and to regard them as "dirty." Families seldom encourage open discussion of sexual feelings or modes of expressing sexuality. These are regarded as private and are rarely talked about, even with friends. Despite the so-called sexual revolution and sex education in schools, most couples have little understanding about their own sexuality or the physical and emotional factors that influence sexual desire and response.

This ignorance is magnified during the childbearing years. Pregnancy, the outward manifestation of the couple's sexuality (Wilkerson and Bing, 1988), is generally viewed as a time for promoting a closer and more intimate relationship between a woman and her partner. Yet many sexual behaviors, including intercourse, have been forbidden by religious taboos, fears, and myths promoted by popular literature.

Expectant women are hesitant to discuss their sexual questions with anyone, least of all their physicians. Traditionally, the only information of a sexual nature that most obstetricians include at regular gynecological visits is that related to contraception. During pregnancy, physicians do not routinely initiate discussions on the topic of sexuality unless the woman asks specific questions or there are medical contraindications to sexual expression. Neither the factors that affect sexual expression nor the possibilities for maintaining sensual and sexual health are introduced by medical caregivers. This may be due in part to the physician's personal discomfort with the subject or the lack of objective information received during medical training. Information on sexuality in most obstetrical texts is still sorely outdated. Midwifery care is more likely to include discussion of sexuality.

Changes in Sexual Response. Patterns of sexual behavior during pregnancy support the trend towards declining sexual desire, interest, frequency, and satisfaction, especially with intercourse in the first and third trimesters of pregnancy. Some studies report increased frequency during the middle trimester (Masters and Johnson, 1968). There is individual variability, depending on many factors, including prepregnant levels of sexual interest, relationship with partner, hormonal influences, responses to the physical and emotional changes of the pregnancy, attitude towards the pregnancy, body image, cultural mores, and religious taboos.

Physical changes in the first trimester, such as nausea, vomiting, fatigue, breast tenderness, and pelvic congestion, with accompanying increased desire for rest and sleep, will often decrease sexual desire and responsiveness. This may be upsetting to the partner or to both individuals as they relish the excitement of the pregnancy. It is not abnormal for couples to experience ambivalence towards the pregnancy, even if planned and desired. Ambivalence may result from worries about the timing of the pregnancy, impending parenthood, finances, careers, and family relationships. For some women, anxiety and sadness in early pregnancy may be related to loss of independence and lifestyle changes that threaten self-esteem, all of which will affect sexual expression. Despite coital desire changes, expectant women and partners need physical contact and emotional closeness. Hugging, holding, caressing, cuddling, kissing, massaging, and oral sex may be pleasuring alternatives for both of them.

Fear of miscarriage, especially in couples who have previously lost a baby in early pregnancy or who have had difficulty becoming pregnant, has a marked effect on the physical expression of sexual desire or capacity to be aroused. Women who feel confident about their sexuality are thought to take the pregnancy more in stride, and may even enjoy sex more as the risk of "getting pregnant" has dissolved.

In the second trimester, lovemaking becomes more comfortable as a greater sense of well-being is experienced. Many of the unpleasant symptoms of the first trimester have disappeared, while increased blood circulation, vaginal lubrication, and engorgement of breasts and labia enhance sexual desire and response. Higher degrees of eroticism in women have been described, many report more intense orgasms, and the woman's fuller shape may make her feel more desirable and provide a source of pleasure for both partners. The male partner may also experience feelings of increased virility; evidence of the enlarging abdomen and these enhanced feelings of couple closeness may translate to heightened mutual pleasuring. Finding new positions for lovemaking that enhance comfort and satisfaction, other than the frequently used "missionary position," can be an interesting challenge. Mutual touching, oral sex, or genital massage (Shrock, 1985) may be other appealing options as pregnancy proceeds.

On the other hand, the woman's changing body shape and weight gain may be perceived as being unattractive and sexually undesirable. Some men are embarrassed or feel guilty approaching their wife's larger and unfamiliar body. The most frequently cited reasons for decreased sexual interest are the male partner's fears that he will injure the fetus or his wife, or that he will cause premature labor. With reassurance from medical caregivers, these fears can be reduced.

When sexual expression is viewed by either or both partners as only a means for procreation, guilt, shame, and repulsion may induce stress in the relationship. This can be exacerbated when men feel lonely and abandoned as their partners become more introspective and preoccupied with the growing fetus. The resultant unhappiness turns some men to extramarital affairs. Honest communication about fears and feelings, reassurance, and expressions of affection and physical loving are important means of maintaining couple closeness.

Outdated medical advice to abstain from coitus for six to eight weeks before the infant's birth may be the reason for consistent findings of decreased sexual activity during the third trimester. However, physical discomfort, including size and weight of the pregnant woman's abdomen, heartburn, fatigue, leg cramps, backache, position of the fetus, leaking breasts, and more intense uterine contractions with orgasm may all play a part in the decreased level of sexual activity during this time. Many women feel less desirable, fat, and misshapen and have lowered self-esteem. Fears and anxieties surrounding the birth and impending parenthood warrant protection of the fetus if the couple believe lovemaking could inflict harm. Religious upbringing may foster confusion of woman as a sexual being and impending mother, responses affecting both men and women.

Health caregivers must discuss valid medical contraindications to coitus and orgasm, such as recurrent miscarriage, bleeding, active herpes, and multiple pregnancy. Healthy couples should be encouraged to maintain a close, loving relationship with emotional and physical pleasuring within the boundaries of safety.

✱ PAMELA SHROCK, Ph.D.

Resources

Bing, E. & Colman, L. (1990). *Making Love During Pregnancy.* New York: Bantam Books.

Colman, A. & Colman, L. (1990). *Pregnancy: The Psychological Experience.* New York: The Seabury Press.

Katchadourian, H. & Lunde, D. (1972). *Fundamentals of Human Sexuality.* New York: Holt, Rinehart and Winston, Inc.

Kitzinger, S. (1980). *The Complete Book of Pregnancy.* New York: Knopf.

———. (1983). *Women's Experience of Sex.* New York: Penguin Books.

Masters, W. & Johnson, V. (1968). *Human Sexual Response.* New York: Little, Brown.

Newton, N. (1982). *Maternal Emotions.* New York: Paul Hoeber.

Schuman, T. (Ed.) (1983). *The Parent Manual: A Handbook for a Prepared Childbirth.* Garden City, NY: Avery Publishing Group, Inc.

Shrock, P. (1985). "Effect of Pregnancy on Marital Relationship and Sexual Expression of Primiparous Expectant Couples." *Dissertation,* Chicago, Northwestern University.

Strong, B. & Devault, C. (1988). *Understanding Our Sexuality.* St. Paul, MN: West Publishing.

Wilkerson, N.N. & Bing, E. (1988). "Sexuality." In F. Nichols and S. Humenick (Eds.) *Childbirth Education: Practice, Research and Theory.* Philadelphia: Saunders, pp. 376-93.

SEXUALLY TRANSMITTED DISEASES

The term "sexually transmitted disease" (STD) is relatively new and replaces the term "venereal disease" (VD). The etymological root of venereal is "venus," the goddess of love, implying a heterosexual and male-centered love and sexual pleasure. Venereal disease was traditionally thought to be punishment derived from men's love and sexual pleasure with women. The stigma remains, providing a barrier to effective preventive education and treatment, which is often complicated by racism, classism, and sexism within the health care system.

STDs range from very mild and benign to life-threatening conditions. More than 20 organisms and syndromes are encompassed by the term "STD," including syphilis, gonorrhea, human immunodeficiency virus (HIV), chlamydia trachomatis, genital herpes, genital warts, and cervical neoplasia. The majority of STD cases are found in individuals under 25 years of age and in medically underserved populations. Women suffer more long-term consequences than men, including pelvic inflammatory disease (PID), ectopic pregnancy, chronic pelvic pain, infertility, and cervical cancer. Because of the "fluid dynamic" of heterosexual intercourse, heterosexually active women are at an increased risk of transmission (Hatcher et al., 1990). Lesbians who engage in exclusive lesbian sex are at very low risk for most STDs, although herpes genitalis and bacterial vaginosus are somewhat common.

Prevention of STDs is similar to HIV prevention. STDs are transmitted via semen, blood, and body fluids. Condoms with a spermicidal cream provide a barrier against heterosexual and/or male homosexual transmission. Latex dental dams provide a barrier against lesbian oral sex transmission. Multiple sexual partners and intravenous drug use both increase the risk of STDs. It is important to know one's partner's sexual history and to practice regular genital self-exam. Education and treatment of sexual partners, along with safer sex practices, are important.

The most common STDs are chlamydia, genital warts, cervical intraepithelial neoplasia, genital herpes, gonorrhea, syphilis, pelvic inflammatory disease, vulvovaginitis, and AIDS.

Chlamydia trachomatis is the most common bacterial STD in the United States. It is both asymptomatic and chronic. It is easily treated with antibiotics. If untreated, it may cause pelvic inflammatory disease (PID) and infertility.

Genital warts (condyloma acuminata) are caused by human papillomavirus (HPV). The most common symptomatic viral STD in the United States is condyloma. Although no therapy has been found to eradicate HPV, topical podophyllin is often applied to remove warts. Podophyllin should not be used during pregnancy or with cervical, urethral, oral, or anorectal warts.

Cervical intraepithelial neoplasia (CIN) is the term to describe early cancerous or precancerous changes of endocervical cells. It is associated with HPV, herpes, and other STDs. It is often asymptomatic and can be diagnosed by Pap smear and colposcopic confirmation. Treatments include surgical excision, cautery, cryosurgery, and/or CO_2 laser therapy.

Genital herpes is caused by herpes simplex virus (HSV) types 1 and 2, a DNA virus that cannot be distinguished clinically. Diagnosis is usually made by clinical evaluation and lab diagnosis. The initial infection may be symptomatic with less symptomatic recurrent infections. There is no known cure; however, the antiviral drug acyclovir may help suppress severe symptoms.

Gonorrhea is caused by the bacterium Neisseria gonorrhoeae. Women may have abnormal vaginal discharge or be asymptomatic. Diagnosis is made microscopically. Antibiotics are the effective treatment of gonorrhea; untreated, PID and sterility may occur.

Syphilis is caused by the spirochete, treponema pallidum. Early diagnosis and treatment with antibiotics can prevent serious later complications including neurosyphilis, cardiovascular syphilis, and localized gumma formation.

Pelvic inflammatory disease (PID) is caused by STD microbial infection. Pain and tenderness of the lower abdominal area are the typical clinical symptoms, assuming that appendicitis and ectopic pregnancy have been ruled out. Combination antibiotic therapy is used since the etiology is usually polymicrobial. PID is potentially life-threatening; complications include involuntary sterility and recurrent pain.

Vulvovaginitis is usually caused by trichomonas vaginalis, bacterial vaginosis, and/or candida albicans. Symptoms may include itching, burning, and characteristic vaginal secretions. Diagnosis is made both clinically and by microscopic examination of a vaginal smear. Flagyl is the usual treatment for trichomonas and bacterial vaginosis; however, Flagyl is a known carcinogen. Yeast can be treated symptomatically with antifungal suppositories. More important is the reacidification of the vagina and reintroduction of healthy acidophilus bacteria. Antibiotic therapy predisposes women to candida infection, which may be prevented by eating yogurt daily during treatment. ✱ LAURA ZEIDENSTEIN, C.N.M., M.S.N.

See also: Pelvic Inflammatory Disease

Resources

American Academy of Pediatrics and American College of Obstetrics and Gynecology. (1988). *Guidelines for Perinatal Care, second edition*. Washington, DC.

Boston Women's Health Book Collective. (1984). *The New Our Bodies, Ourselves*. New York: Simon and Schuster.

Centers for Disease Control. (1989). "Sexually Transmitted Diseases Treatment Guidelines." *Morbidity and Mortality Weekly Report 38* (S-8):1-43.

Hatcher, Robert A. et al. (1990). *Contraceptive Technology 1990-1992, 15th Revised Edition*. New York: Irvington Publishers, Inc.

Holmes, S. et al. (1984). *Sexually Transmitted Diseases*. New York: McGraw Hill Inc.

Missim, Rita. (1986). *Natural Healing in Gynecology: A Manual for Women*. New York: Pandora.

SHOES FOR BABIES

People began wearing protective coverings on their feet around 55 B.C. At that time such coverings were simple shapes of leather or cloth that wrapped or tied around the foot. Over the centuries, footwear construction became increasingly complicated as fashions dictated more tailored styles. In many parts of the world, only the upper classes could afford fitted shoes, and thus they became a status symbol. The advent of the Industrial Revolution made tailored shoes available to

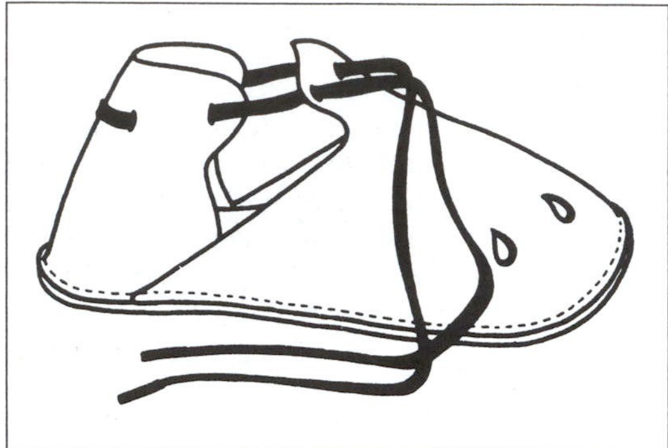

A well-designed children's shoe. Illustration courtesy of Soft Walker Shoes, Colleyville, Texas.

all levels of society, and it was probably at this time that parents began paying more attention to their children's footwear. Parents began to search for the proper shoes to support and nurture their babies' growing feet.

It was once considered mandatory for baby shoes to be stiff and inflexible to properly support the foot and ankle. However, in the last 25 years, public opinion has changed drastically regarding fit and comfort in children's shoes. Today, most doctors agree that comfort and flexibility in shoes allow developing feet to grow naturally.

Understanding the following principles of fitting shoes can alleviate a parent's concern for the proper care of their baby's feet.

When is it appropriate for infants to begin wearing shoes?

It is necessary for infants to wear shoes only when they need protection against their environment. In fact, going barefoot is one of the best ways to encourage the development of strong and healthy foot and leg muscles.

What should one look for in a first pair of shoes?

Children's shoes should be soft and flexible. Growing feet need freedom of movement. They must be allowed to function with shoes just as they function without. Leather uppers are desirable because they absorb moisture and keep the foot dry. Soft rubber soles are advantageous because they provide flexibility, enabling the foot to bend naturally.

How is the child's proper shoe size determined?

Size is best ascertained with the help of a professional shoe fitter. The Brannock device is a measuring tool commonly used at conscientious shoe stores. Once the foot has been measured, a variety of styles should be tried on before determining the best fit. With the child standing, there should be approximately one-half inch of extra length between the end of the large toe and the tip of the shoe. This gives the toes room to move and the foot room to grow. Because children tend to grow in spurts, it is important to remeasure their feet every three to four months.

The most important point to remember regarding children's footwear is fit. Shoes must fit snugly without impeding the natural growth and development of the feet. If care is taken when choosing shoes and fit is monitored during wear, a child's feet will become solid foundations he or she can depend on for life.

Because a baby's first steps are considered to be one of the developmental milestones, parents often want to preserve the memory in some way. Traditionally, bronzing the child's first pair of shoes has been popular, but with today's unusual styles and colors, casting the shoes in clear acrylic is a novel approach to preservation because the details of the shoes remain visible. However, no matter how or when a child begins walking, it will undoubtedly be a memorable occasion for those fortunate enough to stand witness.✱ PAULA HYDE

See **Guide to Related Topics:** Baby Care

Resources

Fast, Julian. (1971). *You and Your Feet.* New York: St. Martin's Press.

Rossi, William A. & Tennant, Ross. (1984). *Professional Shoe Fitting.* New York: National Shoe Retailers Association.

Wikler, Simon J. (1961). *Take Off Your Shoes and Walk: Steps to Better Foot Health.* New York: Devin-Adair Company.

Wilson, Eunice. (1970). *A History of Shoe Fashions.* London: Pittman Publishing.

SHOULDER DYSTOCIA

Shoulder dystocia is the term used to describe the situation when a baby's head has been born, but the shoulders seem to be too big to be born with gentle downward traction. About half of the time, the problem is associated with larger than normal babies, but infants of average size may also have a shoulder impacted behind the pubic symphysis after the birth of the head. Altogether, shoulder dystocia births make up about 1 percent of births.

In many cases, once the forehead emerges, the baby's face does not follow as quickly and easily as usual. Another familiar sign of impending shoulder dystocia is the failure of the baby's head, once born, to turn 90 degrees, as it ordinarily does. Other times, the head will turn with a little gentle manipulation, but with true shoulder dystocia, the baby's neck will not be visible, and the baby's head is actually drawn back deeply against the perineum. Sometimes the mother's contractions will cease at this point; other times she will have the urge to push, but her efforts are not sufficient to deliver the baby's body.

Only a certain degree of traction is safe to put on the baby's head, because of the danger of overstretching the brachial nerve plexus. The longer the baby's head sits on the perineum, the darker and more congested-looking it becomes. Because of compression of the baby's chest, it is harder for blood from the head to return to the baby's body and umbilical cord for renewed oxygenation. If this condition persists too long, the baby can suffer irreparable brain damage. The situation calls for corrective action on the part of the attendant.

Most midwives deal with shoulder dystocia by getting the mother to move into a squat or onto her hands and knees. Both of these positions tend to increase the distance between the pubic arch and the mother's backbone, disimpacting the shoulders. Usually the posterior shoulder will emerge first. Gentle traction with the fingers splinted across the posterior armpit is sometimes necessary, and sometimes the posterior arm is drawn out as well, to ease the delivery of the body.

For women in lithotomy position, the typical obstetrical position, there have been several ways doctors have dealt with shoulder dystocia. One is to have the mother pull her thighs back against her belly. Then an assistant applies suprapubic pressure in an attempt to release the anterior shoulder from behind the pubic arch. Less serious cases may be resolved this way. Authors of some texts advise pushing forward on the anterior shoulder to dislodge it from behind the pubic arch. Another step is to reach for the posterior armpit with the first two fingers and try to pull the baby out with the fingers hooked across the armpit. These maneuvers often work, but they carry the danger of fracture of the baby's humerus or clavicle. Some practitioners try to rotate the baby's torso a little, which, if successful, may bring the baby's anterior shoulder out from under the pubic arch. Another maneuver involves reaching inside to draw out the posterior arm, thereby reducing the diameter across the shoulders. Gentle traction on the head may then be sufficient to complete the delivery.

A couple of more extreme measures have recently been proposed by obstetricians: the Zavanelli maneuver (or cephalic replacement), which involves rotating the baby's head as it was before it emerged, then pushing the baby's head back into the uterus and performing a cesarean. This maneuver obviously carries some risk of injury to mother and baby and, as of 1990, seems to have come into use primarily in the United States. In 1990, a Dutch obstetrician advocated a return

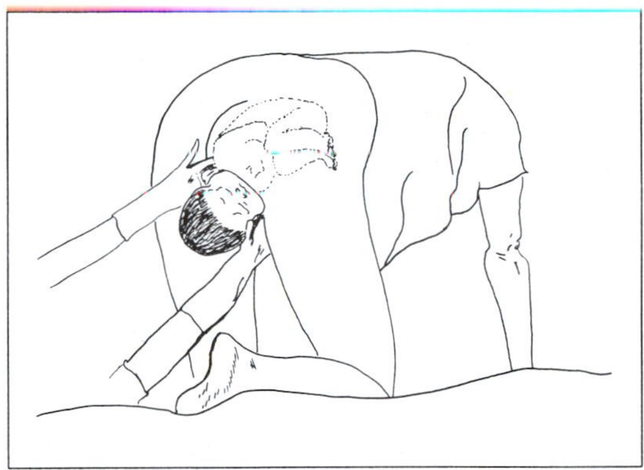

A midwife assisting a mother birthing with shoulder dystocia. Drawing by Ina May Gaskin.

to symphysiotomy (the cutting of the ligament holding the pubic symphysis together). The problem with this approach is that the pelvis is permanently enlarged, and some women will have difficulty walking afterwards.

The complication of shoulder dystocia has begun to receive more attention in recently published medical textbooks, probably because, as the medical profession in North America has come to accept higher rates of cesarean section, medical students and residents have fewer opportunities to see how older, more experienced practitioners deal with the delivery of a large baby. It is also probably true that the degree of panic has risen because of the fear of malpractice suits, now that many women are conscious and aware of what is going on while they give birth, and their partners are much more likely to be with them during labor and birth than was true a generation ago.

Because shoulder dystocia is a complication that is very difficult to predict, some obstetricians advocate a more liberal use of cesarean section to lower its incidence, particularly if they are dealing with mothers with diabetes, who are more likely to give birth to very large babies. But because fully half of shoulder dystocia cases involve babies of average size, the cesarean rate would have to get extremely high to make an appreciable difference in the shoulder dystocia rate. The Farm Midwives' series of 35 shoulder dystocia births out of a total series of 1,750 births shows favorable outcomes for mothers who assumed the all-fours position for delivery of the body. All of these babies were born with high Apgar scores and no injuries.

✷ INA MAY GASKIN

See also: Fetal Presentations

See **Guide to Related Topics:** Pregnancy Complications

Resources

Gabbe, Niebyl. (1986). *Simpson Obstetrics: Normal and Problem Pregnancies.* Churchill Livingstone.

Gaskin, Ina May. (1988, Fall). "Shoulder Dystocia: Controversies in Management." *The Birth Gazette* 5 (1): 14-17.

Iffy, L. et al. (1986). "Abdominal Rescue after Entrapment of the Aftercoming Head." *American Journal of Obstetrics and Gynecology* 154: 623.

Litt, R.L. (1980). "Previous Shoulder Dystocia as an Indication for Primary Cesarean Section." *Collections of Letters of the International Correspondence Society of Obstetrics and Gynecology* 21: 170.

O'Leary, J.A. & Gunn, D.L. (1986). "Option for Shoulder Dystocia: Cephalic Replacement." *Contemporary Obstetrics and Gynecology* 27: 157.

Sandberg, E.C. (1985). "The Zavanelli Maneuver: A Potentially Revolutionary Method for the Resolution of Shoulder Dystocia." *American Journal of Obstetrics and Gynecology* 152: 479.

SIBLINGS AT BIRTH

Ideas about children's participation during labor and birth have undergone many changes during this century. Children whose siblings were born at home were often included in this family event, but when the infant was to be born in the hospital the older siblings were routinely excluded. Not only could they not attend the labor and/or birth but they were not allowed to visit their mother or sibling in the hospital. In the late 1970s, ideas about sibling involvement began to change. Although children began to be more involved in labor and birth, hospital personnel were still wrestling with concerns of infection, disruption, and morality.

Children's participation at birth remains a controversial topic with medical caregivers while, at the same time, more and more families are choosing to include older children in the labor and birth. Families often choose this option because of their desire for a natural transition for the other children in the family, their concerns about sibling rivalry, their desire for family closeness and strong commitment to the family structure, their view of childbirth as a learning experience for all family members, and their belief that birth is a normal, natural life event.

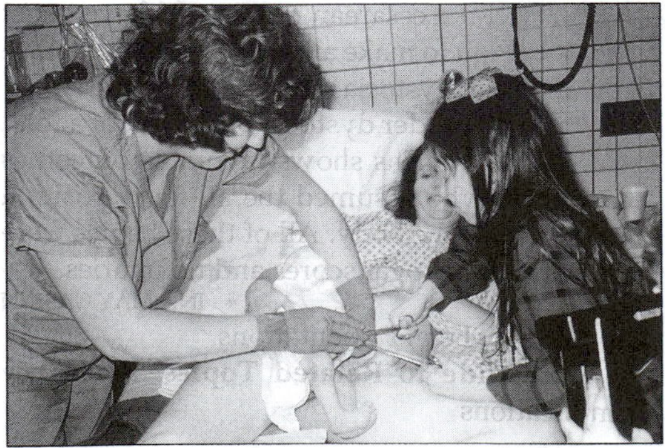

A new sister cutting the cord. Photo courtesy of Paulina G. Perez.

There is overwhelming evidence that siblings benefit from this experience if they are educated about what to expect and supported during the actual birth (Anderson, 1979; Parma, 1979; Perez, 1979; Perez, 1981; Hathaway and Hathaway, 1978; Clark, 1986). Issues to cover during sibling preparation include basic anatomy and physiology of labor and birth, wetness of birth (amniotic fluid, blood, vernix), smells of birth, the hard work and intensity of dealing with labor, pain, episiotomy/laceration and repair, vaginal examinations, perineal massage/support, delivery of the placenta, cutting of the umbilical cord, appearance of the baby, and unexpected events (transfer to hospital, need for forceps/cesarean, etc.). The person who will be giving the sibling support at the birth is invaluable to the success of the experience. Ideally, the sibling support person is someone who is comfortable with both birth and children and who is flexible; this may be a family friend or relative. The support person's job is to be sensitive to the child's needs during the labor and birth. This may mean seeing that the child is fed, taking the child for a walk, answering questions about the labor/birth, or simply holding the child so that he or she can see. The support person must not have a strong desire to personally witness the birth since circumstances may arise where the child will not be in attendance.

It is critical that the events of the day be discussed with the child after the birth. During this discussion it is important to get a sense of how the child interpreted the experience as well as deal with any misconceptions or fears that occurred. Listening to the child is a learning experience for the adults involved as they learn about birth from a child's perspective. Children present at birth show, in a way that no one else can, that birth is an event of great strength, tenderness, pain, love, and dignity. ✱ PAULINA G. PEREZ, R.N., B.S.N. ACCE-R

See **Guide to Related Topics:** Childbirth Practices and Locations

Resources

Anderson, Sandra VanDam. (1979). "Siblings at Birth: A Survey and Study." *Birth and the Family Journal* 6 (2): 80-87.

Anderson, Sandra VanDam & Simkin, Penny. (1981). *Birth Through Children's Eyes.* Seattle, WA: Pennypress.

Clark, Linda. (1986, Aug). "When Children Watch Their Mothers Deliver." *Contemporary OBGYN*: 69-75.

Daniels, M.B. (1983). "The Birth Experience for the Sibling: Description and Evaluation of a Program." *Journal of Nurse-Midwifery 28*: 15-22.

Hathaway, Marjie & Hathaway, Jay. (1978). *Children at Birth*. Sherman Oaks, CA: Academy Publications.

Malecki, Maryann. (1979). *Mom and Dad and I Are Having a Baby*. Seattle, WA: Pennypress.

Mehl, Lewis, Brandsel, C., & Peterson, Gayle. (1977). "Children at Birth: Effects and Implication." *Journal of Sex and Marital Therapy 3*: 274-79.

Parma, Susan. (1979). "A Family-Centered Event? Preparing the Child for Sharing in the Experience of Childbirth." *Journal of Nurse-Midwifery 24* (3): 5-10.

Perez, Paulina. (1979). "Nurturing Children Who Attend the Birth of a Sibling." *Journal of Maternal Child Nursing 4*: 215-17.

———. (1981). "Involvement of Siblings at Birth: A Nurse's Perspective." In Sandra VanDam Anderson & Penny Simkin (Eds.) *Birth Through Children's Eyes*. Seattle, WA: Pennypress.

———. (1982, Winter). "Should Siblings Attend a Birth? Pro." *Childbirth Educator*: 30-36, 49.

SICKLE CELL DISEASE. *See instead* NEWBORN SCREENING

SMOKING IN PREGNANCY

Smoking during pregnancy is probably the most important and readily modifiable cause of poor pregnancy outcomes among women in the United States (U.S. Department of Health and Human Services, 1990). The risks of smoking during pregnancy are well known. In 1936, Sontag and Wallace expressed concern that smoking increased the fetal heart rate, and, in 1957, Simpson reported that smoking during pregnancy resulted in low infant birth weights (about one-half pound less than in infants of nonsmoking mothers). Since that time, a large number of studies have confirmed Simpson's findings and have further identified a broad range of other adverse consequences associated with smoking during pregnancy. These include spontaneous abortion (Kline et al., 1977; McIntosh, 1984), bleeding during pregnancy (Cardoza et al., 1982), placental problems such as early detachment (abruptio placenta) or attachment in the lower portion of the uterus (placenta previa) (Hoff et al., 1986), premature birth (Shiono and Klebanoff, 1986), and increased fetal and infant deaths (Meyer, Jonas, and Tonascia, 1976). There is also a reported association between maternal smoking and incidence of sudden infant death syndrome (SIDS), although in this case, it is not easy to distinguish between the effects of maternal smoking during pregnancy and smoking after pregnancy (Niebyl, 1990).

While there is not universal agreement about the way that maternal smoking adversely affects the fetus, it is proposed that carbon monoxide from the cigarette smoke goes to the fetal blood and decreases its oxygen-carrying capacity (D'Souza et al., 1978). It is also possible that nicotine causes the fetal blood vessels to narrow, thus restricting the amount of oxygen and nourishment reaching the fetus and inhibiting fetal growth (Lehtovirta and Forss, 1978).

If the female smoker stops smoking before she becomes pregnant or during the first three to four months of pregnancy, her infant is likely to be of normal birth weight. Even if the woman stops smoking before the 30th week of pregnancy, her infant will have a higher birth weight than the infant of the woman who continues to smoke throughout pregnancy (U.S. Department of Health and Human Services, 1990).

While the prevalence of smoking has decreased over time, it is still unacceptably high. About 24-30 percent of pregnant smokers continue to smoke during pregnancy even though most of them are aware of the risks associated with the behavior (Juarez & Associates, Inc., 1982; Windsor et al., 1985; Miller, 1990). In general, formal attempts to persuade women to stop smoking during pregnancy have not been very successful (Lumley and Astbury, 1982). Of those who do quit, 70 percent resume smoking within one year after delivery. According to the Surgeon General's report (U.S. Department of Health and Human Services, 1990), recent estimates suggest that elimination of smoking during pregnancy could prevent 5 percent of fetal/infant deaths, 20 percent of low birth-weight births, and 8 percent of the premature deliveries each year in the United States. In groups of women with a high prevalence of smoking (the young, unmarried, and/or un-

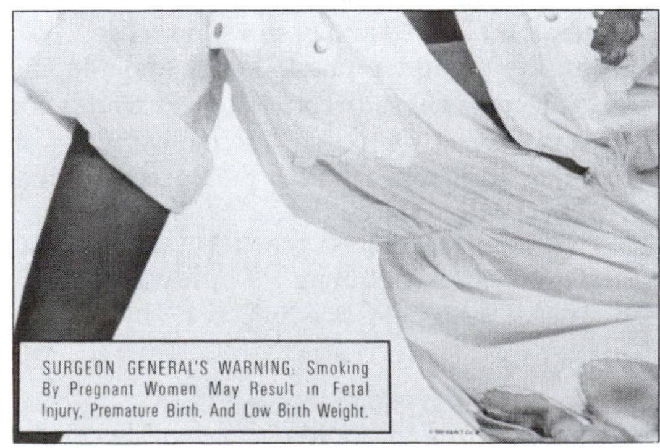

Advertisements such as this one displaying warning labels while simultaneously using images of femininity to sell cigarettes carry a conflicting message to young women. Photo courtesy of Claudia Mann.

educated), elimination of smoking could prevent 10 percent of fetal/infant deaths, 35 percent of low birth-weight births, and 15 percent of premature births.

Many women who continue to smoke during pregnancy may do so because of the highly addictive nature of the habit. Even when motivation to quit is extremely powerful, the physical and psychological process of withdrawal can be very difficult to handle. This is especially true if women do not have sufficient support from their relatives, friends, and others. Contributing to their difficulty in quitting is the tobacco industry's advertising campaigns, which continually tempt people who have quit to resume smoking. Most unfortunate is the fact that such ads, costing billions of tax-deductible dollars for the industry each year, seem to have a powerful appeal for young women and minorities. The ads continue to appear in publications with large female teenage readership such as *Glamour* (25% percent of readers are under 18 years of age). Among people up to age 24, including teenagers, the percentage of female smokers is now higher than male smokers (White, 1988). If present trends continue, by 1995, women smokers of all ages will outnumber men because more girls start smoking and women quit less often ("Tobacco Foes," 1990). This is an ominous prediction for the numbers of females in the future who will approach pregnancy already addicted to cigarettes.

Creating additional confusion over smoking and health issues are the seemingly incongruous federal policies in the United States that mandate removal of asbestos from schools while continuing to allow young students to smoke. In doing this, the government is implicitly condoning cigarettes, thereby creating the impression that they are tolerably safe (Stebbins, 1990). Cigarette advertising and promotion of sport events, simply because it is allowed and even supported, encourages more young women to begin smoking and allays the fears of health consequences in addicted smokers. One way to prevent young women from becoming addicted is to limit their access to cigarettes in the first place.

✱ MARY ANN MILLER, R.N., Ph.D.

See **Guide to Related Topics:** Pregnancy Complications

Resources

Cardoza, L. et al. (1982). "Social and Obstetric Features Associated with Smoking in Pregnancy." *British Journal of Obstetrics and Gynaecology 89*: 622-27.

D'Souza, S. et al. (1978). "Effect of Smoking during Pregnancy upon the Haematological Values of Cord Blood." *British Journal of Obstetrics and Gynaecology 85*: 495-99.

Hoff, C. et al. (1986). "Trend Associations of Smoking with Maternal, Fetal and Neonatal Morbidity." *Obstetrics and Gynecology 68*: 317-21.

Juarez & Associates, Inc. (1982). "Healthy Mothers." *Market Research: How to Reach Black and Mexican-American Women.* Los Angeles: Juarez & Associates.

Kline, J. et al. (1977). "Smoking: A Risk Factor for Spontaneous Abortion." *New England Journal of Medicine 297*: 793-95.

Lehtovirta, P. & Forss, M. (1978). "The Acute Effect of Smoking on Intervillous Blood Flow of the Placenta." *British Journal of Obstetrics and Gynaecology 85*: 729-33.

Lumley, J. & Astbury, J. (1982). "Advice in Pregnancy: Perfect Remedies, Imperfect Science." In M. Enkin & I. Chalmers (Eds.) *Effectiveness and Satisfaction in Antenatal Care.* Philadelphia: Lippincott, pp. 132-50.

McIntosh, I. (1984). "Smoking and Pregnancy: Attributable Risks and Public Health Implications." *Canadian Journal of Public Health 75*: 141-48.

Meyer, M., Jonas, B., & Tonascia, J. (1976). "Perinatal Events Associated with Maternal Smoking during Pregnancy." *American Journal of Epidemiology 103*: 464-76.

Miller, M.A. (1990). "Psychosocial Factors Related to Cigarette Smoking during Pregnancy." Unpublished dissertation. Philadelphia: Temple University.

Niebyl, J. (1990). "Teratology and Drugs in Pregnancy and Lactation." In J. Scott et al. (Eds.) *Danforth's Obstetrics and Gynecology.* Philadelphia: Lippincott, pp. 273-91.

Shiono, P. & Klebanoff, M. (1986). "Ethnic Differences in Preterm and Very Preterm Delivery." *American Journal of Public Health 76*: 1317-21.

Simpson, W. (1957). "A Preliminary Report on Cigarette Smoking and the Incidence of Prematurity." *American Journal of Obstetrics and Gynecology 73*: 808-15.

Sontag, L. & Wallace, R. (1936). "The Effective of Cigarette Smoking during Pregnancy upon the Fetal Heart Rate." *American Journal of Obstetrics and Gynecology 23*: 405-07.

Stebbins, K. (1990). "Transnational Tobacco Companies and Health in Underdeveloped Countries: Recommendations for Avoiding a Smoking Epidemic." *Social Science and Medicine 30*: 227-35.

"Tobacco Foes Attack Ads that Target Women, Minorities, Teens, and the Poor." (1990). *Journal of the American Medical Association 264*: 1505-06.

U.S. Department of Health and Human Services. (1990). *The Health Benefits of Smoking Cessation: A Report of the Surgeon General.* Public Health Service, Centers for Disease Control, Center for Chronic Disease Prevention and Health Promotion, Office on Smoking and Health. DHHS Publication No. (CDC) 90-8416.

White, L. (1988). *Merchants of Death.* New York: Beech Tree Books.

Windsor, R. et al. (1985). "The Effectiveness of Smoking Cessation Methods for Smokers in Public Health Maternity Clinics: A Randomized Trial." *American Journal of Public Health 75*: 1389-92.

SOCIAL SCIENCE RESEARCH ON AMERICAN CHILDBIRTH PRACTICES

At present, approximately 99 percent of childbearing women in the United States give birth in hospitals and 96 percent have physician-attended births (National Center for Health Statistics, 1990). Beginning around 1960, several sociologists and anthropologists have used the naturalistic research techniques of participant observation and open-ended interviewing to examine these prevailing forms of maternity services. Their research reveals fundamental attitudes, constructs, values, motivations, and practices associated with the provision of these services.

Although this research spans several decades, various geographic locations, women of diverse backgrounds, and different types of facilities and levels of providers, the findings are remarkably consistent. The studies seem to reveal widespread and systematic subordination of interests of childbearing women and their families to interests of medical caregivers and institutions. Infrequent exceptions noted in the reports are associated with individuals and are not intrinsic to the delivery system. Seemingly the prevailing patterns of care reflect such core cultural beliefs as the importance of controlling natural processes, the untrustworthiness of nature, the defectiveness of the female body, the validity of patriarchy, and the positive value of science and technology (Davis-Floyd, 1987a).

In inverse proportion to the needs of childbearing women, obstetrical training gives priority to surgical expertise; it devalues and gives minimal attention to normal childbearing, prevention, prenatal care, low-technology interventions, and human relations skills (Rosengren and DeVault, 1963; Shaw, 1974; Scully, 1980). Although women receiving care at training sites may believe that service is the institution's primary mission, residents see their education as the overriding objective (Scully, 1980). Childbearing women are "cases" and "material" to medical students and residents, who routinely "try" or "practice" unnecessary surgery and other procedures to gain experience (Kovit, 1972; Shaw, 1974; Scully, 1980). To obtain surgical experience, residents become adept at stretching or circumventing protocols and at convincing women to accept unnecessary and invasive procedures through frightening and deceptive high-pressure sales techniques (Scully, 1980). Conversely, they regularly avoid care that may be of great value to women (e.g., abortions and tubal ligations or basic preventive information) if they deem it boring and routine (Scully, 1980). Frequently, those providing services lack expertise, and supervision is inadequate (Scully, 1980). The ability to rapidly process patients and successfully maneuver on one's own behalf is highly valued and rewarded (Scully, 1980; Lazarus, 1988a). The training experience involves isolation, hazing, and other classic features of rites of passage that are highly effective in generating personal transformation and unquestioned acceptance of the system one is entering (Davis-Floyd, 1987a, 1987b).

As a consequence of this educational system and of institutionalized classism and racism, conditions for women who lack private insurance and receive care at teaching hospitals are particularly appalling. Onerous barriers to care and powerful sources of indignity for these women include the fragmentation, alienation, and confusion that frequently accompany scheduling and staffing patterns designed to meet training needs (Shaw, 1974; Caro et al., 1988; Scully, 1980; Lazarus, 1988a; Lazarus and Philipson, 1990); a prenatal visit routine that requires from two hours to an entire day, with extensive waiting and only a few minutes of poor-quality time with a physician (Shaw, 1974; Caro et al., 1988; Lazarus, 1988a; Lazarus and Philipson, 1990); a dreary environment that often lacks basic amenities for privacy, comfort, and communication (Shaw, 1974; Scully, 1980; Caro et al., 1988; Lazarus, 1988a); staff attitudes and behavior that often demean and dehumanize (Rosengren and DeVault, 1963; Shaw, 1974; Scully, 1980); a pattern of avoiding providing services to women considered undesirable (Kovit, 1972; Scully, 1980); and inadequate staff language and communication skills (Shaw, 1974; Scully, 1980; Caro et al., 1988; Lazarus, 1988a; Lazarus and Philipson, 1990). A common career pattern involves using clinic-status women as training "material" and then establishing a lucrative private practice (Scully, 1980).

In these studies, medical personnel consistently provide two standards of care, showing more consideration and offering more choices to women with private insurance than to those with clinic status (Rosengren and DeVault, 1963; Kovit, 1972; Shaw, 1974; Scully, 1980). The relationship between private-pay women and their physicians, however, tends to be paternalistic (Shaw, 1974; Danziger, 1980), and these women are adversely affected by pervasive inadequacies of medical maternity care. The nature of medical childbearing arrangements is made particularly mystifying for private-pay women, for example, through their institutional isolation (Shaw, 1974); through their middle-class value system, which encourages submission to expert authority (Scully, 1980); and through experience of subtle coercive socialization during prenatal care (Danziger, 1980). They are thus predisposed to accept overt and misleading justifications for patterns of care that are not in their best interest.

Fundamental inadequacies of medical maternity care affect virtually all childbearing women. These include primary emphasis on pregnancy and birth as pathological states requiring medical intervention (Rosengren and DeVault, 1963; Shaw, 1974; Danziger, 1980; Scully, 1980; Davis-Floyd, 1987a; Lazarus, 1988a); minimal attention to and knowledge of normal childbearing (Shaw, 1974; Davis-Floyd, 1987a; Lazarus, 1988a); a lack of interest in routine care and such preventive measures as nutrition and breastfeeding (Kovit, 1972; Shaw, 1974; Scully, 1980; Lazarus, 1988a); a lack of interest in and disregard for women's wishes, views, and contributions (Shaw, 1974; Scully, 1980; Danziger, 1979, 1980, 1986; Lazarus, 1988b; Caro et al., 1988); a lack of commitment to informed consent (Shaw, 1974; Danziger, 1979); a pattern of blaming women for undesirable occurrences (Shaw, 1974; Davis-Floyd, 1987a); and a narrow physical focus that does not adequately address emotions, family relationships, sexuality, and other areas that are often of deep concern to childbearing women (Shaw, 1974; Danziger, 1979, 1980; Scully, 1980; Lazarus, 1988b). Furthermore, the system tends to treat mothers primarily as means to highly valued infants rather than as individuals in their own right (Rosengren and DeVault, 1963; Shaw, 1974; Davis-Floyd, 1987a).

A major theme of the research reports is a pervasive interest in controlling childbearing women, who are expected to conform to the needs of caregivers and institutions and to a narrow and standardized model of childbearing. Such control makes work routines easier, facilitates educational or financial gain for medical personnel and facilities, minimizes threats to medical authority, and reinforces core cultural values (Shaw, 1974; Danziger, 1979; Scully, 1980; Davis-Floyd, 1987a). Common mechanisms of control include: socialization during prenatal care (Shaw, 1974; Danziger, 1980), muting women's identity through "prepping" in early labor (Rosengren and DeVault, 1963; Shaw, 1974; Davis-Floyd, 1987a); use of medications and numerous other interventions during labor and birth (Rosengren and DeVault, 1963; Shaw, 1974; Danziger, 1979; Davis-Floyd, 1987a); verbal admonition and other authoritative behavior (Danziger, 1979, 1986; Scully, 1980); withholding or distorting information (Spencer and DeVault, 1963; Kovit, 1972; Shaw, 1974; Danziger, 1978, 1979, 1980, 1986; Scully, 1980; Lazarus 1988a); routine processing and ritualization (Rosengren and DeVault, 1963; Shaw, 1974; Danziger, 1979, 1980, 1986; Scully, 1980; Davis-Floyd, 1987a, 1987b); and preoccupation with the pace of prenatal visits and the "progress" of labor (Rosengren and DeVault, 1963; Scully, 1980; Davis-Floyd, 1987a).

The studies also show that clinical decision making for childbearing women is profoundly influenced by many nonmedical factors, including a woman's personal or social characteristics (Kovit, 1972; Shaw, 1974; Danziger, 1980; Scully, 1980); staffing needs (Kovit, 1972; Scully, 1980; Lazarus, 1988a); training needs (Kovit, 1972; Shaw, 1974; Scully, 1980); interpersonal relationships among the staff (Scully, 1980); the availability of technology (Kovit, 1972); a physician's scheduling needs and capacity for patience (Kovit, 1972; Danziger, 1979; Scully, 1980); and a hospital's protocols and routines (Rosengren and DeVault, 1963; Kovit, 1972; Shaw, 1974).

Finally, the studies assess recent changes in medical approaches to childbearing. One analyst concludes that despite some concessions to demands of women, the basic pattern of high-technology intervention remains and has even intensified (Davis-Floyd, 1987a). Physicians who characterize themselves as radical and humanistic nonetheless share many basic traits with their more conventional colleagues, and women seeking humanized birth tend to modify, rather than reject, the technological model of birth (Davis-Floyd, 1987a). Another researcher underscores the similarity in routines imposed upon childbearing women in a hospital noted for its progressive forms of care and in a teaching hospital providing conventional care to indigent women (Danziger, 1979). Any appearance of substantive change may thus be illusory. ✱ CAROL SAKALA, M.A., M.P.H.

See also: Hospital Birth: An Anthropological Analysis of Ritual and Practice; Labor: Overview; Obstetrics, History of

See **Guide to Related Topics:** Caregivers and Practitioners; Childbirth Practices and Locations

Resources

Caro, Francis G. et al. (1988). *Barriers to Prenatal Care: An Examination of Use of Prenatal Care among Low-Income Women in New York City.* New York: Community Service Society of New York.

Danziger, Sandra Klein. (1978). "The Uses of Expertise in Doctor-Patient Encounters during Pregnancy." *Social Science & Medicine 12* (5A): 359-67.

———. (1979). "Treatment of Women in Childbirth: Implications for Family Beginnings." *American Journal of Public Health 69* (9): 895-901.

———. (1980). "The Medical Model in Doctor-Patient Interaction: The Case of Pregnancy Care." *Research in the Sociology of Health Care 1*: 263-304.

———. (1986). "Male Doctor-Female Patient." In Pamela S. Eakins (Ed.) *The American Way of Birth.* Philadelphia: Temple University Press, pp. 119-41.

Davis-Floyd, Robbie E. (1987a). "Obstetric Training as a Rite of Passage." *Medical Anthropology Quarterly 1* (3): 288-318.

———. (1987b). "The Technological Model of Birth." *Journal of American Folklore 100* (398): 479-95.

Kovit, Leonard. (1972, Spring). "Labor Is Hard Work: Notes on the Social Organization of Childbirth." *Sociological Symposium 8*: 11-21.

Lazarus, Ellen S. (1988a). "Theoretical Considerations for the Study of the Doctor-Patient Relationship: Implications of a Perinatal Study." *Medical Anthropology Quarterly n.s. 2* (1): 34-58.

———. (1988b). "Poor Women, Poor Outcomes: Social Class and Reproductive Health." In Karen L. Michaelson (Ed.) *Childbirth in America: Anthropological Perspectives.* South Hadley, MA: Bergin & Garvey Publishers, Inc., pp. 39-54.

Lazarus, Ellen S. & Philipson, Elliot H. (1990). "A Longitudinal Study Comparing the Prenatal Care of Puerto Rican and White Women." *Birth 17* (1): 6-11.

National Center for Health Statistics (1990). "Advance Report of Final Natality Statistics, 1988." *Monthly Vital Statistics Report 39* (4, supplement): 1-48.

Rosengren, William R. & DeVault, Spencer. (1963). "The Sociology of Time and Space in an Obstetrical Hospital." In Eliot Freidson (Ed.) *The Hospital in Modern Society*. Glencoe, IL: The Free Press.

Scully, Diana (1980). *Men Who Control Women's Health: The Miseducation of Obstetrician-Gynecologists.* Boston: Houghton Mifflin Company.

Shaw, Nancy Stoller. (1974). *Forced Labor: Maternity Care in the United States.* New York: Pergamon Press.

SOVIET UNION, FORMER

The former Soviet Union comprised 15 republics and over 100 nationalities which means that aggregate statistics collected before breakup of the Soviet Union into independent states should be used with caution. Presumably, after 1991, data will be collected within each new country independently and the tendency for researchers to speak of the Soviet Union as if it were a single, homogeneous entity will lessen.

According to data collected in 1989, the average national birthrate for the Soviet Union stood at 2.5 children per woman. But the birth rate in the Central Asian and predominantly Moslem areas of the former Soviet Union averaged more than 4 children per woman. At the same time, the birth rate in the Slavic republics (Russia, Ukraine, and Belorussia), as well as in the Baltic republics (Estonia, Latvia, and Lithuania) registered at or below 2.1 children per woman (Naselenie SSSR, 1989). In other words, the Slavic and Baltic republics were experiencing negative or zero population growth.

Medical care in the countries of the former Soviet Union is generally poor, but obstetrical and gynecological care is in a deplorable state. As of 1987, the share of the Soviet Union's national budget devoted to public health was 4 percent. The nations of the former Soviet Union produce only 6 of the approximately 60 different types of obstetric and gynecological equipment needed for normal work. Obstetric and gynecological offices do not have fetal heart monitors and maternity clinics do not have ultrasound equipment. The main tools upon which most obstetricians and gynecologists are forced to rely are a ruler and a wooden tube, the latter serving as a crude stethoscope (*Current Digest of the Soviet Press*, 1987).

In Moscow, the capital of the former Soviet Union, only 12 out of 33 maternity hospitals met present-day standards and sanitary norms in 1987. They continue to be overcrowded, dirty, and inadequately heated. There are no private delivery rooms; most women share a delivery room with three or four other women. It is a standard policy that maternity hospitals do not allow visitors, including the new father. Anesthesia and painkillers are rarely available due to chronic shortages (*Current Digest of the Soviet Press*, 1987). Since 1989 the shortage of medicine has become acute due to the closure of environmentally hazardous pharmaceutical plants.

Every year in Russia, the largest of the former Soviet republics, 600 to 700 women die during deliveries and abortions. One of the main causes of maternal death and one of the major problems for Soviet obstetricians involves preventing toxemia late in pregnancy. In the former Soviet Union toxemia was reported to affect approximately every tenth pregnancy (*Current Digest of the Soviet Press*, 1987).

According to 1989 estimates, seven million Soviet married couples suffered from infertility, yet Soviet infertility research is in its infancy and is not widely available. As of 1989, there had been 17 test-tube babies, and donor insemination programs were available in only 10 major cities. It was reported that one-fourth of all pregnancies did not come to term for "genetic reasons" (*Current Digest of the Soviet Press*, 1989).

The infant mortality rate for the former Soviet Union is high in comparison to other developed nations; in 1986 the rate was 26 per 1,000 births. This broke down into an urban rate of 21.7 and a rural rate of 32.0. The Soviet government counted as newborns children weighing 1,000 grams or more (2.2 pounds), while those weighing less were counted as miscarriages and were not included in infant mortality statistics. The World Health Organization guidelines define babies weighing 500 grams as newborns (Trehub, 1987). Soviet medical experts estimated that about half of the children born weighing 1,500 grams live. It was estimated that premature infants account for between 5 and 10 percent of the children born each year within the borders of the former Soviet Union (*Current Digest of the Soviet Press*, 1987).

Estimates of contraceptive use vary, and availability among former Soviet republics varies as well. However, most forms of contraception are available only sporadically and cannot be relied upon for family planning. Abortion serves as the primary means of limiting family size among the non-Moslem population. The Soviet Union became the first country to legalize abortion in 1920. Though subsequently banned in 1936, abortion as legalized again in 1956. As of 1988, the limit for legal abortions was extended from 12 to 28 weeks and abortions can now be sought for non-medical reasons such as the death of a husband, divorce, imprisonment, or the presence of more than five children. Minors may obtain abortions on the basis of age alone (Bohr, 1988, p. 3). The guidelines for legal abortions are expected to undergo substantial change as each former Soviet republic writes its own legal code.

Few vacuum-suction machines are available in the former Soviet Union; the vast majority of abortions are performed by D&C. According to Soviet sources, most hospitals perform abortions without effective anesthesia. By 1965 the ratio of abortions to births was between 2.5/3.0 to 1, and that ratio has remained stable since that time (Feshbach, 1982, p. 25). One-third of the world total of abortions are performed annually within the territory of the former Soviet Union (Tietze, 1986, p. 29).

Following abortion, condoms and withdrawal are the most common methods of limited family size. The supply of birth control pills is erratic and the side effects seem to be more pronounced in the Hungarian- and Bulgarian-made pills used in the former Soviet Union than in the versions available in the United States. Diaphragms come in a limited number of sizes and the spermicides used with them are difficult to obtain. Though growing in popularity and considered by Soviet doctors to be safer than the Pill, the IUD is used by only 3 percent of those using some form of contraception (Moffet, 1985). Sterilization is extremely rare and prohibited for women except in cases where serious medical complications are expected in the event of future pregnancies. Vasectomies are only obtainable with official consent.

As of 1989 maternity leave benefits included partially paid maternity leave until children reached the age of one and a half. Optional additional unpaid leave is now available until age three. Non-Moslem Soviet women show the highest labor force participation rates during their prime childbearing years. Prior to the expanded maternity leave benefits, the average Soviet woman withdrew from the workforce for a total of less than four years from the time that she began working until retirement (Peers, 1985).

Before the dissolution of the Soviet Union in 1991, the Soviet government made one-time payments to mothers upon the birth of a child. The amount varied with the number of previous children. Monthly payments of between 4 and 15 rubles a month for a total of four years were made to families with four or more children. (This was at a time when the average monthly individual's salary was 200 rubles.)

A 1943 law, still in effect in 1991, allowed any single mother to put her child in a children's home at any time. Adoption is illegal unless the mother agrees to sign papers giving up her rights to the child or unless she is officially deprived of her legal rights. As of 1987, 300,000 children lived in such institutions, while an additional 700,000 children lived in foster homes. Only 4 to 5 percent of these million children are orphans; the rest of the children have parents who are alcoholics, who are incarcerated, or who abandoned the children at the maternity hospital (*Current Digest of the Soviet Press*, 1987). Abandoned and homeless children are a growing social problem.

✷ SUSAN GOODRICH LEHMANN, Ph.D.

See **Guide to Related Topics:** Cross-Cultural Perspectives

Resources

Bohr, Annette. (1988, Sept 13). "Abortion is Still Number One Method of Birth Control in Soviet Union." *Radio Liberty Research 414* (88): 1-4.

Current Digest of the Soviet Press. (1987). 39 (15) (May 13): 19. Columbus, OH: CDSP.

Current Digest of the Soviet Press. (1987). 39 (18) (Jun 3): 18-19. Columbus, OH: CDSP.

Current Digest of the Soviet Press. (1987). 39 (19) (Jun 10): 1-4. Columbus, OH: CDSP.

Current Digest of the Soviet Press. (1987). 39 (19) (Jun 10): 24. Columbus, OH: CDSP.

Current Digest of the Soviet Press. (1987). 39 (32) (Sep 9): 4-6. Columbus, OH: CDSP.

Current Digest of the Soviet Press. (1989). 40 (50) (Jan 11): 23. Columbus, OH: CDSP.

Feshbach, Murray. (1982). *The Soviet Union: Population Trends and Dilemmas.* Washington, DC: Population Reference Bureau.

Hansson, Carola & Liden, Karen. (Eds.) (1983). *Moscow Women: Thirteen Interviews.* New York: Pantheon.

Holland, Barbara. (Ed.) (1985). *Soviet Sisterhood.* Bloomington: Indiana University Press.

Moffett, Julie. (1985, Jul 15). "Contraception in the Soviet Union." *Radio Liberty Research 229* (85): 1-10.

Naselenie SSSR 1988. (1989). Moskva: Finansi i statistika.

Peers, Jo. (1985). "Workers by Hand and Womb." In Barbara Holland. (Ed.) *Soviet Sisterhood*. Bloomington: Indiana University Press, pp. 116-144.

Tietze, Christopher. (1986). *Induced Abortion: A World Review*. 6th edition. New York: Allan Guttmacher Institute.

Trehub, Aaron. (1987, Oct 29). "New Figures on Infant Mortality in the USSR." *Radio Liberty Research 438* (87): 1-3.

SPINA BIFIDA. *See instead* CENTRAL CLOSURE DEFECTS

SPOCK, DR. BENJAMIN

Dr. Benjamin Spock is the well-known author of the self-help guide to parenting *Baby and Child Care* (1945, 1547, 1968, 1976, 1985). Presented in a straightforward, easy-to-read form, this book has been highly influential in shaping cultural images of parenting, mothering, and child care. As a trained pediatrician and psychiatrist, most of Dr. Spock's life has been devoted to issues concerning the biological and psychosocial development of children. His work has served as a rich source of information for many parents.

This alone, however, cannot account for the overwhelming popularity of Spock and his book over the years. Social, political, economic, and historical conditions were also important factors in encouraging Americans to accept Spock and his advice. When *Baby and Child Care* was first published in 1945, World War II was coming to an end, soldiers were returning home, and many women were ending their wartime involvement in the work force. During this period, the marriage rate increased dramatically, followed closely by an increase in the birth rate. This marked the beginning of the baby boom (May, 1988).

In addition to these demographic changes, Americans were becoming increasingly geographically mobile. The likelihood that individuals would marry and settle down in the same community in which they were raised decreased. Ties to extended family, ethnic enclaves, and kin groups were diminished, heralding the era of the nuclear family (Clarke-Stewart, 1978).

These factors contributed greatly to the popular reception of Spock and his book. Mothers in this period were younger, more inexperienced, and less involved in family and kin networks than mothers in previous generations. They were, in many respects, in need of genuine guidance and information about parenting. Spock and his book fulfilled many of these rising needs.

Spock also represented a soothing image amidst uncertain times. The war and the arrival of the atomic age had shaken the nation. McCarthyism and widespread anti-Communist rhetoric were beginning to dominate the public sphere and Americans longed for a sense of security and stability. The reassuring paternalistic wisdom of *Baby and Child Care* was consistent with what many Americans during this period wanted to hear (May, 1988). In his book, Spock offered parents clear and simple instructions for producing happy and healthy children. This approach was especially welcome given the political and social complexities, as well as the technological changes, occurring in this era.

In a variety of ways, Spock encouraged the reinstatement of traditional beliefs. His presentation of home life centered on the mother as dominant caregiver within the family (Spock, 1946). In his warning to working mothers, he suggested that the care of children by others might be damaging, not only to one's child, but also to one's country (Matthews, 1988). Such notions reinforced traditional visions of womanhood and motherhood.

In addition, Spock introduced several new ideas that had not yet found their place in American culture. Most notable among these was the introduction and popularization of Freudian thought (Sulman, 1973). While Freudian thought had already been widely communicated within the academic community, it was not until *Baby and Child Care* that the central themes developed by Freud were presented in a language and in a medium accessible to the general public. The insights provided by Freudian theory drew attention to the importance of childhood as a foundation for stable adult life.

Spock's presentation of these ideas, in combination with an emphasis on permissive child rearing, proved troublesome for many mothers (Weiss, 1977). As Spock drew attention to the significance of the mother-child dyad and further, discouraged strict discipline, he effectively placed a great deal of pressure on American mothers. Problems encountered in daily child rearing could now be perceived as potentially disastrous events with grave implications for the future of one's child. Many women consequently found bringing up their children according to this Spockian tradition a highly anxious and often guilt-ridden experience (Friedan, 1962).

Today Spock's book is now in its fifth edition. While *Baby and Child Care* still enjoys a wide audience, it is only one of a large number of parenting manuals currently available. The impact of

Dr. Spock will not be soon forgotten, however. For not only did Spock influence the rearing of an entire generation of Americans, he influenced American women's conception of themselves and their roles as mothers (Ehrenreich and English, 1978). ✱ DIANA JONES

See also: Pediatrics, History of

See **Guide to Related Topics:** Baby Care

Resources

Clarke-Stewart, K. Alison. (1978). "Popular Primers for Parents." *American Psychologist* 42: 359-69.

Ehrenreich, Barbara & English, Deidre. (1978). *For Her Own Good: 150 Years of the Experts' Advice to Women.* New York: Doubleday.

Friedan, Betty. (1962). *The Feminine Mystique.* New York: Dell.

Matthews, Fred. (1988). "The Utopia of Human Relations: The Conflict-free Family in American Social Thought, 1930-1960." *Journal of the History of the Behavioral Sciences* 24: 343-62.

May, Elaine Tyler. (1988). *Homeward Bound.* New York: Basic Books.

Spock, Benjamin. (1946). *The Common Sense Book of Baby and Child Care.* New York: Duell, Sloan, & Pierce.

Spock, Benjamin & Rothenberg, Michael B. (1985). *Baby and Child Care.* New York: Pocket Books.

Sulman, A. Michael. (1973). "The Humanization of the American Child: Benjamin Spock as a Popularizer of Psychoanalytic Thought." *Journal of the History of Behavioral Sciences* 9: 258-65.

Weiss, Nancy Pottishman. (1977, Winter). "Mother, the Invention of Necessity: Dr. Benjamin Spock's Baby and Child Care." *American Quarterly* 29: 519-46.

S.T.D. *See instead* SEXUALLY TRANSMITTED DISEASES

STILLBIRTH

Every year in the United States, almost 30,000 babies die before birth. The National Center for Health Statistics collects death certificates for all babies who die between the 20th week of pregnancy and the moment of birth; some states use earlier cutoffs, such as 16 weeks, for their data collection. These fetal deaths, or stillbirths, have declined significantly over time, but they still occur in approximately one of every 130 deliveries. Poor women are at greatest risk of having stillbirths, but women of all backgrounds may experience this painful loss.

The most common known reasons for stillbirth are compression of the umbilical cord prior to or during delivery; early detachment of the placenta due to *abruptio placentae* or *placenta previa;* maternal conditions such as toxemia, diabetes, or untreated Rh blood factor; and abnormalities in the fetus. Yet the reasons for as many as half of these deaths are never explained, and this is a source of great concern and frustration to many parents and their caregivers.

The feelings of grief after a stillbirth are very similar to those that people have after any death of a loved one. In addition, family members are shocked by such an unexpected event, and parents may have strong feelings of guilt and failure for not having been able to bring a healthy baby into the world. Many families discover that, while they are grieving for a baby who was already very real to them, others may try to console them by minimizing the event with comments such as, "At least you never knew the baby," or "You're young, you can always have another one." Thus, isolation from friends and family at a time when social support is especially crucial may intensify the depression and anger felt by many parents.

Many (though certainly not all) hospitals and health professionals have greatly improved their care of bereaved families in the last decade or so, in response to parents' efforts individually and through support groups. It is much less common now for babies to be removed automatically before parents can see them. Many hospitals offer parents the opportunity to spend time with the baby, to have pictures taken, and to arrange for the kind of burial or memorial service that best meets their needs. Perinatal bereavement teams attempt to ensure that every family learns what options exist and how they can find help in coping with their loss. Some parents who did not have such opportunities may realize, even years after a stillbirth, that they wish they had been able to do more for the baby. These families are finding ways, on their own or through support organizations, to name or memorialize the baby who was never forgotten.

Although babies who are stillborn are always remembered, the intense pain of the first few months usually diminishes over time. Most women become pregnant again and have a healthy birth, despite the fact that a subsequent pregnancy is often a time of anxiety. There is no fixed waiting period that has been shown to be necessary before a subsequent pregnancy beyond what is needed for the women's physical recovery.

In a longitudinal study of families who experienced pregnancy loss, several characteristics were found to be more common among the men and women who reported the lowest grief scores two years after the loss. These were good mental health prior to the pregnancy, higher social class, the occurrence of the loss earlier in pregnancy, and the pregnancy having been unplanned. Just two months after the loss, grief in this study was also affected by gender (with women reporting higher scores) and was lower among those people who were most satisfied with their partner relationship, who felt supported by their friends, and who already had another child or children in the family (Lasker, 1991).

The findings from this study confirm the idea that family and friends can help to alleviate the most severe effects of the loss. However, some people may have ongoing mental health problems, which can be exacerbated by the loss and which require more intensive follow-up and intervention. Support groups and expressions of concern from available, informative, and caring health professionals also help many people cope with their grief. ✷ JUDITH N. LASKER, Ph.D.

See also: Infant Funerals: Contemporary Practices; Pregnancy after Pregnancy Loss; Support Groups for Infant Loss

See **Guide to Related Topics:** Pregnancy Loss and Infant Mortality

Resources

Borg, Susan & Lasker, Judith. (1989). *When Pregnancy Fails: Families Coping with Miscarriage, Ectopic Pregnancy, Stillbirth, and Infant Death.* New York: Bantam Books.

Callan, Victor & Murray, Judith. (1989). "The Role of Therapists in Helping Couples Cope with Stillbirth and Newborn Death." *Family Relations 38*: 248-53.

Carr, Donna & Knupp, Chaplain Samuel. (1985). "Grief and Perinatal Loss: A Community Hospital Response to Support." *Journal of Obstetric, Gynecologic and Neonatal Nursing 14*: 130-39.

DeFrain, John et al. (1986). *Stillborn: The Invisible Death.* Lexington, MA: Lexington Books.

Kirkley-Best, Elizabeth & Kellner, Kenneth. (1982). "The Forgotten Grief: A Review of the Psychology of Stillbirth." *American Journal of Orthopsychiatry 52*: 420-29.

Lake, Marion et al. (1983). "The Role of a Grief Support Team Following Stillbirth." *Journal of Obstetrics and Gynecology 146*: 877-81.

Lasker, Judith. (1991). "Predicting Grief after Pregnancy Loss: A Two Year Longitudinal Study." Unpublished manuscript, Lehigh University, Bethlehem, PA.

Lasker, Judith & Toedter, Lori. (Forthcoming). "Acute vs. Chronic Grief: The Case of Pregnancy Loss." *American Journal of Orthopsychiatry.*

Stinson, Kandi et al. (Forthcoming). "Gender and Grief: Male and Female Responses to Pregnancy Loss." *Family Relations.*

STRESS IN PREGNANCY

Early animal research on stress and pregnancy focused primarily on the physiological and behavioral responses to differing modalities of stress inducement (e.g., noise, light, restraint, injection, etc.). The primary physiological change that was traditionally measured is the maternal plasma levels of ACTH (adrenocorticotrophin hormone). All of the stress modalities were found to markedly increase maternal levels of corticosterones immediately following acute stimulation (Barlow, Knight, and Sullivan, 1978). When the same stress modalities were applied chronically, adaptation occurred and maternal corticosteroid levels ceased to increase in response to the stress stimulus (Quirce, Odio, and Solano, 1981). Intermittently applied stress (unpredictable) was perceived by the organism acutely, and corticosteroid levels increased accordingly (Fride and Weinstock, 1984; Quirce, Odio, and Solano, 1981). The implications from animal research suggest that adaptation occurs with chronic predictable stress and that chronic unpredictable stress results in a lowered immune system response and poor fetal outcome.

Concurrent with the study of maternal responses to stress stimuli was significant effort to identify infant physical and behavioral responses to maternal stress. As early as 1957, controlled rat experiments were conducted by Thompson, which were designed to look at the emotional and behavioral characteristics of the offspring of stressed rat mothers. In this research, conditioned avoidance training was used prior to mating. During gestation the avoidance component was eliminated with no resultant stressor; the rats' conditioned expectation of stress was used as the stressor. The offspring were cross-fostered, or reared by nontreatment mothers and the behavior of the offspring was compared with nontreatment offspring at 30 to 40 days of age and again at 130 to 140 days of age. Experimental offspring showed a much higher amount and latency of activity (slower response time) at both ages of testing. Experimental offspring were slower to leave their home cage at the first age of testing with no significant difference at the second age of testing.

The work of Sontag (1944), conducted through the Fels Research Institute from 1932 to 1966, focused on exploring the behavior and development of the human fetus: the individual differences in development and response to stimuli during the last four months of pregnancy. A higher maternal basal metabolic rate (BMR) was associated with larger, and slightly more mature, infants at birth, suggesting that maternal thyroid function affects the growth and development of the offspring (Sontag, Reynolds, and Torbert, 1944). Infants of mothers who experienced severe emotional stress during the last trimester of pregnancy were found to be more irritable and hyperactive than normal for weeks or months after birth. Food intolerance and gastrointestinal disturbances (loose stools and frequent regurgitation) were frequent in these stressed infants. Later research by this same group assessed frequency and intensity of fetal movement in late pregnancy. Differences in fetal activity seemed to predict infant activity and behavior (Sontag, 1944).

Stott (1973) conducted a random, longitudinal study on childhood morbidity and maternal stress. The maternal stress interview was retrospective (one month postpartum), which may present a serious limitation to the interpretation of the findings. Childhood morbidity rates through the fourth year of life were significantly higher for the infants of mothers with reported high-anxiety levels during pregnancy.

Since the pioneering work of Sontag, researchers have been examining the effects of maternal stress on infant behavior and development. A severe limitation in research on human populations revolves around the confounding factor of tense or anxious mother/child interactions after birth, which can affect the behavior and development of the infant. The cross-fostering protocol used to eliminate this factor in animal studies is obviously not appropriate for human study. In addition, other components that may affect prenatal/neonatal behavior (e.g., genetic predispositions) are difficult to assess in human populations.

Current research strategies are drawing from various scientific fields. Epidemiologists are establishing that high maternal anxiety or stress may be related to neonatal and infant mortality and morbidity and/or birth complications. Niswander and Gordon (1972) reported results from a massive collaborative perinatal study of more than 10,000 women that widows and unmarried mothers have a much higher incidence of neonatal deaths, neurological impairment, and low birth weight (respectively). Laukaran and van den Berg (1980), after controlling for such factors as maternal health, nutrition, and social class in 8,000 women, found that negative maternal attitudes were associated with a higher incidence of postpartum infections and hemorrhages in the mother and congenital abnormalities and death in the newborn. Psycho-physiologists are establishing the hormonally mediated changes associated with high maternal/fetal stress in animal models. Psycho-biology is attempting to use strategies that integrate social and clinical psychological perspectives to understand stress and reproductive function and dysfunction (Herrenkohl, 1983).

Although the mechanism of prenatal stress has yet to be clearly defined or delineated, the evidence that the structure and function, as well as the behaviors, of fetus and neonates can be altered by negative prenatal environments is strong. As research strategies become more collaborative and sophisticated, the evidence will become clearer. Based even on the current state of knowledge, educational outreach programs that reduce maternal stress and anxiety and promote positive maternal attitudes can be developed and instituted in order to improve maternal and fetal health. The evaluation and assessment of improvements in fetal outcome may reverse the current trend of focusing on technologically advanced methods of decreasing the perinatal morbidity rates in favor of preventative health programs that may do more to improve fetal outcome per dollar spent.

Stress reduction techniques use the basic underlying principle of gaining conscious control over body functions. Benson (1975) and Jacobson (1983) have pioneered the field of various techniques designed to elicit the relaxation response that can help combat the negative consequences of tension and stress. While anecdotal support for using relaxation techniques during pregnancy is high, with many popular books espousing the various benefits, there is a lack of published research or baseline data on the efficacy of practicing relaxation techniques during pregnancy.

✱ DIANE E. DEPKEN, Ed.D.

See **Guide to Related Topics:** Pregnancy, Psychological Aspects

Resources

Barlow, S., Knight, A., & Sullivan, F. (1978). "Delay in Postnatal Growth and Development of Offspring Produced by Maternal Restraint Stress during Pregnancy in the Rat." *Teratology 18*: 211-18.

Benson, H. (1975). *The Relaxation Response.* New York: Avon.

Fride, E. & Weinstock, M. (1984). "The Effects of Prenatal Exposure to Predictable or Unpredictable Stress on Early Development in the Rat." *Developmental Psychobiology 17*: 651-60.

Herrenkohl, L.R. (1983). "Prenatal Stress May Alter Sexual Differentiation in Male and Female Offspring." *Monographs in Neurological Science 9*: 176-83.

Jacobson, E. (1983). *Progressive Relaxation.* Chicago: University of Chicago Press.

Laukaran, V.H. & van den Berg, J.J. (1980). "The Relationship of Maternal Attitude to Pregnancy Outcomes and Obstetric Complications." *American Journal of Obstetrics and Gynecology 136*: 374-79.

Niswander, K.R. & Gordon, M. (1972). *The Women and Their Pregnancies.* Washington, DC: U.S. Department of Health, Education and Welfare.

Quirce, C., Odio, M., & Solano, J. (1981). "The Effects of Predictable and Unpredictable Schedules of Physical Restraint upon Rats." *Life Science 28*: 1897-1902.

Sontag, L.W. (1944). "Differences in Modifiability of Fetal Behavior and Physiology." *Psychosomatic Medicine* 6: 151-54.

Sontag, L.W., Reynolds, E.L., & Torbert, V. (1944). "Status of Infant at Birth as Related to Basal Metabolism of Mothers in Pregnancy." *American Journal of Obstetrics and Gynecology* 48: 208-14.

Stott, D.H. (1973). "Follow-up Study from Birth of the Effects of Prenatal Stresses." *Developmental Medicine in Childhood Neurology* 15: 770-87.

Thompson, W.R. (1957). "Influence of Prenatal Anxiety on Emotionality in Young Rats." *Science* 125: 698-99.

STRETCH MARKS: STRIAE GRAVIDARUM

During the gestational period, the skin is among the many organs undergoing changes. This physiologic change has mainly a cosmetic importance. Irregular, linear, pink-to-violaceous atrophic and finely wrinkled stripes develop opposite the skin tension lines, initially on the abdomen and sometimes on the breasts, the lower portion of the back, the buttocks, the thighs, and the inguinal areas.

The onset of striae usually occurs during the second half of pregnancy, more commonly during the sixth or seventh month. Stretch marks appear to have a hereditary tendency and are uncommon in black and Asian women due to the increased amount of elastin present in the skin. The incidence of this problem is higher in younger women pregnant for the first time (Janine, 1987). There appears to be no correlation between the intensity of striation and the enlargement of body size during pregnancy, although certain physiological factors such as tautness of the abdomen and breasts are probably significant in the localization and the direction of striae. Initially edematous and often itchy, they eventually become atrophic and lighter than normal skin (Sodhi and Sausker, 1988). After pregnancy they will gradually fade and become less noticeable.

Experts do not seem to agree on the exact cause of stretch marks. Possibly a combination of stretching of the skin, adrenocortical hormone, and genetic predisposition are among the causes of stretch marks. Liu, as cited in Wong and Ellis (1984), relates stretch marks to the increase in relaxin, oestrogen, and corticosteroids that occur in pregnancy, therefore acting on the collagen fibers. On the other hand, Shuster, also cited in Wong and Ellis, believes that the stretch with intradermal tears of collagen fibers is the sole factor in stretch marks. Others believe stretch marks are caused by a deterioration of the elastin and an alteration of the collagen fibers brought on by an excessive stretching of the elastic fibers of the skin (Janine, 1987). However, all agree that growth is rapid during pregnancy, and is, in itself, the biggest cause of stretch marks. A women who gains weight rapidly, instead of gradually, increases her chances of developing stretch marks. Also, in the last month, as the baby descends, some stretch marks may appear at the base of the abdomen.

How to prevent stretch marks is a subject of great interest. However none of the available preventive treatments can claim to eliminate all stretch marks. Success in minimizing the number of stretch marks has been obtained using a very methodical approach which involves the application of products that contain elastin and collagen on the abdomen and other probable areas, beginning in the third or fourth month of pregnancy. This treatment is used in addition to massaging, twice daily, with a massage glove or a rough face cloth (Janine, 1987). This preventive treatment is designed to bring a pinkish color to the surface of the skin, therefore activating circulation to the skin and avoiding stretch marks. Doing gentle daily exercises, especially for those who have desk jobs, and avoiding very hot baths or showers will

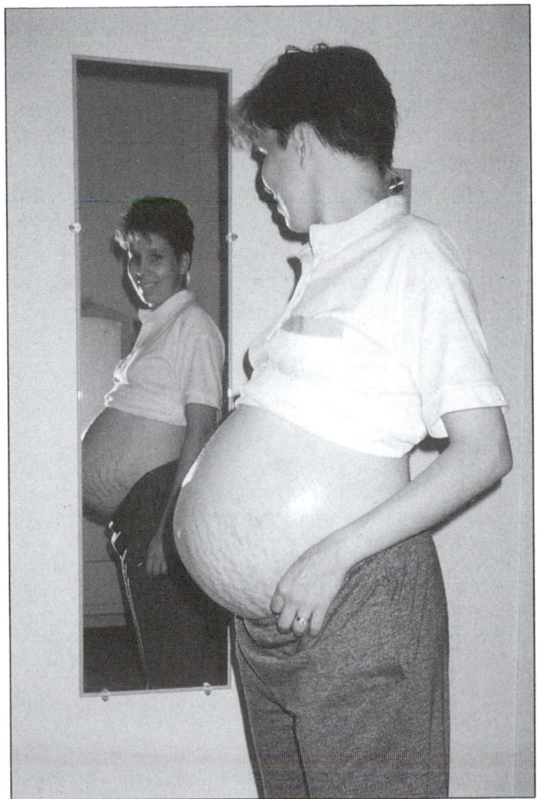

Stretch marks. Photo courtesy of Marie Leduc.

also help. Other centers dealing with therapeutic aesthetics recommend a cream called "Prelude Universal Cream," which is composed mainly of what estheticians refer to as essential oils. However, this particular treatment is quite costly. According to beauticians, this cream can prevent deficiencies in the fatty acids, which lead to problems with keratinization. Another cream manufactured in Switzerland, called "Alphastria" and containing hyaluronic acid, has demonstrated positive results in a double blind study (Buman and DeWeck, 1987). The women were using this cream from the third month of pregnancy until the end of the third month after delivery.

According to DeMarco (1990), daily application of vitamin E during pregnancy (used as a preventive measure), might be helpful to some women. She also recommends daily application of vitamin E oil to the stretch marks, twice daily for three months after birth.

Until recently, the successful treatment of stretch marks was unheard of. However, new methods in aesthetics that are aimed at cellular regeneration (Wade, Wade, and Jones, 1978) are now being discovered. These techniques work better with stretch marks that still show signs of circulation. Although sometimes successful, these methods are costly and require discipline and a holistic approach (including a balanced diet). Treatment may last from six months to three years and involves the application of oils, vials for cellular regeneration, vegetable extracts, treatment with infrared lamps, and balneotherapy.

The war against stretch marks has begun. However, until some of these treatments become more readily available and well researched, the only consolation may be that, with time, stretch marks do fade and become less noticeable.

✱ MARIE LEDUC, R.N.

See **Guide to Related Topics:** Pregnancy, Physical Aspects

Resources

Buman, M. Walther R. & De Weck, Gynak. (1987). "Wirksambert der Alphastria. Creme bei der Vorkengung von Schwangerschafts streigen (Striae distensa). Ergebnisse einer Doppelblind-Studie." *Rdsch 27*: 79-84.

DeMarco, Carolyn. (1990, Apr/May). "How to Handle the Not-So-Joyful Parts of Pregnancy?" *Today's Health*: 15-18.

Clinique de Santé et d'Esthetique Therapeutique de Montréal: Le Concept d'Esthetisme Meridional. *Chronique Journal MERID* - 87 - Corps-22:

Sante, Janine Renaud. (1987, Jul-Aug). (no title). *Health* (30): 19-20.

Sodhi, Vimal K. & Sausker, William F. (1988, Jan). "Dermatoses of Pregnancy." *American Family Physician 37* (1): 131-38.

Wade, Thomas R., Wade, Sylvia L., & Jones, Henry E. (1978, Aug). "Skin Changes and Diseases Associated with Obstetrics and Gynecology." *Obstetrics and Gynecology 52* (2): 233-242.

Winton, Georges B. & Lewis, Charles W. (1982, Jun). "Dermatoses of Pregnancy." *Journal of the American Academy of Dermatology 6* (6): 977-98.

Wong, Reynold C. & Ellis, Charles N. (1984). "Physiologic Skin Changes in Pregnancy." *Journal of the American Academy of Dermatology 10* (6): 929-40.

SUDDEN INFANT DEATH SYNDROME (SIDS)

Sudden infant death syndrome (SIDS) has been defined as the sudden, unexpected, and unexplainable death of an infant or young child. SIDS has in the past also been referred to as "crib death" or "cot death."

SIDS is the number one cause of death in children between the ages of one week and one year in the U.S. (Whaley and Wong, 1983; Shannon, 1984). SIDS claims the lives of two to three infants per 1,000 live births each year (Shannon, 1984; Pillitteri, 1985) and is the second highest cause of death (next to accidents) in children between 7 days and 14 years of age (Shannon, 1984).

Causes. The exact cause of SIDS is unknown. However, many scientists have researched the syndrome and have uncovered some likely correlations between environmental, social, and physiological phenomena and the occurrence of SIDS. Infants and children at risk have been identified as the following: (1) infants of teen mothers; (2) infants born at close interval to previous infant; (3) infants who are small for gestational age; (4) infants who had suffered from respiratory distress syndrome; (5) premature infants; (6) infants born to Native Americans and other nonwhites; (7) infants of low-income families; and (8) siblings of a previous SIDS baby (Shannon, 1984; Pillitteri, 1985; Gabbe, Niebly, and Simpson, 1986). Although many sources state that the increased risk to siblings of a SIDS infant may be as high as five times greater than for the population at large, other researchers state that there is no genetic cause yet known for this increased occurrence. That is, it is not believed to be an inherited disorder (Bergman, 1982; Shannon, 1984).

Some other hypotheses concerning the cause of SIDS include: (1) the possible involvement of viral agents, as 50 percent of all infants who died of SIDS were reported to have had some nasal congestion within the week prior to their death (Bergman, 1982); (2) a positive correlation between maternal smoking in the prenatal and postpartum periods (Gabbe, Niebly, and Simpson, 1986); and (3) the possible association between SIDS and an allergy to cow's milk in infant formula (Robertson, 1986).

Typical Victim. The typical victim of SIDS is a well-nourished child who exhibited symptoms of a head cold within the previous week. There have been reports that no crying or noise accompanied the death. The infant is found often tangled within the covers, which makes the parents wrongly believe that the child died of suffocation. The bed is often found with blood-tinged mucus, leaving the parents with fears of an internal hemorrhage, again a wrong assumption.

Autopsies have revealed that these signs of death do not actually reflect the cause of death. The medical community does not believe that the cause of SIDS is related to suffocation or obstruction of the airway due to sputum (Pillitteri, 1984). However, autopsies consistently reveal petechiae (small blood vessel hemorrhages) in the lungs and mild inflammation in the respiratory tract (Pillitteri, 1985). There is also evidence of chronic hypoxia, that is, a chronic lack of oxygen to the tissues (Whaley and Wong, 1983).

Prevention and Intervention. Due to the unknown cause or causes of SIDS, prevention is difficult. At-home breathing monitoring (apnea monitoring) is encouraged for infants with any documented episodes of apnea or for siblings of previous SIDS infants. At-home breathing monitoring needs to be accompanied by parental training in cardiopulmonary resuscitation (CPR).

Autopsies are recommended for any infant who dies suddenly. These studies can provide families with needed information and can also assist the medical community in uncovering the causes of these sudden deaths.

Emotional Support. Helping families through the loss of a child due to SIDS is probably the most critical intervention. Families who lose an infant or a young child to SIDS are confronted with a sudden, unexpected, and unexplained loss of a child and are often left with feelings of guilt. Parents believe there was something they did to cause the death and certainly feel they should have been able to prevent the death. Siblings of SIDS infants can also have feelings of guilt. Care must be taken with all family members to assure them that none of them was responsible for the death.

Unfortunately, the significant relationship between SIDS and socioeconomic status leads to a large number of families who lack access to a personal healthcare provider, and, consequently, these families may not receive the attention they need.

All families who have suffered a SIDS loss would benefit from a referral to the National SIDS Foundation. This organization consists of families of previous SIDS loss as well as professional staff. The organization has chapters assisting families in many major cities. The address is National SIDS Foundation, 310 S. Michigan Ave., Chicago, IL 60604.

✱ SHANA REED, C.N.M.

See also: Pregnancy Loss: Family Response

See **Guide to Related Topics:** Pregnancy Loss and Infant Mortality

Resources

Bergman, A.B. (1982). In S.S. Gellis & B.M. Kagan (Eds.) *Current Pediatric Therapy 10*. Philadelphia: W.B. Saunders Co.

Gabbe, S.G., Niebly, J.R., & Simpson, J.L. (Eds.) (1986). *Obstetrics: Normal and Problem Pregnancies*. New York: Churchill Livingstone.

Pillitteri, Adele. (1985). *Maternal-Newborn Nursing: Care of the Growing Family, 3rd Edition*. Boston: Little, Brown, & Co.

Robertson, N.R.C. (Ed.) (1986). *Textbook of Neonatology*. New York: Churchill Livingston.

Shannon, D.C. (1984). In S.S. Gellis & B.M. Kagan. *Current Pediatric Therapy 11*. Philadelphia: W.B. Saunders Co.

Whaley, L.F. & Wong, D.L. (1983). *Nursing Care of Infants and Children*. Second edition. St. Louis: C.V. Mosby.

SUPPORT GROUPS

Peer support groups in the childbearing year most likely can trace their beginnings to the founding of La Leche League International in 1956. While La Leche League provided a place for mothers to learn about breastfeeding and share their experiences, the support groups that sprouted during the 1970s focused on dealing with past and future birth experiences. Perhaps the most well-known of these have been those dealing with cesarean and home births and those dealing with infant disabilities and death. While none can duplicate the League's continual growth and success, their activities have raised consciousness and changed attitudes.

Support groups arise out of some consumer dissatisfaction with the status quo and provide a safe place for women (and men) to discuss their common feelings and find out how others have coped in a similar situation. For example, as the prepared childbirth movement gave women control over their births, a surprise cesarean often left a prepared father abandoned in a hallway, and a woman, who expected to feel exhilarated after giving birth, instead feeling physically and mentally off-balance. Support groups were instrumental in the development of family-centered cesareans and a recognition that a cesarean was not just surgery, but also the birth of a baby. As cesarean support groups developed, they also became active in seeking a change in the "once a cesarean, always a cesarean" dictum.

Support groups are generally locally based, although some larger groups provide networking nationally and internationally. They may often be located through local childbirth teaching groups such as childbirth education associations, hospital staffs, or the "meetings" section of the newspaper. As a rule, they should be composed of people sharing similar situations, although some may be led by a professional. There is usually no charge to attend. ✱ JANE C. SZCZEPANIAK, I.C.C.E.

See also: Women's Health Movement

For Further Information

C/SEC, Inc., 22 Forest Road, Framingham, MA 01701. (Information on cesareans and VBAC.)

International Association of Parents and Professionals for Safe Alternatives in Childbirth (NAPSAC), Rt. 1, Box 646, Marble Hill, MO 63764.

International Childbirth Education Association, P.O. Box 20048, Minneapolis, MN 55420.

LaLeche League International, 9616 Minneapolis Avenue, Franklin Park, IL 60131 (Information on breastfeeding.)

Resolve Through Sharing, Lutheran Hospital—LaCrosse, 1910 South Avenue, La Crosse, WI 54601. (Information on miscarriage, stillbirth, and infant death.)

SUPPORT GROUPS FOR INFANT LOSS

> "There were 20 people. I thought a whole maze of thoughts, felt a whole maze of feelings. They, like I, felt like death itself, but we were making no attempts to hide that fact. We were here, smiling, shaking hands, introducing each other, talking about the traffic and it wasn't forced. We weren't talking small talk.
>
> As everyone told their stories, I felt I was watching a sad movie. Things like this don't happen to me. Then it was my turn. "I'm Marion Cohen and my baby girl died on Christmas eve." Here we were, a room full of people, talking about our losses. I left refreshed, regenerated, almost on a high. It was the beginning of control." (Marion Cohen, *Caring Concepts Newsletter, 1990* (Centering Corporation)

There are fewer support groups for infant loss now, primarily because hospitals are doing a much better job encouraging families to see, hold, and name their baby; in facilitating grief; and allowing time to say goodbye. But if nothing else, many parents find one support group meeting is worth attending just to know they are not going crazy, that grief is not a pathological illness but a part of life, and that others understand and share their feelings.

Participants don't have to say anything at a support group. Just listening will help. But participants can and do also share and help others. There are certain ground rules carried out in most support groups, which are self-help, therapeutic but not therapy groups.

1. Everyone's experiences are unique.
2. No one will probe. Participants should share only if they choose to do so.
3. It's OK to cry.
4. Participants may leave at any time.
5. Participants are encouraged to share their feelings about the meeting with their partner if they come alone.
6. Groups are confidential. What goes on at meetings is only discussed among members.
7. Members are encouraged to call each other or the group leader between meetings.

Groups don't last forever. Some have a structure, with a speaker, then discussion and sharing at each meeting. Others are unstructured, with one or more leaders starting the group discussion. As their grief lessens, participants will find that their need to attend lessens, too. However, they will also find they are helping someone else, the newcomers. They will see where they were six months or a year before and see their progress.

Most people come to a group apprehensive and afraid—afraid they'll cry, afraid they'll look stupid, afraid of being rejected. This rarely happens. Usually, people leave as Marion Cohen stated above, refreshed, affirmed, finding a real community of people who finally understand what it means to lose a baby. Groups are not composed of stiff professionals with degrees in group work. They are made up of parents who care. ✱ JOY JOHNSON

See also: Infant Funerals: Contemporary Practices; Pregnancy Loss: Family Response; Stillbirth

See **Guide to Related Topics:** Pregnancy Loss and Infant Mortality

For Further Information

SHARE. *Starting a Parent Support Group.* St. Elizabeth Hospital, Bellevue, IL 62222. SHARE is the international support system for infant death. A complete list of groups available can be obtained from the office listed above.

SWADDLING

The image of the swaddled infant, tightly wrapped, rigid and immobile, is apt to be distressing to American parents, yet the practice of swaddling was widespread in the past and continues today in many parts of the globe. One survey of 139 societies around the world found that 51.8 percent, a surprisingly high number, use some form of infant restraint. Of this 51.8 percent, 30.9 percent simply wrap the infant with strips of cloth or rely on heavy blankets or a tight cradle to limit the infant's ability to move. The other 20.9 percent use a cradleboard or other frame along with swaddling. These practices are usually limited to the first 9 to 12 months of life.

Infant swaddling is more common in colder than in warmer climates. Societies in geographic areas where the mean temperature of the coldest month of the year is less than 50 degrees Fahrenheit are more likely to use restraint than societies where the mean temperature rises above 50 degrees. Thus, societies in North America, Europe, and nontropical Asia are most heavily represented in the group of societies using this form of infant restraint.

To protect infants from the cold is a plausible and intuitively reasonable explanation for the practice of swaddling, but it is not a sufficient explanation since many societies with high summer temperatures swaddle infants all year long. In the American Southwest, the Navaho use cradleboards even when the temperature reaches tropical intensity. Chisholm and Richards (1979) suggest, therefore, that humidity as well as temperature determine how widespread swaddling is. It is possible that tropical peoples avoid swaddling not so much because of the heat but because high humidity promotes bacterial and fungal infections under the swaddling cloths or cradleboard bindings.

In Russia and Eastern Europe, babies raised in the traditional fashion are tightly swaddled in long strips of material that hold their legs straight and their arms down by their sides. This posture is maintained for nine months or so, and the baby is only unswaddled for nursing and bathing. If the mother is very busy, she may nurse the infant without unswaddling him or her.

In the United States, the use of swaddling and cradleboards in Native American tribes, particularly the Navaho, has been widely studied. The Navaho cradleboard consists of three parts: a back of one or two boards about 10 inches wide by 36 inches long, a hinged footrest at one end of the board, and a protective hoop above the baby's face at the other. The baby is placed on a blanket lying on the board and the blanket is quickly wrapped around him or her, immobilizing the torso, arms, and legs. Then the buckskin or cloth covering of the cradleboard is laced up. The result is an almost completely motionless infant, covered right up to the chin by the swaddling material.

The younger the child, the greater the number of hours spent on the cradleboard. At six weeks, fifteen hours each day on the cradleboard is not unusual. By nine months, time on the cradleboard drops to six hours. The Navaho cradleboard is used for about a year; the child decides when to give it up, crying and protesting if the mother attempts to swaddle him or her (Chisholm, 1983).

Much early scholarly interest in the practice of swaddling focused on its possible effect on a child's personality. Gorer (1949), for example, believed that the adult Russian personality is a result of swaddling. He suggested that swaddling creates a personality that alternates between passive acceptance and explosive resistance. According to this theory, adult Russians and East Europeans who were swaddled as children learn the obedience necessary to secure food and love, but this obedience is accompanied by contradictory feelings for the mother who both imprisons and releases the child. Erikson (1963) followed a similar line of reasoning in his analysis of the Oglala Sioux, a stoic group whose tranquil demeanor is periodically rent by outbursts of violence.

Other investigators studied the effect of swaddling on a child's motor development. It was assumed that binding a child's limbs would retard development, but there is no evidence that swaddling has such an effect. In a study of Hopi children, motor development appeared quite normal and such milestones as walking occurred at normal stages.

More recent interest in swaddling has shifted to the infant's physiological responses to swaddling. In an unusual experiment, Lipton, Steinschneider, and Richmond (1965) studied three groups of human infants: one fully swaddled, one swaddled to the armpits, and one unswaddled. The infants' vital signs were recorded before, during, and after swaddling, and after exposure to certain stimuli. The researchers found that the swaddled infants were more content and slept more than the unswaddled infants. They reacted more calmly to loud noises and lights, and their pulse remained steadier in response to stimuli.

In addition to the calming effect of swaddling on the individual child, there appear to be a number of other advantages. The first is safety. The child remains near the mother or caregiver but is not in harm's way. When swaddled, the child is easily portable and makes a pleasant traveling companion. The swaddled child does not demand much attention and is easily incorporated into daily life.

Swaddling can actually eliminate some possibilities for conflict between mother and child. A busy mother's patience is easily strained by a child underfoot, but if her infant is swaddled, the mother can focus on the tasks she has to complete and then turn her attention to her child. Thus when the mother has time for her child, the encounter can be full of love and affection. Such rich episodes of sociability and attention can be thoroughly satisfying interludes for both mother and child and a way to "catch up" during a busy day (Chisholm, 1983).

The resistance of American parents, doctors, and other caregivers to swaddling and similar methods of infant restraint lies in the belief that the child finds immobilization painful and frustrating. Parents are also fearful that swaddling leads to mental and physical impairment. The empirical evidence on swaddling points to significant benefits for both mother and child, but because the adoption of a practice is always dependent on how it fits in with dominant cultural values, there seems little chance that such stringent infant restraint will ever become a mainstream American custom. ✱ PEGGY MCGARRAHAN

See also: Infant Carriers

See Guide to Related Topics: Baby Care

Resources

Barry, H. & Paxson, L.M. (1971). "Infancy and Early Childhood: Cross-cultural Codes." Ethnology 2 (10): 466-508.

Chisholm, J. (1983). Navajo Infancy. New York: Aldine Publishing.

Chisholm, J.S. & Richards, M.P.M. (1979). "Swaddling, Cradleboards and the Development of Children." Early Human Development 2 (3): 255-75.

Dennis, W. (1940). The Hopi Child. New York: Wiley.

Erikson, E. (1963). Childhood and Society. New York: Norton.

Gorer, G. (1949). "Some Aspects of the Psychology of the People of Great Russia." American Slavic and East European Review 8: 155-60.

Lipton, E., Steinschneider, A., & Richmond, J. (1965). "Swaddling: A Childcare Practice: Historical, Cultural and Experimental Observations." Pediatrics 35: 519-67.

Whiting, J.W.M. (1981). "Environmental Constraints on Infant Care Practices." In R.H. Munroe, R.L. Munroe, & B.B. Whiting (Eds.) Handbook on Cross-Cultural Human Development. New York: STPM Press.

SWEDEN

Sweden is a sparsely populated country in northern Europe, its size slightly larger than the state of California with a 1988 population of close to 8.5 million people. Historically, the population has been more homogeneous than in many other countries, but postwar immigration has contributed a large proportion of inhabitants of foreign extraction.

A constitutional monarchy, Sweden has a parliamentary form of government. The Social Democrat Party, alone or in coalition with other parties, has been in power virtually uninterrupted since 1932. It is the Social Democrats who, beginning in the 1930s with the slogan of creating a "people's home," have brought about the existence of the Swedish welfare state. Health care, child allowances, and parental leave policies are key components of the Swedish welfare state, partly developed as childbirth incentives in response to the sharp drop in the birth rate during the economic crisis of the 1930s. Thus maternity insurance benefits were introduced in 1937; in 1939, legislation ensured that gainfully employed women would not be dismissed due to pregnancy or childbirth; in 1947, child allowances were introduced; and in 1974, parents became entitled to share parental allowances associated with the birth of a child.

Publicly employed physicians providing outpatient care existed as early as the 17th century in Sweden, and public hospitals were established in the 18th century. National health insurance, covering medical and dental care and parental and sickness benefits, was established in Sweden in 1955 and is financed by the state and employer contributions. Patients pay a standard charge for public outpatient services, including any x-rays or laboratory work. Prescriptions have a maximum cost, although life-saving drugs needed for chronic and serious diseases are free of charge (Swedish Institute, 1989b). Health care's share of the gross national product (GNP) reached a peak of 9.7 percent in 1982 (Swedish Planning and Rationalization Institute, 1987).

Parental Leave Policies and Child Allowances. Sweden is frequently cited as a model of generous parental leave policies, compensating parents for loss of income when they stay home to look after a baby or sick child. Since the most recent revision of the policy, parents of children born after October 1988 receive benefits for a total of 15 months. For the first 12 months, the compensation received is approximately 90 percent of the parent's normal income, while the subsequent compensation amounts to a fixed daily rate of 60 SEK. There are plans to extend the leave to 18 months. Parents can use this benefit in a variety of combinations; one parent can make use of the full benefit or both parents can share it, combining it with part-time work or staying home full-time. They can also defer using the benefit up until the child's eighth birthday. However, both parents cannot receive compensation simultaneously, and one of them may not take more than 12 months off, reserving the remaining 3 months for the other parent. In addition to the above benefits, fathers are entitled to 10 days of leave with parental benefits when a child is born. Parents are also entitled to share up to 60 days off per child and year with financial compensation if either child or the person who usually looks after the child is sick. Furthermore, parents of children under the age of eight are entitled to an unpaid reduction of their working day by two hours (Swedish Institute, 1989a, 1990a).

About 80 percent of all Swedish women with children under the age of seven are gainfully employed, and a key expectation underlying the system of parental insurance is that parenting should be shared by the mother and father. However, in 1987 the majority (76 percent) of those making use of the childbirth allowance were women, a number that increased during the 1980s. The low number of men taking advantage of their rights to parental leave has been a subject of considerable concern in Sweden. Men were more involved in the care of sick children, composing 41 percent of parents who used sickness leave in 1987 (Statistics Sweden, 1990).

In addition to the benefits described, parents receive a universal cash allowance (SEK 5,820 per child and year in 1990) for children under the age of 16, and families with three or more children receive an additional allowance.

Maternal and Child Health Care. Sweden has increasingly moved toward hospital-based births involving use of medical technology and pharmacology. While most births took place in the home with the assistance of a midwife in 1890, this figure had decreased to six percent in 1950 and to close to zero percent by 1970 (Hofvander, 1984). While home birth is not illegal, it is illegal to deliver a baby without making attempts to procure the assistance of a professionally qualified person (Houd and Oakley, 1986, p. 27). Midwives are responsible for all normal home birth deliveries (Blondel, Pusch, and Schmidt, 1986). Typically, the birth entails use of a sedative, a paracervical or epidural block, a pudendal block, and laughing gas (Ransjö-Arvidson, 1989). In the late 1970s, close to 12 percent of all births took place through cesarean sections (Bergsjø, Schmidt, and Pusch, 1986).

Although the birth typically takes place in a hospital, much maternal and child health care takes place through local primary care districts. Each such district has primary responsibility for the health care of the population in its area, ranging from 5,000 to 50,000 inhabitants. Each district operates one or more health care centers and clinics, staffed by district physicians (normally general practitioners), district nurses, and midwives. Pregnancy tests, pre- and postnatal care, childbirth preparation, family planning, parenthood education, and related services are provided through maternity clinics affiliated with these centers. The services include programs for the early detection of cervical cancer—all women aged 25-60 are called to the clinic once every four years for a Pap smear (Sundström-Feigenberg, 1988).

In the early 1980s, the average number of prenatal visits in Sweden was 14. Midwives play a major role in these visits, taking charge of 10 out of 13 or 14 planned visits (Blondel, Pusch, and Schmidt, 1986). The checkups typically begin in the 12th week of pregnancy and are biweekly until the final month prior to the projected delivery, at which point they take place weekly. At least two consultations with a physician are included. About eight weeks after the delivery, a postnatal checkup is done by the midwife or the physician (Sundström-Feigenberg, 1988).

Child health is further introduced during the mother's stay at the hospital maternity ward, at which time she is provided information about where and how the baby can get regular checkups, vaccinations, and so on during the next few years. These services are free of charge.

Fertility and Mortality Rates. With the exception of temporary increases in the 1940s and the 1960s, the birth rate has been falling steadily during the 20th century. The cumulative fertility rate (the number of children per women) decreased from slightly over 4 in 1890 to 2.0 in 1989. One in seven women does not give birth at all (Statistics Sweden, 1990). Sweden boasts one of the lowest infant mortality rates and highest life expectancies in the world. In 1989 the infant mortality rate (deaths during the first year of life per 1,000 live births) was 5 for girls and 7 for boys, down from 100 and 120 respectively in 1890 (Statistics Sweden, 1990). Perinatal mortality (the number of infants per 1,000 births who die before, during, and up to seven days after delivery) was 7 in 1984 (Sundström-Feigenberg, 1988). Life expectancy for a person born in the late 1980s was 74 years for men and 80 years for women.

The number of maternal deaths (deaths caused by complications during pregnancy and childbirth) has decreased drastically in Sweden from about 360 per 100,000 live births in 1930 to 4 and below per 100,000 live births per year in the 1980s (Nordic Statistical Secretariat, 1988; Sundström-Feigenberg, 1988).

Breastfeeding. Breastfeeding in Sweden reached an all-time low in 1972, with slightly over 30 percent of mothers breastfeeding at two months past delivery and less than 10 percent of mothers breastfeeding at six months (Hofvander, 1984). Since that time, there has been an upward trend. According to the National Board of Health and Welfare (NBHW), 89 percent of mothers were fully breastfeeding for at least one week and 69 percent were fully breastfeeding at two months after delivery in the late 1980s (Ransjö-Arvidson, 1989).

Family Planning. Sweden has a reputation for liberal attitudes toward sexuality that dates back to the 1930s. At that time the Population Commission made proposals concerning abortion, compulsory sex education in the schools, and easy access to birth control information and contraception. Compulsory sex education was implemented in 1956 (Scott, 1982; Brown, 1983). Oral contraceptives and IUDs were introduced in the mid-1960s. Initially high cost and physician gatekeeping limited access; however, when a new abortion act was passed in 1974, birth control was also made more accessible. Today, family planning services are provided at maternity clinics, district physicians' offices, private physicians' offices, and clinics run by the Swedish Association for Sexual Information. Adolescents can receive birth control advice at about 130 special youth clinics and from school physicians or nurses. Furthermore, midwives have been trained to give advice about contraceptives in order to make these more available. At present midwives perform 70 percent of the public health consultations regarding contraception, including insertion of IUDs and necessary prescriptions. The consultations and contraceptives are, to a large extent, free of charge.

Abortion. Abortion was originally permitted for certain medical conditions as early as 1937. The current law went into effect in 1975 and is based on the premise that the woman herself should decide whether or not to have an abortion. Abortion services are designed to avoid a separation between gynecological and other services, and to ensure that abortion is done as early as possible during pregnancy.

According to law, abortion is free upon request through the 18th week of pregnancy. Only if the abortion poses a threat to the woman's life may her request be refused. To obtain an abortion before the 12th week, the woman needs to consult with a physician; past that date she must also consult with a social worker. Abortions past the 18th week of pregnancy require the approval of the NBHW, and may not be given if the fetus is deemed to be viable. Any contacts with the woman's family members by health care workers prior to an abortion decision are to be made only in the woman's own interest and only with her approval. Abortions are only allowed by qualified medical practitioners, at institutions approved by the NBHW.

Abortions performed prior to the 12th week are usually done by vacuum aspiration. In 1989, these composed 92 percent of all abortions, while 0.6 percent were done after the 18th week. The rate of abortions per 1,000 women aged 15-44 was 21.5 in 1989. In the same year, the number of abortions per 1,000 women below the age of 20 was 24.7. In recent years there has been a slight increase in the rate of abortions, possibly attributable to less use of oral contraceptives and women's participation in the labor force (Swedish Institute, 1990b).

Abortion is not likely to be a closed chapter in Swedish reproductive history. New reproductive technologies have prompted debates over the beginnings of life as well as the need to protect "the unborn child." Inevitably, abortion is implicated in these debates.

Teenage Pregnancies. The high pregnancy rate of American teenagers is frequently compared to the much lower rate of Swedish teenagers. Given that the sexual behavior of Swedish teenagers poses equal or greater risk of pregnancy, it is argued that their lower pregnancy rate is to be explained by their contraceptive practices (Jones et al., 1986).

The pregnancy rate of teenage women in Sweden was fairly steady from the mid-1960s to the mid-1970s, while the abortion rate increased dramatically during the same period (Sundström-Feigenberg, 1988). Since the passage of the Abortion Act of 1974 and the associated access to contraceptives, both the pregnancy rate and the abortion rate for teenagers have been decreasing steadily, the former from 57.4 per 1,000 women in 1975 to 34.6 in 1981, and the latter from 28.6 in 1975 to 20.1 in 1981. In contrast, the teenage pregnancy rate in the U.S. was about three times greater (96.0 per 1,000 women) in 1981 (Jones et al., 1986). In 1988 the number of live births per 1,000 Swedish teenage women was 11.4 (Statistical Abstract of Sweden, 1990).

Sterilizations. Sterilizations are performed primarily for birth control (versus medical) reasons in Sweden. Prior to 1976, sterilization of men was not allowed, and for women only on the basis of eugenic, medical, or socio-medical reasons. It became free on demand for those age 25 and over with the enactment of a new law in 1976. Under the new law, those aged 18-24 require the approval of the NBHW. Approval is granted for genetic, or, in the case of women, for medical reasons. No one under the age 18 may be sterilized for the purpose of birth control. With passage of the new law, the number of sterilizations per year doubled. They reached a height in 1981 of about 7,000 per year for women and close to 3,000 per year for men, but have subsequently dropped, especially among men (Statistics Sweden, 1990).

Reproductive Technologies. Around 0.25 percent of the total number of births per year were offspring of donor insemination in the early 1980s. After a court case in which a boy conceived through donor insemination was declared "fatherless" caused a lively debate (Liljestrand, 1990), Parliament passed an Act in 1984 regulating donor insemination. Key features of the law are the following: Insemination may only be undertaken in public hospitals; the child has the right, upon reaching sufficient maturity, to know the identity of the donor; and only heterosexual couples who are married or cohabiting may have access to insemination.

Four years later an In Vitro Fertilization (IVF) Act was passed. This legislation stipulates that IVF may only be undertaken in public hospitals unless a special permit has been given by the NBHW. IVF may not be undertaken with the sperm of any man but only with the woman's husband or cohabitant. Further, an ovum fertilized outside the body may be implanted only in the woman with whom it originated. Finally, the Act prohibits IVF involving a donated ovum as well as surrogacy. ✱ PETRA LILJESTRAND, Ph.D.

See **Guide to Related Topics:** Cross-Cultural Perspectives

Resources

Bergsjø, P., Schmidt, E., & Pusch, D. (1986). "Differences in the Reported Frequencies of Some Obstetrical Interventions in Europe." In J.M.L. Phaff. (Ed.) Perinatal Health Services in Europe: Searching for Better Childbirth. London: Croom Helm, pp. 82-91.

Blondel, B., Pusch, D., & Schmidt, E. (1986). "Some Characteristics of Antenatal Care in 13 European Countries." In J.M.L. Phaff. (Ed.) Perinatal Health Services in Europe: Searching for Better Childbirth. London: Croom Helm, pp. 3-9.

Brown, P. (1983). "The Swedish Approach to Sex Education and Adolescent Pregnancy: Some Impressions." Family Planning Perspectives 15 (2): 92-95.

Hofvander, Y. (1984). "Home-like Post-partum Care and the Promotion of Breast-feeding: The Ringblomman Experience in Sweden." Advances in International Maternal and Child Health 4: 53-58.

Houd, S. & Oakley, A. (1986). "Alternative Perinatal Services." In J.M.L. Phaff (Ed.) Perinatal Health Services in Europe: Searching for Better Childbirth. London: Croom Helm, pp. 17-27.

Jones, E.F. et al. (1986). Teenage Pregnancy in Industrialized Countries. New Haven, CT: Yale University Press.

Jordan, B. (1980). Birth in Four Cultures: A Cross-cultural Investigation of Childbirth in Yucatan, Holland, Sweden and the United States. Montreal: Eden Press Women's Publications.

Liljestrand, P. (1990). Rhetoric and Reason: Donor Insemination Politics in Sweden. Unpublished doctoral dissertation, University of California, San Francisco.

Nordic Statistical Secretariat. (1988). Yearbook of Nordic Statistics, Volume 27. Copenhagen, Denmark: Nordic Statistical Secretariat.

Ransjö-Arvidson, A.B. (1989). Reflections of Maternity Care Routines in Sweden and Zambia (Society and Birth, vol. 3). Stockholm: Department of International Health Care Research, Karolinska Institutet.

Scott, H. (1982). Sweden's "Right to be Human"—Sex-role Equality: The Goal and the Reality. Armond, NY: M.E. Sharpe.

Statistical Abstract of Sweden. (1990). Statistical Abstract of Sweden. Stockholm: Statistics Sweden.

Statistics Sweden. (1990). Women and Men in Sweden: Equality of the Sexes. Stockholm: Statistics Sweden.

Sundström-Feigenberg, K. (1988). "Reproductive Health and Reproductive Freedom: Maternal Health Care and Family Planning in the Swedish Health System." *Women and Health 13* (3/4): 34-50.

Swedish Institute. (1989a). Fact Sheets on Sweden: Equality between Men and Women in Sweden (FS 82 i Ohj). Stockholm: The Swedish Institute.

———. (1989b). Fact Sheets on Sweden: Health and Medical Care in Sweden (FS 76 p Vpb). Stockholm: The Swedish Institute.

———. (1990a). Fact Sheets on Sweden: Child Care in Sweden. Stockholm: The Swedish Institute.

———. (1990b). Fact Sheets on Sweden: Family Planning in Sweden. Stockholm: The Swedish Institute.

Swedish Planning and Rationalization Institute for the Health and Social Services. (1987). Some Facts about Health Care in Sweden. Stockholm: SPRI.

For Further Information

Note: The fact sheets cited, and many others, are produced regularly by the Swedish Institute. They can be obtained free of charge through the nearest Swedish Embassy or Consulate or by writing to one of the addresses below:

The Swedish Institute
Box 7434
S-103 91 Stockholm,
Sweden

The Swedish Information Service
One Dag Hammarskjold Plaza
New York, NY 10017-2201

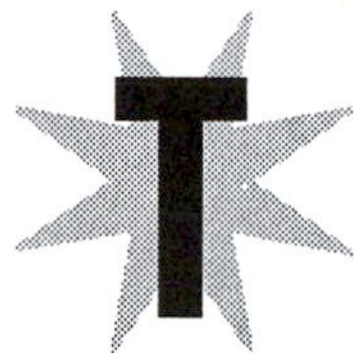

TEENAGE CHILDBEARING: SOCIOECONOMIC ASPECTS

Adolescent pregnancy is a topic that receives much research and media attention in the United States. The rate of adolescent pregnancy in the United States is higher than most other industrialized countries. In 1984, 13.1 percent of all births were to mothers under the age of 20 (Hughes et al., 1987). However, births to teenage mothers represent a disproportionately higher rate of low birth-weight births: 9.4 percent for adolescent mothers compared with 6.7 percent of all births in 1984 (Hughes et al., 1987). Low birth weight (5.5 lbs or less at birth) is the greatest single contributing cause of death among children under the age of one (Rosenbaum, 1985; Children's Defense Fund, 1989). Contrary to popular assumptions, the rate of adolescent pregnancy in the United States has stabilized in recent years, but the tendency for young mothers to remain single has increased substantially.

While adolescent pregnancy is obviously the result of sexual activity with unsuccessful efforts or no efforts to use contraception, *adolescent childbearing* is the conscious and often constrained decision to bear the child.

Early attempts to characterize pregnant adolescents as somehow deviant or maladjusted are not supported by more recent and thorough investigations. Much of the early literature failed to conceptualize the problem in an unbiased manner, choosing instead to assume that pregnant adolescents differed from their cohorts and were deviant and disturbed, and neglecting to control for cultural, economic, or racial differences (Barth, Schinke, and Maxwell, 1983; Winett, King, and Altman, 1989). In general, much of the current literature supports the conclusion that pregnant adolescents do not differ significantly from their nonpregnant counterparts on personality variables when demographic and variables of race and socioeconomic status are controlled (De Anda, 1983).

The etiology of adolescent pregnancy is complex, and the health, social, and economic consequences to the adolescent mother and her children have both short- and long-term repercussions for everyone involved. Because lower socioeconomic status, lower levels of education, and minority status are characteristics of pregnant teenagers as a whole when compared to nonpregnant teens or older pregnant women, this population is more likely to fall into unfavorable categories of nutritional status and less likely to participate actively in institutionalized systems of health care delivery (Rosenbaum, 1985).

Research evidence suggests that it is not the biology of early childbearing that is responsible for the poor birth outcomes that are seen in this population, but rather it is the group characteristics of these young mothers that contribute to the lower birth weights. Adolescents who give birth are more likely to be black, poor, and unmarried than women in older childbearing age groups (National Research Council, 1987). Each of these demographic characteristics (race, poverty status, and marital status) has been identified as a risk factor for poor birth outcomes (Institute of Medicine, 1985).

Although the rate of births to white adolescents is increasing, four out of five teenage births are to black women (Rosenbaum, 1985). Poor adolescents are two-and-a-half times more likely to become parents than are nonpoor adolescents (Children's Defense Fund, 1989). These statistics reflect not only the higher rates of pregnancy for poor and minority youth but also patterns of sexual activity and choices regarding childbearing. Poor adolescents are more likely to become sexually active at an earlier age, with urban teens showing more sexual activity than nonurban teens and ghetto adolescents showing more sexual activity than nonghetto residents (Salguero, 1984; Randolph and Gesche, 1986). In addition, teenagers of low socioeconomic status are less likely to use contraception than other teenagers (National Research Council, 1987).

More poor adolescents carry their fetus to term when compared with middle- and upper-income adolescents (Rosenbaum, 1985; Winett, King, and Altman, 1989). The availability of abortion as an option is different for these populations, both from economic and cultural standpoints.

Receiving public assistance such as Aid to Families with Dependent Children (AFDC) does not appear to induce higher rates of pregnancy (Flick, 1984). Jones et al., (1985) evaluated 36 developed countries and found that all of the countries that had more generous welfare programs than the United States also reported lower rates of teenage pregnancy.

Women who become pregnant at an early age are understandably less likely to complete high school or go on to higher education than those unencumbered with the responsibilities of parenthood. Also in the past decade, young mothers have shown a trend towards remaining single. As a result of these factors, as a group, young mothers show patterns of long-term economic hardship. A young mother is at increased risk for poverty status and reliance on government entitlement programs. This cycle of poverty may have long-term consequences for the health and educational opportunities of children born to young mothers.

Nutritional status and prenatal care are also important factors that contribute to the overall poorer birth outcome seen in pregnant adolescents. Young mothers are more likely to receive late or inadequate prenatal care than their older cohorts. The nutritional needs for teenagers are greater than for women in their 20s or 30s, and pregnancy adds additional nutrition burdens which may not be met by the average teenager's diet.

The factors that lead to poorer birth outcomes for early childbearing are complex and interrelated. The failure to be able to separate the risk factors that contribute to "the problem" of adolescent pregnancy and the individual and societal costs of adolescent pregnancy should encourage integrated, multilevel approaches in school, community, and public health settings (Winett, King, and Altman, 1989). Individuals and organizations concerned with early childbearing in the United States are calling for multilevel, integrated approaches to both the prevention of teenage pregnancy and the enhancement of birth outcomes for young mothers. Also stressed in recent evaluations of the problem is the heterogeneous nature of the population of pregnant teens and the need to tailor programs and efforts to the specific cultural and ethnic backgrounds of the targeted population (Hughes et al., 1987; Institute of Medicine, 1987).

✱ DIANE E. DEPKEN, Ed.D.

See also: Low Birth Weight: United States; Teenage Childbearing: Trends in the United States

Resources

Barth, R.P., Schinke, S.P., & Maxwell, J.S. (1983). "Psychological Correlates of Teenage Motherhood. *Journal of Youth and Adolescence* 12 (6): 471-87.

Children's Defense Fund. (1989). *A Children's Defense Fund Budget*. Washington, DC: Children's Defense Fund.

De Anda, D. (1983). "Pregnancy in Early and Late Adolescence." *Journal of Youth and Adolescence* 12 (1): 33-42.

Flick, L. (1984). *Adolescent Childbearing Decisions: Implications for Prevention*. St. Louis: Danforth Foundation.

Alan Guttmacher Institute. (1987). *Blessed Events and the Bottom Line: Financing Maternity Care in the United States*. New York: Alan Guttmacher Institute.

Hughes, D. et al. (1987). *The Health of America's Children: Maternal and Child Health Data Book*. Washington, DC: Children's Defense Fund.

Institute of Medicine. (1987). *Preventing Low Birthweight*. Washington, DC: National Academy Press.

Jones, E.F. et al. (1985). "Teenage Pregnancy in Developed Countries: Determinants and Policy Implications." *Family Planning Perspectives* 17 (2): 63-68.

National Research Council. (1987). *Risking the Future: Adolescent Sexuality, Pregnancy and Childbearing*. Volume 1. Washington, DC: National Academy Press.

Randolph, L.A. & Gesche, M. (1986). "Black Adolescent Pregnancy: Prevention and Management." *Journal of Community Health* 11 (1): 10-18.

Rosenbaum, S. (1985). *A Manual on Providing Prenatal Care Programs for Teens*. Washington, DC: Children's Defense Fund.

Salguero, C. (1984). "The Role of Ethnic Factors on Adolescent Pregnancy and Motherhood." In M. Sugar (Ed.) *Adolescent Parenthood*. New York: Spectrum Publications, pp. 75-98.

Winett, R., King, A., & Altman, D. (1989). *Health Psychology and Public Health: An Integrative Approach*. New York: Pergamon Press.

TEENAGE CHILDBEARING: TRENDS IN THE UNITED STATES

After rising rapidly during the 1940s and 1950s, teenage birth rates began to fall during the 1960s and 1970s. The birth rate for 15- to 19-year-old women rose from 54 per 1,000 in 1940 to 96 per 1,000 in 1957. By 1975, the rate had dropped to 56. Since 1975, there has been relatively little change in teenage birth rates; the rate in 1988 was 54 (Ventura, 1984; National Center for Health Statistics, 1990).

The trend for young teenagers has been somewhat different than that for all teenagers as a group. Birth rates for 15- to 17-year-old women increased from 36 per 1,000 in 1966 to 39 in 1972 and then fell until 1986, reaching 31. Between 1986 and 1988, the rate rose 10 percent, to 34. Rates for older teens fell by one-third from the mid-1960s to the mid-1970s, from 120 per 1,000 in 1966 to 80 per 1,000 in 1978. The 1988 rate was 82.

Some of the recent increase in rates for young teenagers may be explained by related data from the National Survey of Family Growth (NSFG), conducted by the National Center for Health Statistics. Data from the 1988 cycle of the NSFG show that the proportion of young teenagers who are sexually experienced increased considerably during the 1980s (Forrest and Singh, 1990; Pratt, Eglash, and London, 1990). For example, 26 percent of teens aged 15 years old in 1988 had had sexual intercourse, compared with 16 percent of 15-year-olds in 1980.

Birth rates for black teens have been substantially above those for white teens; since 1970, the rates for black women under 20 have been about 2.5 times those for white women. In 1988, the rate for black teenagers was 106 per 1,000 women aged 15-19 years, compared with a rate of 44 per 1,000 for white teens (Table 1).

The peak year for number of births to teenagers since 1940 was 1970, with 656,000 births reported to mothers under 20 years of age. The number of births fell from 1970 to 1986, to 472,000. The number increased in 1988 to 489,000. The decline in numbers through 1986 reflects the small decline in the birth rates but, to a greater extent, the reduced number of teenagers in the population (U.S. Bureau of the Census, 1990). The teenagers of the mid 1980s were born after the baby boom had ended. While teenage mothers accounted for 19 percent of all births in 1972, they accounted for just 13 percent in 1988.

Table 1. Number of Births and Birth Rates for All Teenagers and for Unmarried Teenagers by Race: United States, 1970, 1980, 1985, and 1988

Age of mother and year	All births						Births to unmarried women[1]					
	Number			Rate[2]			Number			Rate[2]		
	All races[3]	White	Black	All races[3]	White	Black	All races[3]	White	Black	All races[3]	White	Black
10-14 years												
1970......	11,752	4,320	7,274	1.2	0.5	5.2	9,500	2,500	6,800	—	—	—
1980......	10,169	4,171	5,793	1.1	0.6	4.3	9,024	3,144	5,707	—	—	—
1985......	10,220	4,101	5,860	1.2	0.6	4.5	9,386	3,380	5,783	—	—	—
1988......	10,588	4,073	6,182	1.3	0.6	4.8	9,907	3,522	6,111	—	—	—
15-19 years												
1970......	644,708	463,608	171,826	68.3	57.4	140.7	190,400	79,300	107,800	22.4	10.9	96.9
1980......	552,161	388,058	150,353	53.0	44.7	100.0	262,777	127,984	128,022	27.6	16.2	89.2
1985......	467,485	318,725	134,270	51.3	42.8	97.4	270,922	142,131	120,378	31.6	20.5	88.8
1988......	478,353	315,471	146,326	53.6	43.7	105.9	312,499	168,641	133,419	36.8	24.8	98.3
15-17 years												
1970......	223,590	143,646	76,882	38.8	29.2	101.4	96,100	36,200	58,400	17.1	7.5	77.9
1980......	198,222	127,657	65,966	32.5	25.2	73.6	121,900	57,761	61,204	20.6	11.8	69.6
1985......	167,789	106,042	56,809	31.1	24.0	69.8	118,931	61,341	54,136	22.5	14.2	97.0
1988......	176,624	106,907	63,833	33.8	25.5	76.6	136,137	70,501	61,299	26.5	17.1	74.1
18-19 years												
1970......	421,118	319,962	94,944	114.7	101.5	204.9	94,300	43,100	49,400	32.9	17.6	136.4
1980......	353,939	260,401	84,387	82.1	72.1	138.8	140,877	70,223	66,818	39.0	23.6	120.2
1985.....	299,696	212,683	77,461	80.8	70.1	137.1	151,991	80,790	66,242	46.6	30.9	121.1
1988......	301,729	208,564	82,493	81.7	69.2	150.5	176,362	98,140	72,120	52.7	36.4	136.1

[1] For 1970, births to unmarried women are estimated for the United States from data for registration areas in which marital status of mother was reported. For 1980-88, data for states in which marital status was not reported have been inferred from other items on the birth certificate and included with data from the reporting states.

[2] Rates per 1,000 women in specified group.

[3] Includes races other than white and black.

— = Not available.

Childbearing by unmarried teenagers has risen substantially since 1970, continuing a long period of steady increase since 1940, when national data on this topic first became available. The increase in nonmarital childbearing is reflected by all measures used to analyze this topic, including rising birth rates and numbers and proportions of births to unmarried teenaged mothers. The birth rate increased 68 percent, from 22 per 1,000 unmarried women aged 15-19 in 1970 to 37 per 1,000 unmarried women aged 15-19 in 1988. Rates for both younger and older teens have more than doubled (National Center for Health Statistics, 1990) (Table 1).

Although the number of teen births in 1988 was far below what it was in 1972, a sizable proportion of them are to girls under age 18—38 percent in 1988. Very young mothers have the most challenges. Their opportunity to secure a high school diploma is virtually eliminated, at least in the short run, with possible lifetime consequences for their financial security. Partly because their economic and other resources are limited, so is their access to prenatal care and other support services (National Research Council, 1987).

As just indicated, teenaged mothers are considerably less likely to have completed high school than are older mothers. Even if the comparison is restricted to teenaged mothers 18-19, that is, those who should have had an opportunity to complete high school, a sizable differential is observed. Overall, in 1988, 53 percent of mothers aged 18-19, compared with 86 percent of older mothers, had completed high school (Table 2).

Prenatal care initiated early in pregnancy can be beneficial by providing the mother with professional guidance on nutrition and other important matters related to her pregnancy, and by identifying any preexisting medical conditions or other problems that might need special attention during the pregnancy. Birth certificate data demonstrate that teenaged mothers are more likely than older mothers to receive delayed care (beginning in the third trimester) or no care at all. Among white teen mothers, the proportion receiving delayed or no care in 1988 ranged from 11 percent for those aged 18-19 years to 22 percent for those aged 10-14 years, compared with 3-7 percent of mothers in their 20s. Among black mothers, the comparable proportions were 14-20 percent for teens and 9-12 percent for mothers in their 20s. Infants born to mothers receiving no prenatal care at all have a much higher risk of being low birth weight. In 1988, nearly one-fourth of babies born to teenaged mothers who had no prenatal care weighed less than 5.5 pounds at birth compared with 8-12 percent of babies whose mothers had some care.

The proportion of babies weighing less than 5.5 pounds at birth is a key indicator of birth outcome

Table 2. Selected Characteristics of Births to Teenage Mothers: United States, 1988

Characteristic	10-14 years			15-19 years: Total			15-17 years			18-19 years		
	All races[1]	White	Black	All races[1]	White	Black	All races[1]	White	Black	All races[1]	White	Black
	Percent											
Mothers completing high school[2]	—	—	—	37.0	38.0	35.6	8.7	9.0	8.2	52.9	52.4	57.0
Births to unmarried mothers[3]	93.6	86.5	98.9	65.3	53.5	91.2	77.1	65.9	96.0	58.5	47.1	87.4
Mothers who began prenatal care in first trimester	36.5	38.4	35.2	53.5	56.4	47.6	48.9	51.8	44.4	56.1	58.7	50.0
Mothers who had late or no prenatal care[4]	21.0	22.1	20.2	12.7	11.5	15.0	14.2	13.1	15.8	11.8	10.7	14.3

[1] Includes races other than white and black.

[2] Excludes data for California, New York State (exclusive of New York City), Texas, and Washington, which did not require reporting of educational attainment of mother.

[3] For 42 states and the District of Columbia, marital status of the mother is reported on the birth certificate; for 8 states mother's marital status is inferred from other items on the birth certificate.

[4] Care beginning in third trimester or no care.

[5] Birth weight of less than 2,500 grams (5 lb. 8 oz.)

and is closely associated with infant health and survival. Small babies have higher rates of illness and disabling conditions and a greater risk of dying in the first year of life. Infants born to teen mothers are at much greater risk of low birth weight than are those born to older mothers (Table 2). This elevated risk of low birth weight among babies born to teenagers has been observed for many years and is associated in many cases with inadequate diet and nutrition. The 1980 National Natality Survey, conducted by the National Center for Health Statistics, found that mothers under age 20 were much more likely to gain less than 16 pounds during pregnancy. Weight gain of less than 16 pounds is associated with a considerably elevated risk of a low birth-weight outcome (Taffel, 1986). In 1988, young teenaged mothers under 18 were from 61 to 123 percent more likely to have a low-weight baby than mothers in their late 20s (National Center for Health Statistics, 1990).

✷ STEPHANIE J. VENTURA, A.M.

See also: Low Birth Weight: United States; Premature Births: Prevention; Prenatal Care in the United States; Teenage Childbearing: Socioeconomic Aspects

Resources

Forrest, J.D. & Singh, S. (1990). "The Sexual and Reproductive Behavior of American Women, 1982-1988." *Family Planning Perspectives* 22 (5): 206-15.

National Center for Health Statistics. (1990). "Advance Report of Final Natality Statistics, 1988." *Monthly Vital Statistics Report 39* (4) supplement. Hyattsville, MD: Public Health Service.

National Research Council (U.S.). Panel on Adolescent Pregnancy and Childbearing. (1987). *Risking the Future.* Volumes I and II. Washington, DC: National Academy Press.

Pratt, W.F., Eglash, S., & London, K.A. (1990). "Premarital Sexual Behavior, Multiple Partners, and Marital Experience." Paper presented at the annual meeting of the Population Association of America, Toronto, Canada.

Taffel, S. (1986). "Maternal Weight Gain and the Outcome of Pregnancy, United States, 1980." *Vital and Health Statistics*, Series 21, No. 44. Hyattsville, MD: National Center for Health Statistics.

U.S. Bureau of the Census. (1990). "U.S. Population Estimates by Age, Sex, Race, and Hispanic Origin: 1980 to 1988." *Current Population Reports*, Series P-25, No. 1045. Washington, DC: U.S. Department of Commerce.

Ventura, S.J. (1984). "Trends in Teenage Childbearing, United States, 1970-81." *Vital and Health Statistics*, Series 21, No. 41. Hyattsville, MD: National Center for Health Statistics.

THALIDOMIDE

Thalidomide was a drug sold primarily as a sedative, starting in 1957. Although it was advertised as being "completely safe" and having no side effects, it turned out to cause severe birth defects when taken in the first trimester of pregnancy. Between 1958 and 1962, thousands of babies were born with these defects, which included missing, shortened, or misshapen limbs; deafness; severe facial deformities; seizure disorders; dwarfism; and brain damage. Today there are some 8,000 thalidomide-affected adults, and it has been estimated that twice that many babies were stillborn or died shortly after birth because of defects caused by thalidomide. The thalidomide epidemic continued for many months after the withdrawal of the drug in 1961; doctors and pharmacists continued to dispense it despite warnings and headlines.

Thalidomide was formulated in 1953 by Chemie Grunenthal, a German pharmaceutical company. Four years later, thalidomide was released for nonprescription sale. It quickly became Germany's most popular sleeping pill. The miracle of thalidomide was that it acted faster and was more powerful than the other hypnotics of the day, and it didn't kill test animals, despite large doses. However, Grunenthal had little idea how thalidomide worked. Testing was inadequate by the standards of the time and did not include any tests for danger to the fetus, even though it was known in the 1950s that a substance such as thalidomide could cross the placenta. About the same time, in Great Britain, Distillers Company (Biochemicals) Limited, or DCBL, was looking to expand their drug sales. Sleeping pills were a $5 million market, with one out of eight National Health prescriptions being sleeping aids. DCBL started selling thalidomide in Great Britain in 1958, under the trade name "Distaval." In 1959, DCBL sent a notice to doctors advising them of its safety for nursing mothers, pregnant women, and their babies. DCBL got this information from Grunenthal, choosing not to do extensive testing of its own.

Also in the 1950s, Grunenthal decided to expand to the American market. Smith, Kline & French dismissed thalidomide after two years of trials, after discovering that it had no significant hypnotic effect. Lederle also rejected the drug. In 1958, Richardson-Merrell acquired U.S. marketing and manufacturing rights from Grunenthal.

Like DCBL, Richardson-Merrell relied on Grunenthal for much of its testing results, but the FDA did not accept European trials. Richardson-Merrell produced animal tests with similar results to those of Smith, Kline & French. In 1959 Richardson-Merrell started distributing its drug, Kevadon, to doctors to give to their patients, including pregnant women. Because Richardson-Merrell did not demand stringent record keeping for its testing, many victims of Kevadon may have gone unrecognized. In September 1960, Dr. Frances Kelsey of the FDA was assigned the investigation of Kevadon as her first case. Kelsey found several problems with Richardson-Merrell's application. Despite pressure on her and her FDA superiors from Richardson-Merrell, Kelsey continued her demands for complete testing of Kevadon and full disclosure of the results. In 1961, Grunenthal removed thalidomide from the market amidst mounting reports of babies being born with severe deformities. Kelsey had prevented a major American tragedy with her insight and questions.

Compensation claims for thalidomide victims and their families took years to settle and varied greatly from country to country, as lawyers and parents muddled through complex legal systems.

Many reforms in drug regulations around the world resulted from the thalidomide disaster. Still, drug companies continue to produce medications with questionable effects for the pregnant woman. One such drug was Bendectin, which received much negative publicity in the United States and Europe in the early 1980s and was removed from the market.

✱ B. COLLENE STOUT, M.S.W., C.S.W.

See also: DES: Diethylstilbestrol; Research Issues in Childbirth

Resources

Fine, Ralph Adam. (1972). *The Great Drug Deception: The Shocking Story of MER/29 and the Folks Who Gave You Thalidomide.* New York: Stein and Day.

Insight Team of *The Sunday Times* of London (Phillip Knightly, Harold Evans, Elaine Potter, Marjorie Wallace). (1979). *Suffer the Children: The Story of Thalidomide.* New York: Viking Press.

Kelsey, Frances O. (1988). "Thalidomide Update: Regulatory Aspects." *Teratology 38*: 221-26.

McBride, William G. (1977). "Thalidomide Embryopathy." *Teratology 16* (1): 79-82.

Newman, C.G.H. (1985). "Teratogen Update: Clinical Aspects of Thalidomide Embryopathy—A Continuing Preoccupation." *Teratology 32* (1): 133-44.

Quibell, E.P. (1981). "The Thalidomide Embryopathy: An Analysis from the UK." *The Practitioner 225* (1355): 721-26.

THERAPEUTIC ABORTION. *See instead* SELECTIVE ABORTION

TORCH SYNDROME

TORCH Syndrome is an infection of the fetus or newborn with one of the TORCH agents, most commonly diagnosed after a miscarriage or stillbirth, or if the baby exhibits a wide variety of birth defects or symptoms including blindness, hearing problems, fever, or other signs of infection. TORCH is an acronym for toxoplasmosis, other infections, rubella virus, cytomegalovirus, and herpes simplex viruses.

Toxoplasmosis. Toxoplasmosis is an infection caused by a protozoan found in birds and transferred to cats or other animals; thus, pregnant women should be aware of the danger of handling cats and their litter, the need for washing their hands before handling food, and the importance of eating only well-cooked meat.

During pregnancy, toxoplasmosis is asymptomatic in about 90 percent of cases, but if infection is suspected, blood tests showing a high, rising titre (or measure) can confirm recent infection. The infection is passed to the baby via the placenta in 35 to 50 percent of cases, depending on when in the pregnancy the infection occurs. Miscarriage usually occurs if it is contracted during the first trimester. Stillbirth and premature birth are also possible. Toxoplasmosis is a significant factor in causing mental retardation and blindness in the newborn. Sulfadiazone, pyrimethamine, and folinic acids are sometimes given to treat the infection.

Other Infections. Despite the notoriety of rubella and herpes infections, 90 percent of the cases of TORCH syndrome are the result of "other" undetermined infections (Urdang and Swallow, 1983). Pregnant women should therefore make every effort to avoid contact with people who are ill with infectious diseases.

Rubella Virus. Pregnant women are routinely screened during pregnancy for immunity to rubella. If not immune, they should be especially careful to avoid exposure to German measles and should be immunized before future pregnancies. If a pregnant woman contracts rubella during the first eight weeks of pregnancy, the baby is likely to be infected 50 percent of the time and have noticeable birth defects in 85 percent of the cases.

The risk decreases as the pregnancy progresses, and there are no reported defects after 24 weeks.

Cytomegalovirus. Babies born to mothers infected for the first time during pregnancy are much more likely to develop severe congenital anomalies than with a recurring infection. Primary infection during pregnancy is usually asymptomatic but can be diagnosed by blood tests. It is most often first diagnosed by testing a baby who is stillborn or who has severe birth defects, including brain and liver damage.

Herpes Simplex Virus (HSV). Stanford researchers now estimate that newborns have about an 8 percent chance of contracting HSV from passing through an infected mother's birth canal (Arvin and Prober, 1986). If contracted, the disease will cause death about 50 percent of the time, and half of the survivors will suffer serious neurologic damage.

Guidelines. The following new guidelines have been issued by the Infectious Disease Society for Obstetrics and Gynecology (Gibbs et al, 1988):

> Women with a history of genital herpes but no lesions do not need weekly herpes cultures; they may deliver vaginally with mother or baby being cultured after the birth.
>
> Women with genital lesions near their due date should have cultures every 3 to 5 days to increase the likelihood of a vaginal birth. A cesarean is recommended with pre-outbreak symptoms or lesions when labor begins or the membranes rupture.
>
> There is a much higher risk of the baby contracting the disease through the placenta if the mother has her first herpes infection during pregnancy; these babies should be born by cesarean. Newborns can also get herpes from cold sores of staff or relatives after the birth.

✱ RAHIMA BALDWIN

See **Guide to Related Topics:** Pregnancy Complications

Resources

Arvin, Ann & Prober, Charles. (1986). "Neonatal Herpes." *The Helper*. Palo Alto, CA: Herpes Research Center.

Beischer, Norman & MacKay, Eric. (1986). *Obstetrics and the Newborn*. London: Bailliere Tindall.

Gibbs, R.S. et al. (1988, May). "Editorial: Management of Genital Herpes Infection in Pregnancy." *Obstetrics and Gynecology* 71: 779-80.

Urdang, Laurence & Swallow, Helen (Eds.) (1983). *Mosby's Medical and Nursing Dictionary*. St. Louis: C.V. Mosby Co.

TOXEMIA. *See instead* BREWER PREGNANCY DIET

TOXOPLASMOSIS. *See instead* TORCH SYNDROME

TOYS FOR BABIES

Baby toys, that is, playthings made for children in the first year of life, are both a barometer of a culture's economic diversification and a reflection of parents' or families' expectations for infants. Groups economically marginalized in the developed or developing world, whether tribal, peasant, or urban, usually will not expend valuable resources in time or materials creating numerous, enduring toys for infants. Parents in such situations may sustain only modest expectations that their children will survive past the first year or two of life. Baby toys, as well as toys made for older children, will usually be fashioned ingeniously from materials found in the environment, such as wood, stone, straw, seeds, bones, corncobs, shells, gourds, twine, rags, string, used tin cans, old rubber tires, and paper. A Mayan Indian of Mexico may use a dried flower or stalk of grass as a toy to bounce off a baby's nose.

Lack of baby toys in many cultures closely relates to caretakers carrying infants almost constantly until babies walk. Feeding on demand and being surrounded continuously by human contact provide the same stimulation and comfort offered by toys. Baby jumpers, swings, bouncers, rocking horses, and music boxes produced by specialized toy manufacturers today substitute for the comforting movement and ambient voices offered children whose parents expect their babies will be safe and healthy if kept in close physical contact with a caretaker.

Another form of infant care, swaddling, practiced for centuries among Europeans, Native Americans, and others, kept babies' arms and legs immobile to promote healthy growth and discipline, and to ensure safety. Swaddled babies were able to gaze at or hear, but not touch, their toys.

The presence of numerous baby toys indicates growing social stratification, whether among economically deprived or more prosperous peoples. Baby toys indicate growing affluence and mobility. Successful farmers worldwide may forego homemade playthings and buy plastic toys, purchased in markets or cities. Archaeologists have unearthed some of the earliest recognized toys from tombs dating about 1400 B.C. of wealthy ancient Egyptians, including dolls, balls, and animals on rollers (Fraser, 1966, p. 24). In ancient Greece, toys made of bone, wood, leather, lead, and bronze indicate probable use by diverse income groups.

Some toys, particularly rattles and dangling bead-toy ornaments, protect babies from harmful witchcraft, bad spirits, or the evil eye. Rattles in cultures throughout the world may be used by shamans or priests to summon or ward off spirits (Needham, 1967), and at times could be confused with children's toys if not carefully researched. Baby rattles may have been imbued with some of the protective supernatural properties of percussion at the same time they amused and provided a soothing teething object. Rattles of ancient Greece and Rome were likely used both by children and ritualists (Fraser, 1966, pp. 46-49, Jenkins, 1986, pp. 30-37). Ornate silver rattles from Medieval times through the early 20th century in Europe and North America often held a piece of decorative and protective red coral in the shape of a wolf's tooth (Fraser, 1966, p. 62).

Hanging from baby carriers in the Middle East, bright blue beads not only divert a baby's attention but also ward off the evil eye. Among traditional Japanese, a spindle-shaped wooden toy called a Somin-Shorai harks to its protection during an epidemic, while animal heads of clay or papier-mâché on bamboo canes ward off harm (Fraser, 1966, pp. 38-39). Native-American mothers of the Plains encased children's umbilical cords in tiny beaded turtles or lizards, then hung them from the side of the child's carrier. As a toy, the beaded animal visually entertained the immobile child, but as a ritual object, it protected a child from harm, induced longevity, and instilled obedience (Hail, 1980, p. 154). Contemporary parents in Western cultures express similar concerns for their children's welfare, not with beds and rattles, but by using products like Health-Tex clothing and endorsing child safety legislation that protects babies from hazardous toys.

Reasons people offer toys to babies reflect parental and cultural expectations for children. While toys demonstrate affection for and acceptance of infants, assist children and adults to cope with difficulties such as overtiredness or teething, and stimulate a child's intellectual and sensory growth (hence the abundance of "educational toys" in the United States and Europe), early playthings also begin to inculcate in children the values of the parent and the culture. Toy givers may not even be conscious of this inculcation. Values for parents in the United States can include promoting intelligence and independence, celebrating the playfulness and perceived innocence of babies, indicating a family's social status, and in some cases as more children enter day care apart from parents, compensating for time spent away from babies.

Through toys babies learn some of their first lessons about the culture into which they have been born. Materials from which the toys are made will be drawn from the child's physical environment and become associated with early sensory experiences and expectations of status and physical comfort. Shapes and colors reflect the decorative visual arts in a child's life. These arts may have associations with the empowerment of religious figures as in India (Devi and Kurin, 1985, p. 132). Throughout centuries, artisans worldwide have created baby rattles in the art style currently fashionable.

Some toys inculcate concepts about role and gender. Infant boys of India ride an ornate cart, reinforcing the identity between Lord Krishna and the child (Devi and Kurin, 1985, p. 142), while wealthy Victorian babies played with nursery tale figures and animal-shaped toys considered appropriate for children segregated from the cares of adult life (Cohn and Leach, 1987, p. 297). In the United States, toys can be color-coded pink for girls and blue for boys, and can endorse cultural stereotyping of gender, stultifying for individual growth in a country where individualism is admired. Yet individualism itself is a cultural value; the creativity or independence parents foster with toys among some peoples can be associated with witchcraft or other anti-social traits among others. Thus, parents, siblings, and other adults encourage babies to interact with their toys to perpetuate the familiar culture and reinforce the beliefs and experiences that adults transform into political, religious, social, and economic life (Linn, 1987, pp. 181-84). ✱ PRISCILLA RACHUN LINN, D.Phil.

See also: Swaddling

See **Guide to Related Topics:** Baby Care

Resources

Aries, Philippe. (1962). *Centuries of Childhood.* New York: Knopf.

Cohn, Anna R. & Leach, Lucinda. (1987). *Generations: A Universal Family Album.* New York: Pantheon Books; Washington, DC: Smithsonian Institution Traveling Exhibition Services.

Devi, Pria & Kurin, Richard. (1985). *Aditi: The Living Arts of India.* Washington, DC: Smithsonian Institution Press.

Fraser, Antonia. (1966). *A History of Toys.* New York: Delacorte Press.

Hail, Barbara. (1980). *Hau, K La!* Providence, RI: Haffenreffer Museum of Anthropology, Brown University.
Jenkins, Ian. (1987). *Greek and Roman Life.* London: British Museum Publications.
Linn, Priscilla Rachun. (1987). "No Object too Small: A Thought on Babies, Things, and Culture." In Anna R. Cohn & Lucinda Leach (Eds.) *Generations: A Universal Family Album.* New York: Pantheon Books; Washington, DC: Smithsonian Institution Traveling Exhibition Services, pp. 606-14.
Needham, Rodney. (1967). "Percussion and Transition." *Journal of the Royal Anthropological Institute (Man), II* (4): 606-14.

TWILIGHT SLEEP

Twilight Sleep was a hospital-based technique for painless birth, developed in Germany in 1914. This technique involved injecting the woman with morphine at the beginning of labor and then giving her a dose of an amnesiac drug, called scopolamine, which caused her to forget what was happening; once the fetus entered the birth canal, the doctor gave ether or chloroform to relieve the pain caused by the birth of the baby's head. Altogether, the procedure dulled the awareness of pain and, perhaps more important, removed the memory of it. A few American doctors had tried the technique around 1900 and rejected it as unreliable and unsafe, but several American women were so excited by the prospect of a completely painless delivery that they went to Freiburg, Germany, during the opening months of World War I to have such a delivery. They returned to initiate a newspaper and magazine campaign for American women's liberation from suffering.

Women with feminist or suffragist sympathies spearheaded this drive. One such person was Dr. Eliza Taylor Ransom, a homeopathic doctor in Boston. In 1914 Ransom founded her own maternity hospital in Boston's Back Bay in order to provide the painless method for women. She began the New England Twilight Sleep Association in order to force hospitals to offer the procedure. In 1915 she arranged to show healthy babies born under this method to a large group of "stylish" women in a Boston theater; later the association produced films showing the method and featuring the healthy babies. The films were circulated to women's groups throughout the nation.

Brochures of the Twilight Sleep Association advertised the method as the solution to a wide range of problems. It supposedly abolished the need for forceps, shortened the first stage of labor, reduced the time of convalescence and the danger of hemorrhage, and helped the mother produce milk; it was the best method for women with heart trouble and with "nerves." Above all, it removed the fear of pain, which had kept many women from having children. Like other new medical techniques, Twilight Sleep was a panacea for nearly everything.

Many early pioneers in using the method were wealthy society ladies. Mrs. John Jacob Astor's picture appeared in newspaper articles endorsing Twilight Sleep, along with pictures of well-dressed mothers and healthy babies. The social standing of such women made the medical profession take notice.

Women's testimonials for Twilight Sleep claimed that maternity was now a delightful experience. Women insisted that they were healthier and more fit than after earlier deliveries, that their children were more uniformly healthy, beautiful, and intelligent than their earlier children. Some women celebrated Twilight Sleep for allowing them to lapse into feminine passivity, as they said—into the great lap of cosmic forces, the unconscious itself—and to enjoy a birth that earlier, more "natural" women had enjoyed, because they were less nervous and self-conscious creatures of civilization. Since scopolamine was an hallucinogenic, Twilight Sleep may have impressed women as a return to the unconscious, not in a Freudian sense but in the sense of discovering in themselves unknown vitalistic powers that civilization had denied their knowing.

The campaign for Twilight Sleep was successful, for doctors and hospitals came to regard it as safe and even useful. Boston hospitals adopted the method in the early 1920s and, by 1938, used it in all deliveries. Twilight Sleep not only attracted women to the hospital, it made them more manageable during labor and delivery and allowed the routine use of other techniques. In the language of the 1930s, Twilight Sleep "streamlined maternity's miracle." According to the *Boston Traveller* (Feb. 5, 1938),

> Two yellow capsules, a jab in the arm, swiftly blot out the scene, time, knowledge, and feeling for the woman. . . . When she is not aware, sunlight pierces the drapery. And one of the amiable nurses chirps, "It's all over. You've got your baby." With such streamlined ease . . . babies are born.

In the end, however, Twilight Sleep had important disadvantages for birthing women. The method required constant monitoring and could only be used in hospitals. It was responsible for luring many women into giving birth in hospitals, rather than in their homes, after 1920. By the early 1930s, between 60 and 75 percent of urban births took place in hospitals. With the advent of Twilight Sleep, hospital births became more impersonal. Staff, believing that women laboring under scopolamine, or "scoped," would remember nothing, sometimes ignored their patients. Birth became an assembly line. The processing of birth, the smoothing of its rough edges, and the making of all births as predictably similar as possible may have appealed to women who wished an impersonal and speedy delivery. As one of Edith Wharton's characters expressed it in 1927, in the novel *Twilight Sleep*:

> "Of course there ought to be no Pain...nothing but Beauty. It ought to be one of the loveliest, most poetic things in the world to have a baby," Mrs. Manford declared, in that bright, efficient voice which made loveliness and poetry sound like the attributes of an advanced industrialism, and babies as something to be turned out in series like Fords. (pp. 14-15)

In reality, Twilight Sleep was both painful and undignified. The morphine, which had given genuine relief from pain to early advocates of the method, was discontinued after several well-publicized maternal deaths. Scopolamine did not kill pain, only the memory of pain. A woman could scream in agony all night and in the morning remember nothing of her pain. For many women, scopolamine produced temporary symptoms of psychosis that necessitated restrictive measures. But women would not remember thrashing about while strapped to their beds, or perhaps laboring in special "cribs" with high sides covered with canvas to confine them. Unfortunately, scopolamine was also an hallucinogenic. Some women—perhaps one in ten—were left with nightmare memories of the birth.

Under Twilight Sleep, a woman had no control over the birth experience and was unable to find meaning in it, for her participation in it and even her consciousness of it were minimal. She was isolated during birth from family and friends, and even from other women having the same experience. She had to think of herself instrumentally, not as a woman feeling love and fear or sharing in a creative event, but as a body machine being manipulated by others for her ultimate welfare. She played a social role of passive dependence and obedience.

After World War II, Twilight Sleep began to lose popularity. Women sought consciousness at birth, as early as the 1950s, during the years of the "Feminine Mystique." In those years, popular psychology and a reemphasis on domesticity encouraged women to believe once again that motherhood was a woman's fundamental purpose; she therefore should be awake to experience its sublime beginning. Twilight Sleep was gradually supplanted, first by spinal anesthesia (developed in 1942), which allowed the mother to remain conscious, and later, as women sought greater control over birth, by various methods of natural childbirth. By the 1970s, Twilight Sleep, so strongly advocated by feminists early in the century, had become the antithesis of everything that feminists desired in birth. The method is now rarely used. ✱ DOROTHY C. WERTZ, Ph.D.

See **Guide to Related Topics:** Childbirth Practices and Locations

Resources

Leavitt, Judith Walzer. (1986). *Brought to Bed: Childbearing in America*. New York: Oxford University Press.

Sandelowski, Margarete. (1984). *Pain, Pleasure, and American Childbirth: From Twilight Sleep to the Read Method, 1914-1960*. Westport, CT: Greenwood Press.

Wertz, Richard W. & Wertz, Dorothy C. (1989). *Lying-in: A History of Childbirth in America, Expanded Edition*. New Haven, CT: Yale University Press.

TWINS: MYTHS AND LEGENDS

Throughout history, societies have shown a fascination with twins and multiple births. Whereas the prevailing attitudes in Western society today are positive, earlier cultures expressed mixed messages about such births, as is evidenced by the many tales and superstitions various cultures created to explain these events.

Two of the oldest stories about twins appear in Genesis, the first book of the Old Testament. Chapter 25 tells the story of Jacob and Esau, probably fraternal twins. Esau is described as being hairy and Jacob as smooth. Esau, the first born, is favored by his father, Isaac. However, Jacob, with the help of his mother, Rebekah, deceives Isaac into giving his paternal blessing and his birthright to Jacob instead of Esau.

It appears that there was much significance given to the first born of the pair. Genesis, Chapter 38, tells another story about the birth of twins, although this time with a different twist. During labor, the baby Zerah puts out his hand while the midwife ties a scarlet thread around it. Then Zerab withdraws back to allow his brother, Phares, to be the first born. In the New Testament (John 20), it is revealed that the apostle Thomas is a twin called Didymus, the Greek word meaning "twin." "Thomas" actually means "twin" in Aramaic.

Twins are also common in Greek and Roman mythology. Leda, seduced by the Greek god Zeus in the form of a swan, conceives twins Pollux and Helen. On the same night, with her mortal husband, Leda conceives twins Castor and Clytemnestra. The children are hatched from two separate eggs. When grown, the god Neptune grants Castor and Pollux special powers over the weather and the oceans. When the human Castor is killed in battle, he is given immortality and joins his already-immortal brother Pollux, where they become the twin stars of the Gemini constellation. Zeus also fathers the twins Artemis (the virgin goddess of nature, the moon, fertility, marriage, and childbirth) and Apollo (the god of youth and manly beauty). Their Roman counterparts are Diana and Apollo, twins fathered by Jupiter.

Roman mythology tells the story of Romulus and Remus, twin sons of the god Mars, who are abandoned in the countryside, nursed by a wolf, and eventually rescued by a shepherd. They are credited with having founded the city of Rome.

Myths about twins are not limited to biblical and Greek and Roman culture. Indian mythology includes a story about twin gods called the Acvin, who are the protectors of the weak and oppressed. The Aztecs of Mexico attributed their goddess of fertility, Xochiquetzal, with being the first mother of twins. In South American mythology, twins are often important characters in adventure stories in which they are the heroes performing great feats for which humankind will always be indebted.

Some primitive groups received twins with great joy. For example, the Yorubas of western Nigeria, the most prolific producers of twins in the world—one twin birth in every 25 pregnancies—believed twins to be good luck omens. The Yorubas, along with several other tribes, would carve little figures to represent twins. If one died, the other lovingly cared for his or her figure. If both died, it was the duty of the parents or other family members to care for the figurines. The Kwakiutl Indians of British Columbia celebrated the birth of twins as a sign of plentiful hunting and fishing to come. They also believed that twins could cure disease.

On the other hand, not all societies greeted twins so warmly. In fact, in some cultures they were quite unwelcome and considered the product of adultery. In that case, the mothers would be disgraced by the birth and the twins would be killed. As recently as 1946, a special orphanage for twins existed in southern Rhodesia. Rhodesians believed that twins could not come from the same father; therefore, they were abandoned. For Invits, Aborigines, and Native Americans, twinship placed a serious burden on parents and their tribe, whose resources already were scarce. As a result, one twin of the pair was usually killed.

Some cultures believed that one twin was good, while the other was evil. It was up to the shaman, or witch doctor, to decide which was the evil one to be killed. The ancient Incas of Peru regarded twins as the ideal sacrifice for appeasing the gods of pestilence and famine. Oftentimes, the female of a boy-girl pair was killed to prevent incest between them, while in other societies, boy-girl twins were forced to marry. Sometimes a man marrying a twin girl was required to marry her sister as well.

In a number of African tribes, the parents of twins were associated with fertility and were asked to perform rites designed to stimulate the growth of crops or animals. They also believed, along with some American Indian tribes, that twins could control weather and cause thunder, lightning, and rain. In times of drought, women would water the graves of twins in the belief that if the bones were kept moist, the rains would surely come. In some Haitian voodoo cults, twins—both living and dead—were considered powerful beings. They were given special attention due to the belief that they could bring punishment upon their relatives if mistreated.

Today, in most cultures, attitudes concerning twins and multiple births generally are positive. Due to advances in the areas of fertility and neonatal care, multiple births are more commonplace than ever. With this recognition has come many organizations that are researching multiples and social groups that offer support to the families of multiples. ✷ JUDY LOBO FERRY, R.N., B.S.N.

See **Guide to Related Topics:** Literature and the Arts

Resources

Gaddis, Vincent & Gaddis, Margaret. (1972). *The Curious World of Twins*. New York: Hawthorn Books, Inc.

Leach, Maria. (Ed.) (1972). *Funk and Wagnalls Standard Dictionary of Folklore, Mythology and Legend*. New York: Funk and Wagnalls.

Noble, Elizabeth. (1980). *Having Twins: A Parent's Guide to Pregnancy, Birth and Early Childhood*. Boston: Houghton Mifflin Co.

Scheinfeld, Amram. (1967). *Twins and Supertwins*. Philadelphia: J.B. Lippincott Co.

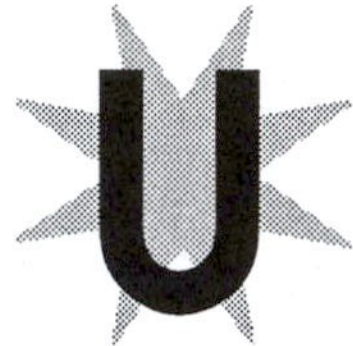

UGANDA

In order to understand the dynamics of childbirth in Uganda, it is necessary to know about the overall national health care system because of its influence on the socioeconomic infrastructure (Dodge and Wiebe, 1985). Until the end of the 1960s, Uganda had the most highly developed and enviable health service system south of the Sahara. But after 20 years of war, health services have totally broken down. Mobile clinics, dispensaries, and other health service posts have ceased running, and all government-run hospitals are under total overhaul.

Uganda is about the size of Oregon and is divided into 33 districts on which the health service system is structured, with a district medical team in each. By 1987, there were 53 government-run hospitals (GRHs) and about 28 private and missionary facilities(PRHs) supplemented by dispensaries and various aid posts. The more developed central and south regions have a higher concentration of PRHs.

Effective service is directly linked with availability of basic medical supplies and equipment. Although PRHs have a "fee-for-service" system (Dodge and Wiebe, 1985; Namazzi, 1989), they have a high percentage of attendance [estimated at 50-60 percent (Asante and Cohen, 1984)] due to an established reputation for high quality of service, reliability, and equipment. They are privately supported and therefore have adequate resources. Urban private clinics are well-stocked and lucratively run by physicians in government and/or private practice. In rural Uganda, private midwives and state-registered nurse-midwives are the backbone of the health care system, charging a minimal fee for treatment of anything from a snakebite to a compound fracture.

The system, coupled with other background factors—ethnic group, religion, education, and economic status—determines the level and type of childbirth care. The educated and economically able have a choice—the private clinic with a physician, which is out of reach of the rural and less-well-to-do; or, if it is near, the government facility (Dodge and Wiebe, 1985). For rural women the private maternity center, usually run by a private midwife only, who will take into consideration family dynamics, is the nearest and best alternative. Traditional beliefs and customs (Kisekka, 1973) are still very much an integral part of childbirth.

Before childbirth, mothers are given a variety of native medicines. One popular practice among the Baganda is "okumenya" a method of softening the pelvic area before childbirth (Namazzi, 1989). Both rural and urban, educated and less educated, practice it to varying degrees. Some women use "akasonko," a tiny shell typically found in banana plantations, to soften the pelvis and lessen childbirth pain. It is crushed into a fine powder and mixed with salve and various native herbs. The mixture is then carefully rubbed around the cervix of the pregnant woman. Others use "enkata"; a warm stone is placed in the center of two head coils of fresh banana leaves. Within a day or two of delivery, the pregnant woman oils the pelvic area and then for about 10-15 minutes, or until the stone is cold, squats above the coils, completely covering them, so that the heat from the stone wafts into her. Many believe that this practice ensures swift and almost painless delivery. While some of these practices in reality do not produce the intended physiological results, they are very psychologically beneficial in that they improve body circulation and muscle control, and prepare the woman emotionally for childbirth.

Many of the herbs have great potential. However, they present potential danger when misused, especially when concurrently used in large doses with Western medicine. Postpartum hemorrhage is very common due to the effects of these herbs. In rural areas that have no hospitals with physician service, it is usually too late to save lives (Namazzi, 1989). Stillbirths are a common result of these native medicines. Commonly used is "emmumbwa" a cylindrical pestle-shaped stone (similar to a mallet) made of a mixture of clay and various herbs and roots. There are many varieties: "balinnoonya" and "mukalakasa" are two of the most popular and are easily obtainable from markets, although their authenticity has to be examined. The more trusted brands are those produced by a well-known and trusted "herbal medicine doctor," who could be any elder in a community.

Childbirth is still very much a woman's domain. Men do not enter the delivery room traditionally even among the more westernized communities; they wait outside for results, or in the event of a long labor, leave a relative to attend to the needs of the mother and child until discharge. In hospitals, childbirth is in the hands of a team of trained personnel; in most rural maternity centers, it is totally in the hands of a private midwife or, in some centers, a private midwife with the assistance of one or two state-registered nurse-midwives. Up to the mid-1950s, in the central region, childbirth attended by traditional birth attendants took place in a well-secluded area of the banana plantation (Mushanga, 1973). Children were not and still are not permitted to witness childbirth because of traditional sexual taboos.

Among some rural Baganda, "muwogo" (a tropical plant with starch roots) and "gonja" (a tropical type of banana fruit) are baked and pounded into a fine dusting powder, which is used on the umbilical cord. Except when stored unsafely, this powder is quite effective in drying the cord when used properly. Otherwise neonatal tetanus infection kills many healthy babies. Frequent bathing of the newborn, three or four times a day, causes chest infections because of exposure (Namazzi, 1989). Many newborns develop respiratory problems and if not given proper medical attention, die. Others are given herbal concoctions from birth in such quantities that they lose their appetite for nourishing food. For example, among some rural Baganda, a newborn drinks from an "olusoggo," a small, ladle-like cup made from banana leaves (Namazzi, 1989). Nine of these hold a different herbal drink and the baby sips from each one. Sanitary conditions, the effects of these drugs, and malnutrition combine to affect newborns adversely, often leading to cases of gastro problems and dehydration. Because they are weakened at such an early stage, many newborns are much more susceptible to other infections.

Available statistics (Dodge and Wiebe, 1985) indicate that the average number of children for an urban educated woman is about five, compared to the rural average of about seven. Many women may have up to 12 or more children.

✷ MARGARET MUWONGE

See **Guide to Related Topics:** Cross-Cultural Perspectives

Resources

Arkutu, A.R. (1984). *Health Risks of Childbearing in East Africa*. Chapel Hill, NC: Carolina Population Center, University of North Carolina: 56-73.

Asante, K. & Cohen, N. (1987). *Primary Health Care, Maternal and Child Health, Family Planning*. African Medical and Research Foundation (AMREF)—IDA Report.

Billington, W.R. et al. (1963). "Custom and Child Health in Uganda: Pregnancy and Childbirth. *Tropical and Geographical Medicine 15*:134-37.

Brown, R.E. (1970). "Attitudes Toward Family Planning among Peri-Urban Africans in Uganda." *Tropical and Geographical Medicine* 22: 87-100.

Dodge, C.P. & Wiebe, P.D. (1985). *Crisis in Uganda: The Breakdown of Health Services*. New York: Pergamon Press.

Kisekka, M.N. (1973). *The Baganda of Central Uganda*. Nairobi, Kenya: East African Publishing House, Cultural Source Materials for Population Planning in East Africa, Vol. 3, pp. 174-86.

A Luganda-English and English-Luganda Dictionary. (1952). London: Society for Promoting Christian Knowledge.

Mushanga, M.T. (1973). *Beliefs and Practices*. Nairobi, Kenya: East African Publishing House, Cultural Source Materials for Population Planning in East Africa, Vol. 3, pp. 174-86.

Namazzi, T.K. (1989). Private Midwife, Masaka, Uganda. (Unpublished private communication.)

ULTRASOUND IN OBSTETRICS: A QUESTION OF SAFETY*

Millions of women and their unborn children are being exposed to diagnostic ultrasound during pregnancy and childbirth without the women being advised prior to exposure that there has been no well-controlled scientific investigation carried out to study the delayed long-term effects of ultrasound on human development. Ova, embryos, and fetuses are often exposed to prolonged sonography because the physician or technician lacks

* Copyright © 1992 by Doris B. Haire.

sufficient expertise to evaluate what he or she is seeing.

Recently the FDA yielded to pressure from industry and organized medicine to relinquish control over the amount of sonic energy that can be emitted by the new ultrasound devices used in obstetrics. The new ultrasound machines will beep at certain levels of energy output but essentially there will be little or no limit on the energy the health care provider may choose to use.

Despite the fact that the FDA's Center for Devices and Radiologic Health acknowledged the potential risks of ultrasound used in obstetrics in its 1982 publication "An Overview of Ultrasound," edited by Stewart and Stratmeyer, there is no evidence that health care providers are obtaining women's truly informed consent to the use of ultrasound in pregnancy.

There are no state or federal regulations which require periodic calibration of ultrasound devices used in osbstetric care. Nor are there any regulations that require a record to be kept of basic information such as:

- The indication for the procedure
- The written consent of the patient
- The name of the manufacturer and the model number of the ultrasound equipment used
- The type of ultrasound employed
- The proposed intensity, as well as the actual intensity of exposure
- The proposed and actual length of exposure
- Maternal height, weight, and temperature
- Identification of the hospital or the office where the procedure is carried out
- Identification and qualification of the sonographer
- Date of exposure

Eight or more major studies have been carried out to evaluate the effectiveness of routine diagnostic ultrasound. None has shown such routine use to improve maternal and infant outcome over that achieved when diagnostic ultrasound was used only when medically indicated.

Are women overly concerned about the safety of ultrasound used in obstetrics? A letter published in the July 1988 issue of the *British Journal of Obstetrics and Gynaecology*, from Dr. Robert Bases, Chief of the Radiobiology Section, Albert Einstein College of Medicine, calls attention to the 1984 review by Stewart and Moore of over 700 publications since 1950 that demonstrate the present chaos in delineating and controlling exposure conditions and the bewildering range of ultrasound bioeffects. Bases states in his letter:

> The increased frequency of sister chromatid exhanges induced by pulsed ultrasound in human lymphocytes, first described by Liebeskind et al (1979), has been amply confirmed in reports from four independent laboratories involving studies of pulsed as well as continuous wave ultrasound. (Haupt et al., 1981; Ehlinger et al., 1981; Ozawa et al., 1984; Stella et al., 1984). Recently further evidence that sister chromatid exchanges in human lymphocytes are induced by high-intensity pulsed ultrasound has been presented by Barnett et al. (1988), who are now able to confirm the previous results.
>
> Free radical production in amniotic fluid and blood plasma by medical ultrasound, probably following gaseous cavitation, has been detected by Crum et al. (1987). This provides a likely mechanism for the origin of the DNA damage. Because of these confirmations and a recent report by Ellisman et al. (1987) that diagnostic levels of ultrasound may disrupt myelination in neonatal rats, the need for regulation, guidance, and properly controlled clinical studies is clear.

The implications of premature ovulation after ovarian ultrasonography, reported by Testart et al., are disturbing. If ultrasound can affect the adult ovary, what then is the effect of ultrasound on the ova of the female fetus?

Even if well-controlled investigations into the delayed long-term effects of obstetric ultrasound begin today, it will be 20 or 30 years before it is known whether ultrasound will be the DES of the next generation. Even where there is a medical indication of need, the woman has a right to be informed, and her health care provider has a legal obligation to advise her of the potential risks and relevant areas of uncertainty regarding the latent effects of ultrasound. "Weasel" wording, which implies that proper research has been carried out and no risks have been found, rather than a clear statement regarding potential risks is still the norm in most health care facilities.

Having each ultrasound candidate sign a consent form would be invaluable in carrying out an investigation into the delayed, long-term effects of ultrasound, not just in the case of obstetrics but for all uses. The consent form offers several benefits.

1. It would help to ensure that women would be advised of the risks and areas of uncertainty before granting consent to diagnostic ultrasound.
2. It would create a database for a long-term follow-up of exposed offspring.

3. It would help to protect the provider from malpractice suits if time proves ultrasound to be harmful to human development.
4. It would shift or share the potential liability by identifying the manufacturer of the device.

American women will not again be so easily deceived into assuming that health care providers always know what is best for them. Information needed by the woman, if her consent is to be truly informed, must include the fact that no properly controlled, scientific investigation has been carried out to evaluate the delayed, long-term effects of ultrasound.

Perhaps time will ultimately prove ultrasound to be safe. However, until well-controlled research has established ultrasound to be without harm, women must be informed of the areas of uncertainty, for themselves and their babies.

✱ DORIS B. HAIRE

See also: Imaging Techniques

See **Guide to Related Topics:** Prenatal Diagnosis and Screening

UMBILICAL CORD

The umbilical cord is the cordlike structure that contains the blood vessels that connect the placenta to the navel of the fetus. It is usually about 50 cm long and about 2 cm wide by the end of pregnancy. It generally contains two arteries and one vein, coated with a light-gray, rubbery substance called wharton's jelly, which protects the blood vessels. A short communicating branch between the two umbilical arteries equalizes the blood flow from the sides of the placenta. About 1 percent of cords contain only one artery; of these, about 30 percent of the infants have some sort of birth defect, usually of the circulatory system. Frequently the blood vessels in the cord are longer than the cord, creating a spiral appearance. The cord generally inserts in the center of the placenta, but it sometimes enters the placenta on the side. This is referred to as battledore placenta or a marginal insertion. In about 1 percent of all cords, the wharton's jelly does not cover the blood vessels all the way to the placenta. This is called a velamentous insertion, and can be dangerous to the fetus because the blood vessels are not protected from being pinched or ruptured, either of which can lead to fetal death.

The function of the umbilical cord is to carry blood from the fetus to the placenta (via the umbilical arteries), where the baby's chemical waste products (carbon dioxide, for example) are released into the mother's blood stream and new elements are picked up (oxygen, calcium, and iron, for example) and brought back to the fetus (via the vein in the umbilical cord).

Some complications that can occur with the cord are different types of cord entanglements. There is an erroneous belief that if a pregnant woman lifts something over her head, the baby will get tangled in the cord. About one in five babies born has the cord wrapped around its neck. Generally the loop is loose and can be pulled over the head; if not, it is clamped and cut. Sometimes in its movements in the uterus, the baby swims through a loop of cord, creating a knot in it. If it is not pulled tight, this presents no problem, but if any tension is put on the cord, the knot tightens and stops the flow of blood to and from the fetus. A very short cord or a cord that is wrapped around the baby can cause the placenta to separate prematurely from the uterine wall as the baby descends down the birth canal.

Occasionally the cord comes down in front of or alongside the baby in the birth canal (most often when the bag of waters breaks). This is referred to as cord prolapse. This happens in about one out of every 400 term pregnancies and is more common in premature births. The cord then gets pinched between the woman's pelvis and the part of the baby that is coming down the birth canal. If part of the cord is actually hanging out of the vagina, the air on the cord usually sets the blood vessels into spasm, decreasing the blood flow. This complication necessitates a speedy delivery or an immediate cesarian section to save the baby.

Generally, the umbilical cord is clamped with a hemostat and a cord clamp and cut with a sterile pair of scissors within three minutes after the birth of the baby. The cord does not appear to have any pain receptors and the baby usually does not cry when the cord is cut. Some birth attendants wait until the cord stops pulsating or until the placenta is delivered before cutting the cord. With delayed clamping and cutting, the baby may receive more blood from the placenta than a baby would if its cord was cut right away, especially if the baby is held below the level of the placenta. There is debate over whether this increased blood flow is healthy or not. Babies who receive more blood this way have more iron in their system and therefore have less anemia, but they also have to break down more red blood cells, which can lead to increased risk of hyperbilirubinemia. If the cord is cut with an unclean pair of scissors or an unclean blade, the baby may get an umbilical infection or tetanus. This is still a significant problem in some

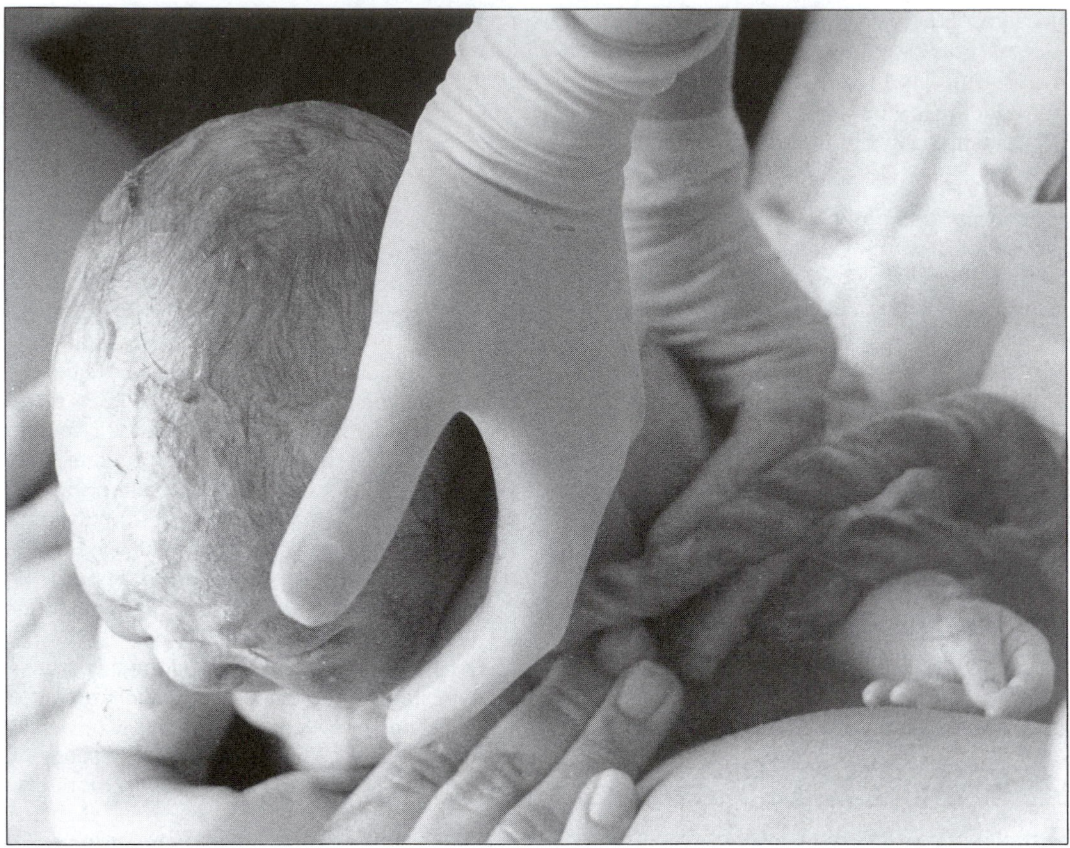

Note the spiral appearance of the umbilical cord. Photo courtesy of Harriette Hartigan/Artemis.

developing countries, for example Haiti, where 145 out of every 1,000 newborns die of tetanus.

After the cord is cut, there are a variety of ways to care for the cord stump. Some people simply leave it alone, in which case it dries up and drops off in about 4 to 14 days. Others use rubbing alcohol to cleanse the cord and the area around it each day, which speeds the drying process. Still others paint on gentian violet or goldenseal powder to kill any bacteria that might get on the cord. In the U.S. in the past (and still among some ethnic groups, including Fillipino and Mexican-American families) a cord binder (a soft, dry cloth tied around the baby's abdomen) is used to protect the cord from cold and to prevent umbilical hernias. Some mothers put a coin over the navel to ensure that the baby does not have a protruding navel.

Some cultures consider the cord stump to have magical powers and have a taboo about the baby going outside before it falls off. It is also believed to be a powerful ingredient in some shamanic medicines. ✱ ALTHEA SEAVER

See also: Placenta

See **Guide to Related Topics:** Pregnancy, Physical Aspects

Resources

Eloesser, Leo, Galt, Edith, & Hemingway, Isabell. (1973). *Childbirth and the Newborn: A Manual for Rural Midwives.* Mexico: Instituto Indigenista Interamericano.

Garrey, Matthew et. al. (1980). *Obstetrics Illustrated.* Edinburgh, Scotland: Churchhill Livingston.

Gaskin, Ina May. (1980). *Spiritual Midwifery.* Summertown, TN: The Book Publishing Company.

Hobbs, Valerie. (1982). *Complications of Labor and Delivery.* New Haven, CT: Informed Homebirth.

Jensen, Margaret, Benson, Ralph, & Bobak, Irene. (1981). *Maternity Care: The Nurse and the Family.* St. Louis: C.V. Mosby.

Moore, Keith. (1974). *Before We Are Born: Basic Embriology and Birth Defects.* Philadelphia: Saunders Company.

Pritchard, Jack, MacDonald, Paul, & Gant, Norman. (1985). *William's Obstetrics.* Norwalk, CT: Appleton-Century-Croft.

Yau, Alice & Lind, John. (1977, Fall). "Cord Clamping Time: Influence on the Newborn." *Birth and the Family Journal* 4 (3).

UNDERWATER BIRTH

A review of the subject of underwater birth in orthodox medical literature would not take long. There was a report on an unplanned birth under water in the proceedings of a French medical society as early as 1805 (Embry, 1805). Then the topic was not mentioned again until the publication of a report describing a series of 100 births underwater (Odent, 1983). On the other hand, underwater birth has been a popular topic in the media since 1980. Millions of women throughout the world have dreamed of giving birth under water.

The Pioneering Work. The use of water during labor developed in parallel in two different places, from two quite different approaches.

- In Moscow, Igor Tcharkovsky was a swimming instructor. He focused his interest on the capacities of human babies in water. He realized that the younger the baby, the better his or her adaptation to water. So he decided that water training should start at birth. Since then he has attended a number of aquatic births at home. It seems that home birth is often confused with water birth in the Soviet Union (Gaskin, 1989). In the West, people's imaginations have been fired by one or two stories about births in the Black Sea among the dolphins.
- In the state hospital at Pithiviers, France, the starting point was different. The main aim was to facilitate the first stage of labor and to avoid the use of drugs. It had been observed that many laboring women were attracted to water, wanting to have a bath or a shower; so the hospital staff introduced first a small paddling pool and then designed a pool in hard material. Thousands of women have used this pool. It is especially efficient when the woman is patient enough not to get into the water until the onset of hard labor when the dilatation is already well advanced. Most women spontaneously get out of the bath when they feel the contractions are not working efficiently any more. Leaving the warm water and returning to a cooler atmosphere often triggers a "fetus ejection reflex" (Odent, 1987) and the baby is born on the floor by the pool.

It is important to know that birth under water is a possibility, though it is not necessarily the aim. In any birthing place where a pool is available, underwater birth is bound to happen every so often. A newborn baby is perfectly adapted to immersion, like a dolphin. There is no risk of inhalation of water. When the birth happens under water, the newborn infant is brought gently to the surface and placed in the mother's arms. This is always done within seconds but without rushing.

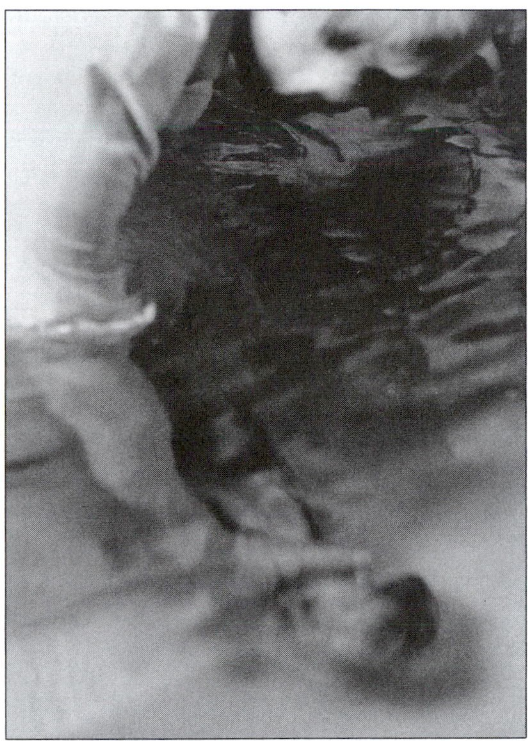

Michel Odent catching a baby at the bottom of the pool. Photo courtesy of Michel Odent.

Practical Advice. The pool should be large enough to allow the woman to adopt any position and deep enough to make complete immersion possible. But if it is too large the sense of privacy is reduced. An ideal size is 3 feet (1m) deep, and the water should be maintained at body temperature.

How Water Works. It is easy to find simplistic physiological explanations:

- Immersion in warm water tends to reduce the level of hormones that belong to the adrenalin family.
- Warm water can have a direct stretching effect on the muscular system by softening the collagen of the tendons.
- Immersion reduces the force of gravity and therefore minimizes stimulation of the inner part of the ear (the vestibular system). When the woman has her ears under water the outside world is cut off completely. This tends to facilitate the reduction of neocortical control and the laboring woman seems to "go off to another planet."

These factors are not sufficient to explain why some women only need to see the blue water and hear the noise of the water to release their inhibitions. One has to recall that water is universally the symbol of the mother and that water can have a mysterious effect on human beings (Odent, 1990). The therapeutic and erotic powers of the element have been used through the ages, and the power of water has always been used by all the world's religions.

The Advantages of Using Water in a Hospital. In a hospital the use of water is an efficient, easy, and economical way to reduce the use of drugs and the rate of other interventions by enhancing the mother's sense of privacy and effectively cutting down on unnecessary stimulations. The mammalian need for privacy is better met. A birth under water guarantees that the germ-free newborn baby will be contaminated first by the germs of the mother rather than by the hospital germs. A newborn baby shares the antibodies that pass through the placenta with his or her mother but is not adapted to the hospital germs.

Advantages of Using Water at Home. Underwater birth at home keeps the baby's father busy. The privacy of the woman in labor is better protected.

Birth underwater at home is happening everywhere in the world in the 1990s. The dangerous fashion of keeping the baby under water several minutes has died out. In London (England) underwater birth at home has become easier thanks to a system of transportable "water birth pools" available for rent (Balaskas and Gordon, 1990). In the United Kingdom several teaching hospitals are installing pools. There are now aquatic birthing centers in most Western countries: Upland (California), Ostend (Belgium), London (England), Malta, Melbourne (Australia), and Toulouse (France).

Concluding Comments. The use of water during labor is a safe way to replace drugs. Birth under water should not become the objective. It is just a possibility; after all, aquatic mammals such as seals go to the land to give birth. However, it is probable that there will be more stories of human births in the sea in the future.

✱ MICHEL ODENT, M.D.

See **Guide to Related Topics:** Childbirth Practices and Locations

Resources

Balaskas, J. & Gordon, Y. (1990). *Water and Birth*. London: Unwin Hyman.

Embry, M. (1805). Observations sur un accouchement terminé dans le bain. (Report of a delivery which ended in a bath). *Annales de la société de medecine pratique de Montpellier* 5:13

Gaskin, Ina May. (1989, Winter). "Report from the USSR." *The Birth Gazette* 6 (1): 12-15.

Odent, M. (1983, Dec 24). "Birth under Water." *Lancet*: 1476-77.

———. (1987). "The Fetus Ejection Reflex." *Birth 14*: 104-05.

———. (1990). *Water and Sexuality*. London: Penguin.

———. (1992). *The Ecology of Birth and Breastfeeding*. Amherst MA: Bergin & Garvey.

UTERINE FIBROIDS

Uterine fibroids are commonly occurring tumors, medically termed "myomas" or "leiomyomas," that affect up to 30 percent of adult females. The growths originate in the myometrium (uterine muscle) and appear to be dense encapsulations of tissue, ranging in size from microscopic to those that cause uterine enlargement. Fibroids most commonly occur in multiples, and their location within the uterus determines the classification of tumor. Intramural fibroids are confined to the middle of the muscular wall and are usually small. Subserous myomas appear on the uterine exterior, while submucous tumors are found inside the uterus beneath the endometrium—the most problematic location.

Although their origin is not fully understood, there appears to be a genetic or inherited predisposition to developing fibroids, as they are commonly found within families. The fact that black women have a greater tendency for fibroid development also lends support for a genetic basis. Most frequently found within the parameters of the childbearing years—menstruation to menopause—it is thought that the nuclei of all fibroids that might develop are established by age 30 (Payer, 1987). Their occurrence and growth are believed to be related to estrogen production; in the presence of high estrogen levels, as may occur during pregnancy, with oral contraceptive use, or in overweight women, fibroids are more frequently discovered and their growth is significantly greater. Conversely, when estrogen levels are decreased (following childbirth or after menopause), the size and presence of the tumors also diminish.

Because fibroids are so frequently asymptomatic, their existence is often discovered by chance during a routine pelvic examination. Occasionally a diagnosis is made in conjunction with related indications, such as an enlarged uterus, pelvic pain, or unusually heavy bleeding. When the presence of fibroids is suspected, their location and size may be established through the use of ultrasound, laparascopy, or hysterosalpingography (all of which permit visualization of internal structures) or surgical procedures such as D & C.

Treatment for uterine fibroids is often unnecessarily aggressive and invasive and, in spite of alternative therapies, has become the most common indication for hysterectomy (accounting for up to 60 percent of all hysterectomies performed) (Hysterectomy Educational Resources and Services [HERS] Foundation). Because the development of myomas is so common and because so few of them present symptoms and no significant difficulties, the most preferable treatment may simply be observation and periodic checkups.

Occasionally, certain symptoms or discomforts may arise that require more active treatment. When rapid growth or persistent pain and bleeding are present, or pressure on other organs causes discomfort, surgery may be considered necessary. The removal of the fibroids (myomectomy) is major abdominal surgery using laser or traditional methods. Because only the tumors are removed and the uterus remains intact, the childbearing potential is preserved, though there is some chance of fibroid recurrence. Submucous fibroids may be removed by hysteroscopic myomectomy, which is performed vaginally and is therefore without the complications of abdominal surgery. Additionally, a drug called GnRH analog has been effective in reducing the size of some fibroids by producing a "reversible menopause" when administered over a period of several months (Payer, 1987).

Hysterectomy, the surgical removal of the uterus, has been described as the only "definitive" therapy as it eliminates all possibility of fibroid recurrence. Hysterectomy is considered appropriate treatment for myomas that enlarge the uterus to a three-month pregnancy size, but this criterion alone should not determine the need for such drastic measures since large fibroids are not necessarily debilitating (Payer, 1987). In the absence of severe symptoms, conservation of the uterus is preferable and observation may be the only course of action necessary.

Fibroids may occasionally be considered contributing factors in certain cases of infertility, although this is generally the exception. Similarly, their presence during pregnancy is usually of little or no consequence, aside from possibly increasing uterine size; complications during birth are infrequent (Pritchard and MacDonald, 1980). Even extensive fibroid growth should not automatically indicate cesarean section, as many women give birth vaginally in spite of fibroids (Cohen and Estner, 1983). ✱ BARBARA URSENBACH LAMB, C.C.E.

Resources

Boston Women's Health Book Collective. (1984). *The New Our Bodies, Ourselves*. New York: Simon & Schuster, Inc.

Cohen, Nancy Wainer & Estner, Lois J. (1983). *Silent Knife*. South Hadley, MA: Bergin and Garvey Publishers, Inc.

Hysterectomy Educational Resources and Services (HERS) Foundation. 422 Bryn Mawr Ave., Bala Cynwyd, PA 19004, (215) 667-7757.

Lauersen, Niels & Whitney, Steven. (1987). *A Woman's Body: The New Guide to Gynecology*. New York: Putnam.

Myles, Margaret F. (1975). *Textbook for Midwives, 8th Edition*. New York: Churchill Livingstone.

Payer, Lynn. (1987). *How to Avoid a Hysterectomy*. New York: Pantheon Books.

Pritchard, Jack A. & MacDonald, Paul C. (1980). *Williams Obstetrics, 16th Edition*. New York: Appleton-Century-Crofts.

Shephard, Bruce D. & Shephard, Carroll A. (1982). *The Complete Guide to Women's Health*. Tampa, FL: Mariner Publishing Co. Inc.

Thomas, Clayton L. (Ed.) (1977). *Taber's Cyclopedic Medical Dictionary, 13th Edition*. Philadelphia: F.A. Davis Co.

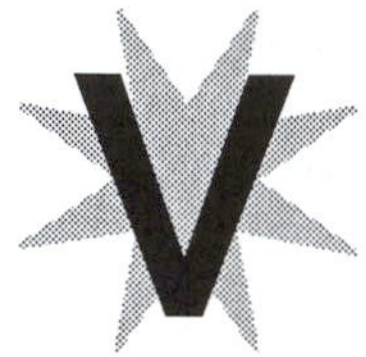

VACCINATIONS

The justification for vaccinating healthy children against specific diseases rests on the twin premises of efficacy and safety: (1) that vaccination simulates true immunity that results in recovery from the natural diseases and (2) that the procedure is in no way injurious to health. But recent evidence indicates that both premises are seriously flawed and deserve closer scrutiny.

The proponents of vaccination demonstrate efficacy in two ways. First, they point to dramatic reductions in the incidence of such diseases as polio and measles since the introduction of the vaccines. Second, by pointing out specific antibodies in the serum of vaccinated children, they can plausibly connect the clinical events to these vaccine-induced microscopic events.

But natural immunity means far more than the presence of specific antibodies in the blood and a lower incidence of the diseases in question. Children recovering from the measles will *never* contract it again, no matter how often they are re-exposed. Yet measles continues to break out in highly vaccinated and serologically "immune" populations (e.g., college students). Vaccinated children are also more likely to develop atypical cases that can be more serious than the "wild type" and are always more difficult to recognize. Finally, once the original vaccine "wears off," there is good evidence that re-vaccination is ineffective. All of these data suggest that the "immunity" conferred by the vaccines may not be genuine.

Second, true immunity also "primes" the immune mechanism to respond optimally to other acute illnesses. Recovering from an acute infection like the measles presupposes the collaboration of lymphocytes, macrophages, serum complement, and the entire immune system. The illness that is called the measles is in fact the process by which the virus is expelled from the blood. Specific antibodies appear only when this outpouring is well under way and persist afterwards as a kind of "memory" for the experience. The technical feat of manufacturing antibodies without the experience of illness to guide them may well prove reckless, since little is understood about how vaccines act inside the body, or how, if at all, the body manages to get rid of them.

The prevailing argument as to the safety of the vaccines rests upon the relative infrequency of severe toxic reactions occurring within a few days of their administration. But this narrow standard overlooks the more likely possibility of chronic, long-term effects.

There can be little doubt that the ability to mount a defense and recover from an acute illness such as the measles is the *sine qua non* for the maturation of a healthy immune system. In this sense, natural immunity is an important overall or net gain for the health of the patient as a whole. Yet vaccinated children appear to be more vulnerable to ear infections, for example, and to develop more relapses, require more antibiotics and more surgery, and show less capacity to recover fully than their unvaccinated counterparts.

These data arouse suspicion, likewise borne out by clinical experience, that vaccinated children are less able to respond acutely to *any* foreign stimulus, i.e., that vaccines act by promoting chronic responses at the expense of acute responses generally. Such a trade-off would be compatible with the hypothesis that vaccine particles can survive as parasites inside the cells of the immune system for decades and thus commandeer their function. "Latency" phenomena of this type are already well-known in microbiology and have been linked to auto-immune phenomena, cancer, and other chronic diseases. To resolve these issues will require studies of a radically new type, comparing the overall health status of vaccinated and unvaccinated children for a whole generation.

For the present, given these major uncertainties, it seems medically, ethically, and politically prudent to make the childhood vaccinations freely available to those who want them, as many European countries have already done. The rationale for compulsory vaccination is simply that the diseases in question pose a clear and urgent threat to the public, and that the public health and welfare would be better served in this way than any other.

It is difficult to see how the conditions for this rationale could be met, since, if the vaccines conferred true immunity, unvaccinated children would then be at risk only to themselves. On the other hand, the equation is sufficiently different for each disease to warrant looking at the individual vaccines one by one.

Seemingly the least popular and the least necessary are the vaccines against diptheria, a disease now rare in the U.S., and measles, mumps, and rubella, now generally viewed as routine diseases of childhood. Measles is actually making a serious comeback in the school-age population, which is already over 90 percent vaccinated, and the current drive for compulsory re-vaccination seems destined for failure.

On the other end of the spectrum, tetanus and polio are still widely feared, even though the risk of actually contracting them remains very small. These vaccines continue to be requested by most parents, and are generally accepted by the public as relatively harmless.

Pertussis, or whooping cough, has become the logical rallying point for the most zealous vaccine proponents and opponents alike, because on the one hand, the disease is still common and troublesome, while on the other hand, the vaccine has been linked with so many serious complications that many pediatricians are beginning to question its use.

At present, nearly half of the states allow parents strongly opposed to vaccinations to waive the requirement for their children. The others exempt only those belonging to a few religious denominations, e.g., Jehovah's Witnesses and Christian Scientists. No state as yet permits parents to choose some vaccines and not others, i.e., to make informed medical decisions for themselves. The growing anti-vaccination movement asserts the more general right of parents to make informed health decisions for their children, while the medical authorities continue to reserve for themselves the prerogatives of technical expertise and the power to make decisions for the public good.

✷ RICHARD MOSKOWITZ, M.D.

See also: Decision Making: Newborn Care
See **Guide to Related Topics:** Baby Care

Resources

Cherry, James. (1980, Jul). "The New Epidemiology of Measles and Rubella." *Hospital Practice*: 49-53.

Mortimer, Edward. (1980, Oct). "Pertussis Immunization." *Hospital Practice*: 103-06.

Moskowitz, Richard. (1983). "The Case against Immunizations." *Journal of the American Institute of Homeopathy 76*(1): 7-25.

———. (1983). "Postscript on Immunizations." *Journal of the American Institute of Homeopathy 76* (3): 101-04.

———. (1987). "Unvaccinated Kids: What Next for Them (and Us)?" *Mothering* (42): 34-39.

VBAC. *See Instead* CESAREAN BIRTH: INDICATIONS AND CONSEQUENCES

VEGETARIANISM AND PREGNANCY

Since pregnancy requires additional calories, vitamins, and minerals to meet the mother's systemic requirements as well as those of the growing fetus, the consideration of maternal diet during pregnancy is important. Maternal age, multiple gestation, and maternal disease all increase the nutrient requirements of pregnancy and affect the nutritional status of the individual. Iron and folic acid anemias are of special concern to pregnant women due to the link in some studies between these deficiences and poor perinatal outcome (e.g., maternal morbidity, fetal neural tube defects, poor levels of iron stores in the infant, toxemia of pregnancy).

The term "vegetarian" is a catchall for a host of dietary types. Vegetarian diets vary widely in nutritional and food item content. Vegan diets are composed primarily of whole grains, fruits, vegetables, and nuts/legumes and herbs. The commonality in vegan diets is nonreliance upon foods of animal origin. Yet one vegan may eat only raw and living foods (e.g., uncooked fruits and vegetables, wheat grass, sea vegetables) while another vegan includes cooked cereal gains (e.g., wheat, rice, barley) in his or her diet. Ovo-lacto diets may include all of the items within a vegan diet, along with egg and milk products such as yogurt, milk, and cheese. Ovo-lacto-pesco diets include egg, milk products, and fish. Macrobiotic diets are strongly rooted in the culturally proscribed/geographically accessible food items of the Japanese islands. However, indigenous animal products that are typically ingested by humans of that region (e.g., fish, shellfish) are often excluded from the macrobiotic diet. Land and sea vegetables common in that region are an important component of the macrobiotic diet (such as the sea vegetables nori, kombu, and arame; the land vegetables carrot, cabbage, and daikon; and whole grains such as rice). In the United States, soy products are readily available protein contributors to the vegetarian diet, which is completely devoid of food products derived from animals. Soy products are complete proteins in that they contain the eight essential amino acids in proportions usable by the human body. Soybeans and soy products such as tofu, miso, soy "milk," and tempeh all contain B vitamins; tempeh, in particular, is one of the rare, nonanimal sources of vitamin B-12.

Vegetable proteins that are less "complete" (do not contain all of the amino acids that cannot be synthesized by the human body) must be combined in order to enhance protein availability/usability to the body. For example, rice and legumes or beans and corn are staple food products in a variety of cultures throughout the world. These combinations are excellent protein companions, with the combination enhancing the body's access to the proteins contained in each single food.

Pregnant vegetarians who are cognizant of the body's additional nutrient requirements during pregnancy are at no greater risk of malnutrition than their omnivorous peers. The pregnant vegetarian can enhance her dietary levels of important nutrients during pregnancy through a combination of food sources and vitamin/mineral supplements. ✱ THAIS R. FORBES

See **Guide to Related Topics:** Pregnancy, Physical Aspects

Resources

Baldwin, Rahima. (1986). *Special Delivery.* Berkeley, CA: Celestial Arts.

Forbes, Thais R. (1987). "Macrobiotics: Diet, Philosophy, Way of Life." Unpublished manuscript, Tampa, FL.

Hoernes, Linda Carol. (1986). "Nutritional Complications during Pregnancy." MPH thesis, New York Medical College, New York.

Lappe, Frances Moore. (1975). *Diet for a Small Planet.* New York: Ballantine Books.

Moore, Keith L. (1982). *The Developing Human.* 3rd edition. Philadelphia: W.B. Saunders Company.

Morreale, Deborah H. (1987). "Nutrition and Women's Health Concerns." MPH thesis, New York Medical College, New York.

Robertson, Laurel et al. (1978). "The Diet during Pregnancy." In *Laurel's Kitchen.* New York: Bantam Books.

Weed, Susan S. (1986). *Wise Woman Herbal for the Childbearing Year.* Woodstock, NY: Ash Tree Publishing.

VERSION. *See instead* EXTERNAL CEPHALIC VERSION

VIOLENCE AGAINST PREGNANT WOMEN

Domestic violence has reached epidemic levels. In the United States alone, approximately four million spouses are beaten annually (Straus, Gelles, and Steinmetz, 1980; Straus, 1986), and 95 percent of these victims are women (Bureau of Justice Statistics, 1983). Physical battery is a leading cause of injuries to women; one Yale study found that battering caused more injuries to women than motor vehicle crashes, rapes, and muggings combined (Rosenberg et al., 1987). More specifically, violence toward pregnant women is an ever increasing public health concern. In 1986, a Surgeon General's workshop identified pregnancy as a high-risk period for battering and recommended that all pregnant women be screened for battering as part of routine prenatal assessments (Surgeon General's Workshop, 1986).

Studies document the increasing prevalence of violence toward pregnant women. In a sample of 290 pregnant women randomly selected from public and private clinics, 23 percent had been physically battered before or during their pregnancy (Helton, McFarlane, and Anderson, 1987). In this study, the primary predictor of battering during pregnancy was prior abuse; 87.5 percent of the women battered during their pregnancy were physically abused prior to being pregnant. Additionally, none of the women had been assessed by a health care provider for battering, nor were they provided with any community resources.

Another study found that as many as 62 percent of 225 women from a battered women's shelter were beaten during pregnancy (Okun, 1986). Unfortunately, these statistics are not unusual in other countries as well. Reports from Great Britain indicate beatings during pregnancy are relatively common ("Britain: Battered Wives," 1973).

Experts have suggested factors that contribute to the battering of pregnant women, including (1) transition and stress, (2) prenatal child abuse, and (3) defenselessness of the women (Gelles, 1975). Pregnancy has been labeled by some as the end of the honeymoon stage of a marriage. For many families, this transition to parenthood creates a number of stresses, including change in family role relations. However, the stresses of pregnancy alone do not cause battering. The crucial point is that the pregnancy stress simply combines with an already high level of structural stress in these families to precipitate violence.

Second, whether on a conscious or subconscious level, violence towards a pregnant woman may be a form of prenatal child abuse or filicide. For example, one woman reported beatings in the stomach whenever she was pregnant, as opposed to her usual beatings in the face. Violence may be a husband's attempt to terminate the pregnancy. Violence is typical of many family relations and is often seen as a normal part of family life. Consequently, for many families, violence that terminates a pregnancy may be more acceptable socially and morally than is an abortion.

Finally, pregnant women may be more vulnerable to violence because their husbands view them as unable or unwilling to retaliate because of their changed physical condition.

Experts have suggested strategies for dealing with violence and pregnancy (Gelles, 1975). Many women are battered because they are carrying unwanted or unplanned-for children. For the battering to cease, avenues must exist to prevent or ease the stress of an unwanted pregnancy. Effective planned parenthood programs, dissemination of birth control, and the removal of legal barriers and social stigma of abortion are all steps in reducing unwanted pregnancies and thus, battering of pregnant women.

A second strategy prepares both men and women for the changes that will occur as a result of pregnancy, childbirth, and the rearing of children. The more knowledgeable people are about pregnancy and the surrounding issues, the better able they are to cope with the changes that accompany pregnancy and children.

Finally, more community networking among social service agencies and medical facilities will help to promote earlier interventions on the woman's behalf. Women who are battered during pregnancy need both medical attention and social service agencies that respond to their physical, emotional, and social needs. If the community can intervene at this point, the cycle of violence may cease to exist.

Overall, because battering during pregnancy is a known problem, it is essential that pregnant women are assessed by caregivers for potential battering. Violence toward pregnant women is a national public health concern that must be responded to accordingly. ✷ DAWN BEVERIDGE, J.D.

See also: Domestic Violence and Pregnancy

See **Guide to Related Topics:** Pregnancy Complications

Resources

"Britain: Battered Wives." (1973, Jul 9). *Newsweek*: 39.

Bureau of Justice Statistics. (1983, Summer). "Report to the Nation on Crime and Justice." U.S. Department of Justice, Office of Justice Programs.

Gelles, Richard. (1975). "Violence and Pregnancy: A Note on the Extent of the Problem and Needed Services." *The Family Coordinator* 24: 81-86.

Helton, A.S., McFarlane, J., & Anderson, E.T. (1987). "Battered and Pregnant: A Prevalence Study." *American Journal of Public Health* 77: 1337-39.

Okun, Lewis. (1986). *Women Abuse: Facts Replacing Myths*. Albany, NY: State University of New York Press.

Rosenberg, M.L. et al. (1987). "Violence: Homicide, Assault and Suicide." In R.W. Amler & H.B. Dull (Eds.) *Closing the Gap: The Burden of Unnecessary Illness*. New York: Oxford University Press, pp. 164-78.

Straus, M.A. (1986). "Domestic Violence and Homicide Antecedents." *Bulletin of the New York Academy of Medicine* 62: 446-65.

Straus, M.A. & Gelles, P.J. (1986). "Societal Change and Change in Family Violence from 1975 to 1985 as Revealed by Two National Surveys." *Journal of Marriage and the Family* 48: 465-79.

Straus, M.A., Gelles, P.J., & Steinmetz, S.K. (1980). *Behind Closed Doors: Violence in the American Family*. Garden City, NY: Doubleday.

Surgeon General's Workshop on Violence: Recommendations on Spouse Abuse. (1986). *Response* 9 (1): 19-21.

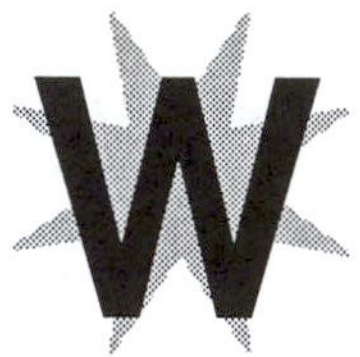

WEANING

Weaning is a term that describes the infant's transition from breastfeeding to bottle feeding or to other food. Weaning begins when the mother makes a decision to stop breastfeeding or accepts her infant's refusal to nurse, and it ends when the infant no longer breastfeeds. Because either the mother may decide to stop breastfeeding or the infant may refuse the breast, weaning is considered to be either "maternal led" (that is, the mother's decision) or "infant led," (the infant's decision to wean, or self-weaning). The mother may decide to wean the infant because she must return to work, she wishes to have more freedom, feels tired, dislikes breastfeeding, desires to become pregnant again, or simply considers the infant "old enough to wean." The infant may suddenly start to refuse the breast because the infant is cutting teeth or becomes distracted and too busy and interested in other things to take the time to nurse. Often, other people, such as friends of the family, parents, or the infant's father, will urge the mother to wean so that they may assist with feeding and caring for the infant or because they feel that the infant is old enough to wean. This is known as "social coercion for weaning" (Morse and Harrison, 1987).

Except in exceptional circumstances, weaning occurs over a period of time. If weaning does occur within one day, this is known as "sudden severance" or "cold turkey." The infant may become very upset with the abrupt change, and the mother may experience some breast engorgement (i.e., fullness); therefore, cold turkey is not generally recommended.

Gradual weaning is the gradual replacement of breastfeeding with formula (in a cup or a bottle) or with solid foods. In a study of 100 mothers who weaned, this method was used by 42 percent of the mothers, and the mean age of the infants was seven months (Williams and Morse, 1989). The mid-morning or mid-afternoon feedings were eliminated first, and once the mothers substituted another source of food for a breast feeding, they did not usually revert back to breastfeeding.

A third method of weaning is to revert to minimal breastfeeding. Minimal breastfeeding is usually a two-step process. First, weaning is initiated

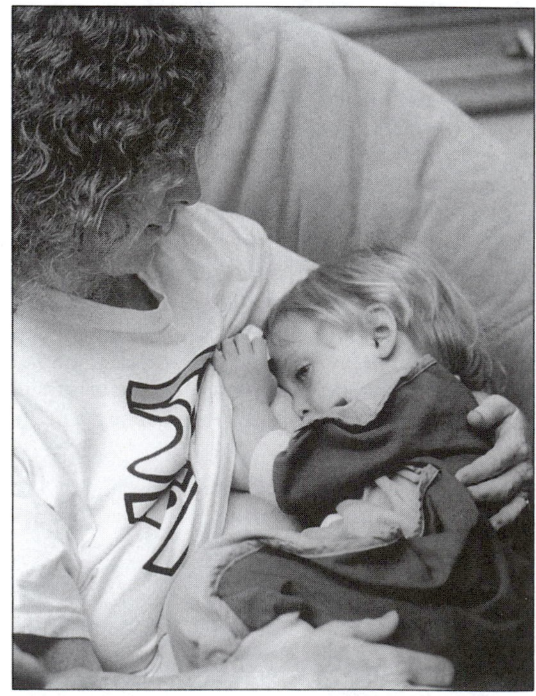

As this three-year-old nursing child illustrates, weaning may take place over a long period, and nursing continues to offer comfort. Photo courtesy of Harriette Hartigan/Artemis.

by gradually reducing the number of feedings until the infant is breastfeeding only in the morning and the evening. This process is easier if the infant's least favorite feeding is eliminated first. Mothers do not express their breasts to relieve engorgement or to maintain lactation: The volume of milk produced appears to gradually adjust to the infant's needs. This pattern may be maintained as long as the infant or the mother wishes it to continue. The second step is the actual weaning or cessation of breastfeeding altogether by gradually weaning the infant from either the night or the morning feed and then, finally, the last feed. In the above study, this method was used by 49 percent of the mothers and was considered preferable because the mothers could retain the nursing bond with their infant, while also having the freedom during the day to work.

When is the best time to wean the infant? There is rarely a "best time" to wean the baby. The time that weaning takes place will depend on many factors, such as the infant's weight gain, contentedness, and satisfaction with nursing; these factors should be balanced against the length of maternity leave or need to return to work, fatigue, the number of other children in the household to care for, and the amount of support the mother has for breastfeeding. However, mothers should continue to breastfeed as long as they can and delay introducing solids or other foods if the infant does not appear to need them.

Many infants continue to nurse as toddlers or beyond. There is no medical or psychological reason to suggest that continuing breastfeeding is harmful, yet many mothers feel awkward and are even reluctant to admit that their nursery-school child is still nursing. Nevertheless, this is a normal practice in many cultures worldwide. The important point is that weaning should not be an unnecessarily difficult period, but rather a gradual relinquishment of a special relationship when the child is ready. ✱ JANICE M. MORSE, Ph.D.

See also: Breastfeeding beyond Infancy; Weaning Food

See **Guide to Related Topics:** Infant Feeding

Resources

Morse, Janice M. & Harrison, Margaret. (1987). "Social Coercion for Weaning." *Journal of Nurse-Midwifery 32:* 205-10.

Williams, Karen Matulonis & Morse, Janice M. (1989). "Weaning Patterns of First-time Mothers." *Maternal Child Nursing 14(3)*: 188-92.

WEANING FOOD

Weaning food is what infants eat during the transition from mother's milk to table food. Cultural systems vary widely in defining weaning food, its entry into the infant diet, and its symbolic significance regarding health, social relations, and cultural values. Weaning food varies from baby foods produced in the United States to foods right off the table in rural Latin America. Premastication, a process in which a woman chews up adult food and then puts it into the infant's mouth, is the means of producing weaning foods in some hunting and gathering and farming societies.

In the middle class of more developed countries (e.g., the United States), infant formula commonly precedes other food in the diet, including breastmilk. Although infant formula is technically a weaning food, laypeople and health professionals instead generally equate it with breastmilk, a view that serves the interests of the infant formula industry. Weaning is thus commonly seen as a shift from infant formula to foods marketed specifically for weaning, commonly called "baby food." Baby food is sold in small jars, with each jar containing a mashed or ground-up vegetable, fruit, or meat. Both infant formula and baby food are produced in factories, marketed by large corporations, and designed to make profits.

Contrary to popular opinion, commercial baby food is not always safe and has caused significant damage to infant health because of errors in composition or manufacturing. Errors in infant formula have periodically caused death and permanent retardation. In addition, commercial efforts have resulted in catastrophic rates of death in less developed countries from the introduction of infant formula to people living in poverty with dangerous water supplies.

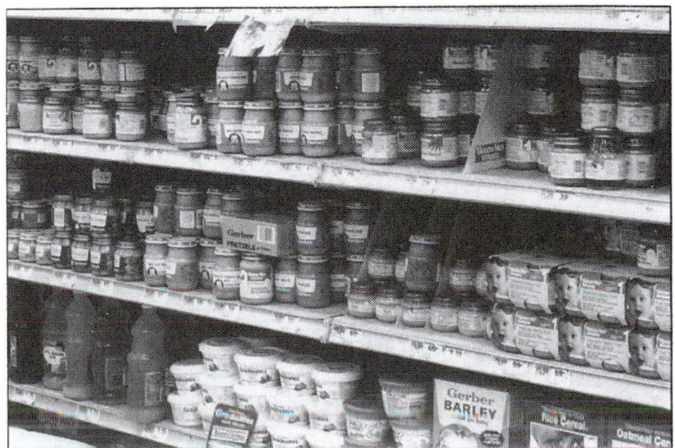

Typical supermarket display of baby foods. Photo courtesy of Jay Rothman.

Recently the use of infant formula in farming societies in less developed countries has increased; traditionally, weaning foods were not purchased but were introduced from the table or made by mothers for their infants. When an agricultural society has a specific weaning food, it tends to be a porridge made of the common staple. In much of rural China, for example, the weaning food is made of rice, and in Tibet, milk and barley flour. In at least some societies (e.g., Malawi and Andean Peru), women make food daily for snacking by children whenever they want, and children eat table foods from the family pot as well. The use of these foods and the manner of introducing them is tied to the age at which infants begin the weaning process.

Technically, infants in farming societies often begin weaning in the first days of life in the sense that they often are given tea (boiled herbs) to drink during the first two or three days after birth, before their mothers' milk supply replaces colostrum, the first fluid produced after birth, which is often prohibited as infant food. Infants may receive teas intermittently for medicinal purposes, particularly for diarrhea.

Excluding tea and focusing on solid and semisolid foods, on the other hand, reveals a pattern of introduction that depends on the child's developmental status. In many Latin American societies, for example, a child who reaches for a food is given a piece of it, and weaning onto solid food proceeds in this fashion at the initiative of the child in response to the food available. The age of the child does not matter particularly, as the developmental stage of the child is what contributes most to the behavior of reaching for food. Children under these circumstances begin to express food preferences immediately, and mothers and other caretakers follow those preferences rather than forcing children onto a regimen of specific foods, quantities, and times for eating, as in the urban middle class.

Pastoralists and nomads tend to wean infants between two and three years of age, and the foods tend to be those derived from herd animals, including mild, meat, and blood, depending on the society. Trade with agriculturalists also can bring grain into the weaning diet, usually mixed with milk in a porridge.

Infant feeding rituals emphasize the cultural significance of weaning foods in some societies, and the weaning food is symbolically charged in all societies on which data are available. The urban middle class views processed baby foods as efficient, nutritious, and safe, and sees other foods generally as dangerous for babies. These views tie to a general confidence in technology and consumer products, whose safety is supposed to be guaranteed by the state.

In societies where a principal weaning food is porridge, it tends to be made of the main staple, which is usually the cultural super food—a food seen as necessary for general well-being and esteemed in religion and myth. The super food is also a product of constraints imposed by ecological and historical forces. The weaning food itself connects the child to the economy and cosmology of the society, and this observation appears to hold across the spectrum of societies, from the urban middle class to hunters and gatherers.

Many societies adhere to weaning food taboos based on kinship relations. The Ponam in Papua New Guinea forbid babies to eat foods that are associated with the mother's clan "on the grounds that they will cause speech impediments, delay toilet training or otherwise hinder the development of a fully social being" (Carrier, 1985, p. 200). How weaning foods are viewed is a composite of cultural knowledge, social organization, and ecological and historical forces; thus the determinants of weaning foods include many more factors than just efficiency and nutritional value.

The approach of the 21st century is a time of flux in weaning foods under pressure from medical professionals, international development agencies, transnational corporations, and changing cultural values, especially those involving prestige. Many health professionals and development agencies continue to reject local weaning foods and press for introduction of industrial products into children's diets. In many respects, these efforts have unwittingly benefitted the commercial sector but have been detrimental to child health and family budgets in impoverished groups throughout the world.

✱ ANN V. MILLARD, Ph.D., and SHERRY HURWITZ

See also: Formula Marketing

See **Guide to Related Topics:** Infant Feeding

Resources

Carrier, Achsah H. (1985). "Infant Care and Family Relations on Ponam Island, Manus Province, Papau New Guinea." In L. B. Marshall (Ed.) *Infant Care and Feeding in the South Pacific.* New York: Gordon and Breach, pp. 189-205.

Chetley, Andrew. (1986). *The Politics of Baby Foods: Successful Challenges to an International Marketing Strategy.* New York: St. Martin's.

Millard, Ann V. & Graham, Margaret A. (1985). "Breastfeeding in Two Mexican Villages: Social and Demographic Perspectives." In V.J. Hull & M. Simpson-Herbert (Eds.) *Breastfeeding, Child Health and Child Spacing.* Dover, NH: Croom Helm, pp. 55-77.

Schieffelin, Bambi B. (1985). "Commentary: The Importance of Cultural Perspectives on Infant Care and Feeding. In L.B. Marshall (Ed.) *Infant Care and Feeding in the South Pacific*. New York: Gordon and Breach, pp. 1-12.

Van Esterik, Penny B. (1989). *Beyond the Breast-Bottle Controversy*. New Brunswick, NJ: Rutgers University.

World Health Organization. (1988) *Weaning from Breast Milk to Family Foods: A Guide for Health and Community Workers*. Geneva: World Health Organization.

WEBSTER v. REPRODUCTIVE HEALTH SERVICES

In January 1989, the United States Supreme Court agreed to decide *Webster v. Reproductive Health Services*, a case involving a Missouri abortion law, one of the most restrictive in the country. Women's rights groups, the medical community, and civil rights groups viewed the case as a substantial threat to a woman's fundamental right to terminate pregnancy as established by *Roe v. Wade*. The Bush administration had urged the Supreme Court to use the *Webster* case to overturn the *Roe* decision. Furthermore, the Supreme Court had become more conservative since *Roe*, making it possible that the Court would abolish or seriously threaten a women's constitutionally protected right to choose an abortion (Kolbert, 1989).

The *Webster* case mobilized the pro-choice majority like never before. Younger women who had grown to depend on reproductive freedom and older women who remembered the deaths and injuries caused by illegal abortions wrote letters to the Supreme Court and took to the streets to support the right to safe and legal abortions. More friends-of-the-court briefs (briefs filed by individuals or organizations not parties to the case but with an interest in its outcome) were filed in the *Webster* case than in any other case in history, reflecting the nationwide interest in the outcome (Tribe, 1990).

The Supreme Court upheld the three provisions of the Missouri law at issue in the *Webster* case: a declaration that life begins at conception; the prohibition on the performance of abortions in public facilities; and the fetal viability testing requirements. The Court found these provisions constitutional without overruling *Roe v. Wade*. (It would take five justices to overrule the case.) However, three justices—Chief Justice Rehnquist, Justice White, and Justice Kennedy (the plurality)—expressly rejected *Roe's* trimester framework. Justice Scalia expressly stated that *Roe* should be overruled (*Webster*, 1989). Justice O'Connor, the first and only woman on the Supreme Court, was the deciding vote in upholding the law. She had attacked the trimester framework in two previous cases, but she declined to do so in *Webster* (Tribe, 1990; *Webster*, 1989).

Justice Blackmun, the author of *Roe* opinion, thought much of the Missouri law was unconstitutional. He believed that the plurality's opinion (which is not the "law of the land" right now but could be in the future) would have a devastating impact on women's lives:

> the plurality . . . casts into darkness the hopes and visions of every woman in this country who had come to believe that the Constitution guaranteed her the right to exercise some control over her unique ability to bear children. . . . [M]illions of women, and their families, have ordered their lives around the right to reproductive choice, and . . . this right has become vital to the full participation of women in the economic and political walks of American life." (*Webster*, at 3077).

Webster did not bring the downfall of *Roe v. Wade*. Neither did the Supreme Court decision or the 1992 Pennsylvania case, which upheld states' ability to restrict access to abortion, including provisions for parental notification and waiting periods, but not husband notification. However, a woman's right to reproductive freedom is now on much shakier grounds than it was in 1973, the year of *Roe v. Wade*.

✱ CAROLE WRIGHT NAPIER, J.D.

See also: Abortion, Politics of; Roe v. Wade

***See* Guide to Related Topics:** Abortion; Legal Issues

Resources

Kolbert, Kathryn. (1989). "Webster v. Reproductive Health Services: Reproductive Freedom Hanging by a Thread." *Women's Rights Law Reporter 11* (3 & 4): 151-62.

Mersky, Roy & Hartman, Gary. (1990). *A Documentary History of the Legal Aspects of Abortion in the United States, Webster v. Reproductive Health Services*. Littleton, CO: Fred B. Rothman & Co.

Tribe, Laurence. (1990). *Abortion: The Clash of Absolutes*. New York: W.W. Norton & Co.

Webster v. Reproductive Health Services, 492 U.S. 490 (1989).

WET NURSING

Wet nursing involves breastfeeding of an infant by a woman who is not the infant's mother. It has been an occupation for women since pre-Christian times. Often it has been a well-paid job with considerable prestige and often it has been the role of enslaved women. It has been an occupation, primarily, of the not-so-distant past except in developing countries where forms of wet nursing still exist. In these situations, wet nursing is generally an informal arrangement between sisters or other female relatives.

Western history has viewed wet nursing in one of two extremes: It is either an "exploitation of women whose own babies were left to die so the woman could sell her milk to survive" or "the wet nurse was a drunken slut who neglected or even murdered her charges" (Palmer, 1988, p. 133). While both of these views were more likely to be true after the Industrial Revolution, these stereotypes do not encompass the history of wet nursing or the women involved.

There are four types of wet nurses; each reflects the social class of both the baby and the wet nurse, as well as cultural norms. The first type is that of royalty or high aristocracy in which a parturient woman of good stock lived in the suckling baby's household and provided infant care beyond just nursing. Her status was greater than that of other household staff. This was respectable employment for a woman that might result in her lifelong care by the employer.

A second more common type was that in which the middle or upper-class nursling was sent to the home of the wet nurse. This arrangement suggests less class distinction between the baby's family and the wet nurse. In these situations, the wet nurse was usually of good stock, married, and had two or three children of her own.

In cultural settings where slavery was prevalent—the American South prior to the 1860s, for example—the slave wet nurse often performed her services at the expense of her own health and that of her children. Despite these disadvantages it is commonly believed that this household work, like other household tasks, was preferable to working in the fields. It was not uncommon for slave wet nurses to stay on to care for the child they had suckled well past weaning. It is curious that throughout much of the history of wet nursing it was been believed that a nursling imbibed the characteristics of its nurse. But, despite the assignment of negative characteristics to the women who nursed, the practice prevailed. In classes that possessed slaves, wet nursing was virtually universal.

The institutional wet nurse was as culturally disenfranchised as the babies she serviced. She was always poor, perhaps diseased, and often unwed, having lost her baby to death or the care of a foundling home not unlike the one that employed her. The foundling hospital provided a means of employment for a class of women who otherwise might have found their only other options to be begging or prostitution.

Wet nurses were employed for a variety of reasons. For women of the middle class a wet nurse made it possible for them to continue to labor outside of the home. Maternal mortality rates in all classes necessitated wet nurses in order to save the lives of the infants. But, beyond necessity, the overwhelming reasons the upper classes utilized wet nurses related to looks and health. It was commonly believed that nursing was disfiguring, inconvenient, and that high-born women were unable to nurse—the abnormal physical demands of high fashion no doubt made this true in many instances.

High infant mortality rates have been associated with wet nursing and have historically been blamed on the wet nurse's character or her diseased body. More likely, infant mortality was high because newborns turned over to a wet nurse were not likely to get the colostrum needed to provide immunity from sickness. Additionally, the temporary passive immunity a newborn enjoys with its own mother is absent when the child is taken into a different environment and suckled by a woman who has been exposed to different infections. Another cause of death to seemingly healthy infants attributed to wet nurses was that of "overlaying," which was said to result when the wet nurse fell asleep and rolled over on the infant and suffocated it. It is likely that many of the deaths attributed to overlaying would now be attributable to Sudden Infant Death Syndrome (SIDS).

By the 1770s it was becoming more fashionable in the industrialized West for mothers to nurse their own babies and for those who did hire wet nurses to have them take up residence in the infant's home. This eliminated the married mother with children of her own as a candidate for wet nursing. Wet nurses were more often single mothers whose situation was not dissimilar to that of the institutional wet nurse. As the century ended, it became more common for wet nursing to be the occupation of lower-class urban women rather than rural women of farmer or artisan stock.

Despite the swing in philosophy in the late 18th century, wet nursing remained a common alternative to maternal breastfeeding in both developing and industrialized countries until after the Second World War. Many foundling hospitals continued to use wet nurses, especially to suckle weak infants or those not thriving on artificial foods. It was common throughout the U.S. for premature infants to be wet nursed or for the infants to drink, from a bottle, milk expressed by wet nurses.

Finally, throughout the history of the world, there have been women who nursed the babies of their relatives, friends, and neighbors. This has usually not been a means of paid employment but rather part of the network of women's caregiving, especially if the baby's life was dependent on human milk. With the resurgence of breastfeeding in industrialized countries, "cross-nursing," in which lactating mothers nurse babies other than their own, is being seen again; however, this is usually a casual and temporary arrangement between close relatives or friends (Kranz, 1981).

✱ AMY KING

See also: Breastfeeding: Historical Aspects; Breastfeeding: Physiological and Cultural Aspects

See **Guide to Related Topics:** Infant Feeding

Resources

Apple, Rima D. (1987). *Mothers and Medicine: A Social History of Infant Feeding*. Madison, WI: The University of Wisconsin Press.

Fildes, Valerie. (1988). *Breasts, Bottles and Babies*. Edinburgh, Scotland: Edinburgh University Press.

———. (1988). *Wet Nursing: A History from Antiquity to the Present*. London: Basil Blackwell.

Kranz, Judith. (1981). "Cross-Nursing: Wet Nursing in a Contemporary Context." *Pediatrics* 57: 715-40.

Palmer, Gabrielle. (1988). *The Politics of Breastfeeding*. London: Pandora Press.

WITCH MIDWIVES

Most of the women accused of witchcraft in medieval Europe were midwives (Ehrenreich and English, 1973). They were cultural descendants of ancient birth-priestesses once everywhere connected with temples of the Mother Goddess. In the old pagan world, no man dared touch a birthing woman for fear of being blasted by her powerful magic. The Bible warns men to keep away from a new mother for 40 days—or 80 days, if her child is a daughter—because she is "unclean" (Leviticus 12:4, 5). "Unclean" originally meant "taboo" in the double sense of frightening and sacred.

It was generally believed that only elder priestesses who were mothers themselves, like the Roman *obstetrix,* could comprehend the primal mysteries of birthing. These traditions passed into folk medicine and witchcraft when Christianity destroyed the Goddess temples and outlawed the priestesses' profession. Lawful or not, witches' midwifery services were still necessary. Women continued to give birth, and men continued to dread and avoid the whole business.

Renaissance witch hunts came down with particular fury on midwives, because of churchmen's resentment of their mysterious knowledge and their intimacy with other women. Official literature of the Inquisition stated: "No one does more harm to the Catholic faith than midwives" (Kramer and Sprenger, 1971). Midwives were consistently accused of witchcraft, tortured and burned. Witch midwives were among the few women who could earn money for themselves in those patriarchal times; moreover, they were often suspected of helping other women to govern their reproductive lives through secret methods of birth control or abortion. This suspected activity stood in direct opposition to the Church's opinion that women's bodies should be entirely at the disposal of men.

From that day to the present, male-dominated establishments have been noticeably hostile toward midwives (Walker, 1983). Around the turn of the last century, the American Medical Association succeeded in legislating women out of their time-honored midwifery profession in order to replace them with men. Some American midwives were imprisoned simply for continuing their lifelong practice, in towns where they had delivered nearly every citizen (Barker-Benfield, 1976).

✱ BARBARA G. WALKER

See also: Midwifery: Overview; Obstetrics, History of

See **Guide to Related Topics:** Caregivers and Practitioners

Resources

Barker-Benfield, G.J. (1976). *The Horrors of the Half-Known Life*. New York: Harper & Row.

Ehrenreich, Barbara & English, Deirdre. (1973). *Witches, Midwives and Nurses: A History of Women Healers*. Old Westbury, NY: Feminist Press.

Kramer, Heinrich & Sprenger, James. (1971). *Malleus Maleficarum*. New York: Dover, pp. 66, 141.

Walker, Barbara G. (1983). *The Woman's Encyclopedia of Myths and Secrets*. San Francisco: Harper & Row, pp. 654-57.

WOMEN'S HEALTH MOVEMENT

The women's health movement developed during the late 1960s and early 1970s, first in North America, then in Europe and around the world. The social conditions of birth and reproductive rights initially brought feminists together to share personal experiences, take political action, and establish alternative services. Women objected to what they saw as the control that men had over their bodies and reproductive functions and believed that reproductive control was a precondition to achieving equal rights in education, politics, employment, and the family. Today, women's health movement activities include empowering women with knowledge; providing woman-centered, culturally sensitive services; and taking political action at the local and national levels to ensure women's health.

Developing and Sharing Knowledge. Initially, women formed study and self-help groups to share experiences and information. The Boston Women's Health Book Collective, one such group, has sold over three million copies of its book, *Our Bodies, Ourselves,* including 14 foreign language editions. Another early group, which grew into the Federation of Feminist Women's Health Centers, promoted cervical self-examination. Women developed and used their self-created knowledge in women's body courses that combined basic anatomy and physiology with women's personal experiences. Many early groups included pelvic self-examination to demystify the body and to help women to recognize gynecological problems. Over time, more specialized self-help groups emerged—for women at a particular life-cycle stage or with a specific problem.

As the movement grew beyond largely white, middle-class participants, groups focusing on the needs of women of color broadened the movement's scope. In the U.S., the National Black Women's Health Project, for example, has over 150 self-help groups in 25 states that address race and gender-specific aspects of infant mortality, teen pregnancy, AIDS, substance abuse, cardiovascular disease, cancer, and stress. The organization provides personal health information and policy material on request. The Native American Women's Health Education Center in Lake Andes, South Dakota, started as a regional, community-based health project offering programs on fetal alcohol syndrome, diabetes, and related health issues. The Center now reaches out to Native American women in the U.S. and Canada with information on a wide array of issues, ranging from toxic waste to racism. The National Latina Health Organization in Oakland, California, distributes information nationally on reproductive health and locally offers prenatal classes in Spanish.

Worldwide efforts at education include the work of hundreds of local and regional groups, many of which have developed material on birth and reproductive health. The Women's Health Reproductive Rights Information Center in London is an example of the type of organization that distributes material nationally and regionally. The Canadian Women's Health Network publishes Health Sharing, a magazine emphasizing regional issues that is distributed throughout Canada.

In 1980, ISIS WICCE (the Women's International Cross-Cultural Exchange) and the Boston Women's Health Book Collective produced *The International Women and Health Resource Guide,* which documented the growth of the women's health movement internationally. Today, ISIS WICCE distributes health information worldwide and provides opportunities for women to learn new skills through placements in other countries. ISIS Internacional in Santiago, Chile, publishes and distributes health information in Spanish and English throughout Latin America and the Caribbean. The Women's Global Network on Reproductive Rights in Amsterdam has member organizations worldwide and sponsors international exchanges and develops health material. Women's Health Interaction in Ottawa, Canada, has strong links with Latin America and engages in international outreach activities worldwide.

Although the women's health movement is less developed in Asia, Africa, the Caribbean, and the Middle East, the Asian and Pacific Women's Action and Resource Center has published a series of health guidebooks. In the Caribbean, health activism is embedded in women's development activities through groups such as the Women and Development Unit at the University of the West Indies in Barbados. In Uganda, groups linked to the Women's Global Network on Reproductive Rights and to other women's organizations throughout Africa are beginning to organize around issues. A Middle Eastern feminist group, Women Living Under Muslim Law, distributes health information.

Medical Services. Some groups provide direct services ranging from medical referral to outpatient medical care, abortion, and midwifery in woman-centered clinics. In addition to the Federation of Feminist Women's Health Centers, the Elizabeth Blackwell Clinic in Philadelphia, the Lyon-Martin Clinic in San Francisco, the Vancouver Women's Health Collective, and the Dispensaire de Femme in Geneva are examples of the type of woman-centered gynecological services feminists established as alternatives to traditional medical care. All emphasize giving women full information, demystifying medical procedures, and using nurses, midwives, and other nonphysician health providers in decision-making roles. In French-speaking Quebec, Regroupement des Francois Centres de Santé de Femme du Québec serves as the coordinating body for women's health centers.

Influencing Public Policy and Health Rights. Feminist health activists are committed to making changes in existing health systems throughout the world. The political "successes" of health movement groups are extensive and impressive. In the U.S., the National Women's Health Network educates the public and monitors legislation and regulatory agencies to protect women's health rights. With a membership of over 11,000 individuals and over 400 organizations, representing a constituency of over half a million people, the Network speaks on behalf of a sizeable interest group. Network expert witnesses testify regularly at congressional hearings and the U.S. Food and Drug Administration (FDA). The Network has also filed class action suits against companies whose products have harmed women, has pressed for better labeling of drugs and devices, and has played a key role in passing the New York Maternity Information Act, which went into effect in 1990 and requires hospitals to make rates of cesarean sections and other surgical procedures public. The Network distributes the "Pregnant Patient's Bill of Rights," developed jointly with the International Childbirth Education Association. Many other groups work at the state and local level.

Growth and Change. While the number of gynecological self-help groups has declined, self-help groups such as those sponsored by the National Black Women's Health Project are increasing in number. Some of the early feminist health organizations suspended operation in recent years, but remaining organizations represent a wide array of women's health interests. The World Health Organization has organized conferences, supported health activist information centers, and encouraged international exchange of feminist information on women's health, including traditional and alternative birth practices. The recent growth of health groups in developing countries reflects the increasingly global character of the women's health movement, although the needs and perspectives of women in developed and developing countries continue to differ significantly. ✱ SHERYL BURT RUZEK, Ph.D., M.P.H.

See also: Support Groups

Resources

Avery, Byllye. (1990). "Breathing Life Into Ourselves: The Evolution of the National Black Women's Health Project. In Evelyn C. White (Ed.) Speaking for Ourselves: The Black Women's Health Book. Seattle, WA: Seal Press.

Boston Women's Health Book Collective. (1984). The New Our Bodies, Ourselves. New York: Simon and Schuster.

Boston Women's Health Book Collective and ISIS. (1980). *International Women and Health Resource Guide.* Boston: BWHBC; Geneva: ISIS.

Doyal, Leslie. (1983). "Women, Health and the Sexual Division of Labour: A Case Study of the Women's Health Movement in Britain." *Critical Social Policy 7*: 21-33.

Federation of Feminist Women's Health Centers. (1981). *A New View of a Woman's Body.* New York: Simon & Schuster.

Ruzek, Sheryl Burt. (1978). *The Women's Health Movement: Feminist Alternatives to Medical Control.* New York: Praeger.

———. (1986). "Feminist Visions of Health: An International Perspective." In Juliet Mitchell and Ann Oakley (Eds.) *What Is Feminism?* London: Basil Blackwell.

Zimmerman, Mary. (1987). "The Women's Health Movement: A Critique of Medical Enterprise and the Position of Women." In Beth B. Hess & Myra Marx Ferree (Eds.) *Analyzing Gender: Social Science Perspectives.* Beverly Hills, CA: Sage Publications.

WRONGFUL BIRTH AND WRONGFUL LIFE

When a medical professional provides negligent care to a pregnant woman and thereby causes injury to her fetus, the law recognizes that the professional should be held liable for the consequences. Thus, the responsible parties may be sued to recover compensation (damages) for the financial burden imposed by the injury, as well as for the resultant physical and emotional harm. Such a lawsuit is known as a malpractice claim for prenatal tort.

Although lawsuits denominating wrongful birth and wrongful life are also malpractice actions concerning the birth of an infant in an impaired condition, they differ dramatically from the typical prenatal tort claim. In such suits it is not asserted that the professional caused or failed to prevent the impairment itself. Rather, in such cases, the negligence consists of a failure to detect or predict the impairment; the claim is that had the defendant not been negligent, the child would not have been conceived, or would not have been carried to term. Thus, whereas in a typical prenatal tort action it is claimed that but for the defendant's negligence, the child would have been born in an unimpaired state, in a wrongful birth or wrongful life suit it is claimed that but for the negligence, the child would not have been born at all.

Such a case might arise, for example, when an obstetrician fails to offer amniocentesis to a pregnant patient who has a known risk of bearing a child with a genetic defect (such as Down's syndrome), or where, prior to conception, a physician fails to detect an inheritable trait in the parents that can manifest itself as a severe defect in the offspring (such as Tay Sachs disease). In this class of cases, the parents will claim either that they would have aborted the fetus or that they would have avoided conception altogether had they been given timely and correct information.

Typically the parents in a wrongful birth or wrongful life suit seek damages for the extraordinary medical and educational expenses of raising the child, and for the emotional harm caused by bearing and raising the child. Claims brought by the parents are known as wrongful birth claims. Wrongful life claims are those brought by or on behalf of the child seeking damages for the costs of his or her care, and for the physical and mental pain and suffering he or she endures.

Although the term "wrongful birth" is sometimes used to describe malpractice cases involving the birth of healthy children following negligently performed sterilization or abortion procedures, such cases are more commonly called "wrongful conception" or "wrongful pregnancy." The issue in such cases are often the same or similar to the issues in wrongful birth and wrongful life cases, but they will not be specifically addressed here.

Wrongful birth and wrongful life suits are a relatively recent development in the law and have not been met with easy or universal acceptance. They raise a variety of difficult legal, social, and philosophical issues. The first reported case of this type was decided in 1967. In Gleitman v. Cosgrove, a physician incorrectly assured a pregnant woman that the rubella (German measles) she had contracted in the first trimester of her pregnancy would not affect her fetus. When the child was born with substantial defects as a result of the rubella, the parents and the child sued the physician, claiming that the pregnancy would have been terminated by abortion if the mother had been given correct information (49 N.J. 22, 227 A.2d 689, 1967). The New Jersey Supreme Court disallowed the child's claim on the ground that it was impossible to prove damages. The general rule is that damages are determined by comparing the injured party's situation with what his or her situation would have been "but for" the defendant's negligence. In this case, but for the defendant's negligence the child would not even exist. The court concluded that it was impossible to "weigh the value of life with impairments against the nonexistence of life itself." The court also denied the parent's claims on the theory that it was impossible to conduct the "but for" comparison required in order to determine damages. Concluding that but for the negligence, the parents would have been denied "the intangible, unmeasurable, and complex human benefits of motherhood and fatherhood," the court held that it was impossible to weigh this benefit against the emotional and financial harm caused by the child's birth.

An additional and probably more important factor in the court's decision was that the abortion would have been illegal in New Jersey and probably everywhere else in the United States at that time. Even if the abortion could have been legally obtained outside the country, the court held that public policy dictated against a claim seeking damages "for the denial of the opportunity to take an embryonic life."

Not surprisingly, courts have been more receptive to wrongful birth claims of parents following the Supreme Court decision in *Roe v. Wade*, which legalized most abortions (410 U.S. 113, 1973). In recent years, most courts that have confronted the issue have permitted the parents to recover damages at least for the expenses attributable to the impairment; a few courts have allowed damages for emotional harm, and some have permitted recovery of all costs of raising the child.

The wrongful life claims of children, however, are still generally precluded. The most frequently cited reasons for the refusal to recognize such claims are that a person's existence, no matter how disabled that person is, does not, in and of itself, constitute an injury to that person, and that even if the law can find that the child's life itself is an injury, it is impossible to measure the damages for such an injury. Notwithstanding these legal and conceptual barriers to recovery, the courts in three states have permitted the child to sue for damages, limited to the extraordinary medical expenses resulting from the impairment.

While the courts continue to grapple with the issues raised in these suits, the legislatures in at least six states have stepped into the arena and passed statutes pertaining to these cases. In several states, any claims based on the negligent prevention of an abortion are prohibited by statute, and South Dakota has a statute that bars all claims related to the birth of a child. ✱ LINDA G. KATZ, J.D.

See also: Eugenics; Prenatal Diagnosis: Overview; Selective Abortion

See **Guide to Related Topics:** Legal Issues; Prenatal Diagnosis and Screening

Resources

Annas, George J. (1988). *Judging Medicine.* Clifton, NJ: Humana Press, pp. 97-107.

Botkin, Jeffrey R. (1988). "The Legal Concept of Wrongful Life." *JAMA 259* (10): 1541-45.

Prosser, William & Keeton, William. (1984). *The Law of Torts.* 5th edition. St. Paul, MN: West Publishing Co., pp. 370-73.

YOGA. *See instead* BODYWORK

Appendix
Organizations and Resources

Abortion and Reproductive Rights

Catholics for a Free Choice
1436 U Street NW
Washington, DC 20009
202-638-1706

The Committee to Defend Reproductive Rights
25 Taylor Street, #704
San Francisco, CA 94102
415-441-4434

Feminists for Life of America
811 East 47th Street
Kansas City, MO 64110
(anti-abortion choice)

International Projects Assistance Services (IPAS)
303 East Main Street
P.O. Box 100
Carrboro, NC 27510
919-967-7052
(abortion)

National Abortion Federation
900 Pennsylvania Avenue SE
Washington, DC 20003
202-546-9060

National Abortion Rights Action League
NARAL
1101 14th Street NW
5th Floor
Washington, DC 20005
202-371-0779

Reproductive Freedom Project
American Civil Liberties Union
132 West 43rd Street
New York, NY 10036
212-944-9800

Women of Color Partnership Program of the Religious Coalition for Abortion Rights
100 Maryland Avenue NE
Washington, DC 20002-5625

Women's Global Network on Reproductive Rights
NWZ. Voorburgwal 32
1012RZ Amsterdam
THE NETHERLANDS

Women's Health Reproductive Rights Information Center
52-54 Featherstone Street
London EC1 8RT
UNITED KINGDOM

Adoption

Adoptees Liberation Movement Association
853 7th Avenue
New York, NY 10019

Adoption Forum
6808 Ridge Avenue (Rear)
Philadelphia, PA 19128

Adoptive Parents for Open Records
P.O. Box 193
Long Valley, NJ 07853

Adoptive Parents of America
OURS Magazine
3333 Highway 100 North
Suite 203
Minneapolis, MN 55422
612-535-4829
(family support groups for transracial adoption)

Concerned United Birth Parents (CUB)
2000 Walker Street
Des Moines, IA 50317
(adoption, birthmothers)

Council for Equal Rights in Adoption
401 East 74th Street
New York, NY 10021

International Soundex Reunion Registry
P.O. Box 2312
Carson City, NV 89702

Medela Breastpumps & Supplemental Nursing System
6711 Sands Road
P.O. Box 386
Crystal Lake, IL 60014
(relactation and induced lactation)

National Adoption Exchange
1218 Chestnut Street
Philadelphia, PA 19107
215-925-0200
(special needs adoption)

National Committee for Adoption
1930 17th Street NW
Washington, DC 20009-6207
202-328-1200

North American Council on Adoptable Children
1821 University Avenue
Suite N 498
St. Paul, MN 55104
612-644-3036
or
810 18th Street NW
Suite 703
Washington, DC 20006
(special needs adoption)

Organization for United Response (OURS)
207 Highway 100 North
Suite 203
Minneapolis, MN 55422
(transnational adoption)

ORIGINS
P.O. Box 444
East Brunswick, NJ 08816
(adoption)

Parents for Private Adoption
P.O. Box 7
Pawlet, VT 05761

AIDS

Body Positive
2095 Broadway, #306
New York, NY 10023
212-721-1346
(women and AIDS resources)

Canadian AIDS Society
170 Laurier Avenue West
Suite 1101
Ottawa, Ontario K1P 5V5
CANADA

Canadian Foundation for AIDS Research (CanFar)
120 Bloor Street East
First Floor
Toronto, Ontario M4W 1B8
CANADA

National Self-Help Clearinghouse
184 5th Avenue
New York, NY 10010

New Jersey Women and AIDS Network
5 Elm Row, Suite 112
New Brunswick, NJ 08901
201-846-4462

Northwest AIDS Foundation
127 Broadway East, Suite #A
Seattle, WA 98102

Sapphex L.E.A.R.N.S.
(Lesbian Education AIDS Resource Network)
14002 Clubhouse Circle, #206
Tampa, FL 33624
813-962-7643

Women's Institute for Mental Health
Women's HIV Project
33 Valencia
San Francisco, CA 94103
415-864-2364

The Women's Project
222 Main Street
Little Rock, AR 72206
501-372-5113

Birth Centers

Maternity Center Association
48 East 92nd Street
New York, NY 10128
212-369-7300

National Association of Childbearing Centers
RD #1, Box 1
Perkiomenville, PA 18074
215-234-8068

Bodywork

Body-Mind Centering
189 Pond View Drive
Amherst, MA 01002
413-256-8615

CONTACT QUARTERLY
P.O. Box 603
Northampton, MA 01061

International Movement Therapy Association
P.O. Box 3701
Stanford, CA 94309
415-525-IMTA

Somatic Learning Associates
8950 Villa la Jolla Drive, #2162
La Jolla, CA 92037
619-436-0418

Breastfeeding

Baby Milk Action (BMAC)
23 Andrew's Street
Cambridge CB2 3AX
UNITED KINGDOM
0223-464420

Breastfeeding Support Consultants
1009 Schoolhouse Road
Pottstown, PA 19464

Geneva Infant Food Association
CP 157 CH 1211
Geneva 19
SWITZERLAND

IBFAN NORTH AMERICA/INFACT
10 Trinity Square
Toronto, Ontario MSG 1B1
CANADA
0101-416-595-9819
(International Baby Food Action Network)

Infant Formula Action Coalition
3255 Hennepin Avenue S
Suite 230
Minneapolis, MN 55408

International Baby Food Action Network (IBFAN)
ACTION
1313 5th Street SE
Suite 302E
Minneapolis, MN 55414
612-379-3905

International Lactation Consultant Associations
201 Brown Avenue
Evanston, IL 60202
708-260-8874

La Leche League Canada
493 Main Street
Winchester, Ontario K0C 2K0
CANADA

La Leche League International, Inc.
P.O. Box 1209
Franklin Park, IL 60131-8209
1-800-LA-LECHE

Medela Breastpumps & Supplemental Nursing System
6711 Sands Road
P.O. Box 386
Crystal Lake, IL 60014
(relactation and induced lactation)

Nursing Mothers Association of Australia
P.O. Box 231
Nunawading, Victoria 3131
AUSTRALIA

Caregivers and Providers, Non-midwife

American College of Obstetrics & Gynecology (ACOG)
600 Maryland Avenue SW
Suite 300E
Washington, DC 20024

Center for Medical Consumers
237 Thompson Street
New York, NY 10012

NAACOG
Nurse Association for the American College of Obstetrics & Gynecology
409 12th Street SW
Washington, DC 20024
800-673-8499

National Association of Labor Assistants
865 Cooper Sage Circle
The Woodlands, TX 77381
713-367-5673

National Association of Neonatal Nurses
191 Lynch Creek Way
Suite 101
Petaluma, CA 94954

National Association of Social Workers
7981 Eastern Avenue
Silver Spring, MD 20910

Simmons College, School of Social Work
Division of Continuing Education
300 The Fenway
Boston, MA 02115
(workshops for pregnant therapists)

Cesarean Births

Cesarean Prevention Movement (CPM)
P.O. Box 152
University Station
Syracuse, NY 13210
315-424-1942

C/SEC, Inc. (Cesareans/Support, Education & Concern)
22 Forest Road
Framingham, MA 01701
508-877-8266

National Center for Health Statistics
U.S. Department of Health & Human Services
6525 Belcrest Road, Room 840
Hyattsville, MD 20782
301-436-8954

VBAC (Vaginal Birth After Cesarean)
10 Great Plain Terrace
Needham, MA 02192
617-449-2490

Childbirth Education

American Academy of Husband-Coached Childbirth
P.O. Box 5224
Sherman Oaks, CA 91413
800-423-2397
(Bradley method)

American Society of Psychoprophylaxis in Obstetrics (ASPO)
1101 Connecticut Avenue NW
Suite 300
Washington, DC 20036
800-368-4404
(Lamaze method)

Birth Resources Training Certification Program
1749 Vine Street
Berkeley, CA 94703

International Childbirth Education Association (ICEA)
P.O. Box 20048
Minneapolis, MN 55420
800-624-4934

The National Childbirth Trust
Education for Parenthood
9 Queensborough Terrace
London W2 3TB
UNITED KINGDOM
01221 3833

Childbirth Education Resources

ARTEMIS
3337 McComb
Ann Arbor, MI 48108
(art and educational materials about the childbirth experience)

Birth & Life Bookstore, Inc.
P.O. Box 70625
Seattle, WA 98107
206-789-4444

BIRTH: Issues in Perinatal Care
43 Oak Street
Geneseo, NY 14454
716-243-0087

Canadian Mothercraft Society
32 Heath Street West
Toronto, Ontario M4V 1T3
CANADA

Childbirth Graphics
P.O. Box 17025
Rochester, NY 14617

Childbirth Resources
327 Glenmont Drive
Solana Beach, CA 92075
619-481-7065

COMPLEAT MOTHER Magazine
Box 209
Minot, ND 58702

Moonflower Birthing Supply Company
P.O. Box 128
Louisville, CO 80027
303-665-2120

MOTHERING Magazine
P.O. Box 1690
Santa Fe, NM 87504
505-984-8116

Children

American Academy of Pediatrics
P.O. Box 927
141 Northwest Point Blvd.
Oak Grove Village, IL 60009-0927

Canadian Council on Children and Youth
2211 Riverside Drive
Suite 14
Ottawa, Ontario K1H 7X5
CANADA

Canadian Institute of Child Health
17 York Street
Suite 105
Ottawa, Ontario K1N 5S7
CANADA

Canadian Paediatric Society
c/o Children's Hospital of Eastern Ontario
401 Smyth Road
Ottawa, Ontario K1H 8L1
CANADA

Canadian Society for the Prevention of Cruelty to Children
356 First Street
P.O. Box 700
Midland, Ontario L4R 4P4
CANADA

Children in Hospitals, Inc.
31 Wilshire Park
Needham, MA 02192

Children's Defense Fund
122 C Street NW
Washington, DC 20001
202-628-8787

International Clearinghouse on Adolescent Fertility
1025 Vermont Avenue NW
Washington, DC 20005

National Institute of Child Health & Human Development
National Institute of Health
9000 Rockville Pike
Building 31, Room 2A32
Bethesda, MD 20205

Soft Walker Shoes
P.O. Box 517
Colleyville, TX 76034
(baby shoes)

Contraception

The Alan Guttmacher Institute (AGI)
111 Fifth Avenue
New York, NY 10003
212-254-5656
(family planning)

Association for Voluntary Surgical Contraception
122 East 42nd Street
New York, NY 10168
212-351-2500

Canadian Coalition on Depo Provera
c/o Winnipeg Women's Health Clinic
419 Graham Avenue
3rd Floor
Winnipeg, Manitoba R3C 0M3
CANADA

Dalkon Shield Information Network
P.O. Box 53
Bethlehem, PA 18016
509-575-6422

International Planned Parenthood Federation (IPPF)
Regent's College, Inner Circle
Regent's Park
London NW1 4NS
UNITED KINGDOM

National Family Planning and Reproductive Health Association
NFPRHA
122 C Street NW
Washington, DC 20001-2690
202-347-1140

National Institute of Child Health & Human Development
Center for Population Research
Executive Plaza North
6130 Executive Boulevard
Room 604
Bethesda, MD 20891
301-496-1101

Planned Parenthood Federation of America
810 Seventh Avenue
New York, NY 10019
212-541-7800

The Population Council
1 Dag Hammarskjold Plaza
New York, NY 10017
212-644-1300

The Population Institute
110 Maryland Avenue NE
Washington, DC 20022
202-544-3300

Womancap
171 East 99th Street, #15
New York, NY 10021
(cervical cap)

Zero Population Growth
1400 16th Street NW
Washington, DC 20036
202-332-2200

DES

DES Action Canada
Snowdon, P.O. Box 233
Montreal, Quebec H3X 3T4
CANADA

DES Action/USA
1615 Broadway
Suite 510
Oakland, CA 94612
or
LIJ Medical Center
New Hyde Park, NY 11040

Disability Issues

Alliance of Genetics Support Groups
38th & R Street NW
Washington, DC 20057

Canadian Association for the Deaf
271 Spadina Road
Suite 311
Toronto, Ontario M5R 2V3
CANADA

Canadian Cleft Lip and Palate Family Association
180 Dundas Street West
Suite 1508
Toronto, Ontario M5G 1X8
CANADA

Canadian Coalition for the Prevention of Developmental Disabilities
c/o Canadian Institute of Child Health
17 York Street
Suite 105
Ottawa, Ontario K1N 5S7
CANADA

Canadian Co-ordinating Council on Deafness
116 Lisgar Street
Suite 203
Ottawa, Ontario K2P 0C2
CANADA

Canadian Council of the Blind
220 Dundas Street
Suite 510
London, Ontario N6A 1H3
CANADA

Canadian Cystic Fibrosis Foundation
2221 Yonge Street
Suite 601
Toronto, Ontario M4S 2B4
CANADA

Canadian Deaf-Blind and Rubella Association
P.O. Box 1625
Meaford, Ontario N0H 1Y0
CANADA

Canadian Down Syndrome Society
5232 4th Street SW
Calgary, Alberta T2V 0Z4
CANADA

Center for Medical Consumers
237 Thompson Street
New York, NY 10012

Coalition of Provincial Organizations of the Handicapped
926-294 Portage Avenue
Winnipeg, Manitoba R3C 0B9
CANADA

Council for Responsible Genetics
19 Garden Street
Cambridge, MA 02138

Disability Information Services of Canada
839 5th Avenue SW
Suite 610
Calgary, Alberta T2P 3C8
CANADA

Federation for Children with Special Needs
95 Berkeley Street
Boston, MA 02116
617-482-2915

International Association of Parents of the Deaf (IAPD)
814 Thayer Avenue
Silver Springs, MD 20910
301-585-5400

March of Dimes Birth Defects Foundation
National Headquarters
1275 Mamaroneck Avenue
White Plains, NY 10605
914-428-7100

National Genetics Foundation
555 West 57th Street
New York, NY 10019

National Self-Help Clearinghouse
184 5th Avenue
New York, NY 10010

National Society of Genetic Counselors
233 Camerbury Drive
Wallingford, PA 19086

Parent-ability
c/o National Childbirth Trust
Alexandra House
Oldham Terrace
London W3 6NH
UNITED KINGDOM

Parent Care, Inc.
101 1/2 South Union Street
Alexandria, VA 22314
703-836-4678
(intensive care infants)

Parents of Blind Children
National Center for the Blind
1800 Johnson Street
Baltimore, MD 21230
301-659-9314

Registry of Interpreters for the Deaf, Inc.
8719 Colesville Road
Suite 310
Silver Spring, MD 20910
301-608-0050

School of Rehabilitation Medicine
Att: Carty & Conine
University of British Columbia
Vancouver, BC V6T 1W5
CANADA

Spina Bifida Association of Canada
633 Wellington Crescent
Winnipeg, Manitoba R3M 0A8
CANADA

Through the Looking Glass
801 Peralta Avenue
Berkeley, CA 94707
(parenting with disabilities)

Turner's Syndrome Society
York University
Administrative Studies Building
Room 006
4700 Keele Street
Downsview, Ontario M3J 1P3
CANADA

Home Birth

American College of Home Obstetrics
P.O. Box 25
River Forest, IL 60305

Friends of Homebirth
103 North Pearl Street
Big Sandy, TX 15755

Homebirth Australia
P.O. Box 107
Lawson, NSW 2783
AUSTRALIA

Informed Homebirth/Informed Birth and Parenting
IH/IBP
P.O. Box 3675
Ann Arbor, MI 48106
313-662-6857

National Association of Parents & Professionals for Safe Alternatives in Childbirth
NAPSAC
P.O. Box 646
Marble Hill, MO 63764-9726
314-238-2010

NEW NATIVITY
P.O. Box 6223
Leawood, KS 66206
(homebirth, unattended)

Infertility and New Procreative Technologies

American Fertility Society
1608 13th Avenue S
Birmingham, AL 35256

Canadian Fertility and Andrology Association
2065 Alexandre de S'eve Road
Suite 409
Montreal, Quebec H2L 2W5
CANADA

Canadian PID Society
P.O. Box 33804, Station D
Vancouver, BC V6J 4L6
CANADA
(Pelvic Inflammatory Disease)

Donors' Offspring
P.O. Box 33
Sarcoxie, MO 64862
(donor insemination)

The Endometriosis Association
P.O. Box 92187
Milwaukee, WI 53202

Ferre Institute
258 Genesee Street
Suite 302
Utica, NY 13502
(infertility)

The Fertility Awareness Network
P.O. Box 1190
New York, NY 10009

FINRRAGE, Europe
Feminist International Network of Resistance to Reproductive & Genetic Engineering, Europe
P.O. Box 201903
D-2000 Hamburg 20
GERMANY

FINRRAGE, USA
Feminist International Network of Resistance to Reproductive & Genetic Engineering, USA
Women's Studies
University of Massachusetts
Amherst, MA 01003

H.O.P.E.
(Helping Offspring Pursue Ethics)
888 Logan, Suite #7D
Denver, CO 80203
303-839-8661
(donor insemination)

New Reproductive Alternatives Society
641 Cadogan Street
Nanaimo, BC V9S 1T6
CANADA

RESOLVE
5 Water Street
Arlington, MA 02174
617-643-2424
(infertility)

Sorono Symposia
100 Longwater Circle
Norwell, MA 02061
(infertility)

U.S.-Canada Endometriosis Association
8585 North 76th Place
Milwaukee, WI 53223
800-426-2362

Interracial Family Issues

Adoptive Parents of America
3333 Highway 100 North
Suite 203
Minneapolis, MN 55422
612-535-4829
(family support groups for transracial adoption)

Biracial Family Network
P.O. Box 489
Chicago, IL 60653-0489
312-288-3644

Interracial Family Circle
P.O. Box 53290
Washington, DC 20009
703-719-9887

North American Council on Adoptable Children
1821 University Avenue
Suite N 498
St. Paul, MN 55104
612-644-3036
or
810 18th Street NW
Suite 703
Washington, DC 20006
(support groups for transracial adoption)

Organization for United Response (OURS)
207 Highway 100 North
Suite 203
Minneapolis, MN 55422
(transnational adoption)

Lesbian and Gay Parenting

Center Kids
The Family Project of the Lesbian & Gay Community Services Center
208 West 13th Street
New York, NY 10011

Custody Action for Lesbian Mothers
Box 281
Narbeth, PA 19072

Lesbian & Gay Parent Project
100 Longwater Circle
Norwell, MA 02061
(infertility)

Maternal and Child Health

American Foundation for Maternal & Child Health
439 East 51st Street
New York, NY 10022
212-759-5510

American Public Health Association (APHA)
1015 15th Street NW
Washington, DC 20025
202-789-5600

Healthy Mothers, Healthy Babies
409 12th Street SW
Washington, DC 20024-2188
202-863-2458

National Center for Education in Maternal & Child Health
38th & R Street NW
Washington, DC 20057

National Maternal & Child Health Clearinghouse
3520 Prospect Street NW
Washington, DC 20057

Maternal Mortality

Maternal Mortality Special Interest Group
American College of Obstetrics & Gynecology
409 12th Street SW
Washington, DC 20024

Maternal Mortality Surveillance
Division of Reproductive Health
Centers for Disease Control
1600 Clifton Road
Mail Stop K21
Atlanta, GA 30033

National Center for Health Statistics
U.S. Department of Health & Human Services
6525 Belcrest Road, Room 840
Hyattsville, MD 20782
301-436-8954

Midwifery

American College of Nurse-Midwives (ACNM)
1522 K Street NW
Suite 1000
Washington, DC 20005
202-289-0171

Association of Radical Midwives
62 Greetby Hill
Ormskirk, Lancaster
L39 2DT
UNITED KINGDOM
0695-72776

THE BIRTH GAZETTE
42, The Farm
Summertown, TN 38483
615-964-2519

Frontier School of Midwifery and Family Nursing
P.O. Box 528
Hyden, KY 41749
606-672-2312

Midwifery Communication and Accountability Project
15 Saxon Terrace
Newton, MA 02161
617-965-8955

MIDWIFERY TODAY
Box 2672
Eugene, OR 97402

Midwives Alliance of North America (MANA)
P.O. Box 1121
Bristol, VT 24203
615-764-5561

Midwives Association of Canada
2043 Ferndale
Vancouver, BC
CANADA

Seattle Midwifery School
2524 16th Avenue S
Room 300
Seattle, WA 98144
206-322-8834

Perinatal Issues

National Perinatal Association
101 1/2 South Union Street
Alexandria, VA 22314

The Perinatal Health and Fitness Network
Box 3092
Stony Creek, CT 06405

Perinatal Support Services
715 Monroe Street
Evanston, IL 60202

Pre & Perinatal Psychology Association of North America
PPANA
13 Summit Terrace
Dobb's Ferry, NY 10522

Postpartum Issues

Depression After Delivery (D.A.D.)
P.O. Box 1282
Morrisville, PA 19067
215-295-3994

National Association of Postpartum Care Services
4414 Buxton Court
Indianapolis, IN 46254
717-293-7763

National Organization of Circumcision Information Resource Centers
NO-CIRC
P.O. Box 2512
San Anselmo, CA 94960
415-488-9883

Pacific Postpartum Support Society
104-1416 Commercial Drive
Vancouver, BC V55 431
CANADA
604-689-9994
(postpartum emotional disorders)

Postpartum Support International
c/o 927 North Kellog Avenue
Santa Barbara, CA 93111
(postpartum emotional disorders)

Pregnancy Loss and Infant Mortality

AMEND
4324 Berrywick Terrace
St. Louis, MO 63128
314-487-7528
(neonatal loss)

Canadian Foundation for the Study of Infant Deaths
P.O. Box 190, Station R
Toronto, Ontario M4G 3Z9
CANADA

Centering Corporation
Box 3367
Omaha, NE 68103
402-553-1200
(pregnancy and infant loss)

The Compassionate Friends, Inc.
P.O. Box 3696
Oak Brook, IL 60522
312-990-0010
(infant and child death)

National Center for Health Statistics
U.S. Department of Health & Human Services
6525 Belcrest Road, Room 840
Hyattsville, MD 20782
301-436-8954

National SIDS Foundation
2 Metro Plaza, Suite 250
8240 Professional Place
Landover, MD 20785
301-459-3388
or
310 South Michigan Avenue
Chicago, IL 60604
(Sudden Infant Death Syndrome)

National Sudden Infant Death Syndrome Clearinghouse
8201 Greensboro Drive
Suite 600
McLean, VA 22102
703-821-8955

Pregnancy & Infant Loss Center
1421 East Wayzata Boulevard
Suite 22
Wayzata, MN 5391
612-473-9372

Resolve through Sharing
LaCrosse, WI 54601
608-785-0530
(neonatal loss)

SHARE National Office
St. Elizabeth's Hospital
611 South Third Street
Belleville, IL 62222
618-234-2415
(miscarriage, stillbirth, and newborn loss)

Twins and Multiple Births

Center for Study of Multiple Births
333 East Superior Street
Suite 476
Chicago, IL 60611
312-266-9093

National Association of Mothers of Twins Clubs, Inc.
12404 Princess Jeanne NE
Albuquerque, NM 87112

National Organization of Mothers of Twins Clubs, Inc.
5402 Amerwood Lane
Rockville, MD 20853

Parents of Multiple Births Association of Canada, Inc.
P.O. Box 2200
Lethbridge, Alberta T1J 4K9
CANADA
403-328-9165

Twinline Services for Multiple Birth Families
P.O. Box 10066
Berkeley, CA 94709
415-644-0861

University of Louisville Twin Study
Department of Pediatrics
Child Development Unit
University of Louisville Health Services Center
Louisville, KY 40292
502-588-5134

Women under Detention

Aid to Imprisoned Mothers, Inc.
61 8th Street NE
Atlanta, GA 303
404-881-8291

CICARWS
Commission on Inter-Church Aid, Refugee and World Service, World Council of Churches
P.O. Box 2100
1211 Geneva 2
SWITZERLAND
011-41-22-791-6316
(Refugee women)

Domestic Violence Hotline
79 Central Avenue
Albany, NY 12206
518-432-4864
914-561-8191 (Spanish speaking)

Women's Health Issues

Asian and Pacific Women's Action and Resource Center
Asian and Pacific Development Center
Persiaran Duta P.O. Box 12224
50770 Kuala Lumpur
MALAYSIA

Black Women's Health Project
1220 North Broad Street
Room 106
Philadelphia, PA 19121

Boston Women's Health Network
Women's Health Sharing
14 Skey Lane
Toronto, Ontario M6J 3S4
CANADA

Center for Medical Consumers
237 Thompson Street
New York, NY 10012

Center for Women Policy Studies
2000 P Street NW
Suite 508
Washington, DC 20036
202-872-1770

Federation of Feminist Women's Health Centers
1680 North Vine Street
Suite 1105
Los Angeles, CA 90028
213-957-4062

Hysterectomy Education Resources & Services
501 Woodbrook Lane
Philadelphia, PA 19119

Inter-African Committee
147 Rue De Lausanne
Geneva CH 1202
SWITZERLAND
(female genital mutilation)

International Women's Health Coalition (IWHC)
24 East 21st Street
New York, NY 10010
212-979-8500

ISIS INTERNACIONAL, Santiago
Casilla 2067 Correo Central
Santiago
CHILE
(international women's health organization)

ISIS WICCE Geneva
3 Chemin des Campanules
CH-1219 Aire (Geneva)
SWITZERLAND
(international women's health organization)

Kav Habriuth: The Women's Health Information Center, Israel
P.O. Box 3667
Tel Aviv
ISRAEL
phone: 03 220 759

National Black Women's Health Project
1237 Gordon Street SW
Atlanta, GA 30310
404-753-0916

National Center for Health Statistics
U.S. Department of Health & Human Services
6525 Belcrest Road, Room 840
Hyattsville, MD 20782
301-436-8954

National Latina Health Organization
1900 Fruitvale Avenue
P.O. Box 7567
Oakland, CA 94601

National Self-Help Clearinghouse
184 5th Avenue
New York, NY 10010

National Women's Health Network
1325 G Street NW
Washington, DC 20005
202-347-1140

Native American Women's Health Education Center
P.O. Box 572
Lake Andes, SD 57356

Regroupement des Francois Centres de Santé de Femme du Québec
CP 1197, SUCC. Place du Parc
Montreal, Quebec H2W 2P4
CANADA

Vancouver Women's Health Collective
1720 Grant Street, #302
Vancouver, BC V5L 2Y7
CANADA

WHAM! (Women's Health Action Mobilization)
P.O. Box 713
New York, NY 10009
212-713-5966

Women's Health Interaction
c/o Inter Pares
58 Arthur Street
Ottawa, Ontario K1R 7B9
CANADA

Women's Health Reproductive Rights Information Center
52-54 Featherstone Street
London EC1 8RT
UNITED KINGDOM

Women's Institute for Childbearing Policy
19 Montfern Avenue
Brighton, MA 02135
617-782-0835

Women's Occupational Health Resource Center
117 St. John's Place
Brooklyn, NY 11217

Index

by Estella Bradley